Interesting Cases in Echocardiography

Interesting Cases in Echocardiography

Editor

Navin C Nanda MD DSc (Hon) DSc (Med) (Honoris Causa) FACC FAHA FISCU (D) FSGC FICA FACA FICP (Hon) FIAE FICMU (Hon) FACIP FCSC (S) FIACS FICC (Hon)

Distinguished Professor of
Medicine and Cardiovascular Disease
University of Alabama at Birmingham
Birmingham, Alabama, USA
President
International Society of Cardiovascular Ultrasound
Editor-in-Chief
Echocardiography: A Journal of Cardiovascular Ultrasound
and Allied Techniques

JAYPEE

JAYPEE BROTHERS MEDICAL PUBLISHERS

The Health Sciences Publisher

New Delhi | London

Jaypee Brothers Medical Publishers (P) Ltd

Headquarters
EMCA House, 23/23-B
Ansari Road, Daryaganj
New Delhi 110 002, India
Landline: +91-11-23272143, +91-11-23272703
+91-11-23282021, +91-11-23245672
e-mail: jaypee@jaypeebrothers.com

Corporate Office
4838/24, Ansari Road, Daryaganj
New Delhi 110 002, India
Phone: +91-11-43574357
Fax: +91-11-43574314
e-mail: jaypee@jaypeebrothers.com

Overseas Office
JP Medical Ltd.
83, Victoria Street, London
SW1H 0HW (UK)
Phone: +44-20 3170 8910
e-mail: info@jpmedpub.com

EU GPSR Authorised Representative
Logos Europe, 9 rue Nicolas Poussin
17000, La Rochelle, France
Phone: +33 (0) 6 67 93 73 78
e-mail: contact@logoseurope.eu

Website: www.jaypeebrothers.com
Website: www.jaypeedigital.com

Interesting Cases in Echocardiography

First Edition: 2017, ***Reprint: 2025***

ISBN: 978-93-86056-94-8

Printed at: Samrat Offset Pvt. Ltd.

Dedicated to

My late parents
Dr Balwant Rai Nanda and Mrs Maya Vati Nanda
My wife
Kanta Nanda MD
Our children
Nitin Nanda, Anita Nanda Wasan MD, and Anil Nanda MD
Their spouses Sanjeev Wasan MD and Seema Tailor Nanda, and
our grandchildren Vinay and Rajesh Wasan, and Nayna and Ria Nanda

Contributors

Elsayed Abo-Salem MD
Assistant Professor of Cardiovascular Medicine
Center for Comprehensive Cardiovascular Care
Saint Louis University Hospital
Saint Louis, Missouri, USA

F Abtahi MD
Echocardiography Laboratory
University of Alabama at Birmingham
Birmingham, Alabama, USA

Ahmed Abuzaid MD
Cardiology Fellowship
Department of Cardiovascular Medicine
Sidney Kimmel Medical College
Thomas Jefferson University/Christiana Care Health System
Newark, Delaware, USA

LG Adarna MD
Echocardiography Laboratory
University of Alabama at Birmingham
Birmingham, Alabama, USA

Olayinka Afolabi-Brown MD
Einstein Medical Center
Division of Cardiovascular Diseases
Philadelphia, Pennsylvania, USA

Aashish Agarwal MD
Echocardiography Laboratory
University of Alabama at Birmingham
Birmingham, Alabama, USA

Kul Aggarwal MD MRCP (UK) FACC
Professor of Clinical Medicine
Division of Cardiology
University of Missouri
Columbia, Missouri, USA
Director
Cardiac Catheterization Laboratory and Chief
Cardiology Section
Harry S Truman Veterans' Hospital
Columbia, Missouri, USA

Masood Ahmad MD
Edward D and Sally M Futch Professor of Cardiology
Director
Echocardiography Laboratory
Division of Cardiology
The University Texas Medical Branch (UTMB)
Galveston, Texas, USA

MI Ahmed MD
Echocardiography Laboratory
University of Alabama at Birmingham
Birmingham, Alabama, USA

Esmat Ahmed AH MD
Echocardiography Laboratory
University of Alabama at Birmingham
Birmingham, Alabama, USA

Ramazan Akdemir MD
Professor
Department of Cardiology
Faculty of Medicine
Sakarya University Training and Research Hospital
Sakarya, Turkey

Murat Aksoy MD
Assistant Professor
Department of Cardiology
Faculty of Medicine
Sakarya University Training and Research Hospital
Sakarya, Turkey

N Alagic MD
Echocardiography Laboratory
University of Alabama at Birmingham
Birmingham, Alabama, USA

Mohsin Alam MD
Senior Cardiologist
Echocardiography Laboratory
Heart and Vascular Institute
Henry Ford Hospital
Detroit, Michigan, USA

Zarina Alam MD
Senior Staff
Department of Internal Medicine
Henry Ford Hospital
Detroit, Michigan, USA

OO Alli MD
Division of Cardiology
University of Alabama at Birmingham
Birmingham, Alabama, USA

Aman M Amanullah MD PhD FACC FASE FASNC FAHA
Section Chief
Noninvasive Cardiology
Albert Einstein Medical Center
Professor of Medicine (Clinical Track)
Sidney Kimmel Medical College of Thomas Jefferson University
Philadelphia, Pennsylvania, USA

Edgar Argulian MD MPH FACC FASE
Assistant Professor of Medicine
Mount Sinai Heart Network
Icahn School of Medicine at Mount Sinai
New York City, New York, USA

José Antonio Arias-Godinez MD
Chief of the Laboratory of Echocardiography
National Institute of Cardiology
Mexico City, Mexico

MJ Arisha MD
Echocardiography Laboratory
University of Alabama at Birmingham
Birmingham, Alabama, USA

Garima Arora MD MRCP
Instructor
Cardiovascular Medicine
University of Alabama at Birmingham
Birmingham, Alabama, USA

Nydia Avila-Vanzzini MD
Physician of the Staff
Laboratory of Echocardiography and Non-Invasive Hemodynamics
National Institute of Cardiologia Ignacio Chavez
Mexico City, Mexico

Mohamed Ayan MD
Resident
Internal Medicine Department
Creighton University School of Medicine
Omaha, Nebraska, USA

Muhammad Soubhi Azzouz MD
Cardiology Fellowship
Cardiovascular Department
Creighton University School of Medicine
Omaha, Nebraska, USA

Sudarshan Balla MD
Assistant Professor of Clinical Medicine
Division of Cardiology
University of Missouri
Columbia, Missouri, USA

Armin Barekatain MD
Cardiology Fellowship
Department of Cardiovascular Medicine
Sidney Kimmel Medical College
Thomas Jefferson University/Christiana Care Health System
Newark, Delaware, USA

K Barssoum MD
Echocardiography Laboratory
University of Alabama at Birmingham
Birmingham, Alabama, USA

Nishchayjit Basra
Fourth-Year Medical Student
Kansas City University of Medicine and Biosciences
Kansas City, Missouri, USA

K Bhagatwala MBBS
Echocardiography Laboratory
University of Alabama at Birmingham
Birmingham, Alabama, USA

Robert WW Biederman MD FACC FAHA FSGC FASA
Professor of Medicine
Director
Cardiovascular Magnetic Resonance Imaging
Temple University School of Medicine
Adjunct Professor of Bioengineering
Carnegie Mellon University and Allegheny Health Network
Allegheny General Hospital
Pittsburgh, Pennsylvania, USA

Francois Bourlon MD
Consultant Cardiologist
Cardiothoracic Centre
Monaco City, Monaco

Christian S Breburda MD PhD FACC FASE FESC
Clinical Professor of Medicine
University of Arizona College of Medicine - Phoenix
Director
Noninvasive Cardiology and Imaging
Maricopa Medical Center
Phoenix, Arizona, USA

Craig Broberg MD
Associate Professor
Cardiovascular Medicine and Radiology
Knight Cardiovascular Institute
Oregon Health and Science University
Portland, Oregon, USA

S Bulur MD
Echocardiography Laboratory
University of Alabama at Birmingham
Birmingham, Alabama, USA

Luke Burchill MBBS PhD
Assistant Professor of Cardiovascular Medicine
Knight Cardiovascular Institute
Oregon Health & Science University
Portland, Oregon, USA

J Burkhart MD
Echocardiography Laboratory
University of Alabama at Birmingham
Birmingham, Alabama, USA

Claudia C Cajas-Morales MD
Physician in Training of Echocardiography
National Institute of Cardiology
Mexico City, Mexico

Maurizio Campaniello MD
Cardiologist
Associate Medical Director
Chest Pain Unit
Cardiology Emergency
University of Bari
Bari, Italy

Angel Lopez Candales MD FACC FASE
Professor of Medicine
Chief
Cardiovascular Medicine
Director
Cardiology Training Program University of Puerto Rico School of Medicine
San Juan, Puerto Rico, USA

Alberto Barón Castañeda MD
Medical Department Director
Clínica de Marly
Bogotá, Colombia

E Celiker MD
Echocardiography Laboratory
University of Alabama at Birmingham
Birmingham, Alabama, USA

Farooq A Chaudhry MD FACP FACC FASE FAHA
Professor of Medicine
Director
Echocardiography Laboratories
Associate Director
Mount Sinai Heart Network
Icahn School of Medicine at Mount Sinai
The Zena and Michael A Wiener Cardiovascular Institute and Marie-Josée and Henry R Kravis Center for Cardiovascular Health
New York City, New York, USA

JR Chahwala MBBS
Echocardiography Laboratory
University of Alabama at Birmingham
Birmingham, Alabama, USA

Soung Ick Cho MD
Fellow
Cardiovascular Disease Fellowship
Echocardiography Laboratory
Heart and Vascular Institute
Henry Ford Hospital
Detroit, Michigan, USA

Rahul Choudhary MD
Senior Resident
Sawai Man Singh Medical College
Jaipur, Rajasthan, India

Jaehoon Chung MD FACC
Cardiologist
Englewood Hospital and Medical Center
Englewood, New Jersey, USA

Marco Matteo Ciccone MD
Professor
Cardiovascular Diseases Section
Department of Emergency and
Organ Transplantation (DETO)
University of Bari
Bari, Italy

Ottavio Di Cillo MD
Cardiologist
Chest Pain Unit
Cardiology Emergency
University of Bari
Bari, Italy

Yudy Miluska Roldan Concha MD
Chief of Cardiology Department
National Hospital Hipolito Unanue
Lima, Peru

WA Crosland MD
Echocardiography Laboratory
University of Alabama at Birmingham
Birmingham, Alabama, USA

Michael J Cuttica MD MS
Assistant Professor of Medicine
(Pulmonary and Critical Care)
Northwestern University Feinburg
School of Medicine
Chicago, Illinois, USA

Saadet Demirtaş MD
Cardiologist
Department of Cardiology
Ankara Dişkapi Research and
Training Hospital
Ankara, Turkey

Fiorella Devito MD
Cardiologist
Cardiovascular Diseases Section
Department of Emergency and Organ
Transplantation
University of Bari School of Medicine
Bari, Italy

Andre Dias MD
Einstein Medical Center
Division of Cardiovascular Diseases
Department of Medicine
Philadelphia, Pennsylvania, USA

M Elguindy MD
Echocardiography Laboratory
University of Alabama at Birmingham
Birmingham, Alabama, USA

Ghazwan Elias MD
Maricopa Medical Center
Phoenix, Arizona, USA

A Elkaryoni MD
Echocardiography Laboratory
University of Alabama at Birmingham
Birmingham, Alabama, USA

M Elsayed MBBCh
Echocardiography Laboratory
University of Alabama at Birmingham
Birmingham, Alabama, USA

Sibel Catirli Enar MD FESC FASE
Associate Professor of Cardiology
Department of Cardiology
Turkiye Hospital and
Istanbul Memorial Hospital
Istanbul, Turkey

MGA Escanuela MD
Echocardiography Laboratory
University of Alabama at Birmingham
Birmingham, Alabama, USA

Nilda Gladys Espinola-Zavaleta MD PhD
Physician and Researcher of the Staff
Laboratory of Echocardiography and
Noninvasive Hemodynamics
National Institute of Cardiology
'Ignacio Chávez'
Mexico City, Mexico

Alfredo Sotomayor Estrada MD
Chief of Cardiovascular Surgery
National Hospital Hipolito Unanue
Lima, Peru

José Carlos Armendáriz Ferrari MD
Chief of Echocardiography Lab
National Hospital Hipolito Unanue
Lima, Peru
Professor of Medicine
National University
Federico Villarreal
Lima, Peru

Francesco Fulvio Faletra MD
Division of Cardiology
Fondazione Cardiocentro Ticino
Lugano, Switzerland

Jose Ricardo FP MD
Cardiology Fellow
Allegheny General Hospital
Pittsburgh, Pennsylvania, USA

Luba Frank MD
Associate Professor of Radiology
Department of Radiology
University of Texas Medical Branch (UTMB)
Galveston, Texas, USA

Leon J Frazin MD FACC
Professor of Clinical Medicine
University of Illinois Hospital and
Health Sciences System
Director of Echocardiography
Jesse Brown VA Medical Center
Chicago, Illinois, USA

Juan Francisco Fritche-Salazar MD
Physician of the Staff
National Institute of Cardiology
Mexico City, Mexico

Nicholas Furiasse MD MS
Clinical Instructor
Cardiovascular Diseases
Bluhm Cardiovascular Institute
Northwestern Memorial Hospital
Chicago, Illinois, USA

S Gaba MD
Echocardiography Laboratory
University of Alabama at Birmingham
Birmingham, Alabama, USA

Julius M Gardin MD MBA
Past Chair
Department of Medicine
Hackensack University Medical Center
Hackensack, New Jersey, USA
Professor of Medicine
Rutgers New Jersey Medical School
Rutgers, New Jersey, USA

Naveen Garg MD
Fellow
Noninvasive Cardiology
Badshah Khan Government Hospital
Faridabad, Haryana, India

Dinesh Gautam MD
Senior Resident
Sawai Man Singh Medical College
Jaipur, Rajasthan, India

GC Giove MD
Echocardiography Laboratory
University of Alabama at Birmingham
Birmingham, Alabama, USA

G Gok MD
Echocardiography Laboratory
University of Alabama at Birmingham
Birmingham, Alabama, USA

Mark H Goldberger MD FACC
Columbia University
New York City, New York, USA

John D Groarke MD MSc
Physician in Heart Failure
Brigham and Women's Hospital
Harvard Medical School
Boston, Massachusetts, USA

Daniel W Groves MD
Cardiovascular Disease Fellow
Department of Medicine
Division of Cardiology
University of Colorado Anschutz
Medical Campus
Colorado, Arizona, USA

EC Guler MD
Echocardiography Laboratory
University of Alabama at Birmingham
Birmingham, Alabama, USA

JC Gulotta MD
Echocardiography Laboratory
University of Alabama at Birmingham
Birmingham, Alabama, USA

N Gupta MBBS
Echocardiography Laboratory
University of Alabama at Birmingham
Birmingham, Alabama, USA

T Guvenc MD
Echocardiography Laboratory
University of Alabama at Birmingham
Birmingham, Alabama, USA

Yuchi Han MD MMSc
Assistant Professor
University of Pennsylvania
Philadelphia, Pennsylvania, USA

Robert Hartman MD
Clinical Assistant Professor
Pediatric Cardiology
Department of Cardiovascular Sciences
East Carolina Heart Institute
Brody School of Medicine at East
Carolina University
Greenville, South Carolina, USA

Mohammed Hasoon MD
Maricopa Medical Center
Phoenix, Arizona, USA

Stephen T Helmke RDCS MPH
Research Echocardiographer
Columbia University Medical Center
(CUMC)
Clinical Cardiovascular Research
Laboratory for the Elderly (CCRLE)
Columbia University Medical Center
New York City, New York, USA

MC Hsiung MD
Division of Cardiology
Heart Center
Cheng-Hsin General Hospital
Taipei, Taiwan

Rachel Hughes-Doichev MD FASE
Assistant Professor of Medicine
Temple University School of Medicine
Medical Director
Department of Echocardiography
Allegheny General Hospital
West Penn Hospital
Pittsburgh, Pennsylvania, USA

Dawn Hui MD
Assistant Professor of Surgery
Department of Internal Medicine
Division of Cardiology
St Louis University Medical School and
Cardiac Surgeon
Center for Comprehensive
Cardiovascular Care
SSM Health
Saint Louis University Hospital
Saint Louis, Missouri, USA

Syed Hussain MD
Cardiology Fellow
Allegheny General Hospital
Pittsburgh, Pennsylvania, USA

Laura Iacuzio MD
Consultant Cardiologist
Cardiothoracic Centre
Monaco City, Monaco

Zeina Ibrahim MD
Advanced Imaging Fellow
Northwestern Memorial Hospital
Northwestern University
Chicago, Illinois, USA

Tevfik Fikret Ilgenli MD
Associate Professor of Cardiology
Chief of Department
Özel Konya Selçuklu Hastanesi
Konya, Turkey

Omer Iqbal MD FACC FESC
Professor
Department of Pathology and
Ophthalmology
Loyola University Health System
Maywood, Illinois, USA

AKM Monwarul Islam FCPS MD FACC FESC FRCP
Assistant Professor
Department of Cardiology
Jessore Medical College
Jessore, Bangladesh

Valentyna Ivanova MD
Cardiology Fellow
Allegheny General Hospital
Pittsburgh, Pennsylvania, USA

Chisato Izumi MD PhD
Cardiologist
Department of Cardiology
Tenri Hospital
Nara, Japan

Rajesh Janardhanan MD MRCP FACC FASE
Associate Professor of Medicine and
Medical Imaging Director
Noninvasive Cardiac Imaging
Director of Echocardiography
Banner - University Medical Center
Phoenix, Arizona, USA

Madeline Jankowski RDCS
Lead Cardiac Sonographer
Echocardiography Accreditation
Laboratory
Northwestern Memorial Hospital
Chicago, Illinois, USA

Kishan Jasti MD
Former Cardiology Fellow
Allegheny General Hospital
Pittsburgh, Pennsylvania, USA

Leng Jiang MD FACC FAHA FASE
Director
Department of Noninvasive Cardiology
Baystate Medical Center
Springfield, Massachusetts, USA
Professor of Medicine
Tufts University
Medford, Massachusetts, USA

Ajay Jindal MD (Medicine) FIAE
Testamur
National Board of Echocardiography
(NBE)
Raleigh, North Carolina, USA
Director
SND Hospital
Rupnagar, Punjab, India

M Joson MD
Echocardiography Laboratory
University of Alabama at Birmingham
Birmingham, Alabama, USA

Amjad Kabach MD
Resident
Internal Medicine Department
Creighton University School of Medicine
Omaha, Nebraska, USA

A Kalla MD
Echocardiography Laboratory
University of Alabama at Birmingham
Birmingham, Alabama, USA

R Kalra MD
Department of Medicine
University of Alabama at Birmingham
Birmingham, Alabama, USA

Megan Y Kamath MD
Fellow
Cardiovascular Disease
Allegheny Health Network
Pittsburgh, Pennsylvania, USA

Kanwal K Kapur MD
Senior Consultant and
Chief of Noninvasive Cardiology
Indraprastha Apollo Hospital
New Delhi, India

Jaroslaw D Kasprzak MD PhD FESC FACC
Professor of Medicine and Head
Department of Cardiology
Medical University of Lodz
Lodz, Poland

Pudussery Kattalan JJ MBBS
Echocardiography Laboratory
University of Alabama at Birmingham
Birmingham, Alabama, USA

Nurgül Keser MD
Professor
Department of Cardiology
Faculty of Medicine
Sakarya University Training and
Research Hospital
Sakarya, Turkey
Professor
Department of Cardiology Clinic
Umraniye Training and Research Hospital
Istanbul Health Sciences University
Istanbul, Turkey

Amber D Khanna MD
Assistant Professor of Medicine
Department of Medicine and Pediatrics
Division of Cardiology
University of Colorado Anschutz
Medical Campus
Colorado, Arizona, USA

Harun Kiliç MD
Professor
Department of Cardiology
Faculty of Medicine
Sakarya University Training and
Research Hospital
Sakarya, Turkey

B Klas BS
TomTec Corporation
Munich, Germany

Ravi Komatireddy MD
Clinical Assistant Professor
Department of Medicine
University of California
San Diego, California

Smadar Kort MD FACC FASE FAHA
Immediate Past Governor
American College of Cardiology
Downstate New York
Professor of Medicine and Director
Valve Center Ltd.
Palmerston North, New Zealand
Director
Noninvasive Cardiac Imaging and
Echocardiography
Stony Brook University
Stony Brook, New York, USA

Nikoloz Koshkelashvili MD
Einstein Medical Center
Department of Internal Medicine
Philadelphia, Pennsylvania, USA

K Kotti MD
Echocardiography Laboratory
University of Alabama at Birmingham
Birmingham, Alabama, USA

Arnav Kumar MD
Rsearch Fellow
Cardiac Imaging
Cleveland Clinic Foundation
Cleveland, Ohio, USA

Raghuveer Kura MD
Clinical Assistant Professor
Department of Medicine
St Louis University School of Medicine
Chief of Medicine
Medical Director
Division of Nephrology
Poplar Bluff Regional Medical Center
Medical Center, Fresenius Kidney Care
Poplar Bluff, Missouri, USA

Susan T Laing MD MSc CPE
Professor of Medicine and Director
Department of Echocardiography
University of Texas Health Science Center at Houston
Memorial Hermann Texas Medical Center
Houston, Texas, USA

Meggo-Quiroz LD MD
Division of Cardiology
University of Alabama at Birmingham
Birmingham, Alabama, USA

Tao Yu Lee MD
Director
Echocardiographic Laboratory
Kaohsiung Veterans General Hospital
Assistant Professor
National Yang-Ming University School of Medicine
Kaohsiung, Taiwan

Marina Leitman MD
Cardiologist
Department of Cardiology
Assaf Harofeh Medical Center
Sackler School of Medicine
Tel Aviv University
Tel Aviv, Israel

Laura Anna Leo MD
Cardiac Imaging Laboratory
Fondazione Cardiocentro Ticino
Lugano, Switzerland

Shoa-Lin Lin MD FACC FESC
Director
Coronary Care Unit
Yuan's General Hospital
Kaohsiung, Taiwan
Professor of Medicine
National Defense Medical College
Saitama Prefecture, Japan

Patricia Lozano-Rodriguez MD
Fellow
Division of Cardiology
University of Texas Medical Branch (UTMB)
Galveston, Texas, USA

Kameswari Maganti MD
Associate Professor
Northwestern University Feinberg School of Medicine
Chicago, Illinois, USA

A Mahajan MD
Echocardiography Laboratory
University of Alabama at Birmingham
Birmingham, Alabama, USA

Tuan V Mai MD
Cardiology Fellow
Knight Cardiovascular Institute
Oregon Health and Science University
Portland, Oregon, USA

Maria Maiello MD
Cardiologist
ASL Brindisi
Cardiology Equipe
Brindisi, Apulia, Italy

Abdullah Al Shafi Majumder MD FACC FESC FRCP FSCAI FCSI
Professor of Cardiology
Popular Medical College
Ex-Director
National Institute of Cardiovascular Diseases
Dhaka, Bangladesh
Senior Visiting Fellow
Cambridge University
Cambridge, UK
Secretary General
Bangladesh Cardiac Society
Dhaka, Bangladesh

Amgad N Makaryus MD FACC FACP FASE FSCCT
Associate Professor
Hofstra Northwell School of Medicine/ Northwell Health
Chairman
Department of Cardiology NuHealth
Nassau University Medical Center
Nassau County, New York, USA

Judy R Mangion MD FASE
Associate Director
Noninvasive Cardiac Laboratory
Brigham and Women's Hospital
Harvard Medical School
Boston, Massachusetts, USA

C Bogdan Marcu MD
Director
Advanced Cardiac Imaging and Imaging Education
Department of Cardiovascular Sciences
East Carolina Heart Institute
Brody School of Medicine at East Carolina University
Greenville, South Carolina, USA

DC McGiffin MD
Cardiac Surgeon
University of Alabama at Birmingham
Birmingham, Alabama, USA

WS McMahon MD
Department of Pediatric Cardiology
University of Alabama at Birmingham
Birmingham, Alabama, USA

Sheridan Meyers MD
Assistant Professor of Medicine
Northwestern University Feinberg School of Medicine
Bluhm Cardiovascular Institute
Chicago, Illinois, USA

J Mishra MD
Echocardiography Laboratory
University of Alabama at Birmingham
Birmingham, Alabama, USA

Shreyas Modi MD
Associate Professor of Medicine
Division of Cardiology
University of Texas Medical Branch (UTMB)
Galveston, Texas, USA

A Mohamed MBBCh
Echocardiography Laboratory
University of Alabama at Birmingham
Birmingham, Alabama, USA

AH Mohamed
Echocardiography Laboratory
University of Alabama at Birmingham
Birmingham, Alabama, USA

Mohamed Morsy MD
Associate Professor of Medicine
Division of Cardiology
The University Texas Medical Branch (UTMB)
Galveston, Texas, USA

Romina Murzilli MD
Cardiac Imaging Laboratory
Fondazione Cardiocentro Ticino
Lugano, Switzerland

IA Mustafa MD
Echocardiography Laboratory
University of Alabama at Birmingham
Birmingham, Alabama, USA

Vidya Nadig MBBS MRCP FACC
Assistant Professor
University of Kentucky
Lexington, Kentucky, USA

Navin C Nanda MD DSc (Hon) DSc (Med) (Honoris Causa) FACC FAHA FISCU (D) FSGC FICA FACA FICP (Hon) FIAE FICMU (Hon) FACIP FCSC (S) FIACS FICC (Hon)
Distinguished Professor of Medicine and Cardiovascular Disease
University of Alabama at Birmingham
Birmingham, Alabama, USA
President
International Society of Cardiovascular Ultrasound
Editor-in-Chief
Echocardiography: A Journal of Cardiovascular Ultrasound and Allied Techniques

Aditi Naniwadekar MD
Fellow
Clinical Cardiac Electrophysiology
Mount Sinai Medical Center
Mount Sinai, New York, USA

Sirikarn Napan MD
Cardiovascular MRI Fellow
Allegheny General Hospital
Pittsburgh, Pennsylvania, USA

Rajasekhar Nekkanti MD
Associate Professor of Medicine
Program Director of Cardiology Fellowship
East Carolina University
Greenville, East Carolina, USA
Program Director of Continuing Medical Education (Cardiovascular Series)
Director of Echocardiography Laboratories
Department of Cardiovascular Sciences
East Carolina Heart Institute
Brody School of Medicine at East Carolina University
Greenville, South Carolina, USA

Ashley L Nickerson DO
Advanced Cardiovascular Imaging Fellow
University of Kentucky and the Gill Heart Institute
Lexington, Kentucky, USA

Paul O'Malley MBA MSP
Stritch School of Medicine
Maywood, Illinois, USA

Ahmad S Omran MD FACC FESC FASE
Consultant Cardiologist
Head
Noninvasive Cardiology Laboratory
King Abdulaziz Cardiac Center
Riyadh, Saudi Arabia
Ministry of National Guard-Health Affairs
Kingdom of Saudi Arabia

Maria del Sol Ordaz MD
Physician in Training of Echocardiography
National Institute of Cardiology
Mexico City, Mexico

Boris Orlov MD
Cardiac Surgeon
Sackler School of Medicine
Tel Aviv University
Department of Cardiac Surgery
Sheba Medical Center
Tel Aviv, Israel

Ibrahim Osman MD
Cardiology Fellow
Department of Cardiovascular Sciences
East Carolina Heart Institute
Brody School of Medicine at East Carolina University
Greenville, South Carolina, USA

Kemaloglu Ozkt MD
Echocardiography Laboratory
University of Alabama at Birmingham
Birmingham, Alabama, USA

Türker Pabuçcu MD
Cardiologist
Department of Cardiology
Sakarya University Training and Research Hospital
Sakarya, Turkey

Ramdas G Pai MD FRCP (Edin) FACC
Director of Cardiac Imaging and Cardiology Fellowship Program
UC Riverside School of Medicine
St Bernardine Medical Center
California, USA
Professor of Medicine
University of California Riverside and Loma Linda University School of Medicine
California, USA

Pasquale Palmiero MD
Adjunct Professor of Cardiology
ASL Brindisi
Cardiology Equipe
Brindisi, Apulia, Italy

Jitendra Pandya MD
Cardiology Fellowship
Cardiovascular Department
Creighton University School of Medicine
Omaha, Nebraska, USA

Jayant Patel MD
Medical Director
Non-Invasive Cardiology Services
Hackensack Meridian Health
Hackensack, New Jersey, USA

Rajiv Patel MD
Staff Cardiologist
Hackensack University Medical Center
Hackensack, New Jersey, USA

Eli Peleg MD
Cardiologist
Department of Cardiology
Assaf Harofeh Medical Center
Sackler School of Medicine
Tel Aviv University
Tel Aviv, Israel

William M Pelton MD
Radiologist
Poplar Bluff Regional Medical Center
Poplar Bluff, Missouri, USA

Nelson Pizzano MD FACC
Head
Cardiovascular Health Program
Hospital Evangelico
Montevideo, Uruguay
Former NIH Research Fellow
Heart Station
University of Alabama at Birmingham
Birmingham, Alabama, USA
Past President
Uruguayan Society of Cardiology
Montevideo, Uruguay

Sourabh Prabhakar MD
Cardiology Fellow
Allegheny General Hospital
Pittsburgh, Pennsylvania, USA

Jyothy J Puthumana MD
Associate Professor of Medicine
Division of Cardiology
Department of Medicine
Northwestern University Feinberg
School of Medicine
Chicago, Illinois, USA

Nishath Quader MD
Washington University School of
Medicine
St Louis, Missouri, USA

Robert A Quaife MD
Professor of Medicine
Departments of Medicine and
Radiology
Divisions of Cardiology and
Cardiothoracic Imaging
University of Colorado Anschutz
Medical Campus
Colorado, Arizona, USA

Supawat Ratanapo MD
Cardiology Fellow
Medical College of Georgia
Augusta University
Augusta, Georgia, USA

Hanumanth K Reddy MD FACC
Clinical Adjunct Professor of Medicine
St Louis University Medical School
Medical Director
Cardiovascular Institute of Southern
Missouri
Poplar Bluff, Missouri, USA
President
American Association of Cardiologists of
Indian Origin
Poplar Bluff, Missouri, USA

Vera H Rigolin MD
Professor of Medicine
Northwestern University Feinberg
School of Medicine
Medical Director
Echocardiography Accreditation
Laboratory
Northwestern Memorial Hospital
Chicago, Illinois, USA

Salomon Rivera-Peralta MD
Physician in Training of
Echocardiography
National Institute of Cardiology
Mexico City, Mexico

Hugo Rodriguez-Zanella MD
Physician of the Staff
National Institute of Cardiology
Mexico City, Mexico

Roberta Romito MD
Associate Medical Director
Chest Pain Unit
Cardiology Emergency
University of Bari
Bari, Italy

Asad Ullah Roomi MD MRCP (UK)
FRCP (Edin) Saudi Board Adult Cardiology
NBE (USA)
Consultant Cardiologist
Prince Sultan Cardiac Center
Prince Sultan Military Medical City (PSMMC)
Riyadh, Kingdom of Saudi Arabia

Angel Romero-Cardenas MD
Physician of the Staff
National Institute of Cardiology
Mexico City, Mexico

Maria Eugenia Ruiz-Esparza MD
Physician of the Staff
National Institute of Cardiology
Mexico City, Mexico

Hyde M Russell MD
Surgical Director
Advanced Heart Failure and
Mechanical Circulatory Support
Attending Surgeon
Cardiac Surgery
NorthShore University Health System
Chicago, Illinois, USA
Clinical Professor of Medicine
Pritzker School of Medicine
University of Chicago
Chicago, Illinois, USA

Juliet Ryan BS RDCS FASE
Lead Cardiology Sonographer
Cardiac Graphics-Echo Lab
Northwestern Memorial Hospital
Chicago, Illinois, USA

Anurag Sahu MD FACC
Assistant Professor and Director
Cardiac Intensive Care Unit
Emory University Hospital
Atlanta, Georgia, USA

Sherif Sakr MD
Professor of Medicine
Department of Cardiovascular Medicine
Mansoura University
Mansoura, Egypt

Ernesto E Salcedo MD
Professor of Medicine
Director of Echocardiography
Department of Medicine
Division of Cardiology
University of Colorado Anschutz
Medical Campus
Colorado, Arizona, USA

Mohsin Salih MD MS
Resident
Internal Medicine Department
St Luke's Hospital
Chesterfield, Missouri, USA

P Sankhyan MD
Echocardiography Laboratory
University of Alabama at Birmingham
Birmingham, Alabama, USA

Shelley Sarson BA RDCS FASE
Cardiac Sonographer
Northwestern University
Northwestern Memorial Hospital
Chicago, Illinois, USA

Alok Saurav MD
Cardiology Fellowship
Cardiovascular Department
Creighton University School of Medicine
Omaha, Nebraska, USA

Daniel R Schimmel MD MS
Division of Cardiology
Department of Medicine
Northwestern University Feinberg School of Medicine
Chicago, Illinois, USA

Roxy Senior MD DM FRCP FESC FACC
Professor of Clinical Cardiology
National Heart and Lung Institute
Imperial College
London, UK
Consultant Cardiologist and Director of Echocardiography
Royal Brompton Hospital
London, UK
Consultant Cardiologist and Director of Cardiac Research
Northwick Park Hospital
London, UK

Arash Seratnahaei MD
Advanced Cardiovascular Imaging Fellow
University of Kentucky and the Gill Heart Institute
Lexington, Kentucky, USA

Sabiye Sevinç MD
Cardiologist
Department of Cardiology
Sakarya University Training and Research Hospital
Sakarya, Turkey

Aijaz Shah MBBS MRCP (UK) FRCP (Edin) NBE (USA)
Consultant Cardiologist Director Cardiac Imaging
Prince Sultan Military Medical City (PSMMC)
Riyadh, Kingdom of Saudi Arabia

Moneal Shah MD
Clinical Assistant Professor of Medicine
Co-Director
Cardiovascular MRI
Allegheny General Hospital
Temple University School of Medicine
Pittsburgh, Pennsylvania, USA

Sangeeta B Shah MD FASE FACC
Associate Professor
Ochsner Clinical School
University of Queensland
Director
Cardiovascular MRI
Co-Director
Adult Congenital Heart Disease
New Orleans, Louisiana, USA

Sanjiv J Shah MD
Professor of Medicine
Division of Cardiology
Department of Medicine
Northwestern University Feinberg School of Medicine
Chicago, Illinois, USA

Gyanendra K Sharma MD FACC FASE
Professor of Medicine and Radiology
Director
Adult Echocardiography Laboratory
Section of Cardiology
Medical College of Georgia
Augusta University
Augusta, Georgia, USA

Rakesh K Sharma MD FACC FSCAI FSCCT
Interventional Cardiologist
Bay Care Medical Group Cardiology
Clearwater, Florida
Adjunct Clinical Professor of Cardiology
University of Arkansas for Medical Sciences
Tampa, Florida, USA

Saurabh Sharma MD
Fellow in Cardiology
Albert Einstein Medical Center
Philadelphia, Pennsylvania, USA

Lubna Ibrahim Siddiqui MBBS
Instructor
Medical Education
Prince Sultan Military Medical City (PSMMC)
Riyadh, Kingdom of Saudi Arabia

Maninder Singh MD (Medicine)
Fellow in Noninvasive Cardiology
Dayanand Medical College & Hospital
Unit: Hero DMC Heart Institute
Ludhiana, Punjab, India

Ravinder Pal Singh MD (Medicine)
Fellow in Noninvasive Cardiology
Dayanand Medical College & Hospital
Unit: Hero DMC Heart Institute
Ludhiana, Punjab, India

Gaurav Singhal MD
Senior Resident
Sawai Man Singh Medical College
Jaipur, Rajasthan, India

I Singla MD
Echocardiography Laboratory
University of Alabama at Birmingham
Birmingham, Alabama, USA

Mara T Slawsky MD PhD
Director
Heart Failure Program
Program Director
Cardiovascular Fellowship
Baystate Medical Center
Springfield, Massachusetts, USA

Aiman Smer MBBCh
Cardiology Fellowship
Cardiovascular Department
Creighton University School of Medicine
Omaha, Nebraska, USA

Beverly Smulevitz BS RDCS
Research Coordinator
Department of Echocardiography
University of Texas Health Science Center at Houston
Houston, Texas, USA

Vincent L Sorrell MD FACC FASE FACP
Anthony N DeMaria Chair of Cardiovascular Imaging
Director of Cardiovascular Imaging
University of Kentucky and the Gill Heart Institute
Lexington, Kentucky, USA

Fabiola B Sozzi MD PhD
Consultant Cardiologist
Ospedale Maggiore Policlinico Instituti di Ricovero e Cura a Carattere Scientifico (IRCCS)
Milan, Italy

A Sungur MD
Echocardiography Laboratory
University of Alabama at Birmingham
Birmingham, Alabama, USA

Martin G St John Sutton MBBS
Professor
University of Pennsylvania
Philadelphia, Pennsylvania, USA

M Tageldin MBBCh
Echocardiography Laboratory
University of Alabama at Birmingham
Birmingham, Alabama, USA

A Taher MBBCh
Echocardiography Laboratory
University of Alabama at Birmingham
Birmingham, Alabama, USA

Rohit Tandon MD (Medicine)
Senior Consultant Physician
Dayanand Medical College & Hospital
Unit: Hero DMC Heart Institute
Ludhiana, Punjab, India

Ersan Tatli MD
Professor
Department of Cardiology
Faculty of Medicine
Sakarya University Training and Research Hospital
Sakarya, Turkey

M Thind MD
Echocardiography Laboratory
University of Alabama at Birmingham
Birmingham, Alabama, USA

MM Townsley MD
Department of Anesthesiology
Division of Critical Care and Perioperative Medicine
University of Alabama at Birmingham School of Medicine
Birmingham, Alabama, USA

Alma Tozaj MD RDCS
Cardiac Sonographer
Echocardiography Laboratory Heart and Vascular Institute
Henry Ford Hospital
Detroit, Michigan, USA

BC Tuck MD
Department of Anesthesiology
University of Alabama at Birmingham
Birmingham, Alabama, USA

NSN Turaga MBBS
Echocardiography Laboratory
University of Alabama at Birmingham
Birmingham, Alabama, USA

B Uygur MD
Echocardiography Laboratory
University of Alabama at Birmingham
Birmingham, Alabama, USA

Inga Vaitenas RCS RCCS
Lead Sonographer
Northwestern Memorial Hospital
Northwestern University
Chicago, Illinois, USA

Anastasia Vamvakidou MBBS MRCP (UK)
Cardiology Specialty Registrar
Northwick Park Hospital
Harrow, UK

Padmini Varadarajan MD
Professor of Medicine
Loma Linda University Medical Center
Loma Linda, California, USA

Archana Vasudevan MD
Resident Physician
Department of Medicine
University of Missouri
Columbia, Missouri, USA

Virginia Michelis Vázquez MD
Former Assistant Professor
National Armed Forces Hospital and Medical Center
Montevideo, Uruguay

Sridhar Venkatachalam MD
Senior Fellow
Division of Cardiology
The University Texas Medical Branch (UTMB)
Galveston, Texas, USA

Zvi Vered MD FACC FESC
Cardiologist and Professor
Department of Cardiology
Assaf Harofeh Medical Center
Sackler School of Medicine
Tel Aviv University
Tel Aviv, Israel

Mustafa Gökhan Vural MD
Cardiologist
Department of Cardiology
Faculty of Medicine
University of Sakarya
Sakarya, Turkey

Ronald B Williams BA RT(R) (MR)
Cardiovascular MRI Technologist
Cardiac MRI Center
Allegheny General Hospital
Pittsburgh, Pennsylvania, USA

June A Yamrozik RT
Cardiovascular MRI Technologist
Cardiac MRI Center
Allegheny General Hospital
Pittsburgh, Pennsylvania, USA

Desiree M Younes MD FACC
Cardiologist
Princeton Healthcare System
A New Jersey Non-profit Corporation
Robert Wood Johnson University Hospital
New Jersey, USA

B Yuzbas MD
Echocardiography Laboratory
University of Alabama at Birmingham
Birmingham, Alabama, USA

Annapaola Zito MD
Cardiologist
Cardiovascular Diseases Section
Department of Emergency and Organ Transplantation
University of Bari School of Medicine
Bari, Italy

Preface

Despite many path-breaking advances in cardiology, echocardiography remains the most cost-effective noninvasive technique in the assessment of various cardiac disease entities. It serves as a valuable tool in the armamentarium of a practicing cardiologist. Throughout the past several decades, various national and international conferences dealing with echocardiography and allied techniques, such as magnetic resonance imaging and computed tomography scans have been held in different countries and many cities of USA. They have served as a forum for exchange of information and have provided updates on the current status and recent advances in echocardiography not only to the practicing echocardiographers and cardiologists, but also to the physicians of various other specialties, such as internists, general physicians, anesthesiologists, emergency room physicians, critical care specialists, and cardiac surgeons as well as technologists and other paramedical personnel. The International Society of Cardiovascular Ultrasound as well as the Echocardiography Laboratory of the University of Alabama, Birmingham, Alabama in co-operation with other organizations have also been in the forefront in conducting these conferences. World Conferences on Echocardiography have been successfully organized practically every year for the past 22 years, and International Conferences on Echocardiography and Allied Techniques have been held at the annual meetings of the American Heart Association and the American College of Cardiology for over three decades. The latter conferences have taken the format of brief interesting and instructive case presentations by a large number of faculties. These case presentations have proven very popular and it was felt by many of us that an effort should be made to publish some of these cases in a book format in both print and internet versions. With this in mind, invitations were sent to the faculty, who had presented cases previously at these meetings and to others to submit their cases for publication. This book, therefore, represents a compilation of more than 280 interesting and instructive cases submitted by several echocardiographers, cardiologists and other physicians from many different parts of the world. The book should prove useful to all physicians, ultrasound technologists and paramedical personnel, who already have some background in cardiac ultrasound, but are interested in learning its usefulness in day-to-day clinical practice.

The book is organized into 11 sections, all of which consist of case presentations. The pattern followed in many cases consists of a brief patient history and relevant clinical findings, echocardiographic images/movie clips, one or more multiple-choice questions with correct answers provided and a short relevant discussion. Pertinent references are also given in some cases. The first three sections of the book deal with the mitral, aortic, tricuspid and pulmonary valves as well as the aorta and pulmonary hypertension. The next two sections cover prosthetic valves, rings, plugs and clips, and infection and endocarditis respectively. These are followed by coronary artery disease, and left/right ventricles and cardiomyopathies. Pericardial disorders, tumors and masses, and congenital heart disease are dealt with next. The last section consists of miscellaneous cases plus a few cases which were submitted late and, hence, could not be accommodated in the relevant sections. Almost all cases predominantly deal with echocardiography with some showing comparisons with other techniques, mainly magnetic resonance imaging and computed tomographic scans. Only magnetic resonance images are shown in a couple of cases.

Navin C Nanda MD

Acknowledgments

I am most grateful to all the contributors who took time off from their busy schedule to send their interesting/instructive cases for publication in this book. I also need to express my heartfelt gratitude to all the current and past echocardiography fellows, researchers, residents and trainees, who helped me edit and, in many cases, labeled the images and movies sent by others as well as those from our Echo Laboratory and Dr Ming Chon Hsiung's Echo Laboratory in Taipei, Taiwan. They are Drs Mohamed Elsayed, Serkan Bulur, Ahmed Taher, Nermina Alagic, Lani Adarna, Emel, Ahmed Mohamed, Neelesh Gupta, Begum Uygur, Tugba Kemaloglu Oz, Jugal Chahwala, Kunal Bhagatwala, Turaga Naga, Pudussery Kattalan, Garima Arora, Burcu Gol, Mustafa Vural, Akhilesh Mahajan, Nurgul Keser, Pratayaksha Sankhyan, Rajat Kalra, Mustafa Ahmed, and Mathew Joson. I am also most appreciative of Dr Ming Hsuing's enormous and heartfelt co-operation in this endeavor. Mr Jitendar P Vij and his team at Jaypee Brothers, which include Ms Chetna Malhotra Vohra, Nedup Denka Bhutia, Saima Rashid and Geetanjali Singh, and their audio-visual team, deserve my deep gratitude for helping publish this book in a timely manner. I am particularly grateful to Mr Jitendar P Vij for his constant encouragement and full support in completing this project. Last but not least, it would not have been possible for me to undertake this work without the enormous support of my wife, Kanta Nanda, who also helped me with editing.

Contents

Section 3: Tricuspid and Pulmonary Valves, Pulmonary Hypertension

Section 4: Prostheses, Rings and Clips

Section 8: Pericardial Disorders

Section 9: Tumors and Masses

Section 10: Congenital Heart Disease

Section 11: Miscellaneous

Abbreviations

- 99m Tc DPD : Technetium diphosphonopropanodicarboxylic acid
- 99m Tc PYP : Technetium pyrophosphate
- 2D : Two-dimensional
- 3D : Three-dimensional
- ABD : Abdomen
- ABG : Arterial blood gases
- ACEI : Angiotensinogen converting enzyme inhibitor
- ACLS : Advanced cardiovascular life support
- AF : Atrial fibrillation
- AICD : Automatic implantable cardioverter-defibrillator
- AML : Anterior mitral leaflet
- Anti CMV : Antibody against cytomegalovirus
- AO : Aorta/aortic
- AR : Aortic regurgitation
- ARB : Angiotensin receptor blocker
- AS : Aortic stenosis
- ASD : Atrial septal defect
- ATVL : Anterior tricuspid valve leaflet
- AV : Aortic valve
- AVR : Aortic valve replacement
- BNP : Brain natriuretic peptide
- BP : Blood pressure
- BSA : Body surface area
- BUN : Blood urea nitrogen
- C/W : Consistent with
- CA : Coronary artery
- CABG : Coronary artery bypass graft
- CAD : Coronary artery disease
- Cath : Catheterization
- CBC : Complete blood count
- CECT : Contrast enhanced computed tomography
- CK : Creatine kinase
- CKD : Chronic kidney disease
- CKMB : Serum creatine kinase MB isoenzyme
- CMRI : Cardiac magnetic resonance imaging
- CO : Cardiac output
- COPD : Chronic obstructive pulmonary disease
- CPK : Creatinine phosphokinase
- CPR : Cardiopulmonary resuscitation
- Cr : Creatinine
- CS : Coronary sinus
- CSA : Cross-sectional surface area
- CT : Computed tomography
- CTA : Clear to auscultation
- CTA : Computed tomography angiography
- CTn : Cardiac troponin
- CV : Cardiovascular
- CVE : Cerebrovascular embolism
- CVP : Central venous pressure
- CVS : Cardiovascular system
- CXR : Chest X-ray
- DA : Descending thoracic aorta
- DCM : Dilated cardiomyopathy
- DD : Diastolic dysfunction
- DM : Diabetes mellitus
- DP : Diastolic pressure
- DTGA : Dextro-transposition of the great arteries
- DTI : Doppler tissue imaging
- DVT : Deep venous thrombosis
- E : Eosinophil
- ECG/EKG : Electrocardiogram
- ED : Emergency department
- EF : Ejection fraction
- EOA : Effective orifice area
- ER : Emergency room
- ESR : Erythrocyte sedimentation rate
- EV : Eustachian valve
- F/U : Follow up
- FAC : Fractional area change
- FHx : Family history
- HB : Hemoglobin
- HCM : Hypertrophic cardiomyopathy
- HCT : Hematocrit
- HF : Heart failure
- HR : Heart rate
- HTN : Hypertension
- HV : Hepatic vein
- Hx : History
- IAS : Inter-atrial septum
- ICD : Intracardiac defibrillator
- ICU : Intensive care unit
- INR : International normalized ratio
- IV : Intravenous
- IVC : Inferior vena cava
- IVRT : Isovolemic relaxation time
- IVS : Interventricular septum
- JVD : Jugular venous distension
- K : Potassium
- KFT : Kidney function test
- L : Left
- L : Liters
- L : Liver
- L : Lymphocyte

- L : Pacemaker lead
- LA : Left atrium
- LAD : Left anterior descending coronary artery
- LCX/CX : Left circumflex coronary artery
- LDL : Low density lipoprotein
- LFT : Liver function test
- Li : Liver
- LTGA : Levo-transposition of the great arteries
- LV : Left ventricle
- LVEF : Left ventricular ejection fraction
- LVH : Left ventricular hypertrophy
- LVO : Left ventricular outflow
- LVOT : Left ventricular outflow tract
- MAP : Mean arterial pressure
- MI : Myocardial infarction
- ML : Mitral valve leaflet
- MPI : Myocardial perfusion imaging
- MR : Mitral regurgitation
- MRI : Magnetic resonance imaging
- MS : Mitral stenosis
- MV : Mitral valve
- MVOA : Mitral valve orifice area
- MVP : Mitral valve prolapse
- N : Neutrophil
- Na : Sodium
- NICM : Non-ischemic cardiomyopathy
- NL : Normal
- NSR : Normal sinus rhythm
- NSTEMI : Non-ST segment elevation myocardial infarction
- NT-Pro BNP: N-terminal pro B-type natriuretic peptide
- NYHA : New York Heart Association
- O_2 : Oxygen
- OA : Orifice area
- OM : Obtuse marginal coronary artery
- OR : Operating room
- PA : Pulmonary artery
- PASP : Pulmonary artery systolic pressure
- PDA : Patent ductus arteriosus
- PE : Pulmonary embolism
- PE : Physical examination
- PE : Pericardial effusion
- PEA : Pulseless electrical activity
- PFO : Patent foramen ovale
- PG : Pressure gradient
- PH : Pulmonary hypertension
- PHT : Pressure half time, Pulmonary hypertension
- PHTN : Pulmonary hypertension
- PISA : Proximal isovelocity surface area
- PL : Pleural effusion
- PLT : Platelet
- PMBV : Percutaneous mitral balloon valvuloplasty
- PML : Posterior mitral valve leaflet
- PP : Pulse pressure
- PR : Pulmonary regurgitation
- PS : Pulmonary stenosis
- Pts : Patients
- PTT : Partial thromboplastin time
- PV : Pulmonary valve
- R : Right
- RA : Right atrium
- RBS : Random blood sugar
- RCA : Right coronary artery
- RCM : Restrictive cardiomyopathy
- Reg Vol : Regurgitation (regurgitant) volume
- RHC : Right heart catheterization
- ROSC : Return of spontaneous circulation
- RRR : Regular rate and rhythm
- RV : Right ventricle
- RVE : Right ventricular enlargement
- RVH : Right ventricular hypertrophy
- RVO : Right ventricular outflow
- RVOT : Right ventricular outflow tract
- RVSF : Right ventricular systolic failure
- RVSP : Right ventricular systolic pressure
- S/P : Status post
- S1 : First heart sound
- S2 : Second heart sound
- S3 : Third heart sound
- SAM : Systolic anterior motion of the mitral valve
- SAX : Short axis view
- SBP : Systolic blood pressure
- SC : Subclavian artery
- SHX : Social history
- SOB : Shortness of breath
- SPECT : Single photon emission computed tomography
- STE : Speckle tracking echocardiography
- STEMI : ST segment elevation myocardial infarction
- STVL : Septal tricuspid valve leaflet
- SV : Stroke volume
- SVC : Superior vena cava
- SVG : Saphenous venous graft
- SVR : Systemic vascular resistance
- T : Temperature
- TAPSE : Tricuspid annulus planar systolic excursion
- TDI : Tissue Doppler imaging
- TEE : Transesophageal echocardiography
- TIA : Transient ischemic attack
- TLC : Total leucocyte count
- TGA : Transposition of the great arteries
- toF : Tetralogy of Fallot
- TPA : Tissue plasminogen activator
- TR : Tricuspid regurgitation
- Trop-T : Troponin T

- TTE : Transthoracic echocardiography
- TV : Tricuspid valve
- UTI : Urinary tract infection
- VC : Vena contracta
- VMAX : Maximum velocity
- V/Q : Ventilation/perfusion
- VS : Ventricular septum
- VSD : Ventricular septal defect
- VTI : Velocity time integral
- WBC : White blood cell
- WMA : Wall motion abnormality

SECTION 1

Mitral Valve

CASE 1

Alagic N, Elsayed M, Uygur B, Adarna LG, Chahwala JR, Bhagatwala K, Bulur S, Turaga NSN, Pudussery Kattalan JJ, Nanda NC

A 46-year-old female with shortness of breath on mild exertion. She had one episode of pulmonary edema in the recent past. There is no definite history of rheumatic fever. 2D TTE, 2D TEE and 3D TEE were done.

1. **What do movies 1–8 show?**
   (a) Rheumatic MS
   (b) MVP
   (c) Lupus erythematosis
   (d) Myxomatous MV
   (e) Severe MV annular calcification producing stenosis

Ans. (a)

The mitral valve (arrow) shows diastolic dooming with a characteristic hockey stick appearance (🎥 1, 4 and 5). Mitral valve (MV) area by Doppler pressure half time (PHT) method measured 0.94 cm^2 consistent with severe stenosis. The most common etiology is rheumatic fever. The LA appendage appears clear on 2D TTE (🎥 2) and this is confirmed by 2D TEE (🎥 7). TR gradient measured 40 mm Hg by TEE suggestive of mild pulmonary hypertension (🎥 6). 3D TEE (🎥 8) shows a narrow MV orifice with commissural fusion indicative of severe stenosis.

The patient underwent successful percutaneous MV annuloplasty.

MOVIES 1 TO 8 🎥

CASE 2

Roomi AU, Shah A, Siddiqui LI, Elsayed M, Bulur S, Nanda NC

A young female with history of rheumatic heart disease in the past who is now presenting with shortness of breath on mild exertion. 2D TEE is done. (9 and 10A and 10B and Figs. 2.1 and 2.2A and 2.2B).

1. **In a patient with mitral stenosis, all the following are contraindicated for balloon valvuloplasty *except*:**
   (a) Spontaneous echo contrast in LA and LAA
   (b) Thrombus in LA or LAA
   (c) Low velocities in LAA
   (d) Marked thickening of mitral subvalvular apparatus
   (e) Severe MR

Ans. (a) and (c)

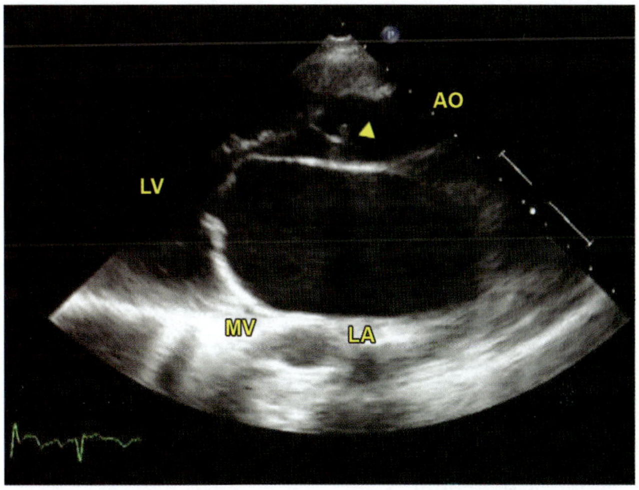

Fig. 2.1: TTE. Parasternal long axis view. Shows restricted motion of thickened MV leaflets presenting with typical hockey-stick appearance indicative of MS. LA is enlarged. Arrowhead shows thickened but mobile AV leaflets.

MOVIE LEGENDS

9: TTE. Parasternal long axis view. Shows restricted motion of thickened MV leaflets presenting with typical hockey-stick appearance indicative of MS. LA is enlarged. Arrowhead shows thickened but mobile AV leaflets.

10A: TEE shows limited opening of the MV (arrow). Arrowhead points to spontaneous echo contrast (SEC) in the dilated LA;

10B: Transesophageal echocardiography. Arrow points to a thrombus in the LAA.

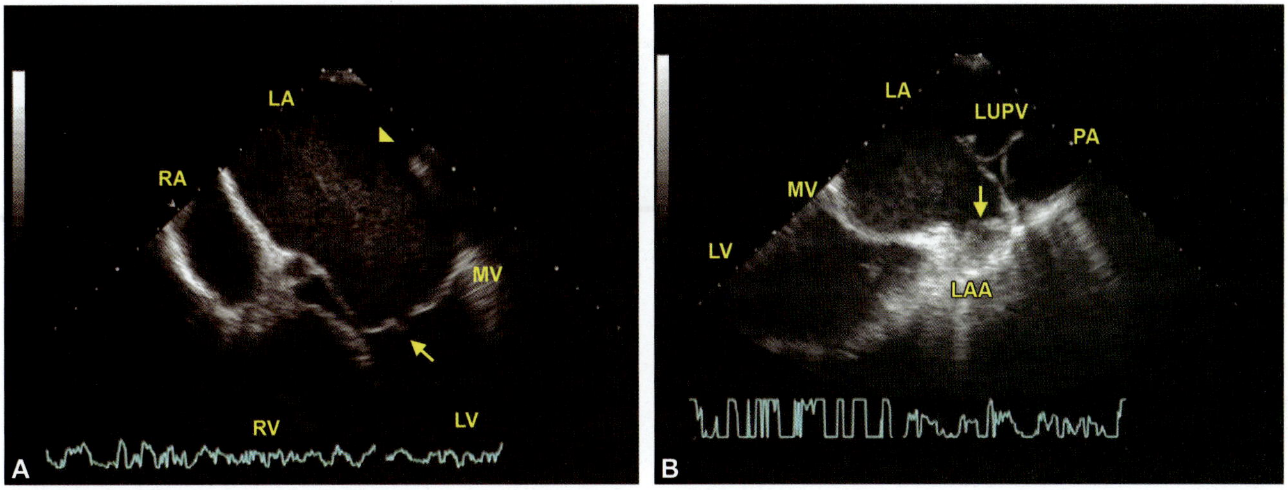

Figs. 2.2A and B: TEE. (A) Shows limited opening of the MV (arrow). Arrowhead points to spontaneous echo contrast (SEC) in the dilated LA; (B) Arrow points to a thrombus in the LAA.

CASE 3

Uygur B, Mohamed A, Gupta N, Elsayed M, Nanda NC

TEEs done in three different patients with mitral stenosis (MS) are shown. Mitral valve is only mildly thickened and LAA is clear in the first patient (🎥 11 to 13). In the second patient, ASD created prior to balloon valvotomy is noted. LAA is clear. 3D TEE was also done showing a narrow mitral orifice (🎥 14 to 17). CW Doppler displaying a flat MV diastolic slope is imaged in the third patient (Fig. 3.1).

1. **All of the following are causes of MS *except*:**
   (a) Mitral valve annular calcification (MAC)
   (b) Rheumatic fever
   (c) Systemic lupus erythematosis
   (d) Turner syndrome
   (e) Large vegetation/tumor
   (f) Congenital

Ans. (d)

2. **All of the following are included in the Wilkin's score which is used to determine suitability for percutaneous MV balloon valvuloplasty *except*:**
   (a) MV thickening
   (b) MV mobility
   (c) MV calcification
   (d) Subvalvular thickening
   (e) Calcification of MV commissures

Ans. (e)

Calcification of mitral commissures, a contraindication for MV balloon valvuloplasty, is a significant omission in the Wilkin's criteria.

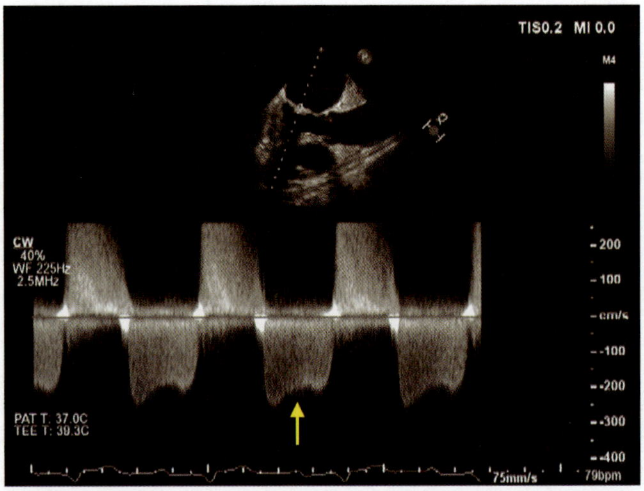

Fig. 3.1: CW Doppler shows a flat MV diastolic slope (arrow)

3. **Which of the following can be used to assess MS severity ?**
   (a) Planimetry
   (b) Continuity equation
   (c) Pressure half time (PHT)
   (d) Proximal isovelocity surface area
   (e) Mean transmitral gradient
   (f) Vena contracta
   (g) All of the above

Ans. (g)

MOVIES 11 TO 17 🎥

CASE 4

Abdullah Al Shafi Majumder, AKM Monwarul Islam

GIANT LEFT ATRIUM

Giant left atrium (LA) is a rare entity with the decreasing incidence of rheumatic heart disease; the reported incidence varies from 0.3–0.6% in those suffering from rheumatic heart disease.[1,2] It was traditionally defined as one where the LA touches the lateral chest wall on chest radiograph.[1,3] With the advent of echocardiography, it has been re-defined variably as the LA having a cardio-thoracic ratio on chest radiograph of >0.7 combined with an LA diameter of >8 cm[4] (or according to some authors >6.5 cm[5]) on two-dimensional transthoracic echocardiography (2D TTE).[5] Giant LA is typically found in patients with rheumatic mitral valve disease, but has also been described in association with mitral valve prolapse, hypertrophic cardiomyopathy, cardiac amyloidosis, heart failure and chronic atrial fibrillation (AF). Giant LA commonly presents with its compression effects on adjacent structures, causing Ortner's syndrome due to left recurrent laryngeal nerve palsy, dysphagia due to esophageal compression, and dyspnea due to atelectasis. Giant LA, specially if accompanied by AF, may facilitate formation of thrombus, or spontaneous echo contrast (SEC), the latter may be the harbinger of the former.

Here, two cases of giant LA have been described, both were in association with predominant mitral stenosis (MS) of rheumatic origin; one showed a large LA mass, either thrombus or myxoma, and the other presented with profuse, dense SEC masking an underlying thrombus in the LA cavity.

CASE A

A 26-year-old female presented with shortness of breath and cough for 6 months. The pulse was irregularly irregular, the 1st heart sound was of variable intensity, and there was a localized mid diastolic murmur in the apical area. ECG showed AF and right ventricular hypertrophy. 2D TTE as well as 2D transesophageal echocardiography (2D TEE) revealed features of severe MS, giant LA, measuring 10 cm, profuse, dense SEC in LA, but no definite thrombus (Figs. 4.1A to D and 🎥 18A to C). For management, initially percutaneous transvenous mitral commissurotomy (PTMC) was thought of, but considering probable technical difficulties in association with a hugely dilated LA, it was abandoned. Peroperatively, during open mitral commissurotomy (OMC), a large amount of thrombus was found in the LA cavity (Fig. 4.1E). Arrowheads in figures and 🎥 point to SEC.

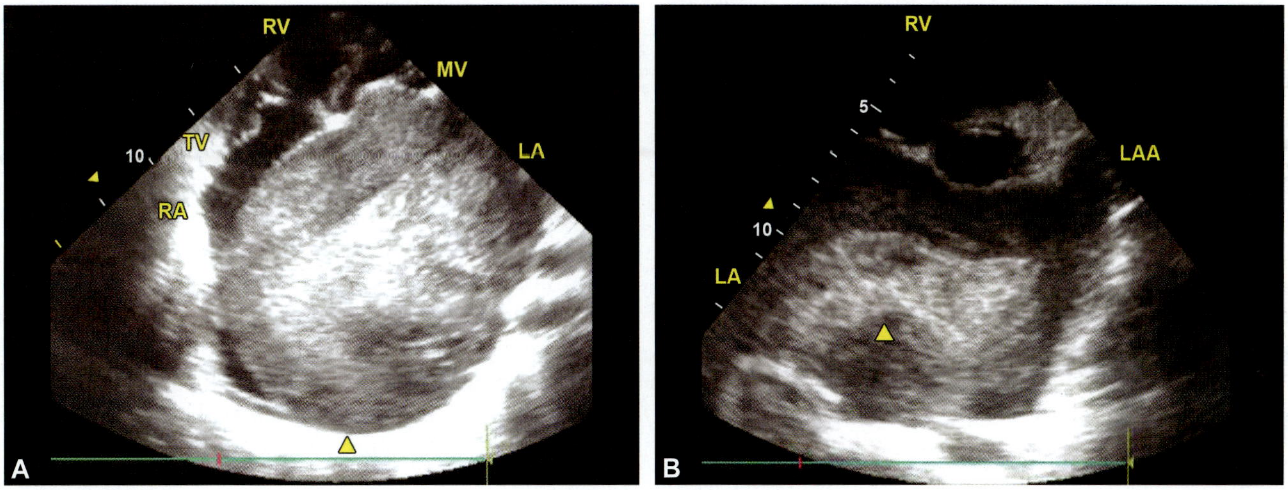

Figs. 4.1A and B

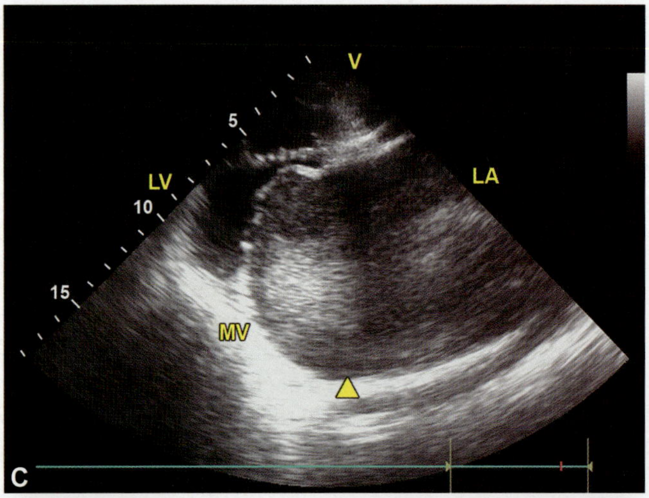

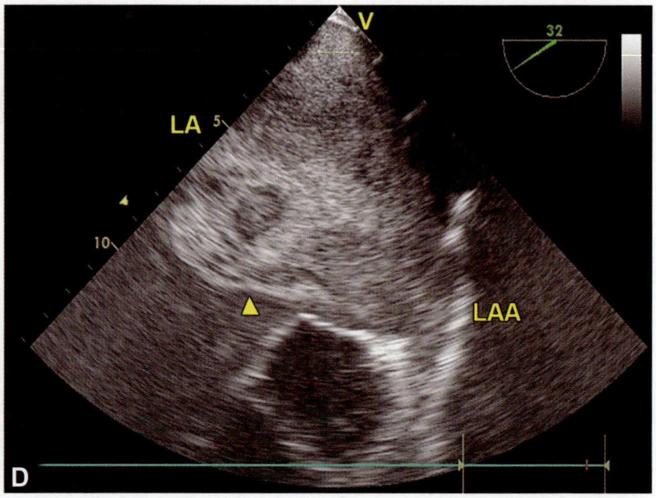

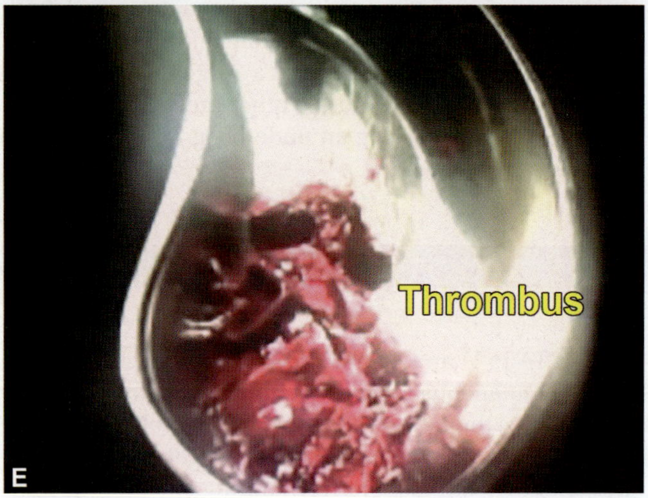

Figs. 4.1A to E: Transthoracic echocardiography apical 4-chamber (A), appendicular (B) and left parasternal long axis (C) views showing features of severe mitral stenosis, dilated left atrium and dense, spontaneous echo contrast. (D) Transesophageal echocardiography mid-esophageal view at 32° showing dilated left atrium, dense, spontaneous echo contrast, and appendage free of definite thrombus. (E) Thrombus extracted from left atrium during open mitral commissurotomy. (LA: Left atrium; RA: Right atrium; LV: Left ventricle; RV: Right ventricle; LAA: Left atrial appendage; MV: Mitral valve; TV: Tricuspid valve).

CASE B

A 32-year-old female presented with shortness of breath and palpitations for 1 year. The pulse was irregularly irregular, the 1st heart sound was of variable intensity, and there was a localized mid-diastolic murmur in the apical area, similar to Case A. 2D TTE revealed features of severe MS, giant LA, measuring 11.2 cm × 12.1 cm, and a large, heterogeneous mass, measuring 6.7 cm × 6.3 cm and 33.1 cm^2, attached to the LA wall, most likely a thrombus (Figs. 4.2A to D and 🎥 19A and B). For management, surgery was planned. Arrows in figures and 🎥 denote the thrombus.

DISCUSSION

Giant LA was first reported by Owen and Fenton as an autopsy finding in a patient with rheumatic fever in 1901.[6] It is most commonly associated with severe, isolated or predominant mitral regurgitation (MR) of rheumatic etiology. In case of isolated MS, giant LA is unusual. Both the two cases presented here have severe MS without significant MR. For giant LA, echocardiography is the imaging technique of choice because of its precision in assessing the heart chambers. Nonetheless, in some cases, echocardiography may not be sufficient to define accurately the atria and adjacent structures; computed tomography and magnetic resonance imaging have been considered as additional techniques for this purpose, particularly in patients with a cardiothoracic ratio > 0.7.[7]

The enlarged LA is associated with blood stasis and thrombus formation and the presence of AF further increases the risk. The incidence of LA thrombus in patients with MS and AF is 7–38%; such an incidence is

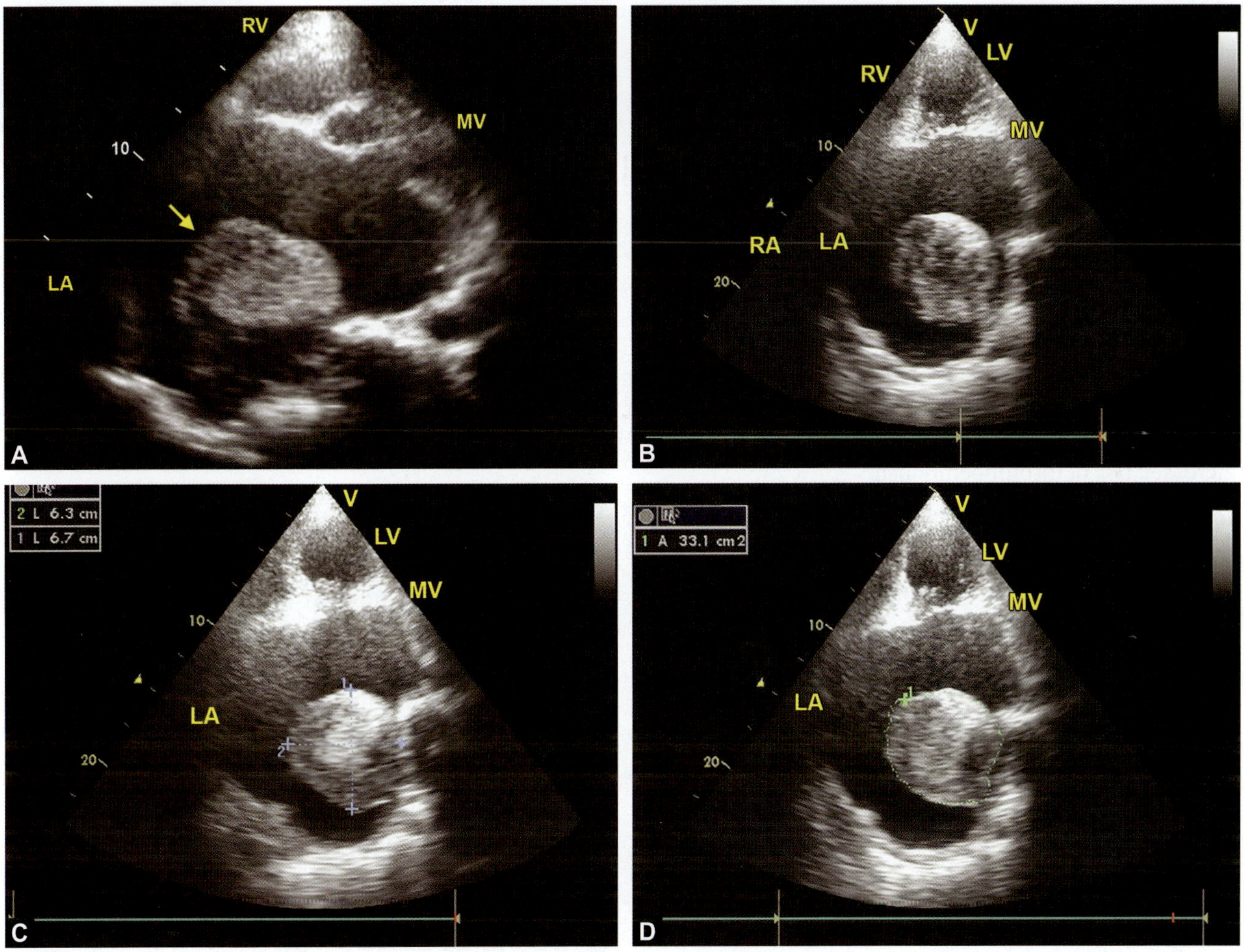

Figs. 4.2A to D: Transthoracic echocardiography off-axis (A) and apical 4-chamber (B, C, D) views showing features of severe mitral stenosis, dilated left atrium and a large, heterogeneous mass (arrow), measuring 6.7 cm × 6.3 cm (C) and 33.1 cm^2 (D), attached to the LA wall. (LA: Left atrium; RA: Right atrium; LV: Left ventricle; RV: Right ventricle; MV: Mitral valve).

directly related to the size of LA.[8-10] The prevalence of SEC in LA may be 54–65% in these patients.[8,11] Dilated LA in association with predominant regurgitant lesion may actually be less prone to stasis in comparison to that resulting from predominant stenosis. Giant LA from underlying MS (with absence of significant MR) and in association with AF created an optimum milieu for the formation of thrombus in Case A and spontaneous echo contrast in Case B. Proper identification of SEC and LA thrombus is of crucial importance since the presence of the latter but not the former is a contraindication for cardioversion and PTMC. 'Coumadin ridge' is a ridge of atrial tissue separating the LA appendage from the left upper pulmonary vein. It can present as a linear structure or even sometimes as a nodular mass that protrudes into left atrium mimicking a thrombus or atrial myxoma. In the past, this structure was often mistaken for thrombus and resulted in the patient being mistakenly prescribed anticoagulation therapy with warfarin (coumadin) and it is because of this it derives its name. Occasionally, extensive SEC can mask a thrombus on 2D TEE as in Case A and in such a case live/real time three-dimensional (3D) TTE/TEE can be helpful in detecting it and also differentiating it from pectinate muscles.[14] A disadvantage of both 2D TTE and TEE is that they provide only a thin slice or section of cardiac structures at any given time limiting their utility in comprehensively assessing the LA appendage. On the other hand, both 3D TTE and TEE can encompass the whole extent of the LA appendage in three-dimensions in the acquired data set, which can then be cropped and sectioned systematically at any desired angulation to more definitively look into the interior. Recently, cardiac computed tomography[13] and cardiac magnetic resonance[14] have been reported to be reliable alternatives to TEE for diagnosing a LA thrombus.

TEE assessment of LA appendage flow velocities by pulsed-wave Doppler examination can also provide incremental information about the risk of clot formation. Of the typical quadriphasic flow pattern thus derived, the late diastolic emptying velocity or LA appendage contraction flow occurring immediately after the P wave on the ECG is a significant predictor of thromboembolic risk. The contraction velocities of ≤ 20 cm/s (normal peak velocities 50–60 cm/s) have been found to be associated with increased risk of thromboembolism.

There may be more than one correct answer.

1. **Definition of a giant left atrium includes:**
   (a) Diameter of left atrium exceeds twice that of aorta
   (b) The cardiac border touches the lateral chest wall on chest radiograph
   (c) Diameter of left atrium is at least twice that of right atrium
   (d) Cardiothoracic ratio >0.6 on a chest radiograph
   (e) Diameter of left atrium exceeds 80 mm

Ans. (b) and (e)

2. **Regarding giant left atrium:**
   (a) Most commonly seen in rheumatic heart disease
   (b) Isolated or predominant stenotic lesion of mitral valve is the usual cause
   (c) Mitral valve prolapse may be a cause
   (d) May lead to Ortner syndrome
   (e) May harbour spontaneous echo contrast, but not thrombus

Ans. (a), (b) and (d)

3. **Spontaneous echo contrast:**
   (a) Always indicates presence of thrombus
   (b) May be seen in the absence of atrial fibrillation
   (c) More commonly found in mitral regurgitation than in mitral stenosis
   (d) Cardiac CT scan is more useful than echocardiography for the diagnosis
   (e) Is a contraindication for percutaneous transvenous mitral commissurotomy

Ans. (b)

4. **Regarding diagnosis of left atrial thrombus:**
   (a) Transthoracic echocardiography is highly sensitive but the specificity is only modest
   (b) Transesophageal echocardiography has high sensitivity and specificity
   (c) Pectinate muscles can produce confusion during transthoracic echocardiography
   (d) Coumadin ridge is a differential diagnosis of an intracardiac mass
   (e) 3D echo cannot differentiate a clot from pectinate muscles in the left atrial appendage

Ans. (b), (c) and (d)

5. **For detection of left atrial thrombus:**
   (a) Spontaneous echo contrast may hide thrombus
   (b) Cardiac computed tomography and cardiac magnetic resonance may be useful
   (c) Cardiac computed tomography is as sensitive and specific as transesophageal echocardiography
   (d) Cardiac magnetic resonance is the gold standard test
   (e) Reduced left atrial appendage velocity may be a useful indicator

Ans. (a), (b), (c) and (e)

MOVIE LEGENDS

18A: Transthoracic 2D echocardiography apical 4-chamber view showing features of severe mitral stenosis, giant left atrium and profuse, dense spontaneous echo contrast in left atrium (arrowhead).

18B: Transthoracic 2D echocardiography appendicular view showing spontaneous echo contrast (arrowhead) in left atrium, but the appendage free of thrombus.

18C: Transesophageal echocardiography mid-esophageal view at 49° showing spontaneous echo contrast (arrowhead) in dilated left atrium, but the appendage free of thrombus.

19A: Transthoracic echocardiography off-axis view showing features of severe mitral stenosis, dilated left atrium and a large, heterogeneous mass (arrow), possibly attached to the left atrial wall.

19B: Transthoracic echocardiography apical 4-chamber view showing features of severe mitral stenosis, dilated left atrium and the thrombus in the left atrium.

REFERENCES

1. DeSanctis RW, Dean DC, Bland EF. Extreme left atrial enlargement. Some characteristic features. Circulation. 1964 Jan;29:14-23.
2. El Maghraby A, Hajar R. Giant left atrium: a review. Heart Views. 2012 Apr;13(2):46-52.
3. Hurst W. Memories of patients with a giant left atrium. Circulation. 2001;104:2630-1.
4. Piccoli GP, Massini C, Di Eusanio G, Ballerini L, Tacobone G, Soro A, et al. Giant left atrium and mitral valve disease: Early and late results of surgical treatment in 40 cases. J Cardiovasc Surg. 1984;25:328–36.
5. Oh JK. Echocardiographic evaluation of morphological and hemodynamic significance of giant left atrium. Circulation. 1992;86:328-30.
6. Owen I, Fenton WJ. A case of extreme dilatation of the left auricle of the heart. Trans Clin Soc London. 1901;34:183-91.
7. Moral S, Fernández-Friera L, Sanz J. Giant left atrium investigated by magnetic resonance imaging. Rev Esp Cardiol. 2011 Mar;64(3):232.
8. Farman MT, Sial JA, Khan N, Rahu QA, Tasneem H, Ishaq H. Severe mitral stenosis with atrial fibrillation—a harbinger of thromboembolism. J Pak Med Assoc. 2010;60(6): 439-43.
9. Apostolakis E, Shuhaiber JH: The surgical management of giant left atrium. Eur J Cardiothorac Surg. 2008, 33(2): 182-90.
10. Di Eusanio G, Gregorini R, Mazzola A, Clementi G, Procaccini B, Cavarra F, et al. Giant left atrium and mitral valve replacement: risk factor analysis. Eur J Cardiothorac Surg. 1988;2(3):151-9.
11. Saha GK, Ali MA, Hossain N, Zaher A, Miah MA, Zaman MA. Incidence of spontaneous echocontrast in left atrium in mitral stenosis detected by transoesophageal echo cardiography and related factors. Bangladesh Med Res Counc Bull. 2000 Aug;26(2):56-60.
12. Kumar V, Nanda NC. Is it time to move on from two-dimensional transesophageal to three-dimensional transthoracic echocardiography for assessment of left atrial appendage? Review of existing literature. Echocardiography. 2012; 29(1):112-6.
13. Romero J, Husain SA, Kelesidis I, et al. Detection of left atrial appendage thrombus by cardiac computed tomography in patients with atrial fibrillation: a meta-analysis. Circ-Cardiovasc Imaging. 2013 Mar 1;6(2):185-94.
14. Rathi VK, Reddy ST, Anreddy S, et al. Contrast-enhanced CMR is equally effective as TEE in the evaluation of left atrial appendage thrombus in patients with atrial fibrillation undergoing pulmonary vein isolation procedure. Heart Rhythm. 2013 Jul;10(7):1021-7.

CASE 5

Ahmad S Omran

RHEUMATIC SEVERE MITRAL STENOSIS PERCUTANEOUS MITRAL BALLOON VALVULOPLASTY (PMBV)

This 39-year-old male presented to our center with acute pulmonary edema. Transthoracic echocardiography (TTE) (Figs. 5.1A and B) showed mitral leaflet thickening, reduced motion of posterior mitral leaflet and typical "hockey stick appearance" of the anterior mitral valve leaflet consistent with rheumatic mitral stenosis (MS). Large pericardial effusion was noted in this study which is not uncommon in severe MS with pulmonary hypertension. This effusion was drained prior to percutaneous mitral valve balloon valvuloplasty (PMBV). Mitral valve area by pressure half time method (PHT) was calculated at less than 1.0 cm^2 and mean gradient across the mitral valve was 15 mmHg. There was trace tricuspid regurgitation with estimated right ventricular systolic pressure of 60–70 mmHg. After initial stabilization of the patient, he underwent transesophageal echocardiography (TEE) for better visualization of the mitral valve and decision- making for PMBV. Transesophageal echocardiography showed marked spontaneous echo contrast (smoke) in the left atrium and appendage (LAA) but no obvious clot was noted. 3D TEE (Figs. 5.2A and B, 20 and 21) clearly showed severely stenotic mitral orifice with fusion of both commissures. Mitral valve area was re-assessed by 3D TEE direct planimetry at the level of the orifice and was repeated by QLAB software which came between 0.7–1.0 cm^2 confirming TTE findings. Echocardiographic Wilkin's score of the mitral valve was calculated as 7–8. There was no contraindication for PMBV based on American and European guidelines for management of patients with valvular heart disease.[1,2] Patient underwent PBMV under general anesthesia and 3D TEE guidance (Figs. 5.3A and B, 22 and 23). Successful PMBV was performed after 2 attempts of balloon inflation with PTMC-28 and 30 (Inoue balloons). 3D TEE en-face view of the mitral valve immediately after PMBV (Figs. 5.4A and B, 24) showed excellent result with mitral orifice area = 1.5 cm^2, both commissures well split and only trace mitral regurgitation. Pre-discharge TTE showed mitral valve area (MVA) by PHT of 2.1 cm^2 and mean gradient of 6–7 mmHg. Follow up TTE after one year showed MVA about 1.9 cm^2 and patient is in good clinical condition.

Percutaneous mitral balloon valvuloplasty (PMBV) was first described by Inoue in 1984. Since its introduction,

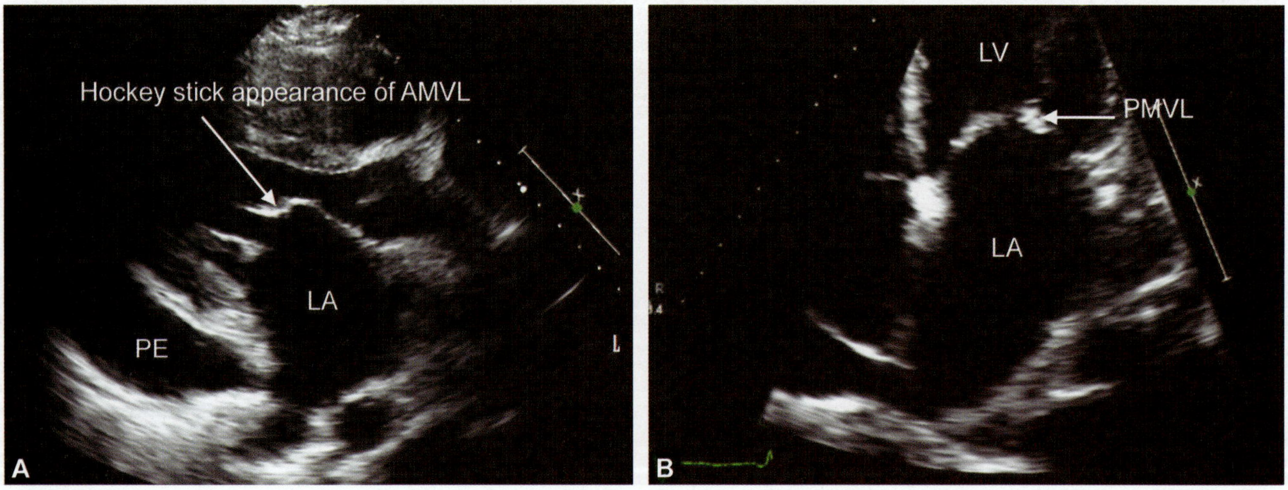

Figs. 5.1A and B: Transthoracic echocardiography (TTE). (A) TTE in parasternal long-axis view shows mitral valve thickening, reduced motion of posterior mitral leaflet and typical "hockey stick appearance" of the anterior mitral valve leaflet (AMVL) consistent with rheumatic mitral stenosis (MS). Large pericardial effusion is noted (PE). (B) Apical 4-chamber view showing diastolic doming of the mitral leaflets. (LV: Left ventricle; LA: Left atrium).

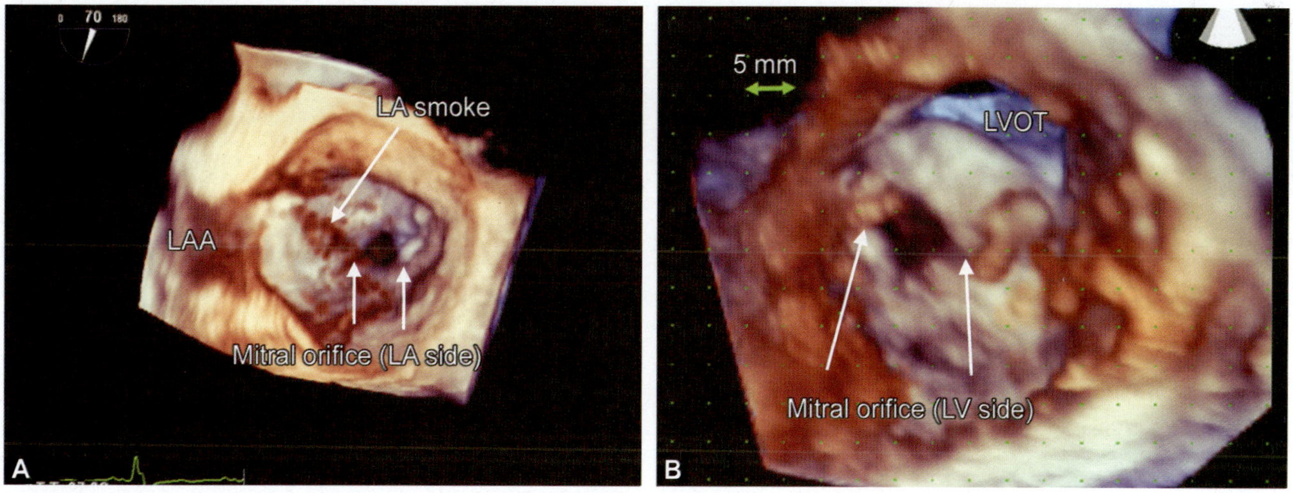

Figs. 5.2A and B: 3D transesophageal echocardiography (3D TEE). (A) 3D TEE zoom mode acquisition of the mitral valve in surgical view shows a severely stenotic mitral valve. Marked "smoke" can be seen in the left atrial appendage (LAA) and left atrium (LA). 3D grid is seen (5 mm) which can be calibrated to calculate mitral orifice area from LA or LV side. (B) 3D TEE zoom mode from left ventricular (LV) perspective showing fish-mouth appearance of the stenotic mitral valve.

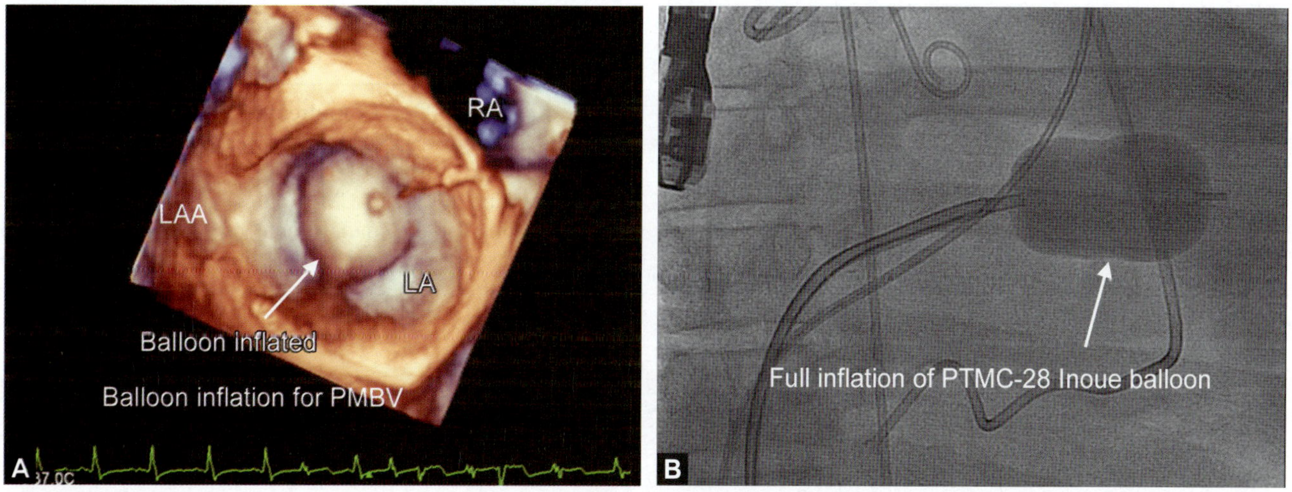

Figs. 5.3A and B: 3D TEE guidance during percutaneous mitral balloon valvuloplasty (PMBV). Patient is under general anesthesia and TEE was done in supine position. (A) Live 3D TEE surgical view of the mitral valve showing full inflation of the balloon within the mitral orifice. (B) Corresponding view by fluoroscopy demonstrating the first attempt by a PTMC-28 Inoue balloon. (LA: Left atrium; LAA: Left atrial appendage; RA: Right atrium).

PMBV has demonstrated good immediate and midterm results and has replaced surgical mitral commissurotomy as the preferred treatment of rheumatic mitral stenosis in appropriate candidates.

1. **In echocardiographic assessment of the mitral valve (MV) for balloon valvuloplasty (PMBV) which of the following statements is correct?**
   (a) A Wilkin score about 10-12 is associated with a successful result
   (b) In a patient with mitral valve area more than 1.5 cm^2, PMBV is contraindicated
   (c) PMBV is indicated in a patient with severe MS and less than moderate mitral regurgitation
   (d) Based on ACC/AHA guideline, PMBV is reasonable (indication IIa) for asymptomatic patients with severe MS (MVA $\leq$1.5 cm^2, stage C) and favorable valve morphology who have new onset of AF in the absence of contraindications

Ans. (b)

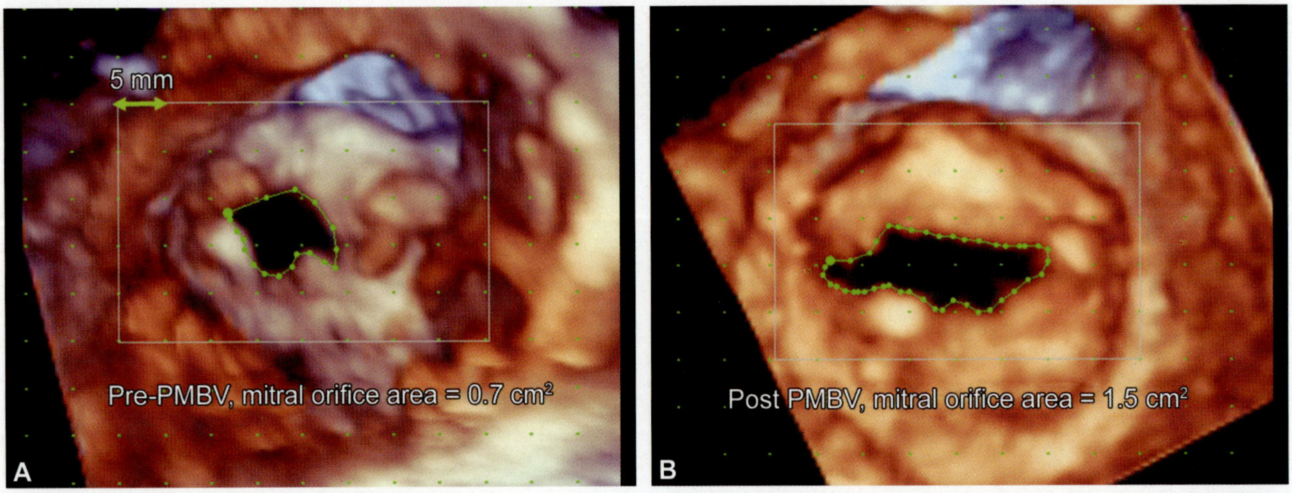

Figs. 5.4A and B: 3D TEE zoom mode of the mitral valve from left ventricular (LV) aspect. (A) Preoperative study showing 3D direct planimetry of the mitral orifice which was calculated as 0.7 cm^2. (B) Immediate post PMBV study in same view using the same method shows mitral orifice area of 1.5 cm^2. This method of calculation of the mitral valve area by 3D is not yet validated by a large study but is very useful in cath lab setting during PMBV where pressure half time (PHT) method is not very accurate. However, one recent study done in our center showed 3D planimetry underestimates mitral valve area compared to the PHT method.

MOVIE LEGENDS

20: 3D TEE zoom mode acquisition of the mitral valve from left atrial perspective.

21: 3D TEE zoom mode acquisition of the mitral valve from left ventricular perspective.

22: Live 3D TEE zoom mode to guide the interventionist to enter the orifice of the mitral valve.

23: Live 3D TEE zoom mode showing full inflation of the Inoue balloon within the mitral orifice.

24: Live 3D TEE zoom mode immediately after PMBV showing mitral valve from left ventricular side with split commissures and acceptable orifice opening. No signs of leaflets avulsion are seen.

REFERENCES

1. Vahanian A, Alfieri O, Andreotti F, et al. Guidelines on the management of valvular heart disease (version 2012). European Heart Journal 2012; 33, 2451-96.
2. Nishimura RA, Otto CM, Bonow, et al. 2014 AHA/ACC Guideline for the management of patients with valvular heart disease: A report of the American College of Cardiology/American Heart Association Task Force on Practice Guidelines. JACC, March 4, 2014.

CASE 6

Adarna LG, Elsayed M, Alagic N, Uygur B, Chahwala JR, Bhagatwala K, Bulur S, Turaga NSN, Pudussery Kattalan JJ, Nanda NC

Elderly patient complaining of shortness of breath. There is no history of prior cardiac surgery. 2D TTE was done.

1. **What do the 🎥 25-31 show?**
   (a) Rheumatic MS
   (b) Congenital MS
   (c) MS produced by degenerative calcific disease
   (d) Mitral annuloplasty ring

Ans. (c)

Mitral annular calcification (MAC, arrow) is easily recognized initially in the parasternal long axis view by high echogenicity posteriorly at the LV-LA junction. This calcification may extend to involve the basal portions of MV leaflets but generally does not produce MV stenosis. Rarely, calcification may extend to the body and tips of the leaflets resulting in stenosis as in this patient. MVA by Doppler pressure half time (PHT) method was 1.38 cm^2 consistent with MV obstruction. Peak and mean MV gradients were also high at 26 and 13 mmHg, respectively (🎥 29 and 30). Calcification may also involve MV chordae and papillary muscles. This is different from rheumatic MS in which commissures are fused. This patient also has degenerative calcific AV disease with mild AR (#1, 🎥 31). #2 in 🎥 31 represents high velocity mitral inflow visualized by color Doppler. 🎥 32 shows shadowing (arrow) produced by MV annular calcification. The structures underneath the calcification are obliterated.

MOVIES 25 TO 32 🎥

CASE 7

Ronald B Williams, Valentyna Ivanova, Sirikarn Napan, June A Yamrozik, Moneal Shah, Robert WW Biederman

A MASS BY ANY OTHER NAME

A 79-year-old Caucasian female was referred for an echocardiogram after having a pre-op chest X-ray for hip replacement surgery. The patient's X-ray had showed a left atrial calcified mass that had increased in size from a 2011 chest X-ray at the time of a right knee replacement. Her past medical history was significant for hypertension, osteoarthritis, dyslipidemia, and family history of coronary artery disease. She was asymptomatic at the time of presentation.

A transthoracic echo was performed which showed a large mass involving the posterior mitral annulus and posterior mitral valve leaflet extending into the left atrium and left ventricle (Figs. 7.1A to D). The mass demonstrated an uneven, irregular surface with peripheral calcifications causing mildly elevated gradients without frank mitral stenosis with a mean 5 mm Hg gradient and 1–2+ mitral regurgitation. The LV was normal in size and systolic function with grade one diastolic dysfunction. The atria bilaterally were dilated. The differential diagnosis was MAC

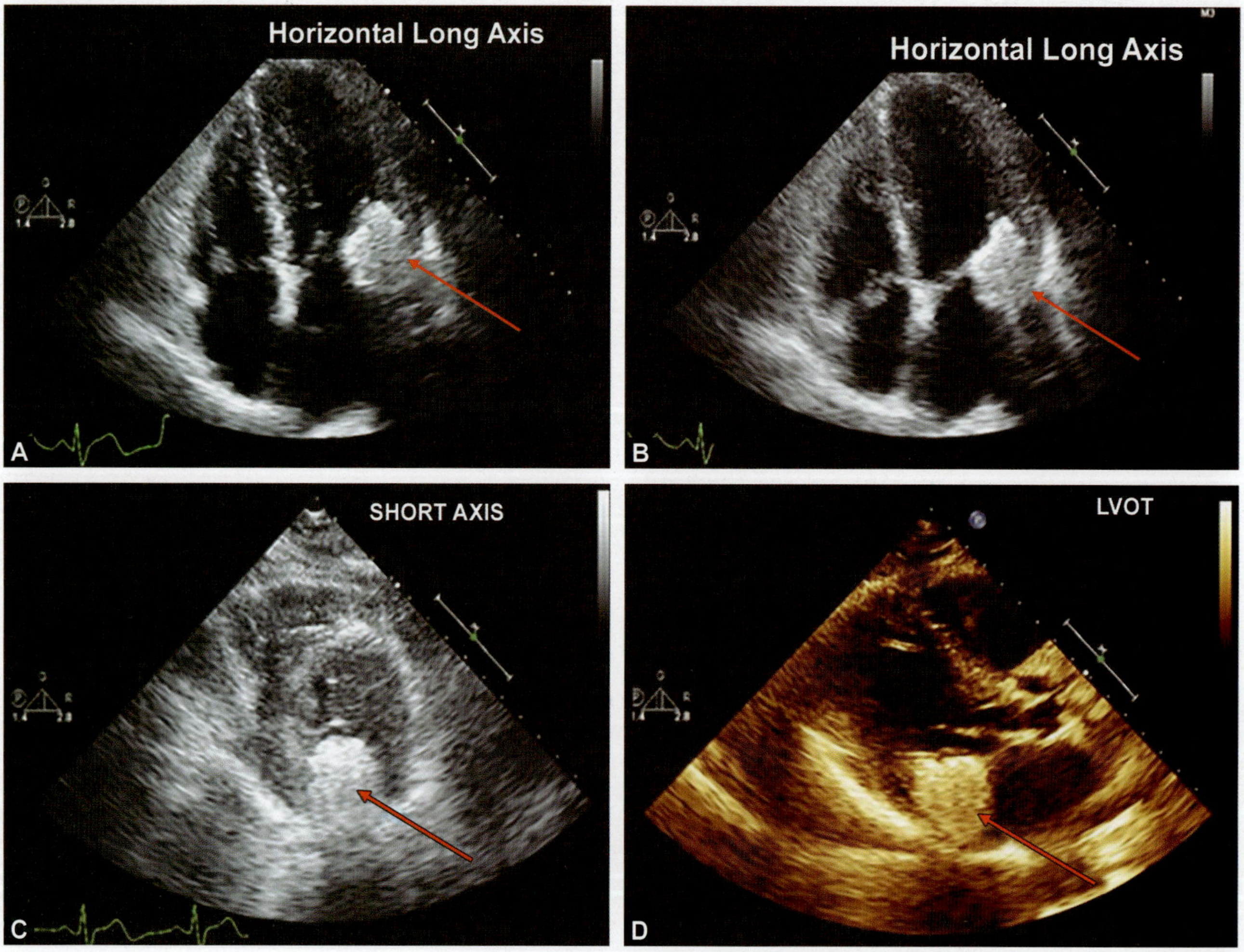

Figs. 7.1A to D: The echo images show the location, calcification, but it is unclear as to whether the extent of the mass is involving the atrium and/or ventricle.

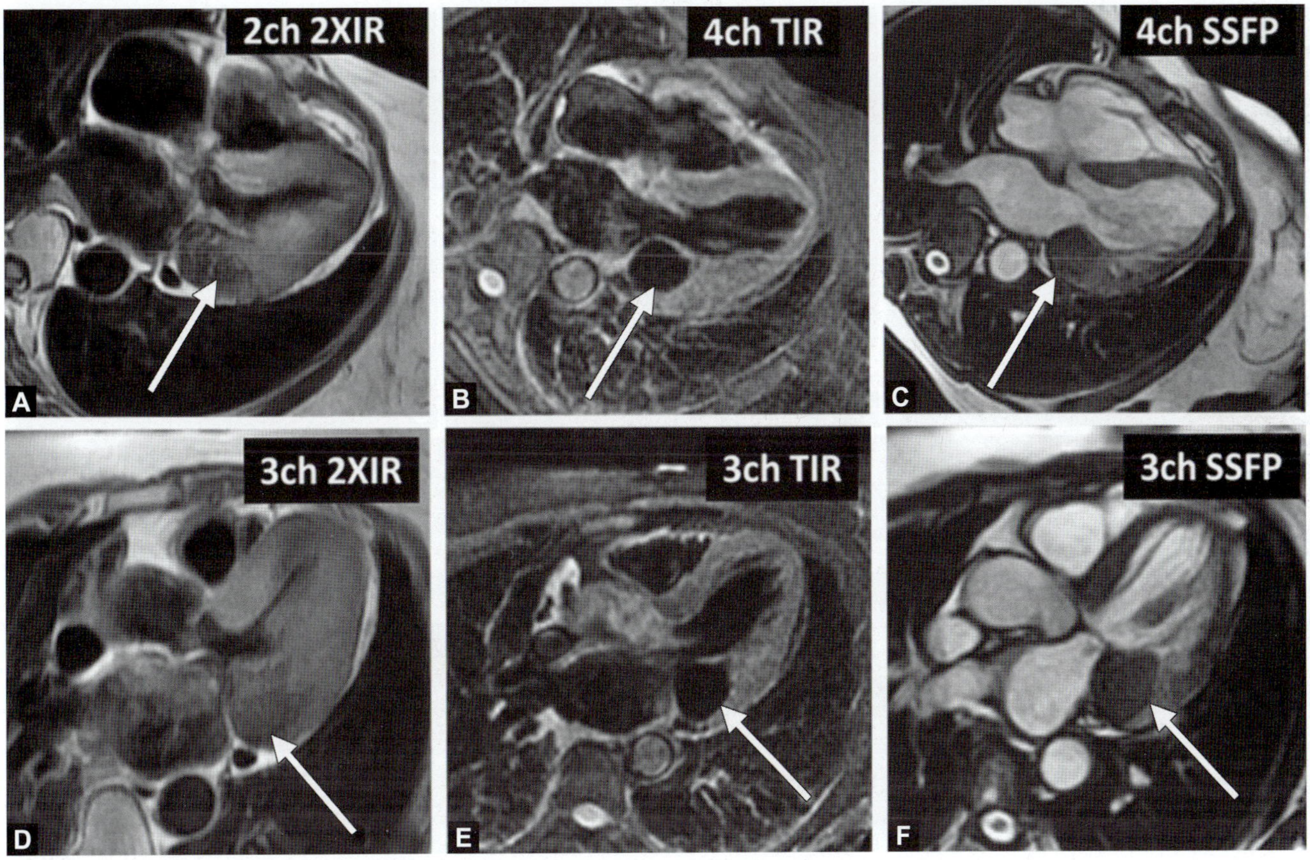

Figs. 7.2A to F: The 2XIR, TIR, SSFP images show the round, well-demarcated mass at the posterior mitral annulus.

(caseous mitral annular calcification), fibroma, or fibroelastoma of the posterior mitral leaflet.

With the broad differential, the patient underwent cardiac magnetic resonance (CMR) imaging. Utilizing Steady State Free Precession (SSFP; dynamic sequence), the patient was imaged in the VLA/HLA views of the heart for structure and function. Black blood (2XIR) images were acquired for anatomical/morphological orientation of great vessels and heart. With the T1W, SSFP, and Triple Inversion (TIR) sequences the mass appeared round, markedly hypointense and well demarcated at the posterior mitral annulus, measuring 36 mm × 29 mm × 37 mm (Figs. 7.2A to F). On first pass perfusion imaging, there was no enhancement noted. On the postgadolinium (late gadolinium enhancement (LGE)) images, the mass shows peripheral ring enhancement without central enhancement (Figs. 7.3A to E). Thus, based on the tissue characteristic and contrast kinetics, the mass was not perfused, had extensive calcification and central proteinaceous material. In the correct setting and location within the posterior wall of the LV, this is pathognomonic for caseous calcification of the mitral annulus, also known as calcific amorphous transformation (CAT), (33 and 34: Echos: HLA, LVOT, SA, HLA (4 = chamber) CMRI, LVOT (3 = chamber) CMRI, SA CMRI).

With the results from the CMR study, her cardiologist placed the patient on aspirin, since there was no evidence supporting systemic anticoagulation in a patient with normal sinus rhythm and mild mitral stenosis. This patient was scheduled for her hip replacement without change in her medical or surgical therapy.

DISCUSSION

Mitral annular calcification (MAC) typically presents as a large, round mass in the region of the atrioventricular groove. Caseous MAC or CAT is a rare variant, typically larger, rounded mass with central necrosis, and when

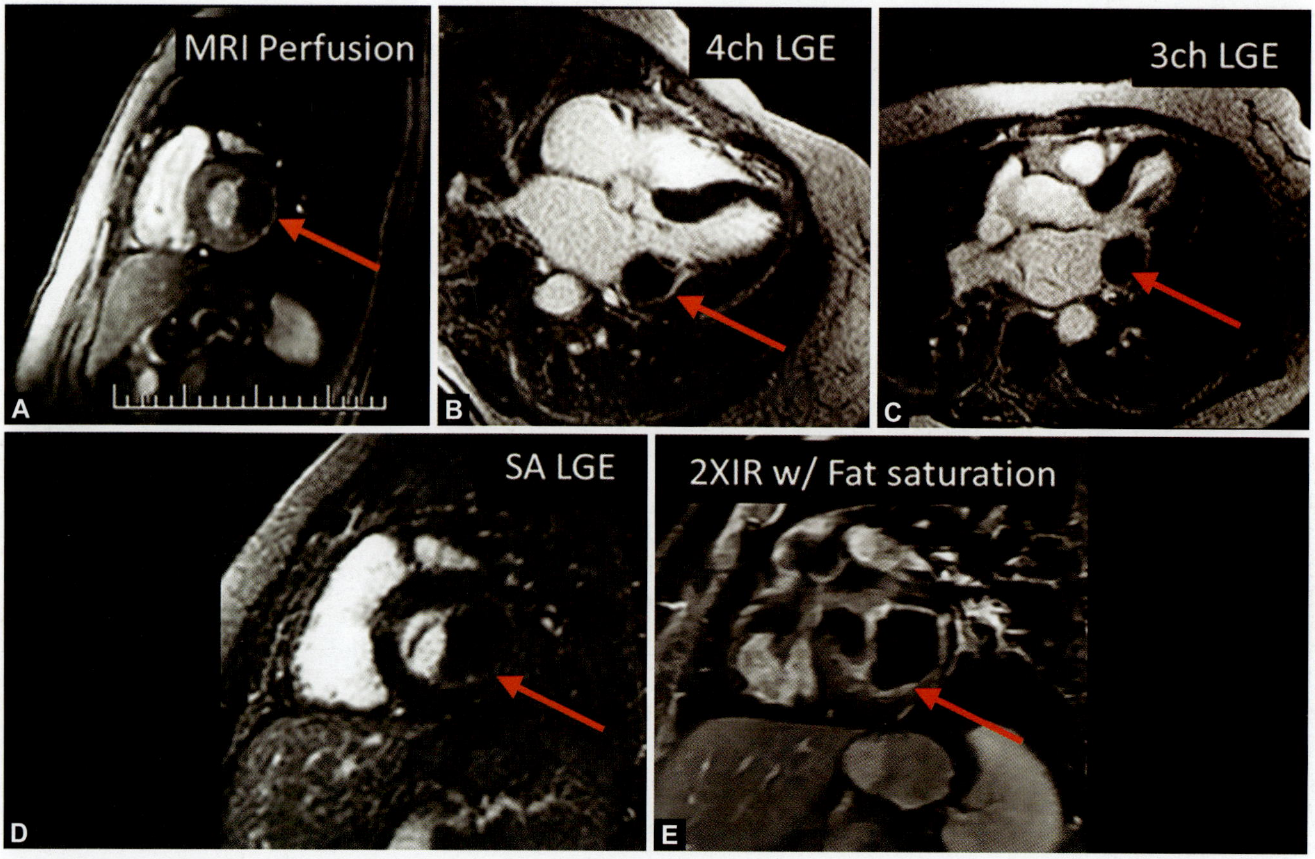

Figs. 7.3A to E: CMR perfusion image showing no enhancement; LGE imaging showing ring/rim enhancement typical of caseous MAC.

incised, has a cream-like mixture with a toothpaste-like texture, consisting of amorphous, acellular and calcific material with a chronic inflammatory reaction. These masses can be several centimeters in size, displacing the mitral valve leaflets, causing valve dysfunction, stenosis, and regurgitation. CMR imaging shows low signal intensity on T1W/T2W images, with rim/ring enhancement on the contrast images.

Caseous MAC, which is associated with increased risk of CVA/TIA, likely due to associated comorbidities, is typically a benign condition with no intervention or medical therapy required.

In the presence of asymptomatic MAC, specific medical treatment other than aspirin therapy, is not required. Some studies suggest there is a strong correlation between MAC and atherosclerosis, valvular heart disease, stroke, renal disease and other vascular diseases. As such, appropriate medical management of cardiovascular risk factors is recommended without specific therapy aimed at MAC (or CAT).

1. **In comparison with CMR, TTE imaging has what general limitations?**
   (a) Limited image quality due to patient's body habitus
   (b) Limited depth of image window
   (c) Reduced spatial resolution
   (d) None of the above
   (e) (a) and (b)
   (f) (a), (b) and (c)

Ans. (f)

2. **The temporal resolution (TR) is typically higher or lower in echocardiography as related to CMR, leading to better or lower ability to resolve highly mobile masses.**
   (a) Echo has higher TR but lower ability to resolve mobile masses
   (b) Echo has higher TR and higher ability to resolve mobile masses
   (c) CMR has lower TR and higher ability to resolve mobile masses

(d) CMR has higher TR and lower ability to resolve mobile masses

Ans. (b)

3. MAC and/or CAT can be recognized on TTE but confirmation that it does not represent a tumor via tissue characterization by CMR (or CT) is advantageous.

(a) True but only by MRI, not CT
(b) True for both MRI and CT
(c) False for both
(d) Calcium is not well represented on MRI from a physical principle but due to its capability to define both T1 and T2, calcium can be inferred.
(e) Hounsfield units via CT accurately and with histological confirmation define calcium
(f) (b), (d) and (e)

Ans. (f)

MOVIE LEGENDS

33A: Echo: Apical four chamber view.
33B: Echo: Parasternal long axis view.
33C: Echo: Parasternal short axis view.
34A: SSFP HLA (4 = chamber) CMRI
34B: SSFP LVOT (3 = chamber) CMRI
34C: SSFP SA CMRI

CASE 8

Chahwala JR, Elsayed M, Alagic N, Adarna LG, Bhagatwala K, Bulur S, Turaga NSN, Nanda NC

Adult patient with MR. 2D TTE was done.

1. **Factors that need to be taken into account when semi-quantitatively assessing MR severity during echocardiographic examination are all of the following *except*: (35–38)**
   (a) Nyquist limit
   (b) Color gain
   (c) Color M-mode to check whether MR is pansystolic or not
   (d) Family history
   (e) Multiple plane examination
   (f) Blood pressure
   (g) LA and LV dilatation
   (h) Eccentricity of MR jet

Ans. (d)

Nyquist limit is best standardized around 50 cm/sec since a lower Nyquist limit such as 23 cm/sec will increase MR jet size and produce artifacts extending beyond the cardiac borders (38). Very high Nyquist limit will reduce the jet size and result in underestimation of severity. Changes in Nyquist limit also change the color wall filter and that is the reason for changes in jet size. Color gain is also an important factor. In 37, the color gain was reduced from 67 to 46 and the MR jet shows a considerable decrease in size. When the color gain was further decreased to 27, severe MR completely disappeared. Color gain should be gradually increased till speckles and artifacts appear and then it should be gradually decreased till they just disappear. MR should also be assessed using multiple planes and the maximum jet size taken.

2. **What does the arrow in 39 point to?**
   (a) Trabeculation
   (b) Leading edge of a thrombus
   (c) Vestigeal membrane
   (d) False tendon

Ans. (d)

This patient also has a hypertrophied papillary muscle.

MOVIES 35 TO 39

CASE 9

Alagic N, Adarna LG, Elsayed M, Chahwala JR, Bhagatwala K, Bulur S, Turaga NSN, Mohamed A, Gupta N, Nanda NC

This is an adult patient with a murmur and shortness of breath. 2D TTE was done (🎥 40–42)

1. **What is the abnormality (🎥 40–42)?**
   (a) Prolapse of anterior MV leaflet
   (b) Prolapse of posterior MV leaflet
   (c) Prolapse of both MV leaflets
   (d) MV is redundant but does not prolapse beyond MV annulus

Ans. (c)

There is marked prolapse of both MV leaflets (arrow in 🎥 40) with severe MR. The MV chordae also appear to be redundant.

MOVIES 40 TO 42 🎥

CASE 10

Naveen Garg, Kanwal K Kapur

EVALUATION OF MITRAL REGURGITATION

A 51-year-old male, a known case of diabetes mellitus, systemic hypertension and triple vessel disease (CT-angiography done a few days ago showed LAD 90%, LCx 100% and RCA 100% blocked) reported with complaints of dyspnea on exertion. Troponin-T was negative. He came for echocardiography evaluation before CABG.

PREOPERATIVE (43. PRE-CABG)

Preoperative analysis revealed posteriorly directed MR jet with dense CW-Doppler signals, color Doppler flow signals from MR reaching the roof of LA (Figs. 10.1A to E).

Table 10.1: Echocardiographic and Doppler Data

LV end diastolic diameter = 4.38 cm	*MV annular diameter = 2.51 cm*	*MR jet velocity peak = 466 cm/s*
LVOT diameter = 2.09 cm	MV inflow VTI = 13.1 cm	MR VTI = 79.3 cm
LVOT VTI = 16.9 cm	E = 95.3 cm/s	MR mean V = 322 cm/s
LVEF= 73%	A = 68.6 cm/s	Heart rate = 84/min
LAVol. = 28 ml	e' = 10.1	BSA = 1.87 kgm^2

1. Is severe MR the cause of patient's symptoms?
2. Does this patient need MV replacement/MV repair along with CABG?
   Further hemodynamic analysis shows in Table 10.1.

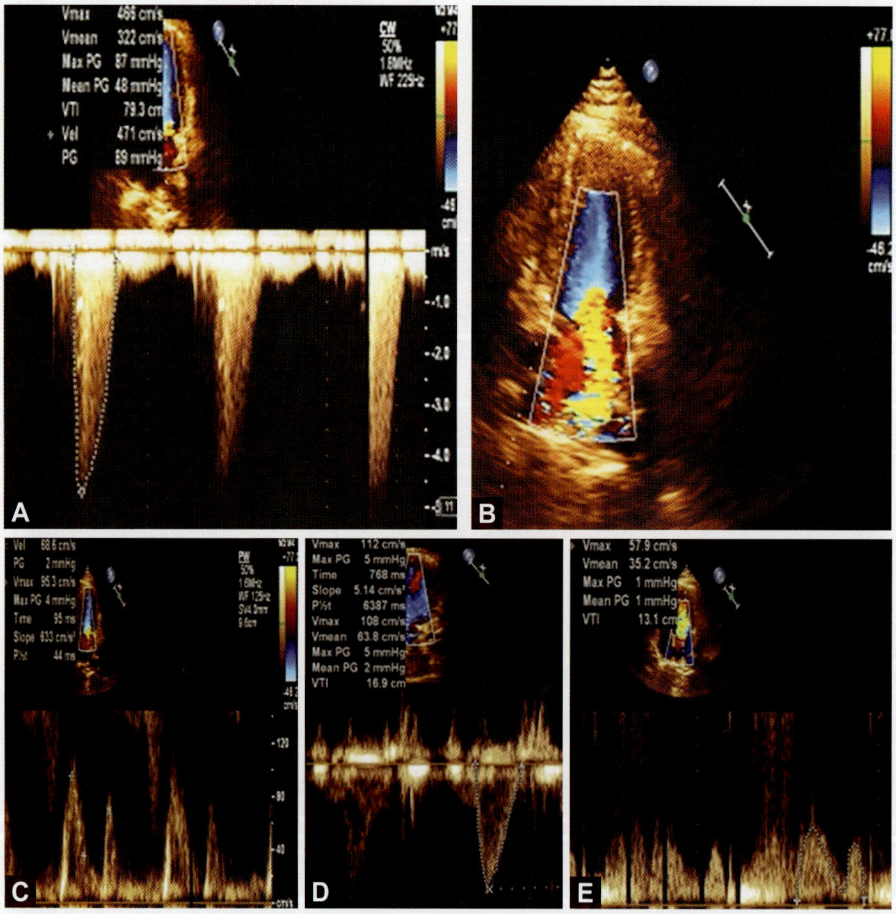

Figs. 10.1A to E: (A) Jet of MR VTI = 79.3 cm; (B) MR jet touching roof of LA; (C) Mitral Inflow velocity; (D) LVOT VTI = 16.9 cm; (E) MV inflow VTI = 13.1 cm

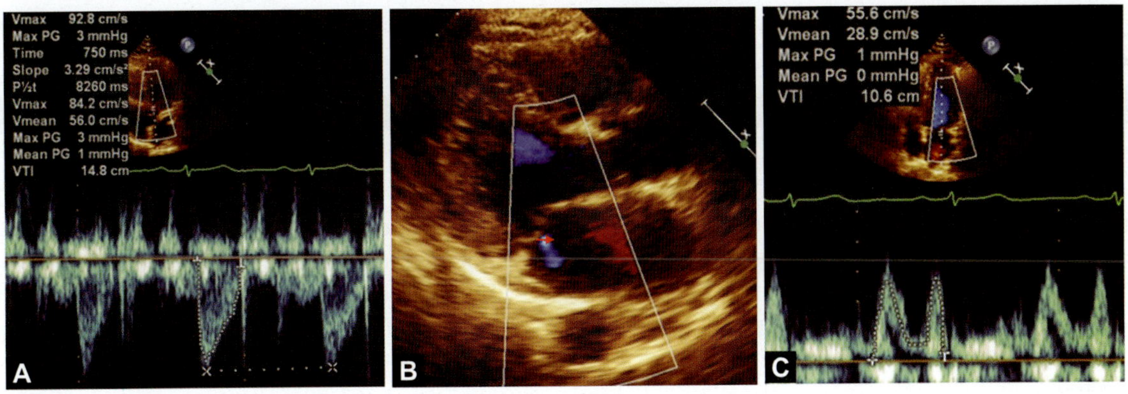

Figs. 10.2A to C: (A) LVOT VTI = 14.8 cm; (B) MR jet (Plax view); (C) Mitral inflow VTI = 10.6 cm.

Mitral inflow (Total SV) = 0.785 × 2.52 × 2.51 × 13.1 = 64.78 ml

Forward Stroke Volume = 0.785 × 2.09 × 2.09 × 16.9 = 57.94 ml

MR volume and fraction = 6.84 ml and 10.56% respectively.

Thus, in spite of color Doppler and CW-Doppler findings indicative of severe MR, MR volume and fraction done by the stroke volume method suggest only mild MR precluding the need for associated MV replacement or repair.

Patient underwent off pump CABG and was followed up by a color Doppler study after 6 months......(44 POST CABG) (Figs. 10.2A to C).

LVOT VTI = 14.8 cm; MV VTI= 10.6 cm

Forward SV= 50.7 ml ; Mitral Inflow (Total SV) – 52.4 ml MR volume and fraction = 1.72 ml and 3.2% respectively.

DISCUSSION

1. The symptoms in this patient were due to three vessel coronary artery disease which considerably improved after CABG. The significant reduction in MR jet area was likely due to amelioration of papillary muscle ischemia.
2. Color flow imaging and CW-Doppler signal density are widely used indices in the assessment of MR severity. However occasionally, as was the case in this patient, significant errors could occur if additional quantitative parameters are not performed.
3. However, quantitative estimation involves diameter assessment across two valves and this could lead to significant interobserver variability and also significant errors in estimation of MR volume.

COMMENTS

Although the estimated regurgitant volume by the Doppler calculation is negligible (only 6.8 ml), the semi quantitative estimation by jet area method shows that this regurgitation could actually be moderate to severe. The small LA size in this patient who never had pulmonary edema is consistent with relatively mild MR. This case therefore illustrates the limitations in the Doppler computation (diameter assessment errors for LVOT and mitral annulus) as well as the possible overestimations by jet area method. This case however does show that decision to avoid mitral valve repair procedure during CABG was justified as the MR practically disappeared after the revascularization procedure.

Editor's note: Prominent flow acceleration (PISA) and the large vena contracta also suggest that MR was significant and might have improved after CABG. LA volume is normal in this patient and that can provide a clue that MR, if it was chronic, was less severe. MR volume of only 6.84 ml calculated by the output method is definitely grossly erroneous.

MOVIES 43 AND 44

CASE 11

Bulur S, Nanda NC

This is a 70-year-old male with known murmur of MR for several years who came for a follow-up examination. 2D TTE was done.

1. **(Fig. 11.1 and 45): How would you grade the severity of MR?**
   (a) Mild
   (b) Moderate
   (c) Severe because the VC dimension is 0.88 cm (more than 0.7 cm) and the MR jet occupies more than 40% of LA

Ans. (c)

MR does appear severe in this apical four chamber view.

2. **(Figs. 11.2 and 11.3): MR is found only in mid to late systole using color M-mode with minimal MR occurring very early in systole due to the closing motion of MV (Fig. 11.2). Also, the LA is not enlarged (Fig. 11.3). Would these findings make you reconsider the severity of MR?**
   (a) Yes
   (b) No

Ans. (a)

Both of these findings are important when considering MR severity specially in patients with classical mid to late systolic MV prolapse in whom the MR may not be pan-systolic. Also, LA would be expected to be enlarged in patients with chronic (but not acute) severe MR. Arrow in Figure 11.3 points to posterior MV leaflet prolapse.

3. **What is the best method to calculate MR volume in this patient?**
   (a) Multiplying 2D TTE VC (taking 0.88 cm as the diameter and assuming the VC to be circular or elliptical) by MR VTI obtained by continuous wave Doppler
   (b) Using the standard PISA method
   (c) Multiplying the VC obtained by 3D TTE and MR VTI assessed by continuous wave Doppler
   (d) Using the volume method by subtracting the stroke volumes obtained from LVO and RVO using PW Doppler

Ans. (c)

The exact size of the VC which is necessary to calculate MR volume, can be assessed by 3D TTE (or 3D TEE). It cannot be generally obtained reliably by 2D TTE (or 2D TEE) because at any given time the 2D provides only a thin slice-like view of the MV and MR. On the other hand, the full extent of the MV and MR VC is

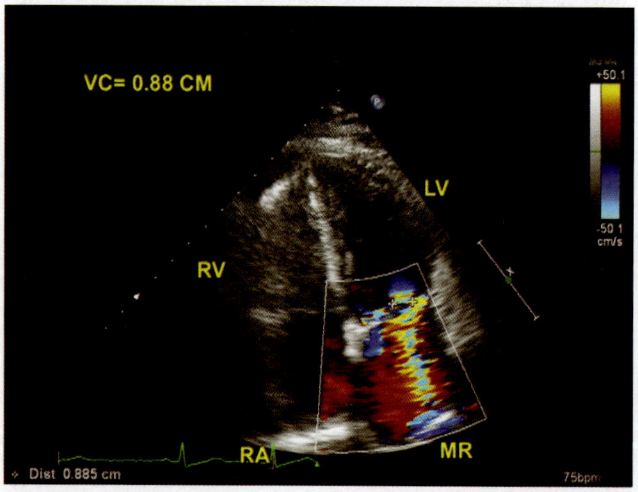

Fig. 11.1: Apical four chamber view. MR vena contracta (VC) measured 0.88 cm.

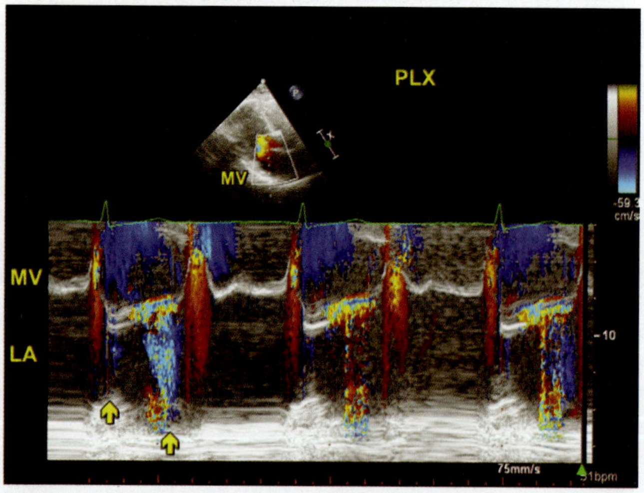

Fig. 11.2: Color M-mode examination. Left arrow points to minimal MR resulting from closing movement of the MV. Right arrow shows mid to late systolic MR. (PLX: parasternal long axis view).

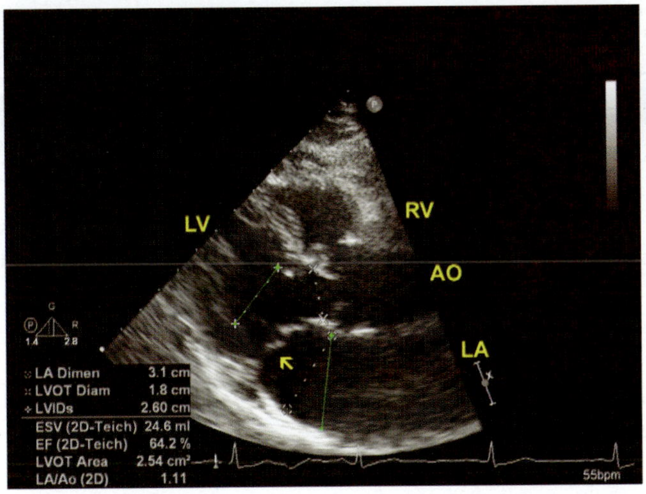

Fig. 11.3: Parasternal long axis view. LA size is normal, measuring 3.1 cm.

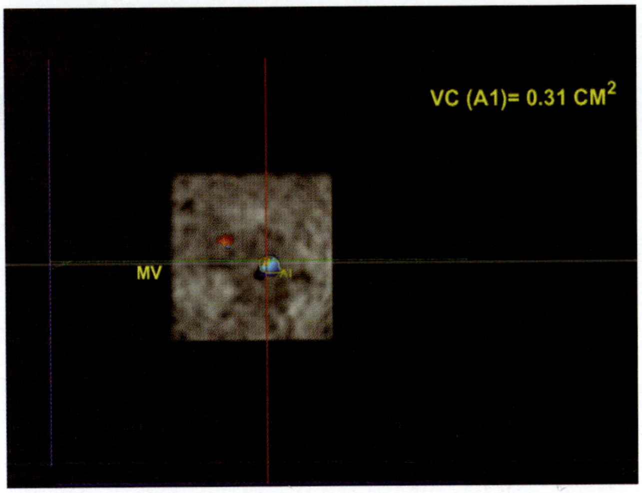

Fig. 11.4: Vena contracta (VC) area (A1) of the mid to late systolic MR by 3DTTE measured 0.31 cm^2. VC of early systolic MR produced by the closing movement of MV was negligible.

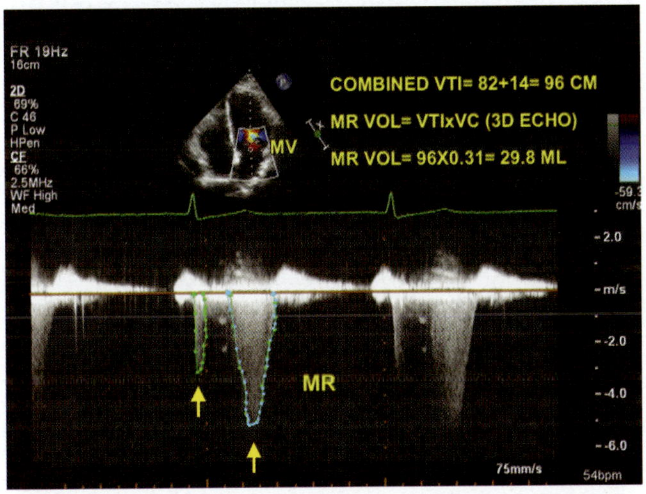

Fig. 11.5: Shows calculation of MR volume (VOL) by multiplying the combined velocity time integrals (VTI) of the two MR jets by the vena contracta (VC, 0.31 cm^2) of MR obtained by 3DTTE. Left arrow shows measurement of VTI (14 cm) of MR produced by closing movement of the MV and right arrow VTI (82 cm) of the mid to late systolic MR. Total MR volume measured 29.8 ml.

encompassed in the 3D data-set facilitating accurate viewing of the shape and size of VC. The PISA method is less reliable because it assumes the PISA to be hemispherical which is not the case in most patients. The volume method is also unreliable because of errors in correctly measuring the LVO and RVO diameters. Also, associated regurgitation of other valves will affect the results. In this patient, MR volume was calculated as 29.8 ml consistent with only moderate MR (Figs. 11.4 and 11.5 and 46).

MOVIES 45 AND 46

CASE 12

Alagic N, Elsayed M, Adarna LG, Chahwala JR, Bhagatwala K, Bulur S, Turaga NSN, Mohamed A, Gupta N, Pudussery Kattalan JJ, Nanda NC

1. What is the severity of MR in this patient? (🎥 47)

(a) Mild

(b) Moderate

(c) Severe

Ans. (a)

MR appears moderate only with a PVC otherwise it appears mild. It is important to take into account the presence of arrhythmia when evaluating valve regurgitation severity.

MOVIE 47 🎥

CASE 13

Adarna LG, Chahwala JR, Elsayed M, Alagic N, Bhagatwala K, Bulur S, Turaga NSN, Mohamed A, Gupta N, Nanda NC

1. **What does the arrow point to in this adult patient with MR (🎥 48)?**
   (a) Minimal lower velocity MR occurring during MV closure before real MR.
   (b) Artifact produced by CW Doppler.

Ans.(a)

The peak MR velocity is very high reflecting the gradient between LV and LA pressures during systole.

MOVIE 48 🎥

CASE 14

Ahmad S Omran

FLAIL ANTERIOR MITRAL VALVE LEAFLET

This 61-year-old woman presented to our ER with acute coronary syndrome. Emergency coronary intervention was done for LAD stenosis. Transthoracic echocardiography (Figs. 14.1A and B 49, 50) showed flail anterior mitral valve leaflet and severe eccentric posteriorly directed jet of mitral regurgitation (MR). Preoperative transesophageal echocardiography (TEE) confirmed the diagnosis of myxomatous mitral valve with at least two ruptured chordae of the anterior leaflet and severe MR (Figs. 14.2A and B 51, 52).[1,2] Patient underwent cardiac surgery for mitral valve repair (MV repair). Ruptured chordae tendineae were

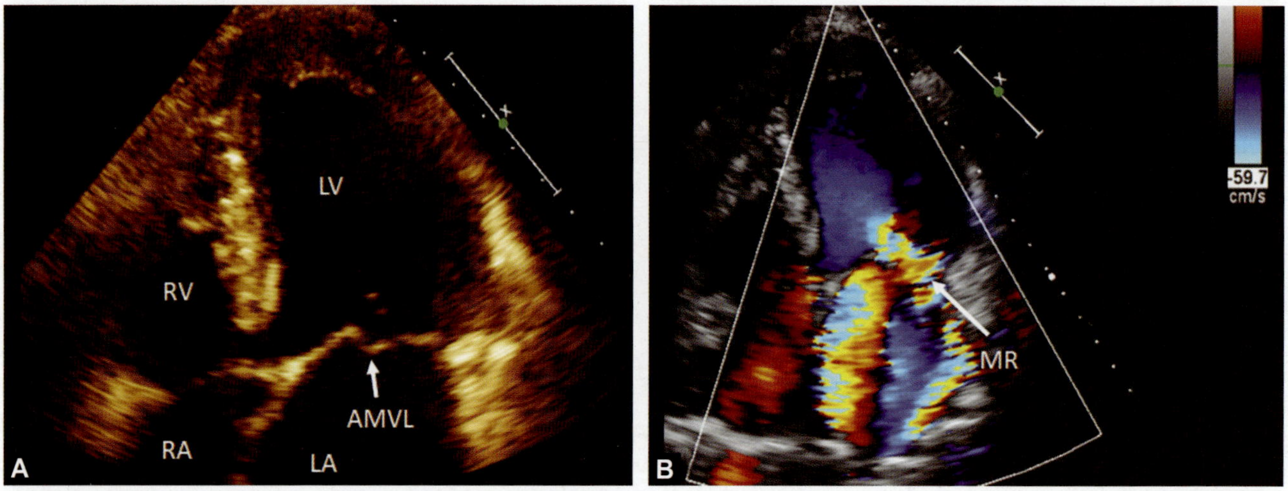

Figs. 14.1A and B: Transthoracic echocardiography (TTE). (A) TTE in apical 4-chamber view shows anterior mitral valve leaflet (AMVL) with flail tip. (B) Same view with color Doppler demonstrates severe eccentric posteriorly directed jet of mitral regurgitation (MR) with flow signals swirling around the left atrium. (LV: Left ventricle; LA: Left atrium; RA: Right atrium; RV: Right ventricle).

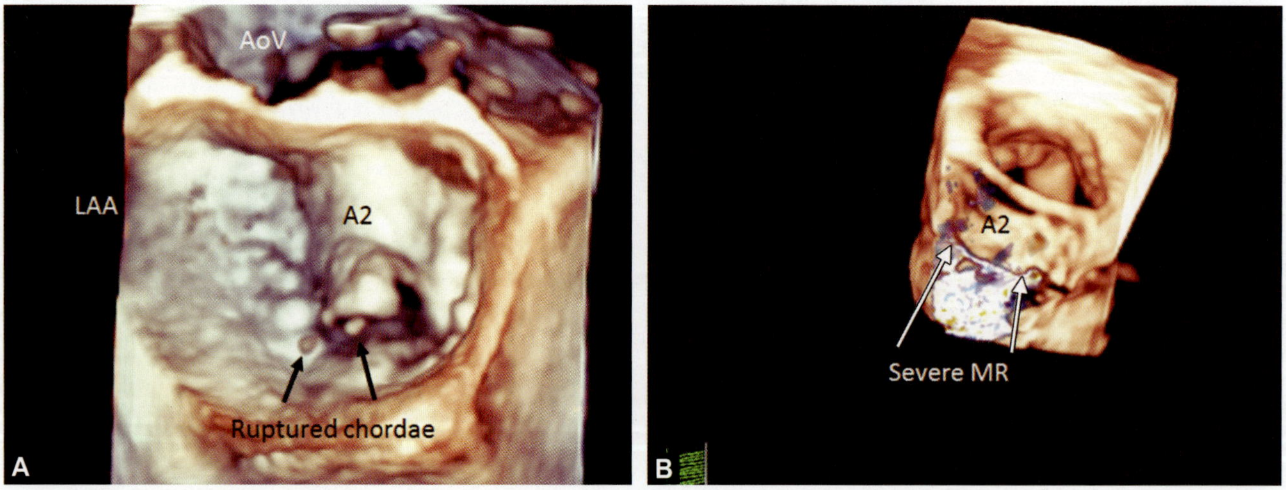

Figs. 14.2A and B: 3D Transesophageal echocardiography (3D TEE). (A) 3D TEE zoom mode acquisition of the mitral valve in surgical view shows middle segment of the anterior mitral leaflet (A2) with 2 ruptured chordae. (B) Same view with full volume color Doppler acquisition demonstrates severe eccentric posteriorly directed jet of mitral regurgitation (MR). (AoV: Aortic valve; LAA: Left atrial appendage).

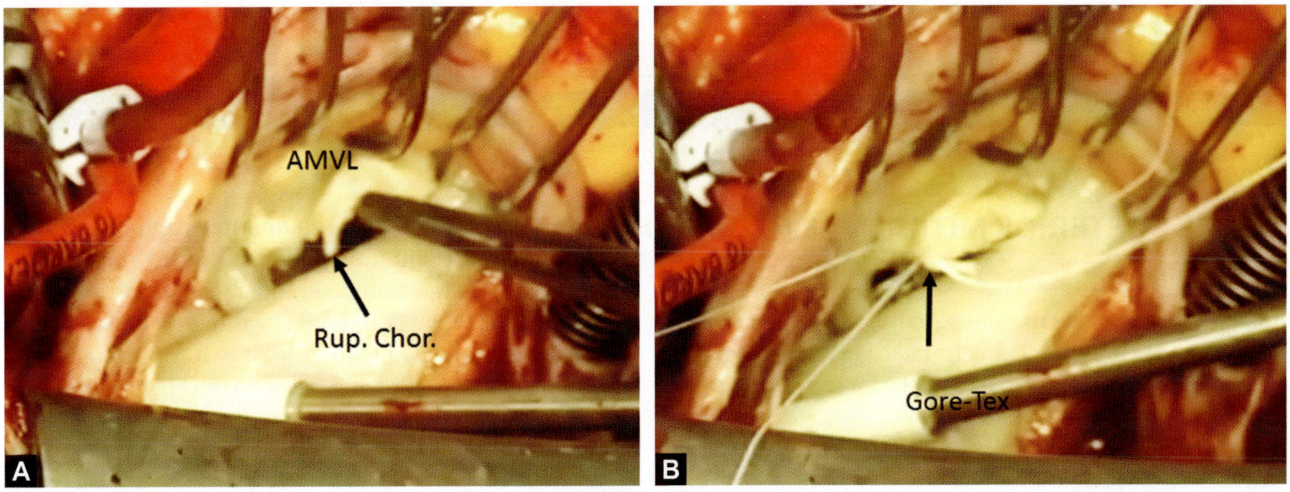

Figs. 14.3A and B: Surgical exploration of the mitral valve via the left atrium. (A) Two chordae of the middle segment of the anterior mitral valve leaflet were ruptured. (B) Ruptured chordae (Rup. Chor) were replaced with Gore-Tex sutures. A size 30 complete ring (Physio ring) was used for mitral annuloplasty. (AMVL: Anterior mitral valve leaflet).

replaced with two pairs of artificial Gore-Tex sutures (Figs. 14. 3A and B). An annuloplasty ring was used to stabilize the repair and improve leaflet coaptation (size 30 Physio ring). Intraoperative TEE immediately after repair showed an excellent result with no evidence of mitral stenosis or regurgitation. Patient was discharged home and follow up echocardiography 2 years after MV repair showed no residual MR.

1. **In cchocardiographic assessment of the mitral valve which of the following statements is correct?**
   (a) Anterior mitral valve leaflet consists of 3 scallops with distinct indentation between the scallops.
   (b) Ruptured chordae in myxomatous mitral valve are more common in the female.
   (c) Bileaflet prolapse may cause central MR. Degree of MR can be underestimated in this pathology.
   (d) Interrogation of left upper pulmonary vein inflow is adequate for assessment of MR severity.

Ans. (c)

MOVIE LEGENDS

49: Intraoperative TEE in 4-chamber view showing flail anterior mitral leaflet.
50: Same view of previous movie demonstrates severe posteriorly directed jet of MR.
51: 3D TEE surgical view of the mitral valve showing 2 ruptured chordae tendineae.
52: Postoperative 3D TEE showing Physio ring annuloplasty.

REFERENCES

1. Tsang W, Lang RM. Is 3-Dimensional echocardiography essential for intraoperative Assessment? Circulation, Aug 2013; 643-52.
2. Faletra FF, Demertzis S, Pedrazzini G, et al. Three-Dimensional transesophageal echocardiography in degenerative mitral regurgitation. J Am Soc Echocardiogr 2015;28: 437-48.

CASE 15

Ahmad S Omran

FLAIL POSTERIOR MITRAL VALVE LEAFLET

This 45-year-old male presented to our center with severe shortness of breath. Transthoracic echocardiography (Figs. 15.1A and B) showed flail posterior mitral valve leaflet at middle scallop (P2) with multiple ruptured chordae. Severe eccentric anteriorly directed jet of mitral regurgitation (MR) was noted. Preoperative transesophageal echocardiography (TEE) confirmed the diagnosis of myxomatous mitral valve with at least two ruptured chordae of the posterior leaflet and severe MR (Figs. 15.2A and B,

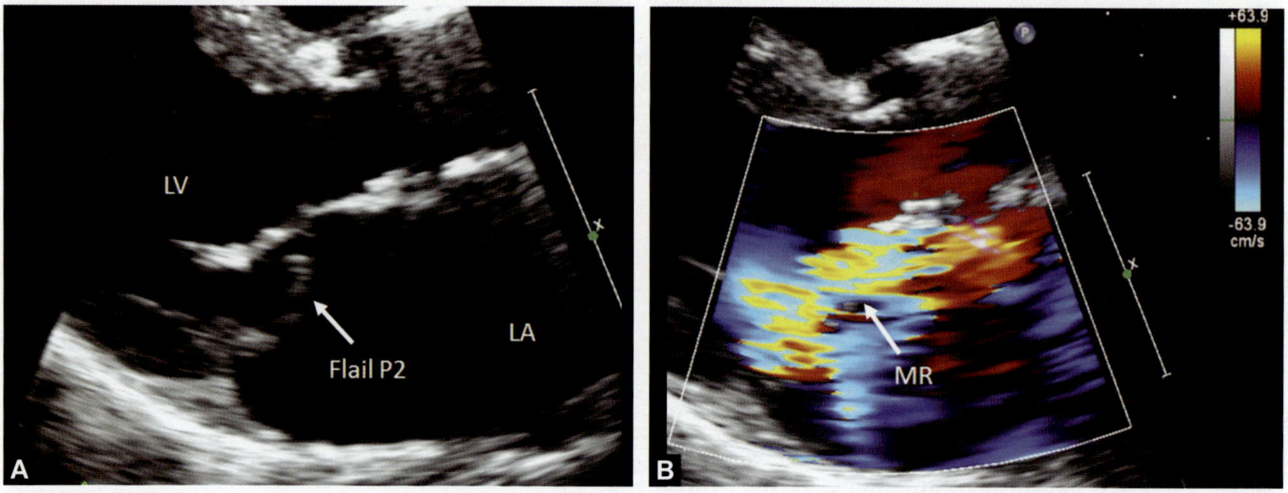

Figs. 15.1A and B: : Transthoracic echocardiography (TTE). (A) TTE in parasternal long-axis view shows posterior mitral valve leaflet (PMVL) with flail middle scallop (P2). (B) Same view with color Doppler demonstrates severe eccentric anteriorly directed jet of mitral regurgitation (MR). (LV: Left ventricle; LA: Left atrium).

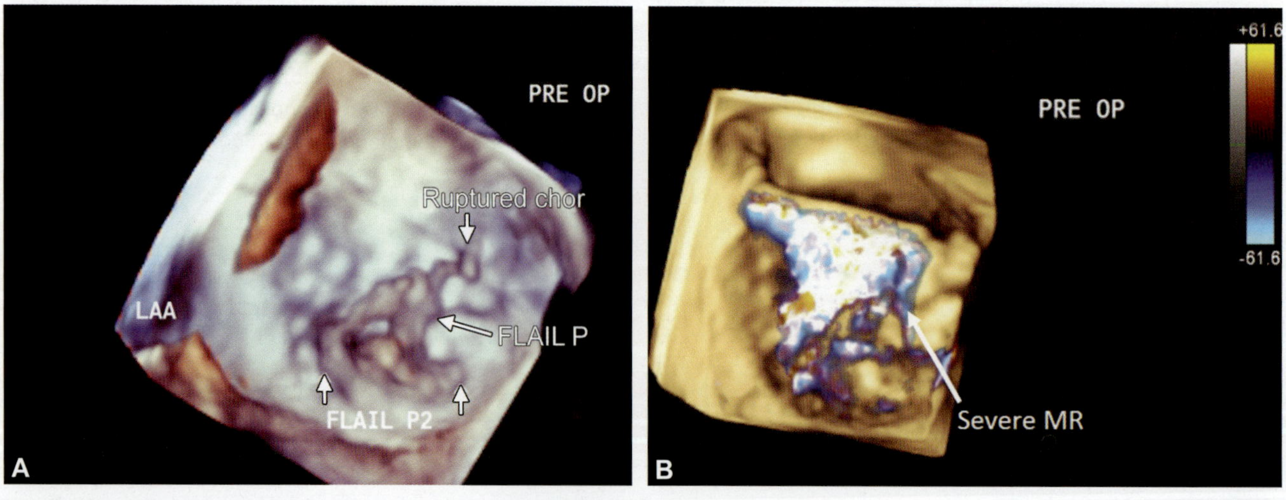

Figs. 15.2A and B: 3D Transesophageal echocardiography (3D TEE). (A) 3D TEE zoom mode acquisition of the mitral valve in surgical view shows middle scallop of the posterior mitral leaflet (P2) with multiple ruptured chordae. (B) Same view with full volume color acquisition demonstrates severe eccentric anteriorly directed jet of mitral regurgitation (MR). (LAA: Left atrial appendage).

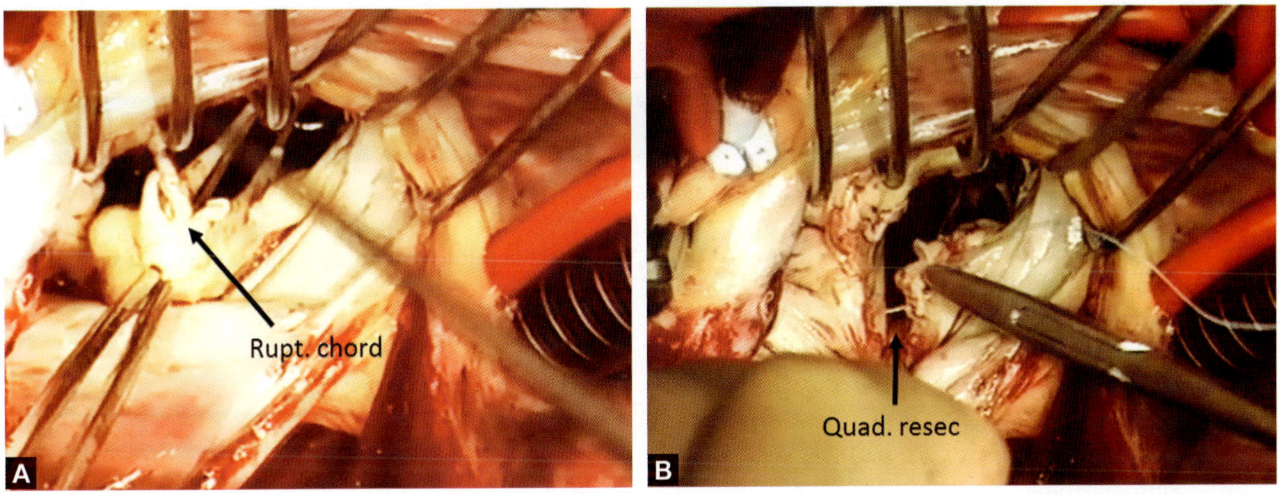

Figs. 15.3A and B: Surgical exploration of the mitral valve via the left atrium. (A) At least two chordae of the middle segment of the posterior mitral valve leaflet were ruptured (Rup. chord). (B) Quadrangular resection of the P2 (Quad. Resec) was performed with sliding plasty of other scallops to prevent postoperative SAM (systolic anterior motion). A size 32 complete ring (Physio II ring) was used for mitral annuloplasty.

53-56).[1,2] Patient underwent cardiac surgery for mitral valve repair (MV repair). Posterior leaflet had quadrangular resection at P2 and sliding plasty of medial and lateral scallops (P3 and P1). An annuloplasty ring (C-E Physio II ring size 32) was used to stabilize the repair and improve leaflet coaptation (Figs. 15.3A and B). Intraoperative TEE immediately after repair showed excellent result with no signs of mitral stenosis, residual MR or mitral systolic anterior motion (SAM). Patient was discharged home and follow up echocardiography 2 years after MV repair showed no residual MR.

1. **In echocardiographic assessment of the mitral valve (MV) which of the following statement is correct?**
   (a) Accuracy of 2D TEE in identifying MV segments is about 90-97%.
   (b) In 3D TEE with surgical view of the mitral valve, anterior mitral leaflet is adjacent to the right coronary cusp of the aortic valve.
   (c) 3D TEE zoom mode acquisition provides the image with the highest frame rate for assessment of the mitral valve.
   (d) In surgical view of the mitral valve by 3D TEE, aortic valve should be positioned at the bottom of the image and left atrial appendage to the right of the image.

Ans. (a)

MOVIE LEGENDS

53: Intraoperative TEE in 4-chamber view showing flail middle scallop of posterior mitral leaflet (P2).

54: Same view of previous movie demonstrates severe anteriorly directed jet of MR.

55: 3D TEE surgical view of the mitral valve showing multiple ruptured chordae tendineae.

56: Same view of previous movie with full volume color acquisition showing severe anteriorly directed jet of mitral regurgitation (MR).

REFERENCES

1. Omran AS, Woo A, David, et al. Intraoperative transesophageal echocardiography accurately predicts mitral valve anatomy and suitability for repair. J Am Soc Echocardiogr. 2002;15(9):950-7.
2. Lang RM, Badano LP, Tasang W, et al. EAE/ASE Recommendations for image acquisition and display using three-dimensional echocardiography. J Am Soc Echocardiogr. 2012;25: 3-46.

CASE 16

Nilda Espinola-Zavaleta, Salomon Rivera-Peralta, Hugo Rodriguez-Zanella, Jose Antonio Arias-Godinez, Maria Eugenia Ruiz-Esparza, Nydia Avila-Vanzzini, Juan Francisco Fritche-Salazar, Angel Romero-Cardenas

A 39-year-old male with history of blunt chest trauma and sudden onset of dyspnea. Physical exam revealed an apical holosystolic murmur grade IV/VI radiating to the axilla. 2D and 3D echocardiography was done (Figs. 16.1, 16.2 and 57–59)

1. **The most likely diagnosis is:**
   A. Vegetation
   B. Fibroelastoma
   C. Flail MV
   D. Thrombus

Ans. (c)

Mitral regurgitation can be explained by multiple causes such as endocarditis, ischemia, tumor, myxomatous disease, trauma, hypertrophic cardiomyopathy, among others. However, blunt chest trauma rarely causes mitral regurgitation. In this clinical scenario, it is caused by papillary muscle, chordae tendineae and/or MV rupture.[1] The most frequent reason is rupture of the anterior mitral leaflet, followed by rupture of chordae tendineae. The latter structures are thinner and more fragile, making them susceptible to rupture.[2] In the present case, blunt trauma resulted in a flail posterior MV leaflet with severe MR as evidenced by 2D TTE and 3D TEE.

MOVIE LEGENDS

57: Zoomed view of the mitral valve in four chamber view, showing a flail posterior mitral leaflet.

58: 2D TTE and color flow four chamber view with severe mitral regurgitation.

59: 3D TEE showing enface view of the flail posterior MV leaflet.

REFERENCES

1. Hajime K, Yoshiharu H, Shinji H, Norimasa M, Taira K. Mitral valve plasty for Mitral regurgitation after blunt chest trauma. Ann Thorac Cardiovasc Surg. 2001;7:175–9.
2. Selzer A, Kelly JJ, Vannitamby M, Walker P, Gerbode F, Kerth WJ. The syndrome of mitral insufficiency due to isolated rupture of the chordae tendineae. Am J Med. 1967;43:822–36.

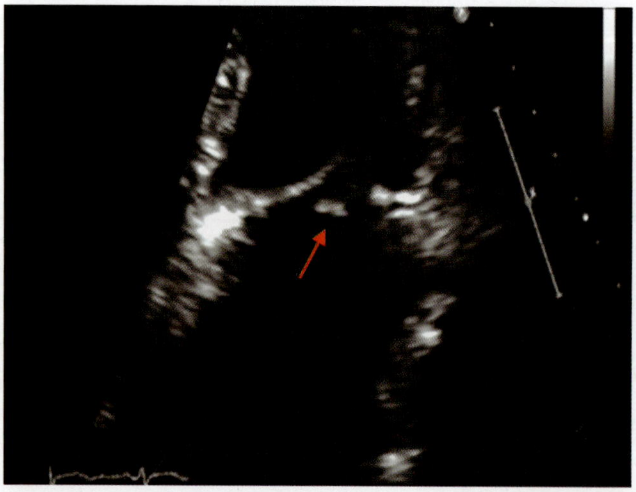

Fig. 16.1: Zoomed view of the mitral valve in four chamber view, showing a flail posterior mitral leaflet (arrow).

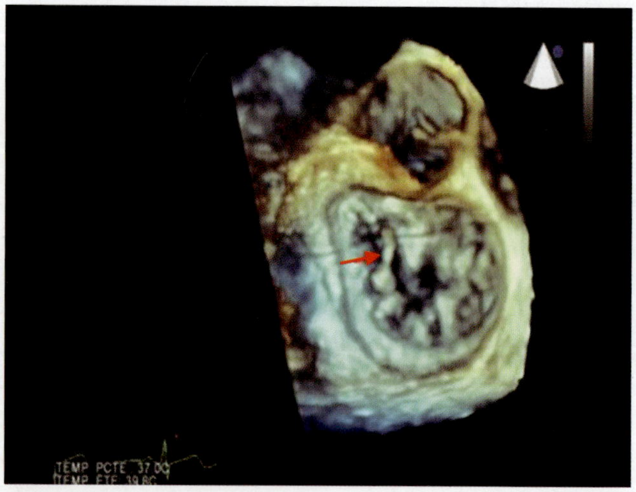

Fig. 16.2: 3D TEE showing enface view of the flail posterior MV leaflet (arrow).

CASE 17

Mohamed A, Gupta N, Elsayed M, Nanda NC

This patient is a 48-year-old male referred for a murmur. 2D TTE showed mitral valve prolapse with moderate MR.

1. **What does the arrow in 🎥 60 show?**
    - A. Membrane in LV
    - B. MV chordae rupture
    - C. Redundant MV chordae
    - D. Membranous cyst in LV

Ans. (c)

Redundant MV chordae are more often seen in patients with myxomatous MV and prolapse as in this case. They are occasionally seen as an isolated finding.

MOVIE 60 🎥

SECTION 2

Aortic Valve, Aorta

CASE 18

Bulur S, Nanda NC

Elderly male with non-specific chest pain. 2D TTE was done.

1. **What does the arrow in 🎥 61 point to?**
   (a) Vegetations
   (b) Lamble's excrescences
   (c) Fibroelastomas
   (d) Something else

Ans.(d)

Localized thickening is noted in the mid portion of the right and non-coronary cusps of AV. These represent thickened nodules of Arantius. These nodules are normally present on all three cusps of AV but are well visualized when they are thickened as in this patient. The nodule on the left cusp was not detected. There is no clinical evidence of endocarditis and no oscillating masses consistent with vegetations are seen on the AV. Fibroelastomas are also nodular structures but they are typically attached to the AV by a stalk and the surface has fronds. Lamble's excrescences are linear and mobile.

MOVIE 61

CASE 19

Adarna LG, Elsayed M, Chahwala JR, Bhagatwala K, Bulur S, Mohamed A, Gupta N, Nanda NC

This is an elderly patient complaining of shortness of breath. 2D TTE was done (62–64).

1. **All the following statements are true *except*:**
    (a) AV shows decreased motion on both M-mode and 2D
    (b) The mean AV gradient of 43 mm Hg suggests severe AS
    (c) AVA by continuity equation of less than 1 cm^2 indicates severe AS
    (d) The mean AV gradient of 43 mm Hg suggests moderate AS

Ans. (d)

Please see the next case for discussion regarding AS severity.

MOVIES 62 TO 64

CASE 20

Bulur S, Alagic N, Elsayed M, Uygur B, Turaga NSN, Chahwala JR, Adarna LG, Nanda NC

This patient is a 66-year-old female with end stage renal disease who was sent for an echocardiogram as part of work up for renal transplant evaluation. Her body surface area (BSA) is 1.4 m^2. See Figures 20.1-20.5 and 🎥 65-67.

1. Parasternal long and short axis views show an essentially normal AV (arrow in 🎥 66) with good opening and closing movements and no evidence for stenosis. Peak and mean AV gradients were 22 and 13 mmHg, respectively. The LVO tract measured 1.6 cm at the LV-AO junction.

(a) True
(b) False

Ans. (a)

Not only the AV opening is completely normal, the gradients are also trivial.

2. Using the continuity equation, aortic stenosis is falsely graded as:

(a) Mild
(b) Moderate
(c) Moderately severe
(d) Moderately severe to severe
(e) Severe

Ans. (d)

Aortic stenosis is graded as severe when the mean AV gradient is >40 mm Hg or the AVA by the continuity equation is <1.0 cm^2 (<0.6 cm^2 when indexed to body surface area, BSA). Aortic stenosis is considered moderate if the mean AV gradient is 20–40 mm Hg or AVA is 1.0–1.5 cm^2 (0.6–0.85 cm^2 indexed). Mild aortic stenosis is denoted by a mean gradient of <20 mm Hg or AVA >1.5 cm^2 (>0.85 cm^2 indexed). AVA of this patient measured 1.06 cm^2 using the VTI method and 1.02 cm^2 (0.73 cm^2 indexed) using peak velocity. These values are consistent with almost severe stenosis, even though this patient in reality has no significant stenosis. This case clearly shows the limitation of using the continuity equation to calculate AVA especially when the LVOT is borderline or narrow (20 mm or less). In this patient, LVOT measured 1.6 cm.

The ratio of peak LVOT velocity (120 cm/s) to peak AV velocity (227 cm/s) is 0.53 which is also consistent with no significant stenosis (moderate AS = 0.25-0.50 and severe AS <0.25).

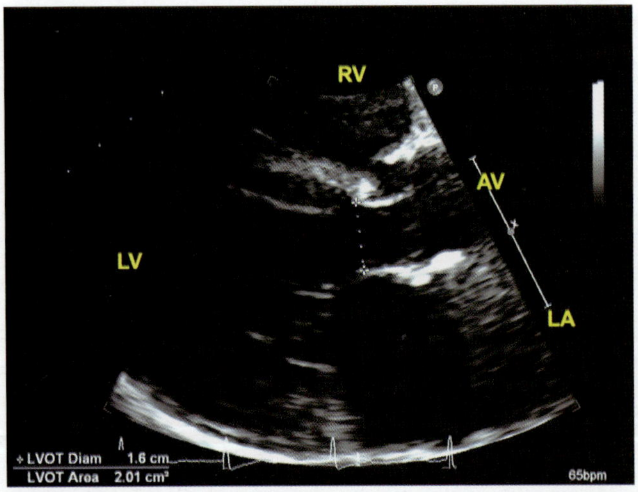

Fig. 20.1: Parasternal long axis view.

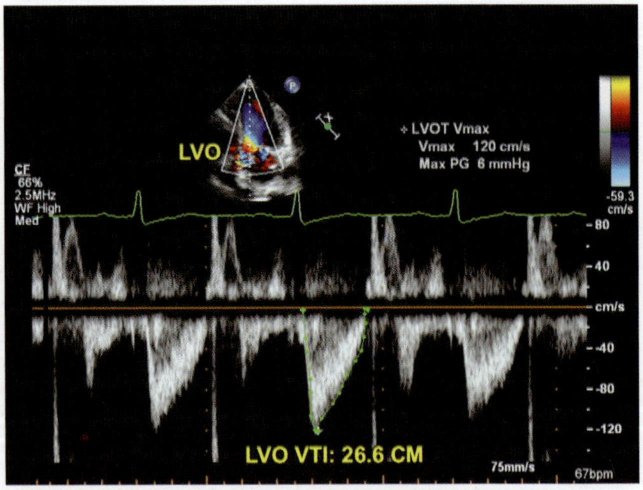

Fig. 20.2: Apical five chamber view. Pulsed Doppler examination of left ventricular outflow tract (LVOT). VTI = Velocity time integral.

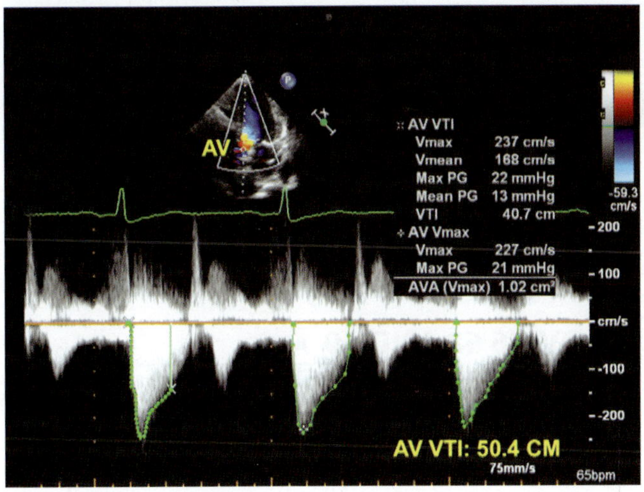

Fig. 20.3: Apical five chamber view. Continuous wave Doppler examination of the AV.

Calculation of Aortic Valve Area Using the Continuity Equation

- $AVA = \pi r^2 \times VTI_{LOVT} / VTI_{AV}$
- $AVA = 3.14 \times 0.8 \times 0.8 \times 26.6 / 50.4$
- $AVA = 1.06\ cm^2$
- $AVA = \pi r^2 \times$ Peak Vel_{LVOT}/ Peak Vel_{AV}
- $AVA = 3.14 \times 0.8 \times 0.8 \times 120 / 237$
- $AVA = 1.02\ cm^2$

Fig. 20.5: AV area using the continuity equation in this patient.

Calculation of Aortic Valve Area Using the Continuity Equation

- $SV_{AV} = SV_{LVOT}$ (continuity of flow)
- $AVA \times VTI_{AV} = CSA_{LVOT} \times VTI_{LVOT}$ (Doppler principle)
- $AVA = CSA_{LVOT} \times VTI_{LVOT} / VTI_{AV}$
- $AVA = \pi r^2 \times VTI_{LOVT} / VTI_{AV}$

Or

- $AVA = \pi r^2 \times$ Peak Vel_{LOVT} / Peak Vel_{AV} (simplified)

- AVA = Aortic valve area
- CSA = Cross-sectional area
- LVOT = Left ventricular outflow tract
- SV = Stroke volume
- VTI = Velocity time integral

Fig. 20.4: AV area using the continuity equation.

MOVIES 65 TO 67

CASE 21

Bulur S, Alagic N, Elsayed M, Uygur B, Turaga NSN, Chahwala JR, Adarna LG, Nanda NC

Movies 68 and 69 represent another patient with AS in whom the AV area was over estimated using the continuity equation. LVOT width was 18 mm. Peak and mean AV gradients were 39 and 19 mm Hg consistent with mild AS. AV area by continuity equation measured 0.62 cm^2 falsely indicative of severe AS. The dimensionless index (76.7/312 = 0.246) also erroneously suggested severe stenosis.

MOVIES 68 AND 69

CASE 22

Chahwala JR, Adarna LG, Mohamed A, Gupta N, Elsayed M, Bulur S, Alagic N, Nanda NC

This is a 74-year-old male with coronary artery disease. 2D TTE was done (🎥 70).

1. **What does the arrow point to?**
   (a) Normal AV
   (b) Bicuspid AV
   (c) AV prolapse
   (d) Bioprosthetic AV

Ans. (c)

Prolapse of the right coronary cusp of AV is clearly seen. AR was only trace. LV function was normal with no wall motion abnormalities. There is also borderline MV prolapse.

MOVIE 70 🎥

CASE 23

Gupta N, Mohamed A, Elsayed M, Nanda NC

This is a 66-year-old female who was referred for a treadmill exercise echo study because of chest pain. Baseline 2D TTE was done. LV and RV functions were normal without any wall motion abnormalities.

1. **What do Figure 23.1 and 71 and 72 show?**
   (a) Normal AV with mild AR
   (b) Thickened AV with mild AR
   (c) AV prolapse with mild AR
   (d) Thickened AV with moderate AR

Ans.(c)

Arrow in 71 shows intermittent prolapse of the AV. Arrow in 72 points to mild AR which is also noted on color Doppler M-mode examination (arrow in Fig. 23.1). This patient's stress echo study was normal.

MOVIES 71 AND 72

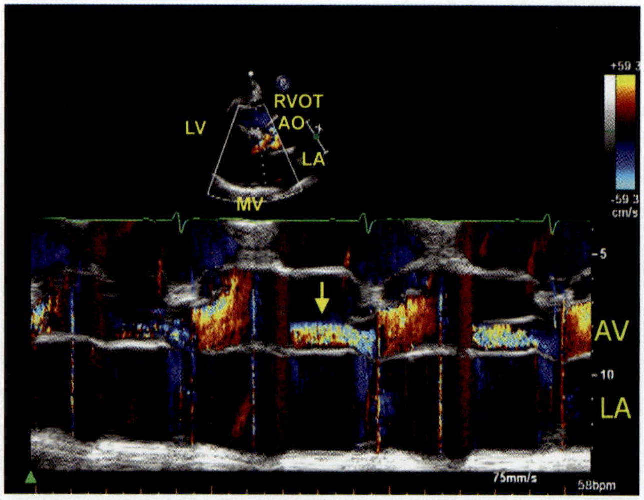

Fig. 23.1: Color M-mode examination.

CASE 24

Bulur S, Nanda NC

The patient is a 53-year-old male in whom an early diastolic murmur was heard in the aortic area. His BP was 140/85 mm Hg. 2D TTE was done (Fig. 24.1 and 🎥 73-75).

1. **How severe is AR in this patient?**
   (a) Mild because the AR jet width (height, two small arrows) measured at the point of its exit from the AV is less than 25% of the LVO dimension taken at the same point in the cardiac cycle. Parasternal long axis view.
   (b) AR is at least moderate in severity because the jet width is much larger further downstream.
   (c) AR is at least moderate, if not severe because the jet extends a long way towards the LV apex
   (d) AR is trivial because I see no evidence of turbulent flow signals in the jet which should be present if AR was more significant

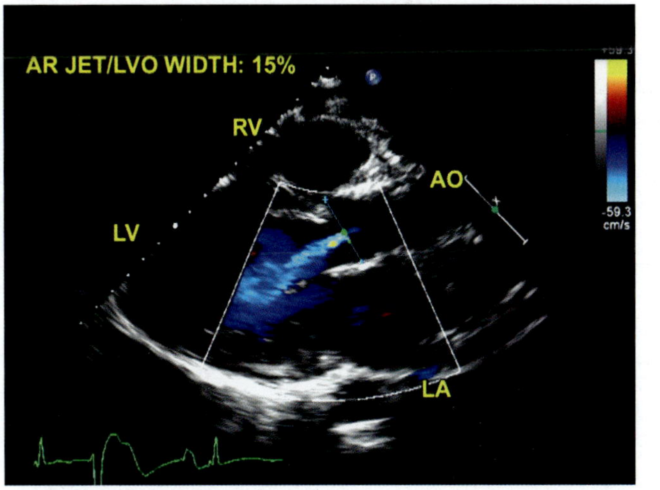

Figs. 24.1: Parasternal long axis view.

Ans. (a)

As shown by the small arrows, the Jet width (or height as it is often called) should be measured at the point of exit from the AV, practically on the ventricular side of the AV. This virtually represents the vena contracta width. The LVO is measured at the same point in the cardiac cycle as the inner dimension. A jet width/LVO width ratio less than 25% represents mild AR and over 65% (2/3 of LVO width) denotes severe AR. The jet size is also influenced by the Nyquist limit control knob on the instrument panel because increasing or decreasing the Nyquist limit also changes the color filter.

🎥 76 and 77 are from another patient with mild AR. The color M-mode shows a small pandiastolic AR jet (arrows).

MOVIES 73 TO 77 🎥

CASE 25

Chahwala JR, Elsayed M, Alagic N, Uygur B, Turaga NSN, Adarna LG, Taher A, Mohamed A, Gupta N, Bulur S, Nanda NC

Adult patient with a murmur. 2D TTE was done.

1. **Estimate the severity of AR (Fig. 25.1 and 🎥 78 and 79):**
   (a) Severe AR
   (b) Moderate AR
   (c) Mild AR
   (d) Very severe AR
   (e) Unable to differentiate between severe and less severe AR

Ans. (e)

The width of AR jet at its exit from AV measured 2 cm and the LVOT measurement at the same point was 3 cm. Therefore, proximal AR jet occupied practically 2/3 of LVOT suggesting severe AR. When the Nyquist limit was increased to 83.7 cm/sec it became more clear that the AR jet was eccentric and originated more anteriorly at the level of right coronary cusp. It then coursed down along the AV possibly giving a false impression of severe AR. In such cases, it is important to do a suprasternal examination to differentiate between severe and less severe AR. Arrow in Figure 25.1 points to flow acceleration at the origin of the AR jet.

2. **To further assess AR severity, PW Doppler examination from the suprasternal notch was done. What does it show (Fig. 25.2)?**
   (a) Severe AR
   (b) Not severe AR

Ans. (b)

Large pandiastolic flow signals would be consistent with severe AR. In this patient reversed diastolic flow signals (solid arrow) are not pandiastolic and occupy only earlier part of diastole suggesting AR is not severe. Ideally, the color Doppler should be first turned on and then the PW Doppler sample volume should be placed within the reverse diastolic red flow signals at the aortic isthmus (junction of aortic arch with descending aorta, level of left subclavian artery origin). Hollow arrow in Figure 25.2 shows Doppler "noise" which is of same magnitude above and below the baseline.

3. **🎥 80 (from another patient) represents pressure half time (PHT) measurement of CW Doppler tracing of AR jet obtained from apical 5 chamber view. Estimate the severity of AR:**
   (a) Severe AR
   (b) Not severe AR

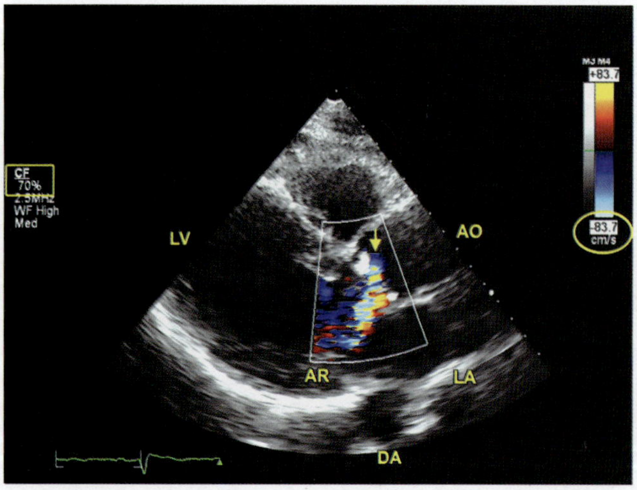

Fig. 25.1: Parasternal long axis view showing eccentric AR.

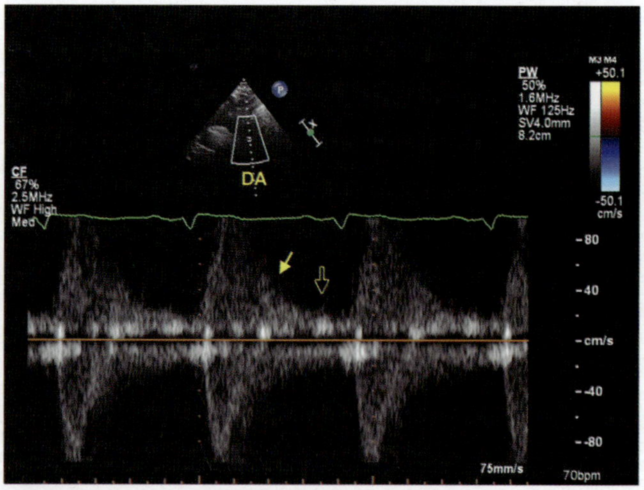

Fig. 25.2: Suprasternal examination demonstrating absence of pandiastolic reverse flow at the junction of the aortic arch and descending thoracic aorta.

Ans. (b)

A flat slope (PHT > 500 ms) is consistent with mild AR, while a steep slope (PHT < 200 ms) correlates with severe or acute, decompensated AR.

Color M-mode echo taken in the aortic root short axis view from another patient (81) with mild to moderate AR. Shows initially mild/moderate AR turning into severe AR filling the whole LVOT lumen completely towards the end of diastole. This results from motion of the aortic root such that the ultrasound beam which initially interrogated the proximal AR at its exit from the AV (essentially the vena contracta) later examines the AR jet further downstream where its width has become much larger because of the large diastolic gradient between the AO and LV. This highlights the limitation of assessing AR in the AO/LVOT short axis view. AR is best evaluated in the parasternal long axis and apical 5 chamber/long axis views.

MOVIES 78 TO 81

CASE 26

Mohamed A, Gupta N, Elsayed M, Nanda NC

This is an 84-year-old female with a murmur heard by her referring physician. She is asymptomatic with new onset of hypertension. 2D TTE was done (82).

1. **What do the arrows in 82 show?**
   (a) Mild AR (right arrow) with fistula into LV (left arrow).
   (b) Mild AR (right arrow) with a septal perforator opening into LV (left arrow).
   (c) Mild AR, no fistula.
   (d) Mild AR (right arrow) with small fistula into LV, unknown origin.

Ans. (c)

The narrow AR jet initially moves anteriorly (red color, right arrow) towards the ventricular septum and then turns posteriorly (blue color, left arrow) after impinging on it.

MOVIE 82

CASE 27

Gupta N, Mohamed A, Elsayed M, Nanda NC

The patient is a 69-year-old female being followed in the Outpatient Clinic for aortic regurgitation (AR). 2D TTE was done (83 to 87).

1. **What is the severity of AR in this patient?**
   (a) Mild
   (b) Moderate
   (c) Severe
   (d) Cannot determine severity reliably, need more views

Ans. (b)

The ratio of AR jet width taken at its exit from AV to LVOT width taken at the same point was 29% consistent with moderate AR (ratio for mild AR < 25%, moderate AR 26–50%, moderately severe AR 51–64% and severe AR ≥ 65%).[1] The pressure half time (PHT) is 432 ms also consistent with moderate AR (PHT for mild AR >500 ms, severe AR <200 ms). Suprasternal examination with the PW Doppler sample volume carefully placed at the aortic isthmus (junction of ascending and descending AO, level of origin of left subclavian artery) in the red (reversed) diastolic color flow signals (hollow arrow) revealed only early diastolic back flow (solid arrow) ruling out severe AR which would have shown prominent pandiastolic back flow. Arrow heads denote low frequency Doppler "noise" on both sides of the baseline. MV diastolic flutter (arrow) produced by the AR jet impinging on the MV is noted on the M-mode in 87.

MOVIES 83 TO 87

REFERENCE

1. Nanda NC, Karakus G, Degirmencioglu A (Editors): Manual of Echocardiography. Jaypee Brothers Medical Publisher, Philadelphia, New Delhi, London and Panama. 2016.

CASE 28

Gupta N, Mohamed A, Elsayed M, Nanda NC

The patient is a 48-year-old male complaining of shortness of breath (NYHA Class II-III). His blood pressure was 151/69 mm Hg. 2D (Figs. 28.1 to 28.4 and 88 to 92) and 3D (Fig. 28.5 and 93 to 95) TTEs were done.

1. **Regarding the severity of AR in this patient by 2D TTE (90 and 91), which of the following is an incorrect statement?**
   (a) The Nyquist limit in this patient was increased from 50 to 80 cm/s (circles in 90 and 91) in an attempt to detect the origin of the eccentric AR jet. Higher Nyquist limits tend to remove lower velocity flow signals facilitating detection of AR origin where the velocity is much higher. In this patient, AR jet appears to originate posteriorly with subsequent anterior direction.
   (b) The severity of eccentric AR may be difficult to estimate using the color Doppler jet width/LVOT width criteria and hence suprasternal examination becomes all the more important.
   (c) Suprasternal examination is standardized by placing the PW Doppler sample volume at the junction of aortic arch and descending aorta (aortic isthmus, Fig. 28.2). Before doing this, it is advisable to first turn the color Doppler on looking for reversed red diastolic flow signals and then placing the Doppler sample volume in the middle of these signals (Fig. 28.3, 92).
   (d) Prominent pandiastolic reverse red flow signals at the level of the aortic isthmus are indicative of severe AR (Fig. 28.2). These should not be confused with much lower frequency Doppler "noise" recorded on both sides of the baseline. Color M-Mode may also show pandiastolic reversal (Fig. 28.4)
   (e) Attention should be paid to both the Nyquist limit and color Doppler gain when using the methodology given in (b) above.
   (f) Pressure half time (PHT) measurement of AR jet using CW Doppler may also help in assessing AR severity (Fig. 28.1). Pressure half time less than 200 ms denotes severe AR and more than 500 ms is consistent with mild AR.
   (g) Quantitative assessment of AR severity may be provided by 3D echo which views the vena contracta (VC) en face facilitating planimetric measurement of its area (A1 in Fig. 28.5 and 95). A VC area of ≥0.6 cm^2 denotes severe AR (mild AR: VC <0.2 cm^2, moderate AR: VC 0.2-0.4 cm^2, moderately severe AR: 0.4-0.6 cm^2).[1] VC width of ≥6 mm by 2D TTE suggests severe AR (VC <3 mm denotes mild AR).[1]
   (h) PHT measurement of AR jet is most reliable in grading AR severity.

Ans.(h)

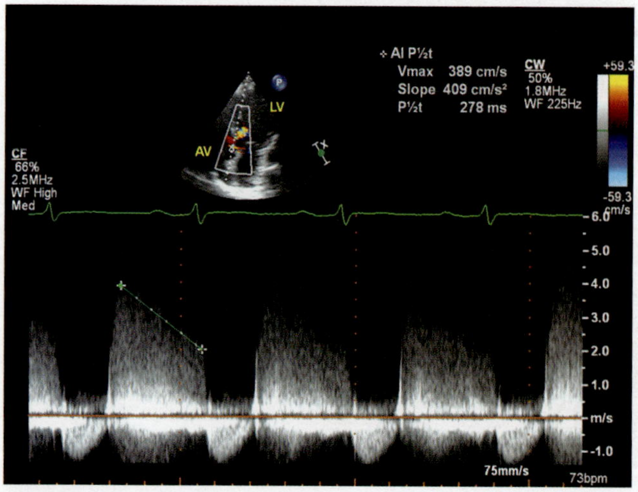

Fig. 28.1: AR pressure half time measured 278 ms suggesting that AR was not severe.

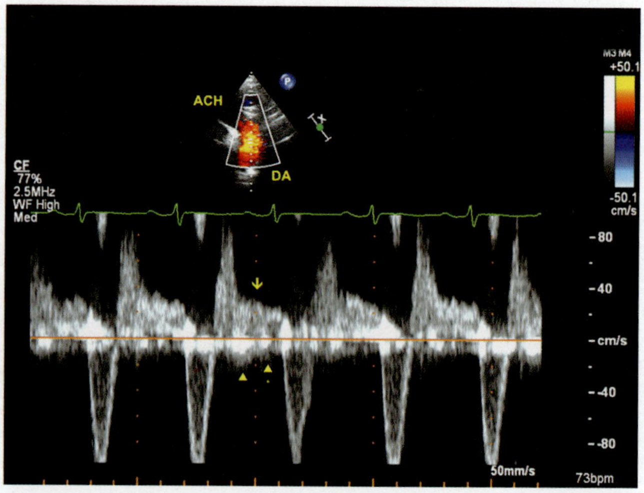

Fig. 28.2: Suprasternal examination shows pandiastolic flow reversal indicative of severe AR.

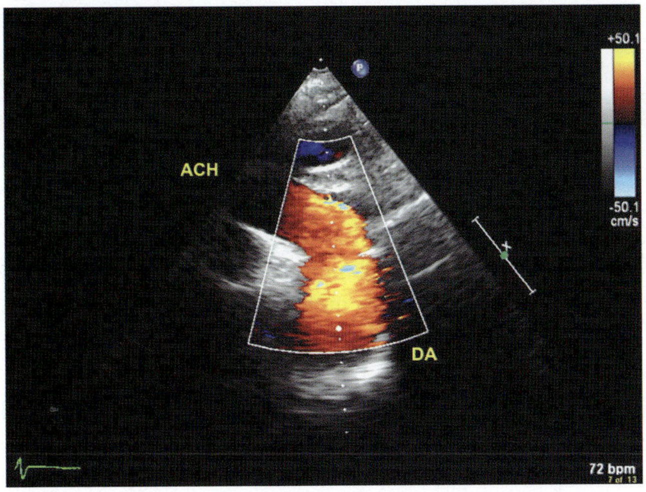

Fig. 28.3: Prominent red signals indicative of backflow are noted in the aortic arch (ACH), isthmus and proximal descending aorta (DA).

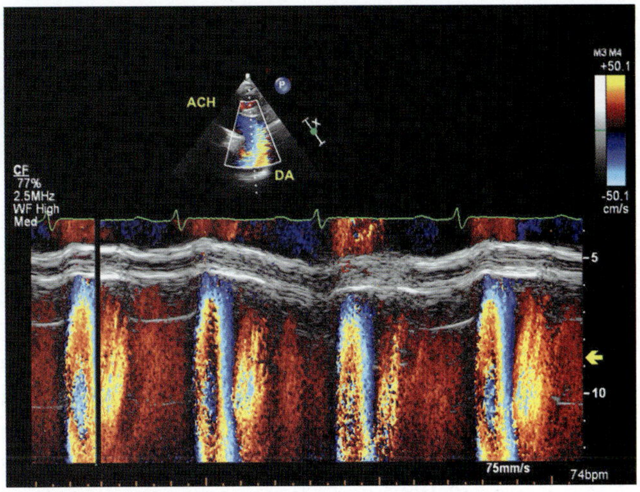

Fig. 28.4: Color M-mode examination showing diastolic backflow (arrow) in the ACH, isthmus and DA.

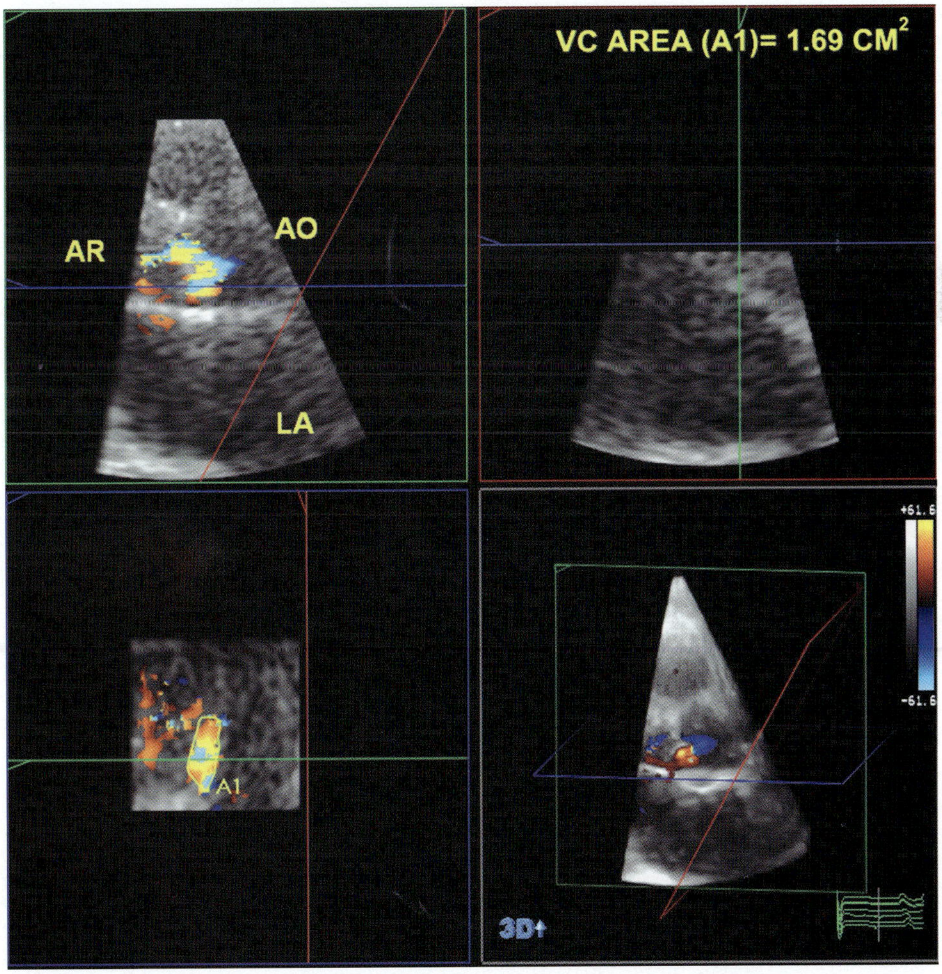

Fig. 28.5: 3D TTE assessment of AR vena contracta which measured 1.69 cm^2 indicative of torrential AR.

In this patient, PHT was 278 m/s which is not consistent with severe AR. However, all other 2D and 3D TTE parameters indicated severe AR. It is thus important to assess all clinical and echo criteria when grading AR severity. In this patient, LV was enlarged measuring 66 mm and LVEF was 50%. Also, LA was mildly enlarged at 44 mm. These findings show the deleterious effect of severe AR on the left heart. This patient has been scheduled for AV replacement.

2. **Regarding AV morphology, all of the following statements are correct *except*:**
   (a) The morphology of AV may be difficult to assess correctly by 2D TTE in some patients because at any given time it images only a thin slice of the AV. On the other hand, with 3D echo the AV in its entirety is captured and stored in the 3D dataset permitting interrogation using multiple plane angulations. Thus, a bicuspid AV can be more easily differentiated from tricuspid morphology by 3D echo as compared to 2D modalities (88 and 89).
   (b) Presence of a raphe (hollow arrow in 94, 3D MPR Mode) in a bicuspid AV which may mimic a third leaflet is more easily identified by 3D echo.
   (c) Bicuspid AV with equal sized leaflets will always result in significant stenosis unless the leaflets are redundant with multiple folds (arrow in 88). This is because the cusp diameters are much smaller than the aortic root circumference.
   (d) All bicuspid AVs are associated with coarctation of the aorta.
   (e) Some of the redundant folds in a bicuspid AV may prolapse into the LVOT (arrow in 88 and 94).

Ans. (d)

Bicuspid AV syndrome has been recently described. It incorporates many abnormalities which may be associated with a bicuspid AV. These include AS, AR, aortic dilatation and aneurysm, aortic dissection and aortic rupture. Other lesions which may occur with a bicuspid AV include MV prolapse, VSD, PDA and coarctation of aorta. Bicuspid valves may also get infected. However, these conditions are not always present. 96 shows the technique of 3D TTE cropping.

MOVIES 88 TO 96

REFERENCES

1. Nanda NC, Karakas G, Degirmencioglu A. Manual of echocardiography. Pages112-127 and 372. Jaypee Brothers Medical publishers. Philadelphia, New Delhi, London, Panama. 2016.
2. Yuan SM, Jing H. The bicuspid aortic valve and related disorders. Sao Paulo Med J. 2010;128(5):296-301. Review. PubMed PMID: 21181071.

CASE 29

Roomi AU, Shah A, Siddiqui LI, Elsayed M, Bulur S, Nanda NC

A 42-year-old male is a known case of hypertension and diabetes mellitus. He is also a heavy smoker. Stress test was positive for myocardial ischemia on low work load. He then was admitted for catheterization.

Post cath. patient became hypotensive and 2D TTE and 2D TEE were done (Figs. 29.1 to 29.3 and 97 to 99).

SURGICAL FINDINGS

Torn non and left coronary cusps resulting in severe aortic regurgitation caused by percutaneous angioplasty were found. Aortic valve replacement was subsequently done.

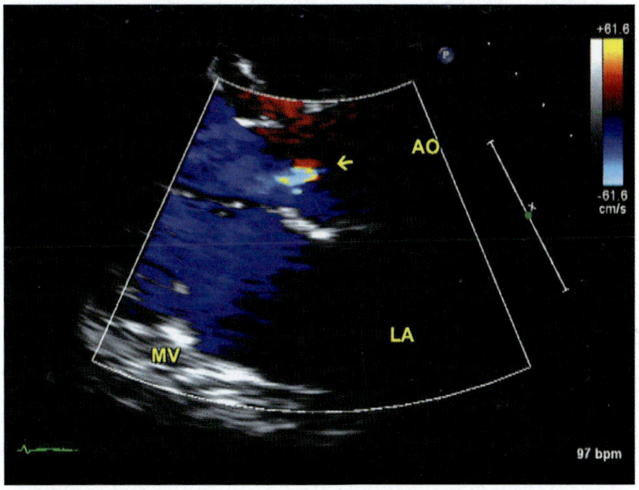

Fig. 29.1: Transthoracic parasternal long axis view. Arrow points to aortic regurgitation.

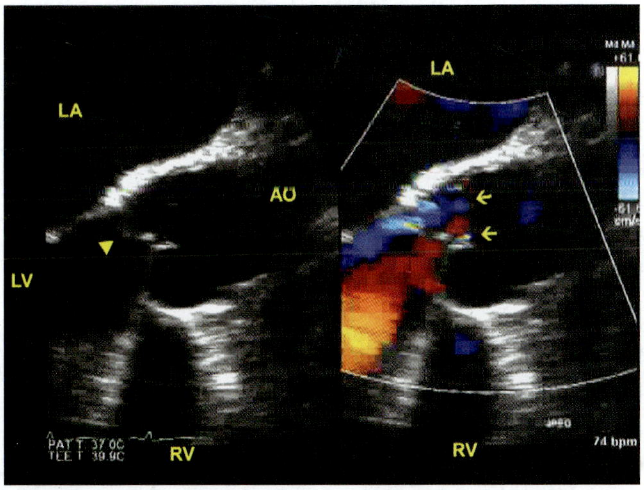

Fig. 29.2: Transesophageal echocardiography. Arrows point to 2 jets of aortic regurgitation. Arrowhead points to a prolapsed leaflet.

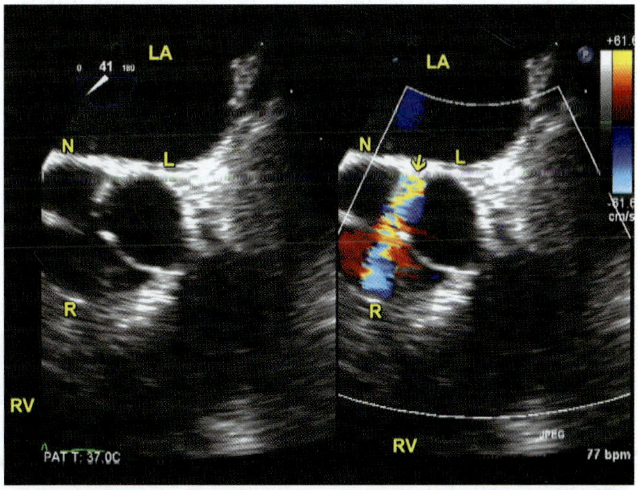

Fig. 29.3: Transesophageal echocardiography. Arrow points to aortic regurgitation. L, N and R correspond to left, non and right coronary cusps of AV.

MOVIE LEGENDS

97: Transthoracic parasternal view. Arrow points to aortic regurgitation.

98: Transesophageal echocardiography. Arrows point to 2 jets of aortic regurgitation. Arrowhead points to prolapsed leaflet.

99: Transesophageal echocardiography. Arrow points to aortic regurgitation. L, N and R correspond to left, non and right coronary cusps of AV.

CASE 30

Hanumanth K Reddy, Raghuveer Kura, Dawn Hui, William M Pelton, Nishchayjit Basra

A PATIENT WITH SEVERE CHEST PAIN

A 51-year-old man presented to a community hospital with severe chest pain radiating to the inter-scapular region associated with nausea and mild diaphoresis. Past medical history includes hypertension and smoking.

Nitroglycerin partially relieved the pain. Narcotic analgesics were required to alleviate the chest pain.

Physical Examination showed a moderately built, well nourished individual with pulse rate 110 bpm, blood pressure 150/90 mm Hg and respirations 18 per min.

Cardiac examination revealed normal heart sounds without any gallop or murmur. Lungs were clear to auscultation without any adventitious sounds. Rest of the examination was unremarkable. Laboratory data revealed normal cardiac enzymes and comprehensive panel. Chest X-ray was normal. Computed tomography angiography (CTA) of the chest is shown in Figures 30.1 and 30.2. Transesophageal echocardiography (TEE) shows longitudinal and cross-sectional views of the ascending aorta in Figures 30.3 and 30.4 respectively.

1. **Etiology of this patient's chest pain is:**
   (a) Acute coronary syndrome
   (b) Pulmonary embolism
   (c) Aortic intramural hematoma (IMH)
   (d) Reflux esophagitis

Ans.(c)

2. **The next step in the management of this patient is:**
   (a) Cardiac catheterization
   (b) Beta blockers, nitrates and heparin
   (c) TEE and consult CT surgeon
   (d) Proton pump inhibitor and morphine

Ans.(c)

3. **Appropriate management of Type A - Intramural hematoma includes:**
   (a) Surgical repair
   (b) Medical therapy
   (c) Pericardiocentesis
   (d) Medical therapy with frequent monitoring for complications
   (e) (a) and (d)

Ans.(e)

Figure 30.5 is an intra-operative image of the aortic intramural hematoma presenting as hemorrhagic aneurysmal aorta. Interestingly, this hemorrhage extends onto the RV myocardium.

DISCUSSION

The symptoms and CT of the chest findings are suggestive of aortic intramural hematoma. CT chest showed peri-aortic cuff of high attenuation without intimal flap. A TEE showed eccentric aortic wall thickening.

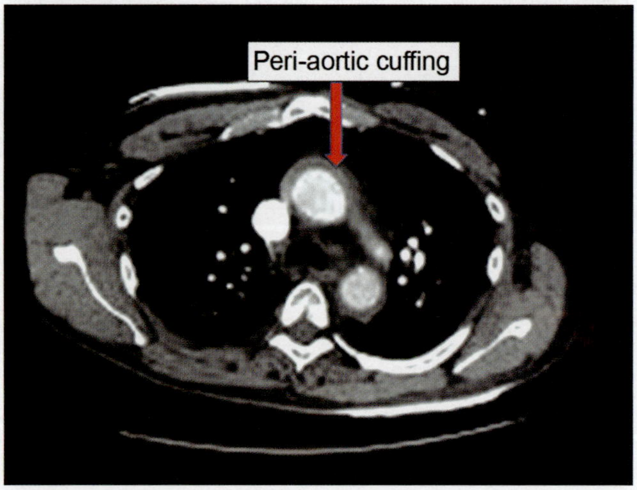

Fig. 30.1: Noncontrast computed tomography of the chest.

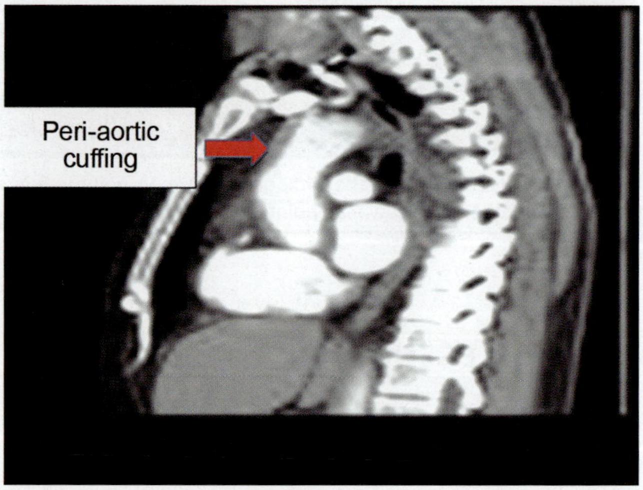

Fig. 30.2: Noncontrast computed tomography of chest.

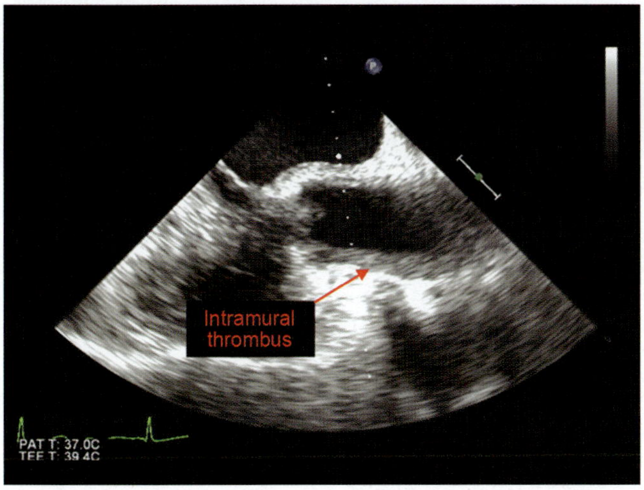

Fig. 30.3: Transesophageal echocardiography (TEE) showing longitudinal view of the ascending aorta.

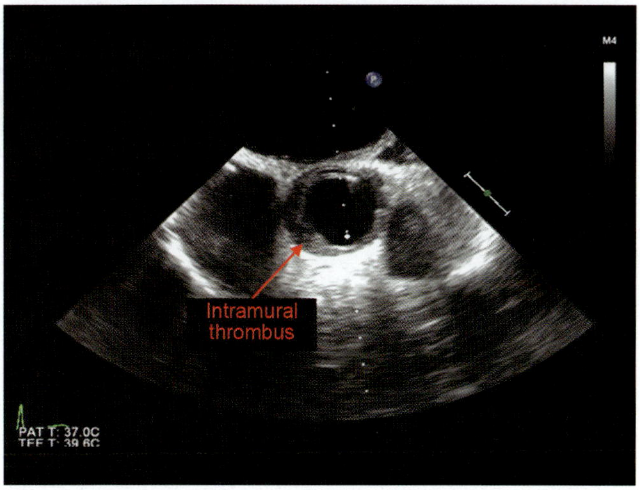

Fig. 30.4: Transesophageal echocardiography (TEE) showing a cross-sectional view of the ascending aorta.

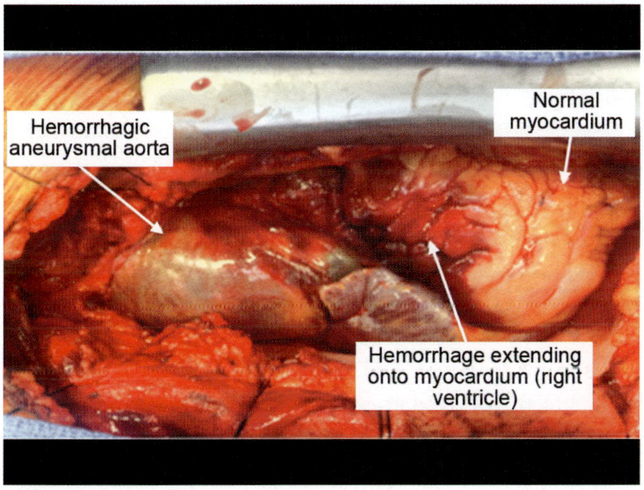

Fig. 30.5: Intraoperative image of IMH.

Aortic intramural hematoma (IMH) is a variant of acute aortic syndrome with clinical presentation similar to that of aortic dissection (AD). Intramural hematoma (IMH) begins with spontaneous rupture of the vasa vasorum, the small blood vessels traversing the outer half of the aortic media and supply blood to the aortic wall. The small IMH then spreads along the medial layer of the aorta. Subsequently, the intramural hematoma weakens the aorta and may progress to either outward rupture of the aortic wall or to the inward disrupting the intima, the latter leading to communicating aortic dissection (AD). In an international registry of acute aortic dissection (1996-2011), 6.2% of patients out of 2830 had IMH. The patients with IMH were older than those with AD.

NATURAL HISTORY AND MANAGEMENT OF IMH

Intramural aortic hematomas are usually seen in the older hypertensive patients. Intramural hematoma may occur in patients with blunt chest trauma by aortic wall injury or penetrating atherosclerotic ulcer.

Similar to proximal aortic dissection, acute IMH of proximal ascending aorta as in this patient is managed by surgery. However, recent reports from Japan favor medical treatment in some patients with proximal IMH. Overall in-hospital mortality is similar in IMH compared to AD (26.6 versus 26.5). Medically managed type - A IMH patients had mortality (40%) much less than that of classic AD (61.8%; p = 0.195).[1]

Distal IMH is managed conservatively with medical therapy.

In very elderly patients with proximal IMH, surgical repair poses a high risk for mortality and morbidity. The recommended strategy in this high risk group is supportive medical treatment with frequent non-invasive monitoring for complications and reserve surgery for patients with complications.[2]

REFERENCES

1. Harris KM, Braverman AC, Eagle KA, Woznicki EM, Pyeritz RE, Myrmel T, et al. Acute aortic intramural hematoma: an analysis from the International Registry of acute aortic dissection. Circulation. 2012;126(suppl I):S91-S96.
2. Evangelista A, Dominguez R, Sebastia C, Salas A, Permanyer-Miralda G, et al. Prognostic value of clinical and morphologic findings in short-term evolution of aortic intramural haematoma: therapeutic implications. Eur Heart J. 2004;25:81–87.

CASE 31

Elsayed Abo-Salem, Angel Lopez-Candales

A 39-year-old pregnant female, 35 weeks, presented to the hospital with uncontrolled hypertension and chest pain. She had a history of hypertension, chronic kidney disease and syphilis with poor compliance of therapy. Examination revealed a diastolic murmur at the base radiating to the right sternal border. ECG showed nonspecific ST-T wave changes in the anterior leads. Echocardiography showed a dilated aortic root (Fig. 31.1), severe aortic regurgitation and moderate left ventricular hypertrophy. There was an echodense linear structure in the aortic root (Fig. 31.1).

1. **What is the most appropriate next step in the evaluation of this linear structure?**
    (a) Report as artifact and no further work up is recommended
    (b) Chest computed tomography
    (c) Contrast echocardiography
    (d) Chest X-ray
    (e) Cardiac catheterization

Ans. (c)

DISCUSSION

Echocardiographic contrast agent was injected intravenously and filled the true lumen rapidly with slower filling of the false lumen (Fig. 31.2, 100). A diagnosis of proximal aortic dissection was made and chest computed tomography was done to assess its extension. Patient refused surgery and was discharged 2 weeks later. A major challenge for echocardiographic evaluation of ascending aorta is the presence of linear reverberation artifacts. The use of color flow Doppler and contrast echocardiography can enhance the sensitivity and specificity of transthoracic echocardiography for the diagnosis of type A aortic dissection. Contrast study may also help to differentiate true and false lumens.[1] Chest computed tomography is a reasonable option for cases with a high probability of aortic dissection, but associated with fetal radiation exposure.

MOVIE LEGEND

100: Apical 5 chamber view. Contrast injection clearly delineates the aortic dissection flap (arrow) and both true (T) and false (F) lumens.

REFERENCE

1. Abo Salem E, López-Candales A. Diagnosis of asymptomatic aortic dissection during pregnancy using contrast echocardiography. Journal of Cardiology Cases, 2014; 9(5): 200–202.

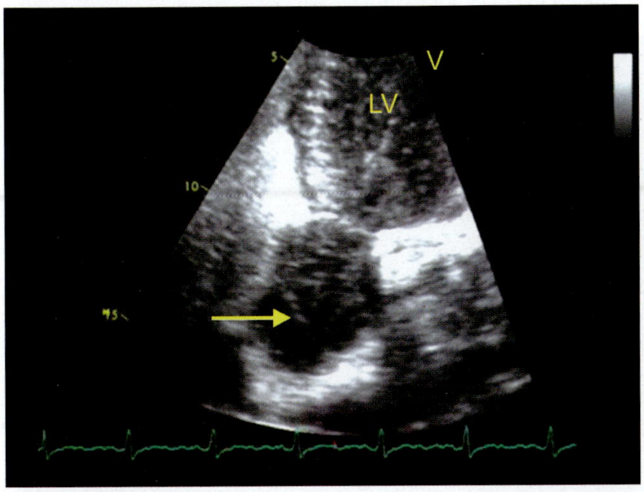

Fig. 31.1: Transthoracic Echocardiography modified apical view, showing left ventricle (LV) and dilated aortic root with a possible intimal flap (arrow).

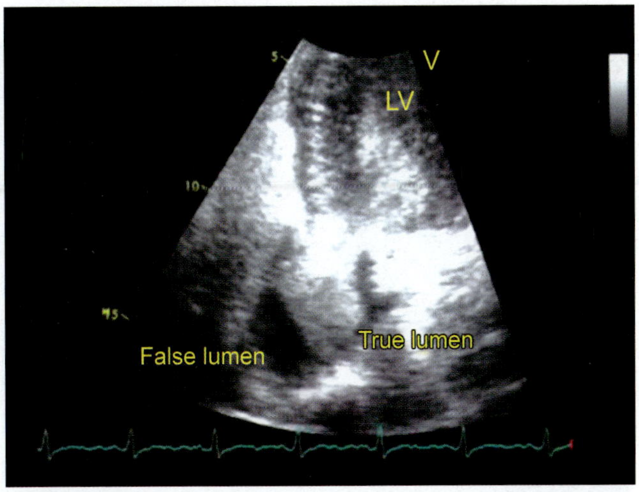

Fig. 31.2: Apical 5 chamber view. Contrast injection clearly delineates the aortic dissection flap and both true (T) and false (F) lumens.

CASE 32

Inga Vaitenas, Zeina Ibrahim, Kameswari Maganti

A PRESENT FROM NIGERIA

A 72-year-old male with history of hypertension presented to the emergency room with intermittent chest pain for 3–4 weeks. The pain was sharp, substernal, and occurred at rest when he laid down in the right lateral decubitus position. He was otherwise healthy until about 5 months prior to admission when he developed a cough that was persistent. On evaluation in Nigeria, he was found to have a thoracic mass that was determined to be an enlarged aorta. He was deemed not to be a surgical candidate due to lack of ICU facilities in his hometown where he spends part of the year. He came back to his home in USA for further evaluation.

A chest X-ray (Figs. 32.1A and B) revealed a large, lobulated mass in left hemithorax that measured approximately 11.5 cm that was favored to represent the aorta (red bar with arrowheads). This extends from the posterior arch of the thoracic aorta to the midthoracic level with mild rightward deviation of the trachea.

A CT angiogram that was performed demonstrated extensive type B dissection which originates immediately distal to the left subclavian artery and involves the descending thoracic aorta and abdominal aorta extending into the proximal right common iliac artery. The descending thoracic aorta is aneurysmal measuring approximately 10.3 cm × 9.0 cm and shows a large false lumen and a narrow true lumen. In the lower thoracic aortic false lumen there is irregular soft tissue consistent with thrombus. The lower thoracic aorta measures 5.4 × 5.9 cm. At the level of the diaphragmatic aortic hiatus, the aorta measures 9.4 × 7.0 cm with celiac artery originating at this level. The SMA and IMA arise from the true lumen and opacify normally. Both renal arteries arise from the true lumen (Figs. 32.2 to 32.4).

The echocardiogram demonstrated normal left ventricular size and systolic function. The enlarged descending aorta with a dissection flap was once again seen. (Figs. 32.5 and 32.6, 101 to 103)

The patient underwent resection and replacement of the thoracoabdominal aneurysm with reattachment of celiac artery, superior mesenteric artery and bilateral renal arteries. Five years later, he is doing well without any complaints.

DISCUSSION

Aortic aneurysmal disease is now recognized as a distinct degenerative process involving all layers of the vessel wall. The pathophysiology of aortic aneurysms is characterized by four events: infiltration of the vessel wall by lymphocytes and macrophages; destruction of elastin and collagen in the media and adventitia by proteases, including matrix metalloproteinases; loss of smooth-muscle cells with thinning of the media; and neovascularization.

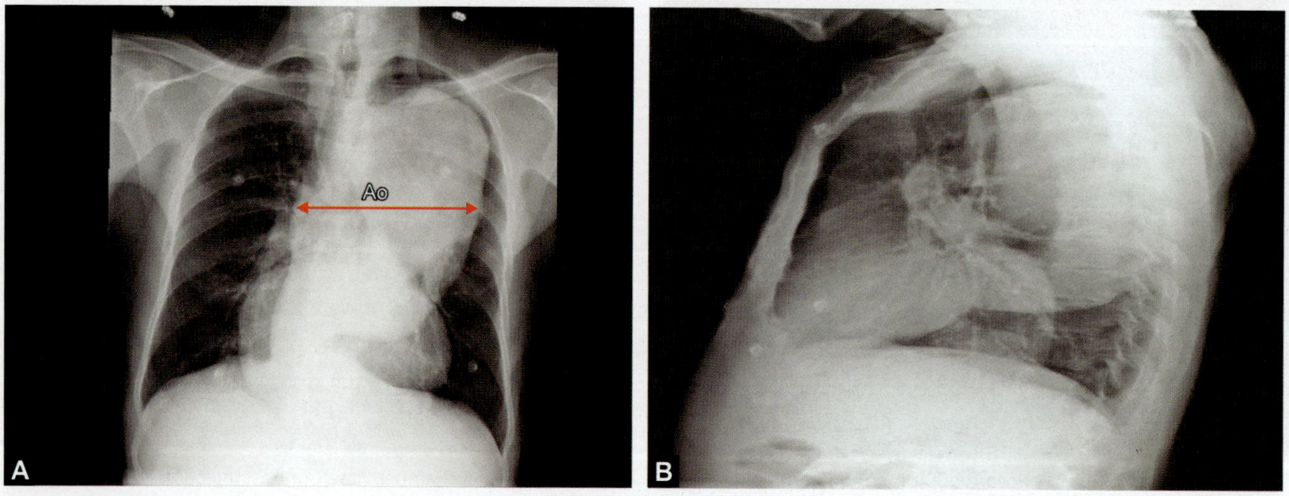

Figs. 32.1A and B: Large soft tissue mass in the left hemithorax as indicated by arrow heads is most indicative of a thoracic aorta aneurysm.

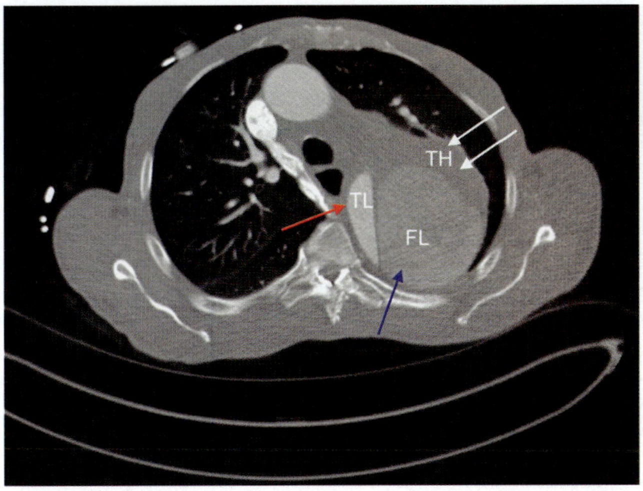

Fig. 32.2: Axial plane of CTA revealing a small true lumen (red arrow), a large false lumen (purple arrow) and a large burden of thrombus (two white arrows).

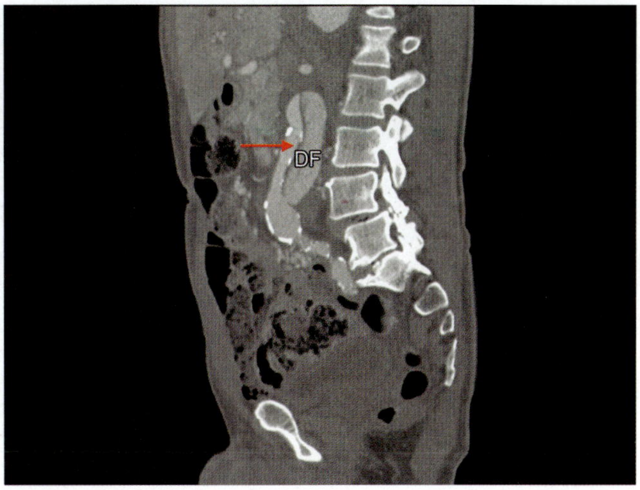

Fig. 32.3: Sagittal plane of CTA demonstrating the extensive dissection flap (red arrow).

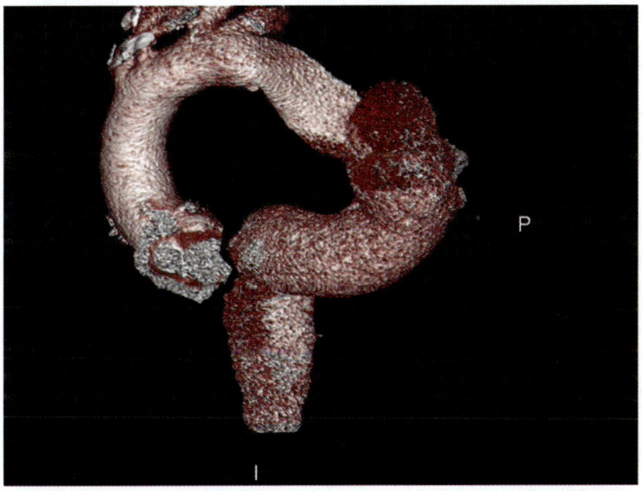

Fig. 32.4: 3D reconstruction of abdominal aorta that reveals aneurysmal aorta which is irregular and tortuous.

Dissection is a distinct process that most often involves the ascending, thoracic, or thoracoabdominal aorta.

The risk factors for abdominal aortic aneurysm[1] include older age, male sex, and a family history of the disorder. The risk of abdominal aortic aneurysm is approximately four times as high among men as among women and four times as high among people with a family history of the disorder as among those without a family history. Smoking, hypertension, hyperlipidemia, obesity, and PAD are other risk factors. Race plays a role as well with abdominal aortic aneurysms more prevalent among whites.[1-4]

Small abdominal aortic aneurysms (3.0 to 5.4 cm in diameter), when identified, should be monitored for expansion. In accordance with Laplace's law, the larger the aneurysm, the higher the rate of expansion. Current guidelines regarding the frequency of monitoring are as follows: for aneurysms with a diameter of 3.0 to 3.4 cm every 3 years; 3.5 to 4.4 cm yearly; and 4.5 to 5.4 cm every 6 months. US Preventive Services Task Force recommendations support screening in men 65 to 75 years of age with a history of smoking and selective screening in men 65 to 75 years of age without a smoking history, although the optimal cohort to be screened remains controversial.

Abdominal aortic aneurysms are usually asymptomatic[1,4] until they rupture, with an ensuing mortality of 85 to 90%. Symptomatic patients require urgent repair. Treatment should always include risk factor modifications.[3] Medical therapy typically includes beta-blockers, ACE-inhibitor, or antibiotics. However, none of the medical therapies have been shown to prevent aneurysm expansion. The usual threshold for elective repair is an aortic diameter of 5.5 cm in men and 5.0 cm in women. Endovascular repair results in lower perioperative morbidity and mortality than open repair, but the two methods are associated with similar mortality in the long term.

1. **In patients with Type B[1,2,4] dissections, what specific findings predicts complicated dissections?**
   (a) Primary entry tear on concavity of distal arch
   (b) Primary entry tear on convexity of distal arch
   (c) Both
   (d) None

Ans. (a)

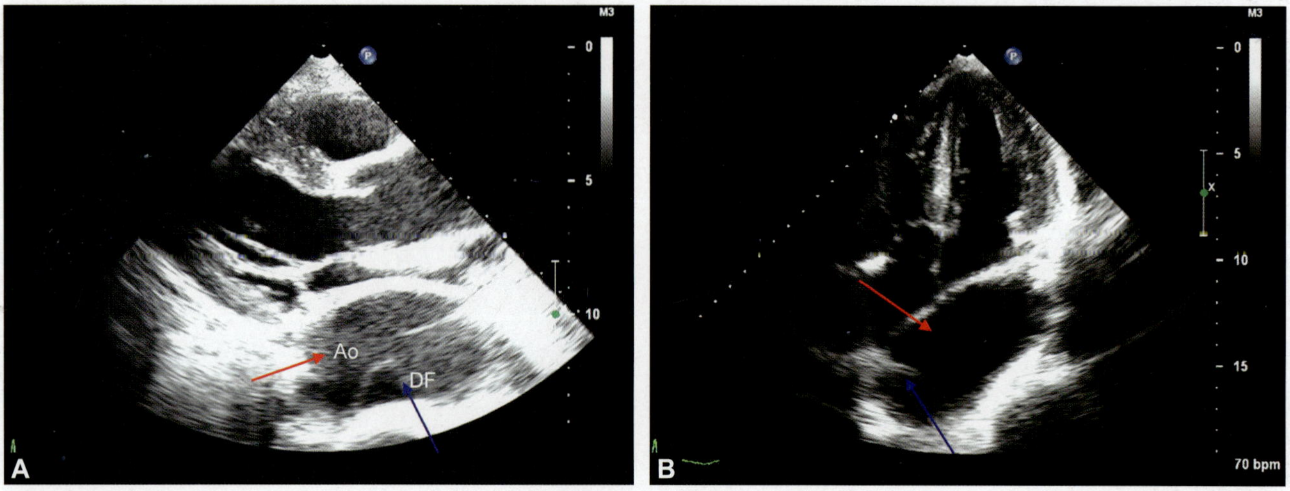

Figs. 32.5A and B: 2D TTE. Parasternal long axis (A) and apical 4 chamber (B) views demonstrating the aneurysmal descending aorta (red arrow) with encroachment on left atrium. The dissection flap is visualized (purple arrow).

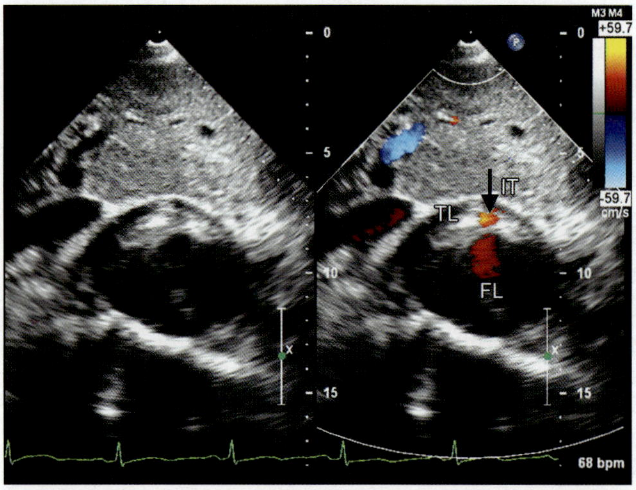

Fig. 32.6: Subcostal view demonstrating an intimal tear (arrow, IT) with blood flow going from a very small true lumen (TL) to a large false lumen (FL).

Complicated dissections are dissections associated with development of shock, periaortic hematoma, spinal cord ischemia, mesenteric ischemia/infarction, acute renal failure, limb ischemia, recurrent or refractory pain, or refractory hypertension. It is felt that dissections that involve concavity of arch tend to have more extensive involvement and often are associated with complicated dissections. Independent predictors of in-hospital mortality for type B dissection were age >70, preoperative limb ischemia, periaortic hematoma, and need for surgical management.

2. **What is the test of choice for a patient with suspected type B acute aortic dissection?**
   (a) Computed tomographic angiography
   (b) Magnetic resonance angiography
   (c) Transesophageal echocardiogram
   (d) All of the above

Ans. (d)

All of the choices above have excellent sensitivity and specificity to diagnose acute aortic dissection with a high sensitivity (>95%) and specificity (>95%). If one of the diagnostic tests is suboptimal, a second test can be used to arrive at the accurate diagnosis.

MOVIE LEGENDS

101 and 102: 2D TTE. Parasternal long axis and apical 4 chamber views demonstrating the aneurysmal descending aorta (red arrow) with encroachment on left atrium. The dissection flap (purple arrow) is visualized.

103: Subcostal view demonstrating an intimal tear (black arrow) with blood flow going from a very small true lumen to a large false lumen.

REFERENCES

1. Kent KC. Clinical Practice, Abdominal aortic aneurysms. N Engl J Med. 2014;371(22):2101-8.
2. Hughes GC. Management of acute type B aortic dissection; ADSORB trial. J Thorac Cardiovasc surg 2015;149:S158-62.
3. Tsai TT, Nienaber CA, Eagle KA. Acute aortic syndromes. Circulation. 2005;112:3802–13.

4. Hiratzka LF, Bakris GL, Beckman JA, et al. 2010 ACCF/AHA/AATS/ACR/ASA/SCA/SCAI/SIR/STS/SVM guidelines for the diagnosis and management of patients with thoracic aortic disease: a report of the American College of Cardiology Foundation/American Heart Association Task Force on Practice Guidelines, American Association for Thoracic Surgery, American College of Radiology, American Stroke Association, Society of Cardiovascular Anesthesiologists, Society for Cardiovascular Angiography and Interventions, Society of Interventional Radiology, Society of Thoracic Surgeons, and Society for Vascular Medicine. Circulation. 2010;121:e266–369. This consensus guideline document provides comprehensive recommendations for the diagnosis and treatment of patients with acute aortic syndromes.
5. Harris KM, Strauss CE, Eagle KA, et al. Correlates of delayed recognition and treatment of acute type A aortic dissection: the International Registry of Acute Aortic Dissection (IRAD). Circulation. 2011;124:1911–8.
6. Harris KM, Braverman AC, Eagle KA, et al. Acute aortic intramural hematoma: an analysis from the International Registry of Acute Aortic Dissection. Circulation. 2012;126:S91–6.

CASE 33

Adarna LG, Nanda NC

This is a 70-year-old female with previous aortic valve and ascending aortic graft replacement for aortic dissection several years ago. She came for a follow-up in the outpatient clinic. She is asymptomatic. 2D TTE was done.

1. Which of the following statements is correct (104, R = prosthetic reverberations):

(a) Both leaflets of the mechanical aortic prosthesis move well
(b) Only one leaflet of the prosthesis is visualized and it moves well
(c) It is not possible to comment on the motion of the prosthetic valve
(d) It is more important to assess the gradients than motion of a prosthetic valve

Ans. (c)

Two leaflets of the prosthetic valve are well seen next to each other in diastole but in systole they go out of view making it difficult to assess whether they opened fully and briskly. Viewing the prosthetic valve from different planes and angulations or using 3D TTE may help detect its motion in systole. Full and brisk (90 degree) opening indicates absence of any obstruction caused by pannus or a thrombus. Variable pressure gradients are noted with practically all types of aortic prosthetic valves specially mechanical ones but high gradients in the presence of normally moving leaflets would suggest obstruction elsewhere such as in the LVO/subaortic/supravalvar region, severe AR or prosthetic patient mismatch particularly when a small prosthesis is implanted.

2. What does the arrow in 105 show?

(a) Descending thoracic aorta aneurysm with dissection
(b) Descending thoracic aorta aneurysm with no dissection but an artifact since what appears to be the dissection flap shows very little motion during the cardiac cycle
(c) Descending thoracic aorta aneurysm with probable chronic dissection
(d) This is not aorta since I have never seen it imaged behind the LV viewed in short axis

Ans. (c)

In most but not all cases of acute aortic dissection, the dissection flap shows typical chaotic, irregular motion ("a worm wiggling in the aorta"). However, in chronic dissection, the dissection flap may show little or no motion such as in this patient who had aortic dissection several years ago. This patient's aorta is however, markedly enlarged and would need consideration for intra-aortic repair or open graft replacement if there is compromise of blood flow to vital organs such as the intestines, kidney and the spinal cord. An artifact is generally parallel to the walls of the aorta and may have an arc-like shape which aids in its recognition.

MOVIES 104 AND 105

CASE 37

Elsayed M, Gupta N, Mohamed A, Nanda NC

This is a 36-year-old male with previous IVC filter with concern for embolus. 2D TTE done.

1. **What does the arrow in 117 indicate?**
   (a) Pericardial effusion behind RA wall
   (b) Pericardial cyst
   (c) Raised diaphragm possibly from liver enlargement

Ans. (c)

There was no evidence of obstruction to RA flow. The arrow in 118 points to the IVC filter.

2. **Which of the following statements is incorrect (119)?**
   (a) Both celiac and superior mesenteric branches of abdominal aorta can be visualized subcostally.
   (b) Proximal abdominal aortic aneurysm and dissection can be identified by subcostal/abdominal examination
   (c) Iliac branches can also be well examined using subcostal/abdominal approaches

Ans. (c)

The distal abdominal aorta and distal branches such as iliac vessels cannot be examined by ultrasound scanning of the abdomen. Two proximal aortic branches (#1 and #2) are visualized in 119. The aorta is not enlarged and there is no dissection. The celiac trunk is a large branch originating just below the diaphragm. It is short in length, about 1–2 cm, and divides into left gastric, hepatic and splenic branches. The superior mesenteric artery is a large vessel arising about 1.25 cm below the celiac artery.

MOVIES 117 TO 119

SECTION 3

Tricuspid and Pulmonary Valves, Pulmonary Hypertension

CASE 38

Chahwala JR, Elsayed M, Alagic N, Uygur B, Turaga NSN, Adarna LG, Mohamed A, Gupta N, Bulur S, Nanda NC

This is an adult patient with a cardiac murmur on physical examination. 2D TTE was done.

1. **What does the arrow show (120)?**
   (a) Mouth of the coronary sinus (CS)
   (b) Body of the CS
   (c) A portion of the TR jet entering CS

Ans. (c)

TR jet extending into the CS is considered a sign of severe regurgitation.

MOVIE 120

CASE 39

Ahmad S Omran

SEVERE SECONDARY TRICUSPID REGURGITATION

This 34-year-old man with a known history of congenital heart disease presented to our center due to shortness of breath and easy fatigability. He had a history of cardiac surgery to repair Tetralogy of Fallot (TOF) 15 years ago in another hospital. Transthoracic echocardiography (TTE) showed severe pulmonary regurgitation, and previous ventricular septal defect (VSD) patch repair dehiscence with a large shunt. Right ventricle was severely dilated. Severe tricuspid valve regurgitation (TR) was present with hepatic vein inflow systolic reversal (Figs. 39.1A and B). Patient was investigated for possible infective endocarditis as a cause for VSD patch dehiscence which was negative. Patient was taken to the operating room for redo-surgery. Preoperative 3D transesophageal echocardiography (3DTEE) confirmed the diagnosis of severe TR due to lack of leaflet coaptation (Figs. 39.2A and B, 121 and 122). Patient underwent redo VSD patch repair, tricuspid valve repair and pulmonic valve replacement (Figs. 39.3A and B, 123 and 124). Tricuspid valve was repaired with a size 34 Medtronic contour annuloplasty ring with only trace postoperative TR. Pulmonic valve was replaced with a size 27 Magna bioprosthetic valve. Patient was discharged home in good condition.

1. **In echocardiographic assessment of patient with tricuspid valve regurgitation (TR), all of the followings are correct *except*:**
   (a) A small degree of TR is present in approximately 70% of normal adults.
   (b) 90% of patients with moderate to severe TR have primary tricuspid valve pathology.
   (c) Ebstein's anomaly is the most common form of congenital heart disease affecting the tricuspid valve.
   (d) Risk of post-operative TR is lower with a prosthetic ring than with suture repair procedures.

Ans. (b)

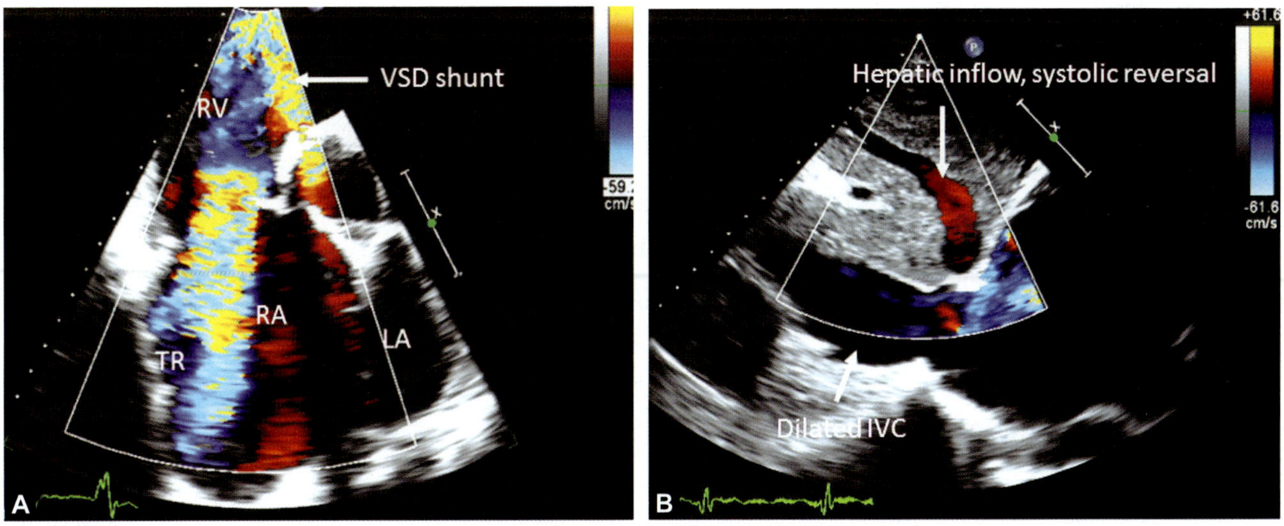

Figs. 39.1A and B: Initial transthoracic echocardiography (TTE). (A) Parasternal short-axis view shows a large VSD shunt through the dehisced previous patch. Severe tricuspid valve regurgitation (TR) is noted as well. (B) Subcostal view shows severely dilated hepatic vein with reduced respiratory collapsibility. Hepatic vein inflow color Doppler shows severe systolic reversal flow (red color) supporting diagnosis of severe TR. (RA: Right atrium; LA: Left atrium; RV: Right ventricle).

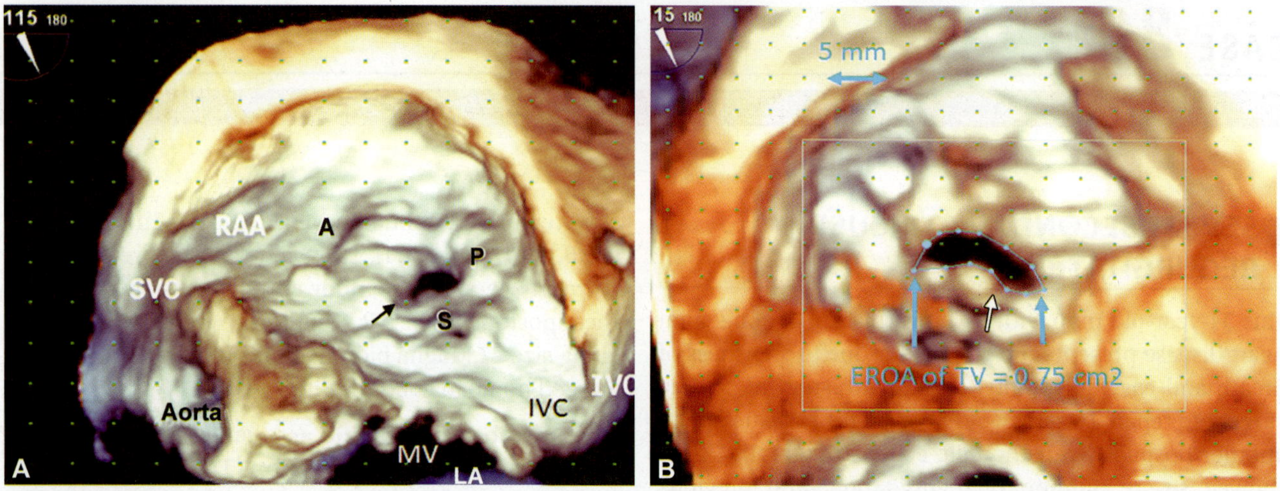

Figs. 39.2A and B: Preoperative 3D transesophageal echocardiography (3DTEE). (A) 3D zoom mode acquisition of the tricuspid valve in surgical view showing severely dilated tricuspid annulus, all 3 leaflets of the tricuspid valve and a large gap during systole. This large gap (lack of leaflet coaptation) is the cause for severe tricuspid regurgitation. Internal landmark for identification of the tricuspid septal leaflet (S) is interatrial septum, ostium of the coronary sinus. Landmark for tricuspid anterior leaflet (A) is aortic root and right atrial appendage (RAA), and landmark for tricuspid posterior leaflet (P) is inferior vena cava (IVC). (B) 3D zoom mode of tricuspid valve from right ventricular (RV) aspect showing three leaflets with a large coaptation gap. Effective regurgitation orifice area (EROA) by 3D planimetry calibrated with 3D grid was calculated as 0.75 cm^2. This EROA is consistent with very severe TR. (MV: Mitral valve).

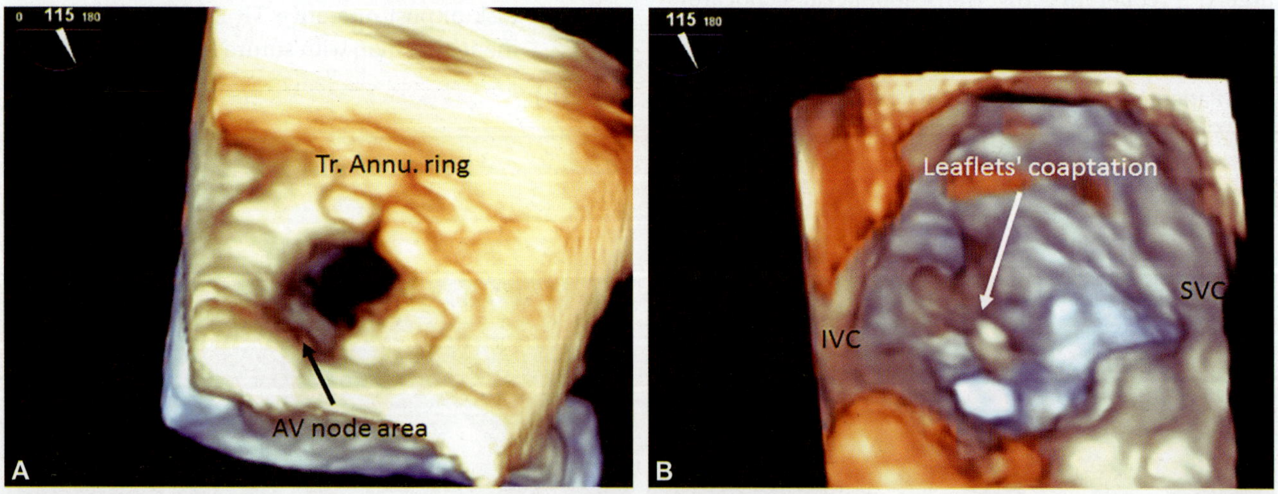

Figs. 39.3A and B: Postoperative 3D TEE in the operating room. (A) 3D TEE zoom mode acquisition in surgical view of the tricuspid valve showing the annuloplasty ring (Tr. Annu. Ring) seated well. Note: these rings are C-shaped and the open part of the ring should be towards the area of the atrioventricular node (AV node) to decrease the risk of AV block. (B) 3D TEE of the tricuspid valve from right ventricular side showing good coaptation of the three leaflets consistent with no residual TR. (IVC: Inferior vena cava; SVC: Superior vena cava).

MOVIE LEGENDS

121: Preoperative 3D TEE, surgical view of the tricuspid valve showing a large systolic gap (white arrow) resulting in severe TR.

122: Preoperative 3D TEE showing tricuspid valve from right ventricular aspect (white arrow shows large systolic gap).

123: 3D TEE immediately after tricuspid valve repair showing tricuspid valve from RV side with good leaflet coaptation.

124: Pulmonic valve replacement with a Magna bioprosthetic valve viewed from pulmonary artery side.

CASE 40

Chahwala JR, Elsayed M, Alagic N, Uygur B, Turaga NSN, Adarna LG, Mohamed A, Gupta N, Bulur S, Nanda NC

This is an adult patient who underwent cardiac transplantation a few years ago. 2D TTE was done.

1. What does the arrow in 🎥 125 show?

(a) Flail anterior TV leaflet
(b) Flail septal TV leaflet
(c) Flail posterior (inferior) TV leaflet

Ans. (b)

The septal leaflet clearly prolapses below the anterior leaflet with noncoaptation. The mobile component on the septal leaflet represents a ruptured chord. These patients with cardiac transplantation undergo several ventricular septal biopsies with a bioptome inserted intravenously which can damage the TV and the subvalvular apparatus.

2. What is the severity of TR in this patient (🎥 126)?

(a) Severe
(b) Moderately severe
(c) Moderate
(d) Mild to moderate

Ans. (a)

The turbulent TR jet is eccentric, loses its high velocity when it strikes the lateral wall of the RA (Coanda effect) and takes on red color as it swirls around the RA. Red color occurs because the velocity of the TR jet has now decreased below the Nyquist limit of 54.2 cm/s. Therefore, it is important to take into account both the turbulent and the non-turbulent color flow signals moving in the same phase in systole when assessing regurgitation severity, fully realizing that a part of those low-velocity signals will be due to SVC and IVC inflow and entrainment. In this patient, the combined turbulent and non-turbulent laminar red flow signals occupy a large portion (>33%) of the RA indicative of severe TR.

MOVIES 125 AND 126 🎥

CASE 41

Gupta N, Mohamed A, Elsayed M, Nanda NC

This is a 66-year-old male who had cardiac transplantation 20 years ago. He is asymptomatic and came for a routine follow up. 2D (Fig. 41.1 and 127 and 128) and 3D TTE were done (129 to 131).

1. **What does the arrow in 127 show?**
   (a) Flail anterior TV leaflet
   (b) Flail posterior TV leaflet
   (c) Flail septal TV leaflet
   (d) TV vegetation

Ans. (c)

Generally, in the RV inflow view, anterior and posterior (inferior) TV leaflets are detected. However, 3D cropping (130) in which the blue cursor line is passing through the flail TV leaflet (both upper panels) shows the cut section of this leaflet located adjacent to the VS and MV (lower left panel) identifying it as the septal TV leaflet. Both the anterior and posterior TV leaflets in the left lower panel do not show any evidence of chordae rupture.

2. **What is the etiology of flail TV leaflet in this patient?**
   (a) It is fairly common in cardiac transplantation patients and may be related to the operative technique used.
   (b) May be related to the trauma caused to TV by frequent right-sided biopsies done to assess cardiac rejection.
   (c) The patient may have subclinical TV endocarditis.
   (d) May be related to cardiac rejection which can cause damage to all three TV leaflets.

Ans. (b)

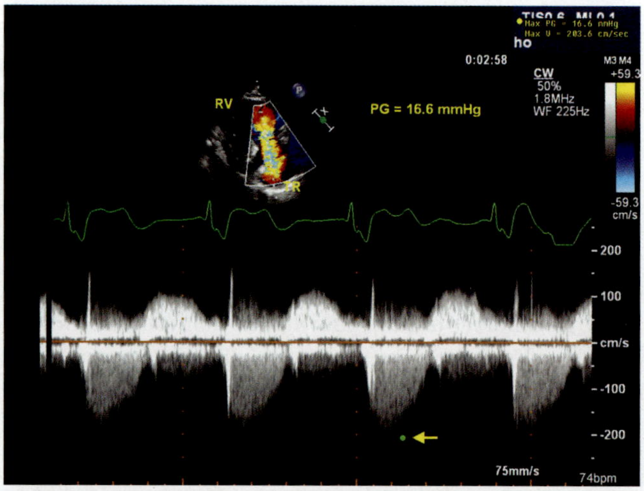

Fig. 41.1: Color Doppler guided continuous wave recording shows a low gradient across the TV consistent with normal PA pressure.

In this patient, the TR jet occupies most of the RA shown, indicating severe TR. Also TR jet is seen entering the coronary sinus (CS), another reported sign of severe TR (128). In addition, TR vena contracta (VC) area by 3D echo is large measuring 0.85 cm^2 consistent with very significant regurgitation. RV/PA systolic pressure is normal suggesting that TR is not secondary to pulmonary hypertension (PHT) but is related to primary TV pathology (Fig. 41.1).

MOVIES 127 TO 131

CASE 42*

Elsayed M, Thind M, Nanda NC

This is a 64-year-old female with previously diagnosed gastric adenocarcinoma, MVP and severe MR who was referred for a follow up echocardiogram. She complained of worsening shortness of breath but denied chest pain or any other symptoms. Physical examination was normal except for an apical pansystolic murmur of MR. 2DTTE was done and showed as before prominent MVP and severe MR.

1. **What does 2D TTE show (Figs. 42.1A to C and 132)?**
   (a) Minimal TR (b) Severe TR
   (c) TVP (d) MVP

Ans. (c)

Mid to late systolic TR on color M-mode and also mid to late systolic CW Doppler of TR jet is highly suggestive of mid to late systolic TVP.

The maximum TR jet area occupies 20.5% of the RA area taken in the same frame where the maximum TR was found which is consistent with mild-to-moderate TR. However, since TR does not occur throughout systole, TR would be expected to be less severe than found by color Doppler. 3D TTE would be ideal for quantification of TR. This was subsequently done (Figs. 42.2A to D and 133A to D) and the TR vena contracta (VC) by 3D TTE measured 0.50 cm^2. TR volume was calculated by multiplying the

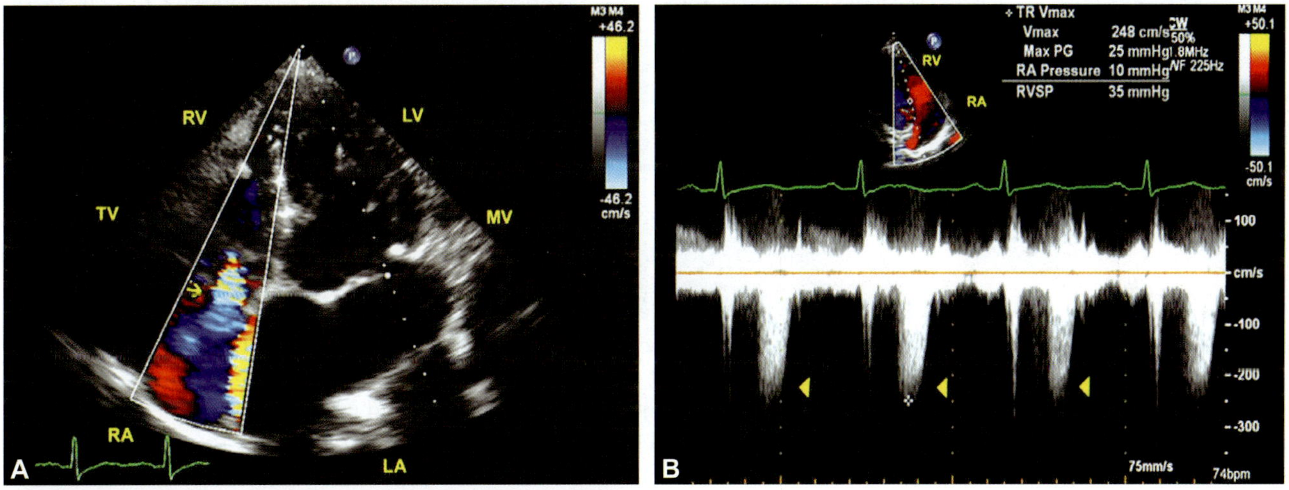

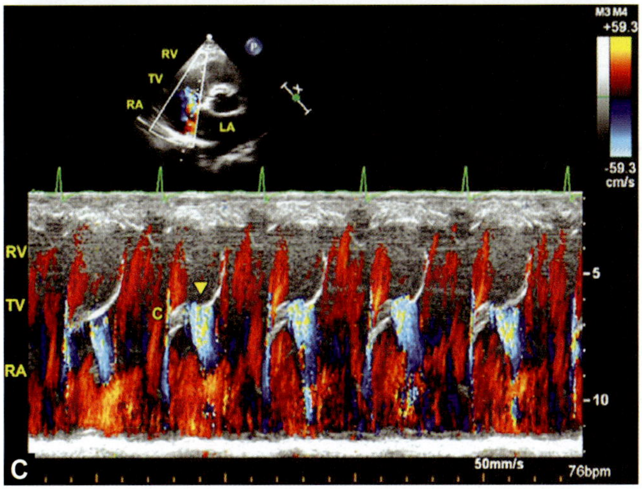

Figs. 42.1A to C: Two-dimensional transthoracic echocardiography in tricuspid valve prolapse with mid-to-late systolic regurgitation. (A) Apical four-chamber view. Arrow points to tricuspid regurgitation jet from right ventricle (RV) into right atrium (RA). Tricuspid valve (TV), left atrium (LA), mitral valve (MV), and left ventricle (LV) are also seen. (B) Color Doppler-guided continuous wave Doppler. Arrowhead points to mid-to-late tricuspid regurgitation jet velocity waveform. (C) Color M-Mode. Arrowhead points to tricuspid regurgitation jet confined to mid-to-late systole. C points to tricuspid valve closure. 132.

*This case is reproduced with permission from: Elsayed M, Thind M, Nanda NC. Two- and Three-dimensional Transthoracic Echocardiographic Assessment of Tricuspid Valve Prolapse with Mid-to-Late Systolic Tricuspid Regurgitation. Echocardiography. 2015 Jun;32(6):1022–5.

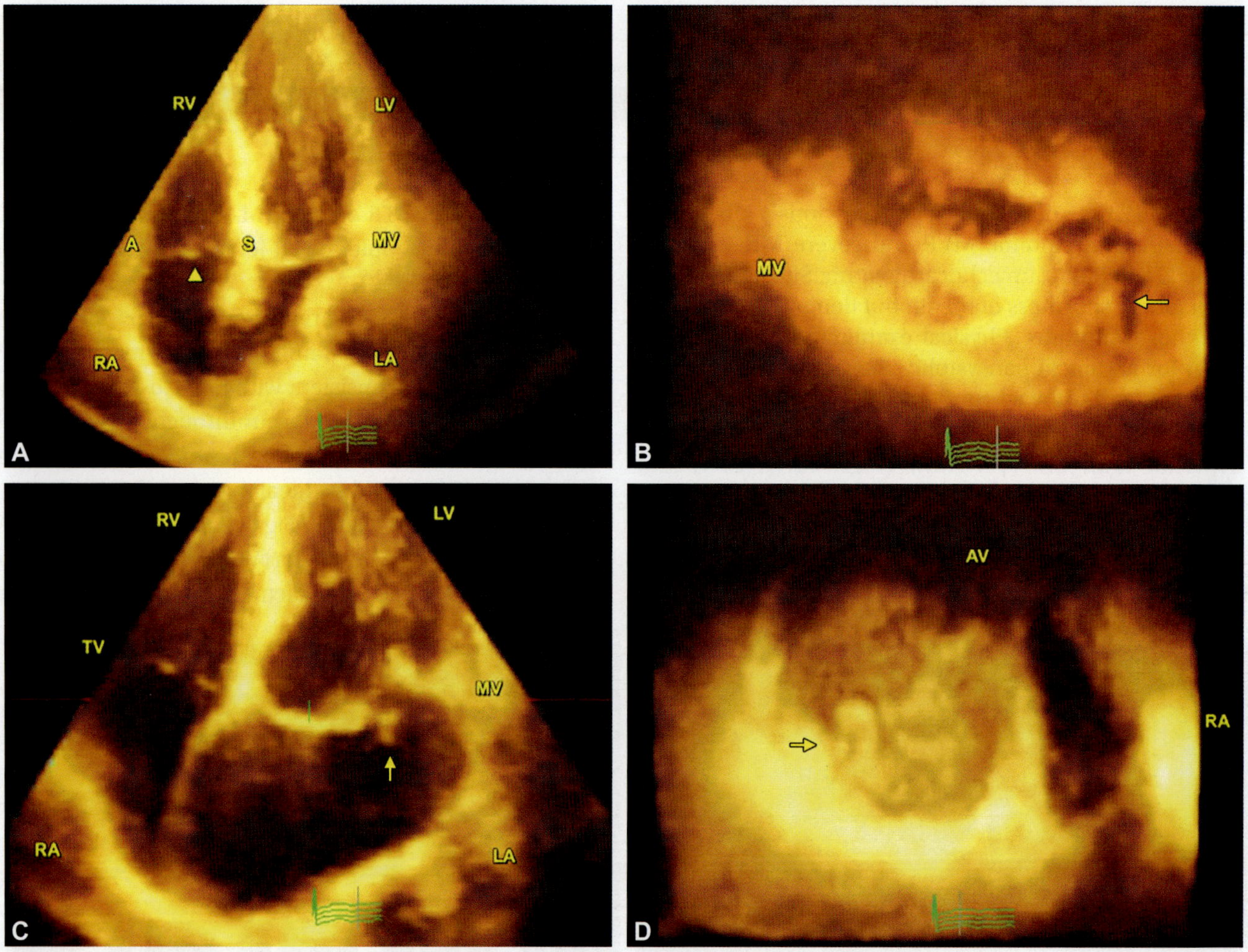

Figs. 42.2A to D: Live/real-time three-dimensional transthoracic echocardiography in tricuspid valve prolapse with mid-to-late systolic regurgitation. (A) Apical four-chamber view. Arrowhead points to anterior leaflet (A) of tricuspid valve prolapsing into right atrium behind the septal leaflet (S). (B) En face view of tricuspid valve. Arrow points to prolapsed mid-segment of anterior leaflet of tricuspid valve. (C) Apical four-chamber view. Arrow points to a flail segment of posterior leaflet of mitral valve with chordae rupture. (D) En face view of mitral valve. Arrow points to prolapsed mid (P2) segment of posterior leaflet of mitral valve with chordae rupture. Aortic valve (AV) is also seen. 133A to D. Abbreviations as in Figures 5.1A to C.

3D VC with TR VTI (35.7 cm) obtained by CW Doppler. This was found to be only 17 cc, indicative of only mild TR.

The TR volume was small because TR occurred only in mid-to-late systole. If we were to extend the TR waveform to include all of systole assuming TR to be pansystolic, the TR VTI would have been much higher (94.6 cm) leading to more than double the TR volume (47.3 cc) consistent with severe TR.

2. What did 3D TTE add to 2D TTE in this patient (Figs. 42.2A to D and 133A to D)?

(a) Showed the exact segment of anterior TV leaflet which was prolapsing
(b) Showed the exact scallop/segment of prolapsing MV
(c) Only B is correct
(d) Only A is correct
(e) Both A and B are correct

Ans. (e)

MOVIES 132 AND 133A TO D

REFERENCE

1. Lancellotti P, Moura L, Pierard LA, et al: European Association of Echocardiography recommendations for the assessment of valvular regurgitation. Part 2: Mitral and tricuspid regurgitation (native valve disease). Eur J Echocardiogr J Work Group Echocardiogr Eur Soc Cardiol 2010;11: 307–332.

CASE 43

Adarna LG, Elsayed M, Alagic N, Uygur B, Turaga NSN, Chahwala JR, Mohamed A, Gupta N, Bulur S, Nanda NC

Color M-mode and CW Doppler in an adult with TR.

1. **What do movies 134 and 135 show?**
   (a) Pansystolic TR
   (b) Pansystolic plus late diastolic TR
   (c) Normal PA pressure
   (d) Normal EKG

Ans. (b)

This patient has a prolonged PR interval (heart block, seen well on the EKG tracing in 134) which causes the TV to close in late diastole resulting in lower velocity late diastolic TR (#1 in 134 and arrow in 135). The patient also has pansystolic TR (#2 in 134) and a high-peak gradient of 71 mm Hg indicative of high RV systolic pressure, which will be the same as PA systolic pressure in the absence of obstruction in RV or RVOT.

MOVIES 134 AND 135

CASE 44

Adarna LG, Elsayed M, Alagic N, Uygur B, Turaga NSN, Chahwala JR, Bulur S, Nanda NC

CW Doppler velocity waveform was obtained in a patient with TR (136).

1. **How would you assess the PA systolic pressure assuming there is no obstruction to flow in the RV?**
   (a) Add the estimated RA pressure by imaging IVC
   (b) Add the actual RA pressure obtained by right heart catheterization.

Ans. (a)

IVC can be imaged noninvasively in most patients using the subcostal approach. On the other hand, cardiac catheterization is an invasive procedure.

2. **The maximum TR gradient in this patient was 49 mm Hg. RA pressure would need to be added to this to obtain the PA systolic pressure. There is no obstruction in the RV or PV. How would you assess RA pressure by inspecting the IVC? All statements below are correct except:**
   (a) If the internal diameter of IVC is 2.1 cm or less (at least 1 cm upstream from IVC-RA junction) and it collapses > 50% during respirations or sniff, add 3 mm Hg
   (b) Same as above but if IVC collapses less than 50%, add 8 mm Hg
   (c) If IVC is large (> 2.1 cm) and collapses > 35%, add 13 mm Hg
   (d) Same as C but collapses 0–35%, the actual number could not be determined but it will be more than 13 mm Hg
   (e) All of the above statements are highly accurate

Ans. (e)

These statements are only a rough guide to measure RA systolic pressure in day-to-day clinical practice. Caveats include congenital and acquired abnormalities of IVC and patients on ventilators. Young athletes may also have a dilated IVC, even though the RA pressure is normal. There are also problems in correctly estimating PA pressures during cardiac catheterization.

MOVIE 136

CASE 45

Bulur S, Nanda NC

The patient is a 65-year-old female with suspected pulmonary hypertension. 2D TTE was done.

1. **Regarding Figure 45.1:**
   (a) Both peak (Max G) and mean (Mean G) TR gradients are correct
   (b) Both peak (Max G) and mean (Mean G) TR gradients are incorrect
   (c) Only mean TR gradient is incorrect
   (d) Only peak TR gradient is incorrect

Ans. (c)

Peak TR velocity appears to be measured correctly but the tracing does not follow the TR velocity waveform faithfully. Hence, the TR mean velocity and, therefore, the TR mean gradient have been overestimated.

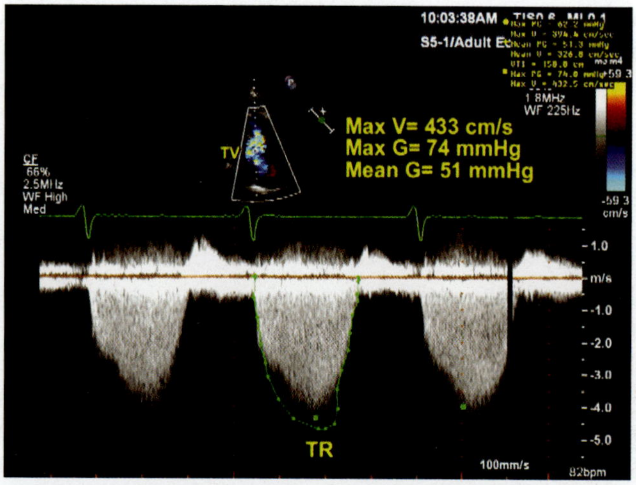

Fig. 45.1: Tricuspid regurgitation (TR) waveform.

CASE 46

Bulur S, Nanda NC

This is an adult patient with suspected pulmonary hypertension.

1. **How severe is TR in this patient (137)?**
   (a) Moderately severe to severe TR
   (b) Moderate TR
   (c) Severe TR
   (d) TR severity cannot be estimated because no attention is given to color gain and Nyquist limit.

Ans. (c)

Even though the Nyquist limit is rather high at 59 cm/s (should ideally be around 50 cm/s), the TR jet occupies more than 33% of the RA indicating severe TR. We cannot be sure whether the color gain was optimized. The color gain should be increased until one visualizes stationary artifactual echoes and then decreased till they just disappear.

2. **What is the PA systolic pressure in this patient (138A and B)?**
   (a) PA systolic pressure is 68 mm Hg
   (b) Both PA systolic and mean pressures are less than 68 mm Hg because Doppler generally overestimates
   (c) PA systolic pressure is 83 (68+15) mm Hg because the IVC is dilated to 3.0 cm (normal 2.1 cm) and collapses very little during respiration. This means RA pressure is 15 mm Hg and, therefore, you have to add this number to the peak Doppler gradient.
   (d) PA systolic pressure is at least 83 mm Hg.

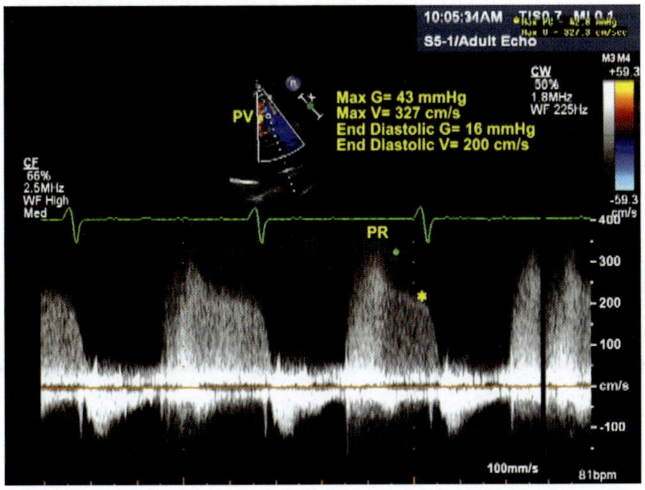

Fig. 46.1: Pulmonary regurgitation (PR) waveform. Maximum (Max) and end diastolic gradients (G) and velocities (V) are shown.

Ans. (d)

When the IVC is dilated and does not collapse, or collapses only minimally as in this patient, the RA pressure is more than 15 mm Hg but an exact number cannot be determined which may be very high. Therefore, PA systolic pressure could be higher than 83 mm Hg.

Estimation of mean PA pressure by adding the RA pressure obtained from inspection of IVC to the mean TR gradient or the peak PR diastolic gradient can be done but may need further validation. Peak end diastolic PR gradient plus RA pressure gives PA end diastolic pressure. The technique for measuring peak (maximum) and end diastolic velocities and gradients of the PR jet is shown in Figure 46.1 from a different patient. Pulmonary hypertension is diagnosed if the mean PA is 25 mm Hg or more at rest. Mild pulmonary hypertension is categorized by mean PA pressures of 30–40 mm Hg, moderate 40–70 mm Hg and severe t>70 mm Hg. This patient, therefore has moderate pulmonary hypertension.

MOVIES 137 AND 138

REFERENCE

1. Chopra HK, Nanda NC, Fan P, et al. Can two-dimensional echocardiography and Doppler color flow mapping identify the need for tricuspid valve repair? J Am Coll Cardiol. 1989 Nov 1;14(5):1266-74.

CASE 47

Taher A, Elsayed M, Nanda NC

A 42-year-old male was referred for an echocardiogram prior to renal transplantation. PV prolapse was noted as an incidental finding (🎥 139 A-C).

1. **Which of the following is correct?**
   (a) PV prolapse is always isolated.
   (b) Only one leaflet of the PV can prolapse in any given patient.
   (c) All these leaflets of the PV can never be identified by 2D echo. You need 3D echo to do this.
   (d) PV prolapse may be isolated or may be associated with prolapse of other cardiac valves.

Ans. (d)

It is very difficult to visualize all three leaflets of the PV in a normal adult. However, if the PA is enlarged and in children, all three leaflets can be detected. More than one leaflet may be noted to prolapse in some patients and PV prolapse may occur in association with prolapse of other valves as a manifestation of myxomatous disease. This patient also has MV prolapse.

2. **How are the three leaflets of the PV named?**
   (a) Right, left and anterior leaflets.
   (b) Right left and noncoronary leaflets.
   (c) There are no specific names except the left leaflet, which is imaged next to the aortic root.
   (d) Right anterior, posterior and left anterior leaflets.
   (e) Right, left and septal leaflets.

Ans. (a) and (d)

(a) is based on the location of the leaflets in the fetus and (d) is based on their location in the adult. Both the terminologies are given in Gray's Anatomy but (a) is more commonly used.

MOVIE LEGENDS 🎥

139A: Aortic short axis view demonstrating all three leaflets of the AV and the PV which does not appear to prolapse.

139B: Aortic short axis view with long axis of the PA (reverse orientation). Arrow points to prominent prolapse of one leaflet of PV into the RVO. The other leaflet does not show prolapse.

139C: Color Doppler examination shows trivial PR (reverse orientation).

CASE 48

Bulur S, Nanda NC

The patient is a 74-year-old female with ischemic heart disease and chronic renal failure. 2D TTE was done (140).

1. What does the arrow point to?

(a) Normal flow signals in the RVO
(b) Small patent ductus arteriosus
(c) Mild PR
(d) Eccentric mild PR jet

Ans. (d)

Normally PR jets are red in color (arrowhead) since they are directed to the transducer. There is an additional PR jet which is eccentric and directed somewhat away from the transducer. Therefore, it appears blue in color. The jet is very small in proximal width, indicative of mild PR.

MOVIE 140

CASE 49

Adarna LG, Elsayed M, Alagic N, Uygur B, Turaga NSN, Chahwala JR, Mohamed A, Gupta N, Bulur S, Nanda NC

This is an adult patient who underwent left ventricular assist device (LVAD) placement for dilated cardiomyopathy and heart failure.

1. **What does 141 (P = pacing lead) show?**
   (a) Mild/mild to moderate PR
   (b) Severe PR
   (c) Moderate AR
   (d) PDA
   (e) Anomalous left coronary artery origin from PA (ALCAPA)

Ans. (a)

The PR jet width at its origin occupies 25–30% of RVOT diameter measured at the same point. A ratio of < 25% signifies mild PR, > 65% severe PR, intermediate values moderate PR. Also, PR jet extending to within 1 cm of TV signifies severe TR. This patient also has mild AR.

MOVIE 141

CASE 50

Mohamed A, Gupta N, Elsayed M, Nanda NC

The patient is an 18-year-old male complaining of vague chest pain. 2D TTE was done. All valves appeared to be structurally normal and both ventricles showed normal function.

1. **What is the severity of PR in this patient (Fig. 50.1 and 142)?**
   (a) Mild
   (b) Moderate
   (c) Severe

Ans. (c)

The width of the PR jet at its exit from PV occupies 73% of the RVOT inner diameter measured in the same frame. This is suggestive of severe PR.

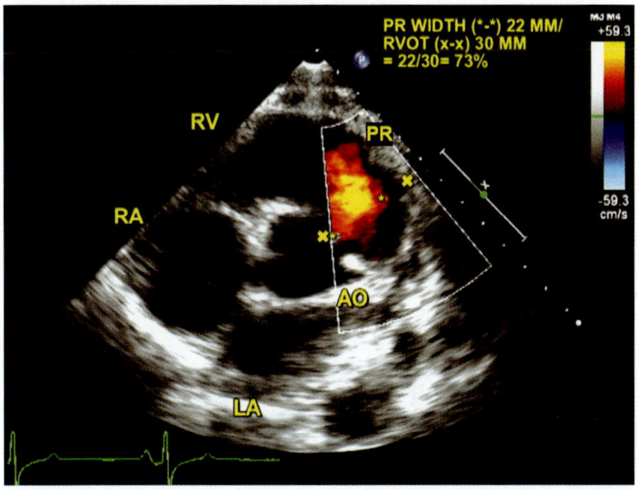

Fig. 50.1: The pulmonary regurgitation (PR,+-+) jet at its origin occupies 73% of the right ventricular outflow tract (RVOT) width (x-x) taken in the same frame indicative of severe PR.

MOVIE 142

SECTION 4

Prostheses, Rings and Clips

CASE 51

Chahwala JR, Celiker E, Bulur S, Nanda NC

An adult patient underwent metallic mitral valve replacement (MVR). 2D TTE was done (Fig. 51.1 and 143 and 144, arrow = reverberation from MVR).

1. **Given only M-mode and 2D echoes and no Doppler gradients, how confident would you feel that the MVR is well seated and there is no obstruction?**
   (a) Very confident
   (b) Not confident at all, I must have gradients
   (c) Mildly confident

Ans. (a)

In the parasternal long axis view, both leaflets of metallic MVR are clearly seen opening very well. Also, the M-mode shows brisk (90 degrees) opening (1) and closing (2) movements. Therefore, obstruction can be ruled out. Most of the time, only one leaflet of metallic MVR is visualized moving well and in that case, the confidence level is reduced since the status of the second leaflet is uncertain. In these cases, 3D TTE is often helpful in detecting both leaflets and their motion.

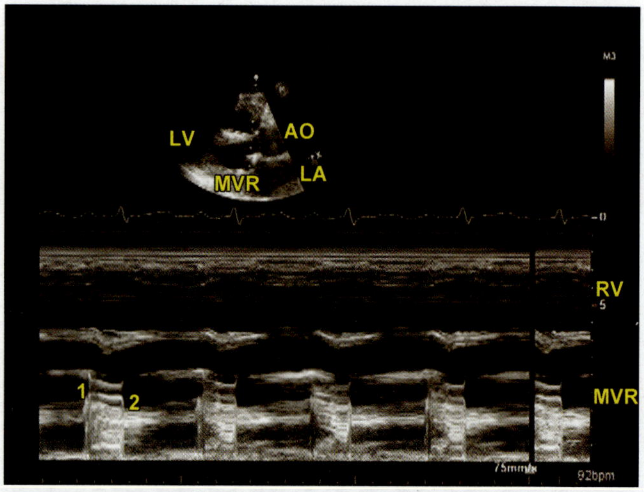

Fig. 51.1: Normal vertical opening and closing motion of a mechanical mitral prosthetic valve.

MOVIES 143 AND 144

CASE 52

Sibel Catirli Enar

A PROSTHETIC MITRAL VALVE CASE WITH FEVER AND LBBB

A 67-year-old woman who had undergone mechanical prosthetic valve replacement 11 years ago presented with fever and dyspnea. She was in NYHA class III. Her ECG showed LBBB with a widened QRS (>130 ms).

TTE (145 and 146): Her LVEF was 25%. LV end diastolic diameter was 5.9 cm, and left atrium was 4.8 cm. She had mild MR and mild AR. In addition, she had intraventricular dyssynchrony. Septal to lateral wall delay > 65 ms (Long axis dyssynchony).

Thorax CT: Increase in pleural density and in high abdominal cross-sections, 2 stones were detected in the gallbladder.

1. **What is the diagnosis and how should she be treated?**
   (a) Infective endocarditis, medical therapy
   (b) Infective endocarditis, surgical therapy
   (c) Not endocarditis, medical therapy
   (d) Not endocarditis, medical and ICD therapy
   (e) Not endocarditis, surgical therapy.

Ans. (d)

Diagnosis was cholecystitis. She responded well to antibiotics. Based on echo and ECG criteria, CRT therapy was planned, and CRT-D device was implanted.

DISCUSSION

Infective endocarditis is a serious complication of prosthetic heart valves. Detection of vegetations or regurgitation by echocardiography confirms the diagnosis.

CRT therapy is useful in patients with advanced heart failure who are symptomatic despite optimal medical therapy. Various echocardiographic methods such as tissue Doppler imaging, speckle tracking imaging and 3D imaging have been developed to identify patients who can benefit from this therapy.

In summary, this case is an example of a patient with MVR who developed dilated cardiomyopathy. Although the patient presented with fever, examination revealed that it was not due to infective endocarditis but due to cholesystitis. Based on clinical findings, ECG and echo criteria CRT therapy was planned and a CRT-D device was implanted.

According to the US (2012) and ESC (2010) guidelines, in symptomatic heart failure patients indications for CRT therapy are:[1]

1. LVEF ≤35%, LBBB, QRS duration ≥ 150 ms, sinus rhythm is class I recommendation and class IIIA recommendation is present if QRS is 120–149 ms (US guidelines).
2. LVEF ≤ 35%, QRS duration ≥ 120 ms, sinus rhythm is class I recommendation (ESC guidelines).

Echo Parameters for CRT therapy:[2]

For intraventricular dyssynchrony, long axis dyssynchrony is mostly accepted. With TDI from four chamber and long axis views, opposing wall delay (or septal to lateral wall delay) in ejection phase should be ≥ 65 ms. For short axis dyssynchrony, septal to posterior wall delay with speckle tracking from short axis mid-LV view should be ≥ 130 ms.

For interventricular dyssynchrony, interventricular mechanical delay should be ≥ 40 ms using Doppler echo QRS to the onset of aortic flow minus QRS to the onset of pulmonary flow from LV and RV ouflow tract views.

MOVIES 145 AND 146

REFERENCES

1. Cardiac resynchronization therapy: who benefits? Chinitz JS, d'Avila A, Goldman M, Reddy V, Dukkipati S. Ann Glob Health. 2014 Jan-Feb;80(1):61-8.
2. Cardiac resynchronization therapy: state of the art 2013. Yu CM, Hayes DL. European Heart Journal, 2013 May; 34(19):1396-403.

CASE 53

Elsayed M, Nanda NC

A 56-year-old male with past history of mitral valve replacement (MVR) returned for a follow-up study. 2D TTE done.

1. **What does the arrow in the parasternal long axis view point to: (147 and Fig. 53.1)**
   (a) Normal motion of mitral valve prosthesis
   (b) Left ventricular outflow tract
   (c) Hypertrophied ventricular septum
   (d) Prosthetic valve is in contact with the ventricular septum in systole

Ans. (d)

The arrow points to the anterior strut of the mitral bioprosthetic valve, which appears to make contact with the ventricular septum in systole. However, there was no evidence of obstruction by continuous wave Doppler.

2. **This finding may potentially result in all of the following *except*:**
   (a) Left ventricular outflow tract obstruction.
   (b) Serious ventricular arrhythmia.
   (c) This is a normal finding in many patients because of the anterior position of the prosthetic valve.
   (d) Localized thickening and fibrosis of the left side of the ventricular septum.

Ans. (c)

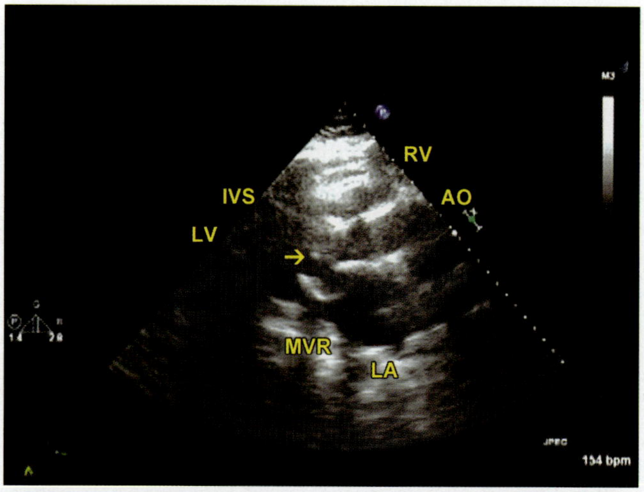

Fig. 53.1: Arrow points to MVR in contact with the VS.

This patient is asymptomatic without any arrhythmia, LV outflow tract obstruction or thickening of the ventricular septum. Therefore, he continues to have regular clinical and echocardiographic follow-up.

MOVIE 147

CASE 54

Padmini Varadarajan

HISTORY

A 72-year-old male with history of mechanical mitral valve replacement for rheumatic heart disease.

- On therapeutic dose of warfarin and had subdural hemorrhage
- Warfarin was discontinued by his treating physicians
- Cardiologist paged for assistance as patient went into flash pulmonary edema, atrial fibrillation with rapid ventricular response, was intubated emergently and imaging was performed.

1. **What do Figures 54.1A and B show?**
   (a) Vegetations
   (b) Pannus
   (c) Thrombus
   (d) Tumor masses

Ans. (c)

Thrombus. The images show thrombi attached to the mitral valve sewing ring (arrows in figures 54.1B and 54.2). The thrombi are preventing the prosthetic valve from opening (see accompanying 🎥 148 and 149). Arrowhead points to immobile prosthetic leaflet (🎥 149).

2. **Which of the values indicates that the mitral valve is obstructed?**
   (a) VTI prMV/VTI LVOT of < 2.2
   (b) VTI prMV/VTI LVOT > 2.2
   (c) VTI prMV/VTI LVOT of 1
   (d) VTI prMV/VTI LVOT < 1.5
   VTI = velocity time integral
   prMV = prosthetic mitral valve
   LVOT = left ventricular outflow tract

Ans. (b)

VTI prosthetic MV/LVOT of > 2.2 is indicative of significant valve stenosis.

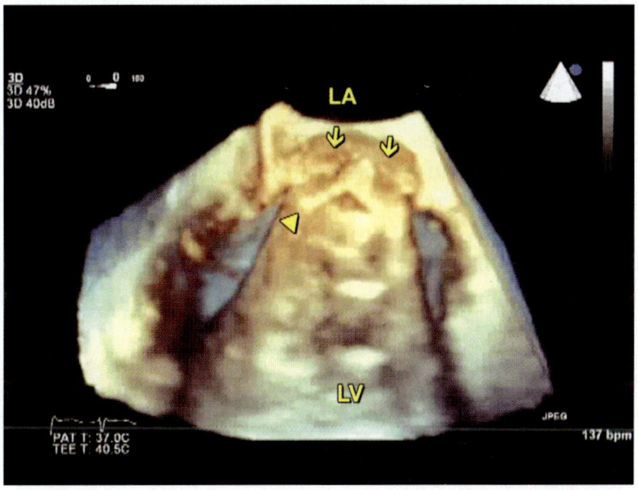

Fig. 54.2: 3D of the mitral prosthetic valve showing the thrombus.

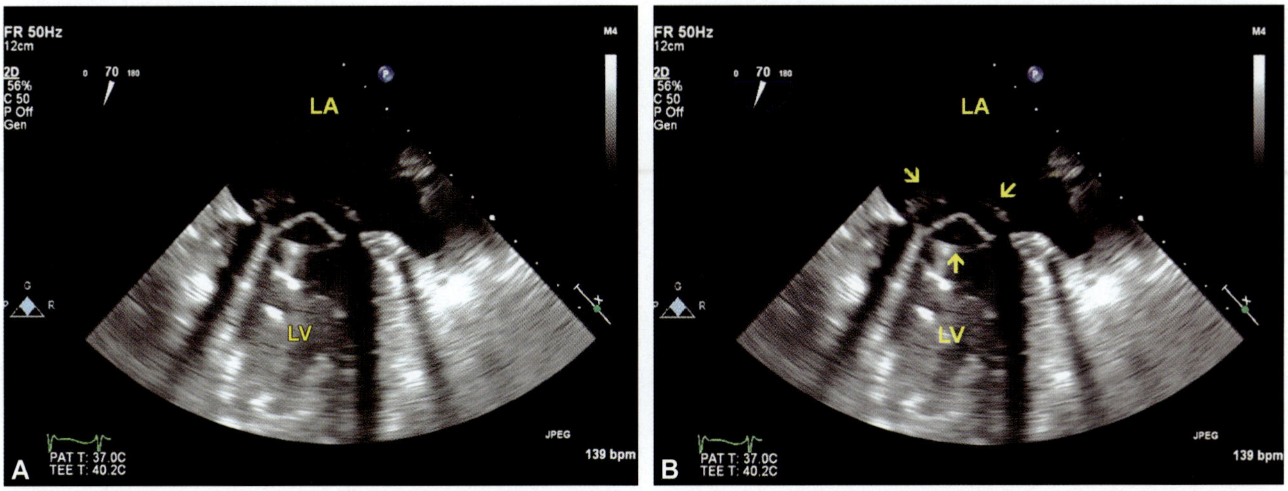

Figs. 54.1A and B: 2D images of the prosthetic valve showing thrombi attached to the valve ring, protruding into the left atrium (top 2 arrows show thrombus and the bottom arrow show prosthetic leaflet).

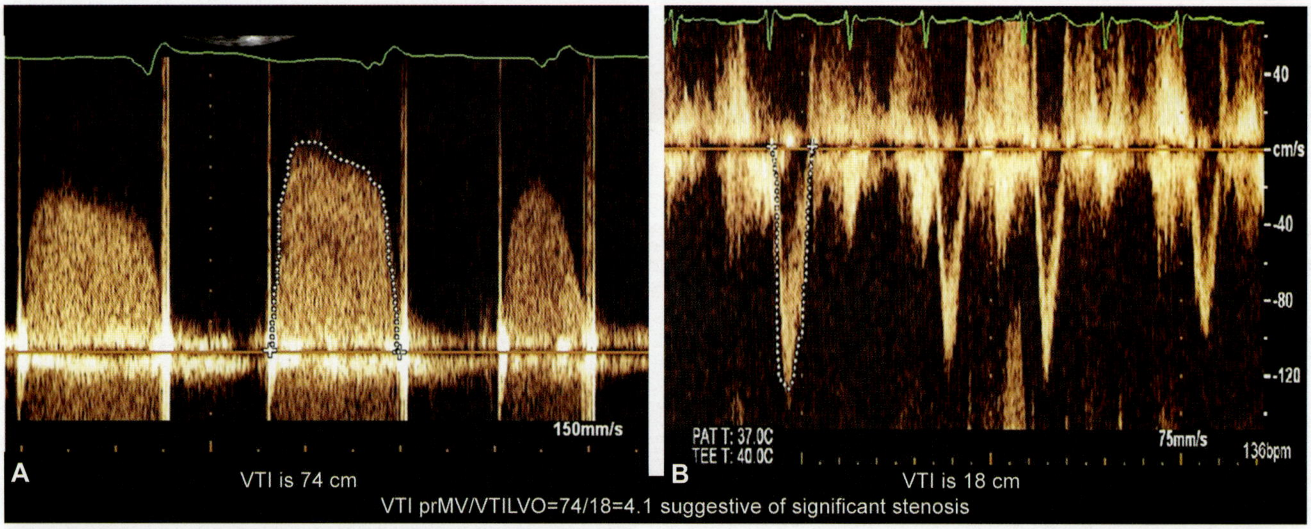

Figs. 54.3A and B: (A) CW Doppler across mitral valve; (B) PW across aortic valve.

Arrows in figures and movie clips show the thrombus and the arrowhead shows the immobile prosthetic leaflet.

The Vmax 2.7 m/sec, PHT 270 ms and mean gradient across the valve was 32 mm Hg. All these along with VTI-prMV/VTILVO of 4.1 are indicators of significant prosthetic valve stenosis (Figs. 54.3A and B). Please refer to Table 54.1.

Table 54.1: Doppler parameters of prosthetic mitral valve function.

	Normal	*Possible stenosis*	*Significant stenosis*
Peak velocity	< 1.9	1.9–2.5	> 2.5
Mean gradient (mm Hg)	≤ 5	6–10	> 10
C (see previous slides)	< 2.2	2.2–2.5	> 2.5
EOA (cm^2)	≥ 2.0	1–2	< 1
PHT (ms)	< 130	130–200	> 200

Ref: Zoghbi W, Chambers JB, Dumesenil JG et al. Recommendations for Evaluation of Prosthetic Valves With Echocardiography and Doppler Ultrasound. *J Am Soc Echocardiogr 22:975,2009.*

SUMMARY

- Patients with mechanical valves need to be on warfarin and baby aspirin
- When anticoagulation is withdrawn suddenly, the chances for valve thrombosis are very high, especially with mechanical mitral valves
- Usual presentation is flash pulmonary edema with atrial fibrillation with rapid ventricular rate
- Treatment includes thrombolytics, surgery
- This patient was taken to OR and the valve was debrided with recovery of valve function. He was not given thrombolytics due to recent bleeding. Post surgery, prosthetic valve gradient dropped to 4 mm Hg.

MOVIES 148 AND 149

CASE 55

Nishath Quader, Hyde M Russell, Sheridan Meyers, Vera H Rigolin

PROSTHETIC VALVE THROMBOSIS: A COMPLEX DISORDER THAT REQUIRES CAREFUL IMAGING

History

A 67-year-old female with history of mechanical bileaflet prosthetic valves in the aortic and mitral positions presented to the hospital with dyspnea on exertion in the setting of a subtherapeutic International Normalized Ratio. Her transthoracic echocardiogram demonstrated significantly elevated mitral prosthetic gradients (Figs. 55.1, 55.2, 150) compared to a prior baseline study. Due to suspicion for prosthetic valve thrombosis, the patient underwent cinefluoroscopy that demonstrated immobility of one of the mitral prosthetic leaflets (Fig. 55.3). Since the patient was hemodynamically stable with New York Heart Association (NYHA) class II symptoms, she was initially conservatively managed with high-dose intravenous unfractionated heparin therapy. However, due to persistence of symptoms and elevated prosthetic gradients, she underwent cardiac surgery for re-do replacement of both the mitral and prosthetic valves.

Pre-operative two-dimensional and three-dimensional transesophageal echocardiogram confirmed an immobile leaflet of the mitral valve (Figs. 55.4, 55.5 and 151, 152A and B). Intraoperative findings included a large burden of organized thrombus obstructing the normal function of one of the prosthetic mitral valve leaflets (Fig. 55.6). She underwent valve replacement of both the mitral and aortic valves with bioprosthetic valves and recovered uneventfully postoperatively.

Comment

Prosthetic valve thrombosis is a dreaded complication of mechanical valves. The incidence of valve thrombosis is reported to be as high as 20% overall in patients with tricuspid mechanical valves and 0.2–6%/patient-year in those with aortic or mitral prosthesis.[1,2] In left-sided valve thrombosis, patients may present with a myriad of symptoms: from silent thrombosis, strokes/transient ischemic attacks, peripheral embolism, hemodynamic instability from valve obstruction, and heart failure, thus often making diagnosis difficult. Noninvasive imaging is useful, but each imaging modality has its own set of limitations.

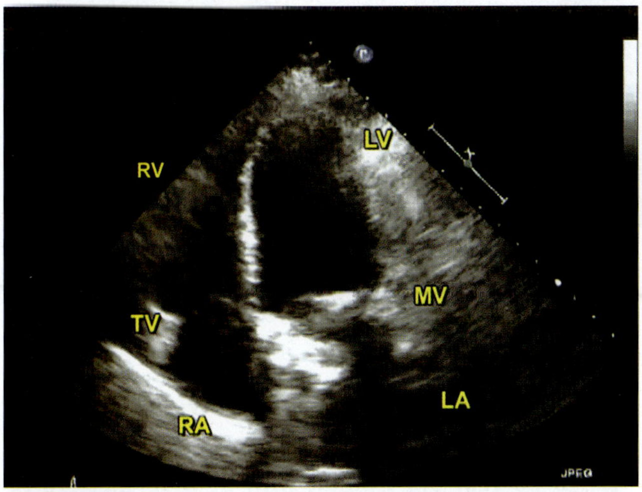

Fig. 55.1: This image demonstrates a transthoracic echocardiographic apical four-chamber view of this patient with a prosthetic mitral valve. As is evident in this image, transthoracic echo can be limited in the diagnosis of prosthetic valve thrombosis given acoustic shadowing of the left atrium and poor image quality. (LA: Left atrium; LV: Left ventricle; RA: Right atrium; RV: Right ventricle).

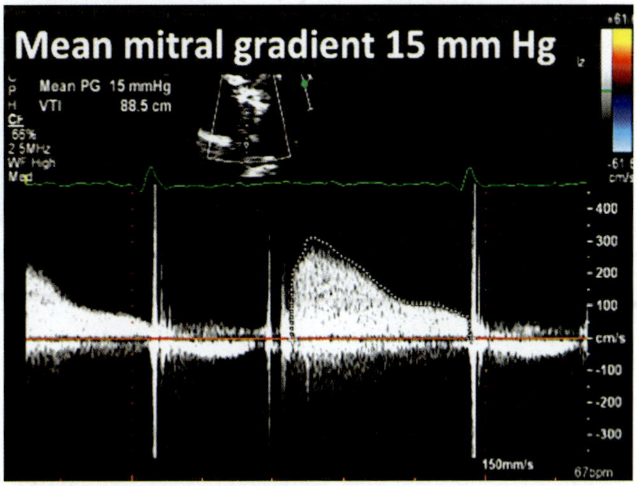

Fig. 55.2: Continuous wave Doppler of the prosthetic mitral valve. One clue to prosthetic valve thrombosis is elevated prosthetic gradients. Continuous wave Doppler of the prosthetic mitral valve demonstrates a gradient of 15 mm Hg, consistent with severe mitral stenosis.

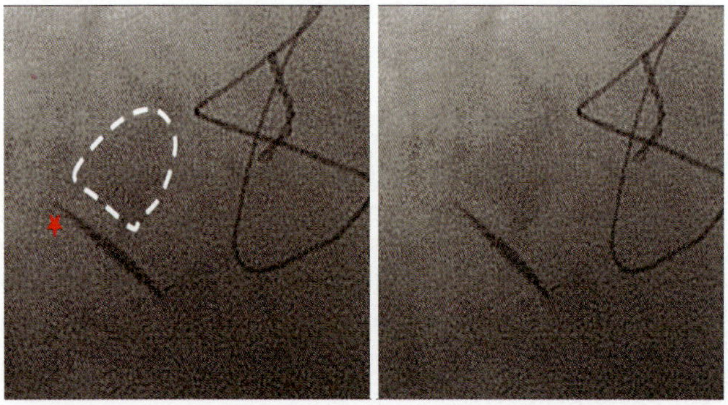

Fig. 55.3: Fluoroscopy is another method used to diagnose prosthetic valve thrombosis. In this fluoroscopic image of the prosthetic valve, there is an immobile leaflet as demonstrated by the white hemisphere in comparison to the mobile leaflet (red asterisk).

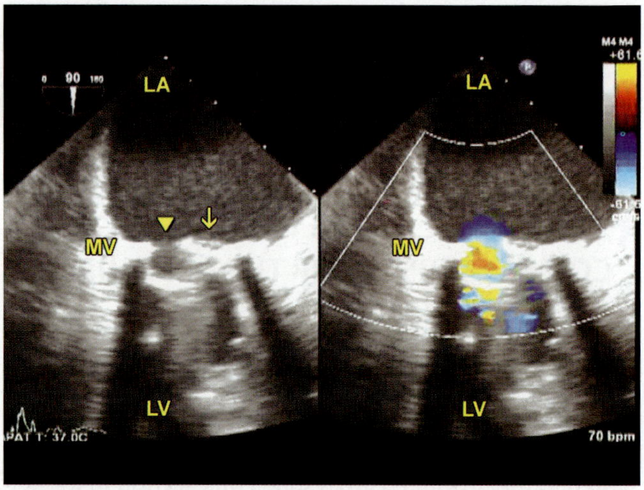

Fig. 55.4: Transesophageal echocardiogram of the valve is crucial in this disease. On the right side of the image, color Doppler demonstrates flow acceleration at the valve plane consistent with mitral stenosis. The left side of the panel demonstrates the immobile leaflet (arrow) and mobile leaflet (arrowhead).

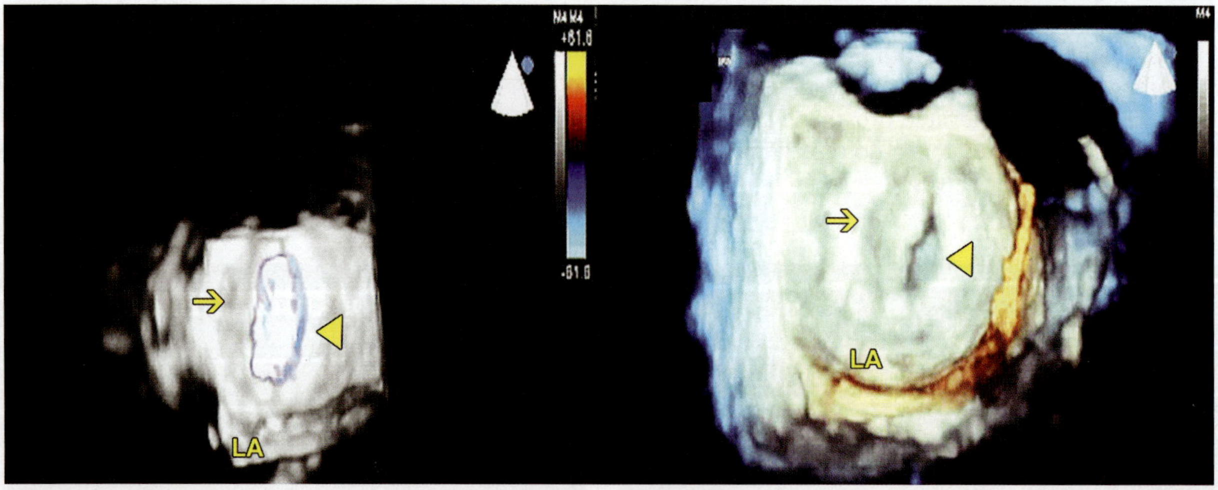

Figs. 55.5A and B: Three-dimensional echocardiography can be useful in the diagnosis of this disease since it gives an en-face view of the mitral valve. The mobile leaflet is demonstrated by the arrowhead while the arrow points to the immobile leaflet.

Diagnosis of prosthetic valve thrombosis often requires integration of clinical history, cardiac auscultation, fluoroscopy, transthoracic and transesophageal echocardiography. This comprehensive approach to the patient allows for the appropriate and timely diagnosis of prosthetic valve thrombosis. Once the diagnosis of prosthetic valve thrombosis has been made, the decision to proceed with surgical management depends on the patient's functional class, hemodynamic stability, overall surgical risk, and center experience.[3]

1. **An 80-year-old woman with St Jude mechanical aortic valve presents with shortness of breath and NYHA class III heart failure symptoms. She lives independently and recently ran out of her medications. She presents to the Emergency Department where her physical exam reveals diffuse rhonchi**

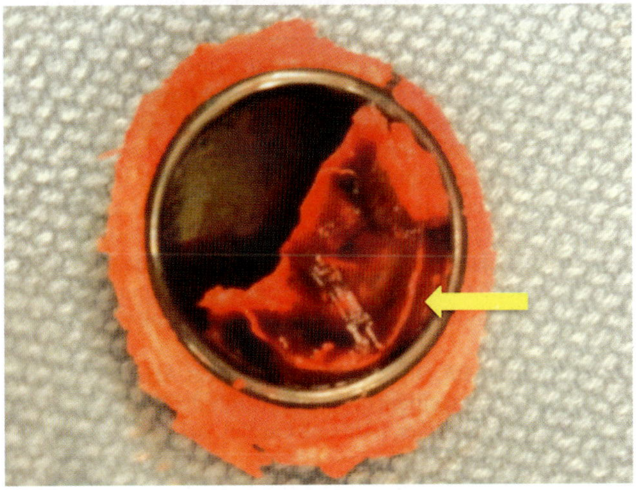

Fig. 55.6: This image demonstrates the intraoperative findings on explant of the mitral prosthesis. The yellow arrow demonstrates a large amount of organized thrombus obstructing an entire leaflet.

in bilateral lung fields. Her labs reveal an international normalized ratio (INR) of 1.5. Prosthetic valve dysfunction and/or thrombosis are suspected.

1A. What is the next step in management?

(a) Transthoracic echocardiogram (TTE) to confirm diagnosis (prosthetic valve stenosis) and to assess hemodynamic severity
(b) Transesophageal echocardiography (TEE) to assess leaflet motion and thrombus size
(c) Fluoroscopy to assess leaflet motion
(d) Gated CT scan to assess thrombus burden and leaflet motion
(e) Both (a) and (b)

Ans. (e)

TTE and TEE are indicated in the initial assessment of patients with suspected prosthetic valve stenosis or thrombosis not only to assess hemodynamic severity but also to assess leaflet motion and thrombus size. This is a class I recommendation set forth by the ACC/AHA guidelines.[4] CT and fluoroscopy are given a class II recommendation.

1B. TEE revealed a 1.0 cm^2 thrombus on the aortic valve restricting leaflet motion. What is the next step in management?

(a) Fibrinolytic therapy
(b) Anticoagulate with IV heparin
(c) Emergency surgery
(d) Fibrinolytic therapy and heparin

Ans. (c)

Emergency surgery is recommended in patients with left-sided valve thrombosis with NYHA class III-IV symptoms or a mobile or large thrombus (> 0.8 cm^2).[4]

2. A 55-year-old male with a mechanical St Jude aortic valve replacement is scheduled to undergo elective inguinal hernia repair. How should his oral anticoagulation be managed?

(a) Patient should be admitted a few days before his surgery for interruption of his oral anticoagulation. He should then be placed on intravenous unfractionated heparin as a "bridge" until his surgery.
(b) Patient's oral anticoagulation cannot be interrupted due to his mechanical AVR.
(c) Temporary interruption of oral anticoagulation is reasonable in this patient.
(d) The risk of undergoing an elective procedure is too high and thus the patient should be discouraged from doing so.

Ans. (c)

Temporary interruption of oral anticoagulation is acceptable in those with low risk of valve thrombosis. Risk factors for valve thrombosis include atrial fibrillation, previous thromboembolism, left ventricular dysfunction, hypercoagulable conditions, older generation mechanical aortic valves, mechanical mitral valve.[4]

3. Which of the following anticoagulation strategies is accurate in prosthetic valves?

(a) Mechanical MVR: INR goal 3; aspirin 75 mg–100 mg
(b) Mechanical AVR: INR goal 2.5; aspirin 75 mg–100 mg
(c) Mechanical AVR with risk factors: INR goal 3.0; aspirin 75 mg–100 mg
(d) TAVR: Clopidogrel 75 mg; aspirin 75 mg–100 mg for first 6 months
(e) All the above

Ans. (e)

Refer to the ACC/AHA valvular heart disease guidelines.[4]

MOVIE LEGENDS

150: This image demonstrates a transthoracic echocardiographic apical four-chamber view of this patient with a prosthetic mitral valve. As is evident in this movie, transthoracic echo can be limited in the diagnosis of prosthetic valve thrombosis given acoustic shadowing of the left atrium and poor image quality. (LA = left atrium; LV = left ventricle; RA = right atrium; RV = right ventricle).

151: Transesophageal echocardiogram of the valve is crucial in this disease. On the right side of the image, color Doppler demonstrates flow acceleration at the valve plane consistent with mitral stenosis. The left side of the panel demonstrates the immobile leaflet (arrow) and mobile leaflet (arrowhead).

152A,B: Three-dimensional echocardiography can be useful in the diagnosis of this disease since it gives an en-face view of the mitral valve. The mobile leaflet is demonstrated by the arrowhead while the arrow points to the immobile leaflet.

REFERENCES

1. Cannegieter SC, Rosendaal FR. Thromboembolic and bleeding complications in patients with mechanical heart valve prostheses. Circulation 1994; 89: 635-41.
2. Thorburn CW, Morgan JJ, Shanahan MX, et al. Long-term results of tricuspid valve replacement and the problem of the prosthetic valve thrombosis. Am J Cardiol 1983; 51:1128-32.
3. Ledain LD, Ohayon JP, Colle JP, et al. Acute thrombotic obstruction with disc valve prosthesis: diagnostic considerations and fibrinolytic treatment. J Am Coll Cardiol 1986; 7:743-51.
4. Nishimura RA, Otto CM, Bonow RO, et al. AHA/ACC Guideline for management of patients with valvular heart disease: executve summary. J Am Coll Cardiol. 2014; 63 (22):2438-88.

CASE 56

Rajesh Janardhanan

PROSTHETIC MITRAL VALVE OBSTRUCTION: REAL-TIME THREE-DIMENSIONAL TRANSESOPHAGEAL ECHOCARDIOGRAPHY-GUIDED DIAGNOSIS AND MANAGEMENT

A 55-year-old female presented with progressive exertional dyspnea, orthopnea and profound fatigue on minimal activity for 5 days. Her medical history was notable for rheumatic fever with severe mitral regurgitation. She had undergone mitral valve repair 5 years earlier. Following the failure of that mitral repair two years later, she underwent a repeat sternotomy and mechanical mitral valve replacement (26 mm Carbomedics valve) due to worsening symptoms. She endorsed nonadherence to warfarin therapy. She denied any recent infection or drug abuse. Examination on arrival revealed bi-basilar pulmonary crackles and bipedal edema. Her cardiovascular exam was notable for a diastolic murmur at the apex with absence of audible prosthetic valve clicks.

The results of routine biochemical tests were within normal limits with the exception of a subtherapeutic International Normalized Ratio (INR) of 1.2. A fluoroscopic view of the prosthesis indicated absent opening and closing of one mechanical disc (153). A transthoracic echocardiogram (TTE) revealed mitral valve obstruction with an increased mean transmitral gradient of 24 mm Hg. 2D-transesophageal echocardiography (2D-TEE) revealed an immobile disc with haziness noted on its atrial side (Fig. 56.1). Images obtained using real time (RT)3D-TEE demonstrated the presence of a mass, with texture and appearance suggestive of a partially obstructive thrombus attached to the atrial side of the mechanical valve restricting the anteromedial disc of the valve (Figs. 56.2 and 56.3, 154).

Due to the patient's comorbidities, two prior sternotomies, and high STS score of 17%, our multidisciplinary team recommended that she undergoes thrombolysis with systemic tissue plasminogen activator (tPa). She received 10 mg IV bolus alteplase, followed by 90 mg infused over one-and-a-half hours and subsequently IV heparin infusion. Post-thrombolysis, her symptoms resolved and a

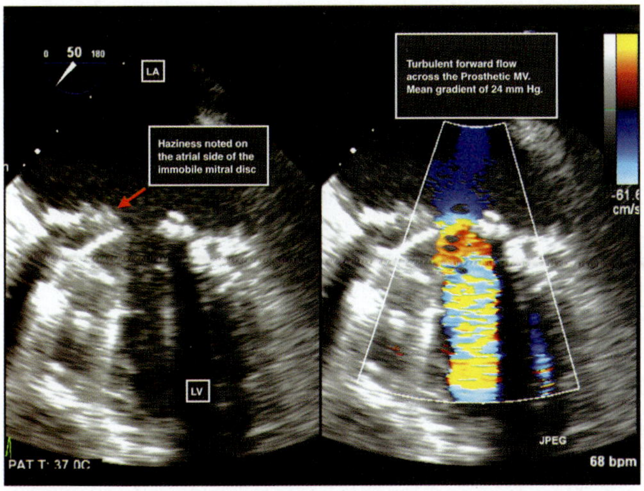

Fig. 56.1: 2D transesophageal echocardiographic view of the prosthetic mitral valve. Haziness noted over the atrial side of the prosthesis (left). Turbulent forward flow across the prosthetic mitral valve with measured mean gradient of 24 mm Hg (right).

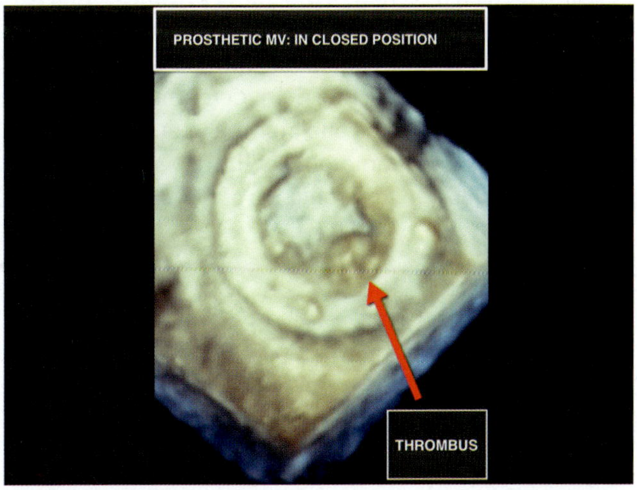

Fig. 56.2: Real-time 3D transesophageal echocardiogram of prosthetic mitral valve in closed position showing a mass suggestive of a partially obstructive thrombus attached to the atrial side of the mechanical valve, restricting the anteromedial disc of the valve.

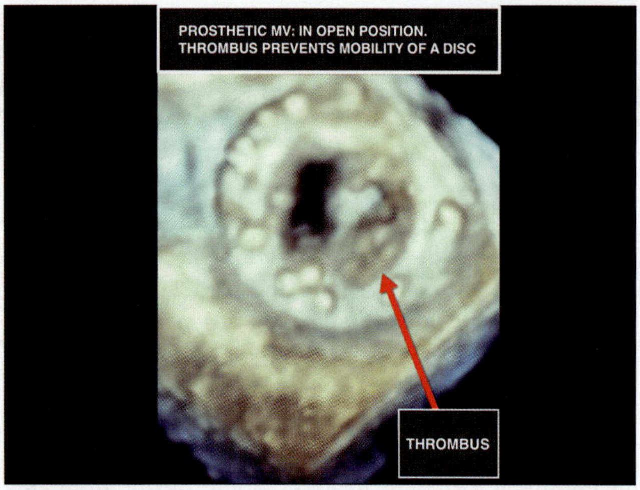

Fig. 56.3: Real-time 3D transesophageal echocardiogram of prosthetic mitral valve in open position showing a mass suggestive of a partially obstructive thrombus (arrow) attached to the atrial side of the mechanical valve, restricting the anteromedial disc of the valve.

follow-up TTE revealed reduction in mitral valve gradient to 6 mm Hg. The full excursion of the disc was confirmed on fluoroscopy suggesting resolution of obstruction (🎥 155). She was discharged home under stable condition. During the 4-week outpatient follow-up, she reported resolution of all her symptoms. An outpatient TTE was performed 4 weeks after the thrombolysis confirming full excursion of the discs and a normal mitral valve gradient.

In summary, we present a case of an acute thrombus causing obstruction of a mechanical mitral valve. RT3D-TEE provided en face view of the mitral prosthesis that was otherwise not obtainable with routine 2D-TEE. Accurate diagnosis and confirmation of the partial thrombus using RT3D-TEE, was crucial in determining the best management strategy for our high-risk patient, who had undergone two prior sternotomies. The decision to attempt thrombolysis allowed for avoidance of high-risk surgery.

1. **The standard therapy for acute prosthetic valve thrombosis of left-sided valves is:**
   (a) Thrombolysis
   (b) Urgent surgery
   (c) Thrombolysis followed by surgery
   (d) Conservative management

Ans. (b)

2. **The major risk factors for prosthetic valve obstruction include:**
   (a) Mitral location of the prosthesis
   (b) Inadequate anticoagulation therapy
   (c) Aortic location of prosthesis
   (d) Tricuspid location of prosthesis
   (e) (a) and (b)

Ans. (e)

3. **The following imaging modalities can help in the diagnosis of prosthetic valve thrombosis:**
   (a) TTE
   (b) TEE
   (c) Cine-fluoroscopy
   (d) EKG-gated CTA
   (e) All of the above

Ans. (e)

MOVIE LEGENDS 🎥

153: Cine-fluoroscopic view of the prosthesis (prethromboysis) indicated absent opening and closing of one mechanical disc.

154: Real time 3D transesophageal echocardiography of the prosthetic mitral valve (view from the atrial side) showing restricted movement of the anteromedial disc due to a partially obstructing thrombus (red arrow).

155: Fluoroscopic video of the opening and closing of the prosthetic mitral valve, postthrombolysis. The full excursion of the valve is appreciated here.

CASE 57

Ahmad S Omran

ACCELERATED BIOPROSTHETIC MITRAL VALVE DEGENERATION RESULTING IN SEVERE MITRAL STENOSIS

This 24-year-old woman with 35-week pregnancy presented to our center with acute pulmonary edema. She was intubated and admitted to ICU. Patient had a history of mitral valve replacement 5 years previously with a bioprosthetic pericardial valve. In her last follow-up echocardiography about one year ago, the mean gradient across the bioprosthetic mitral valve was slightly higher than normal but she was totally asymptomatic. Transthoracic echocardiography (TTE) during current admission showed thickened, calcified mitral leaflets with mean gradient of about 28 mm Hg (Figs. 57.1A and B). Patient was treated medically and extubated the day after admission. She underwent Cesarean section one week later. Transesophageal echocardiography (TEE) was done after delivery and showed severe pannus formation on the sewing ring of the bioprosthetic mitral valve with thickening and calcification of the leaflets. Mitral valve was severely stenotic. 3D TEE showed the bioprosthetic mitral valve with two leaflets totally immobile and one cusp with limited opening (Figs. 57.2A and B, 156–161). Patient was taken to the operating room 10 days after Cesarean section. During surgery, the bioprosthetic valve showed pannus formation on the sewing ring and immobile leaflets exactly as was described by preoperative 3D TEE (Figs. 57.3A and B). Mitral valve was replaced by a mechanical prosthetic valve. Patient was discharged home one week later in good general condition.

1. **All of the following are risk factors for accelerated structural bioprosthetic valve deterioration in the mitral position *except*:**
   (a) Less than 40 years of age
   (b) Systemic hypertension
   (c) Hyperparathyroidism
   (d) Renal insufficiency

Ans. (b)

MOVIE LEGENDS

156: Preoperative 2D TEE in commissural view showing a severely calcified and stenotic bioprosthetic mitral valve. Pannus formation and calcification of the sewing ring are noted.

157: Same view as previous movie with color Doppler showing severe mitral inflow diastolic turbulence due to stenosis. Mild mitral regurgitation is noted.

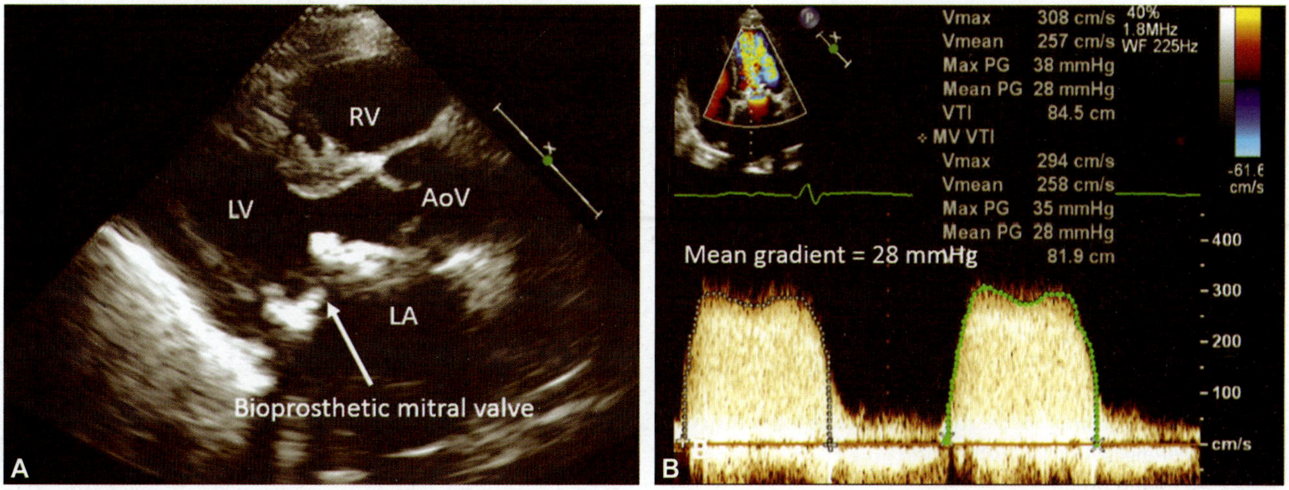

Figs. 57.1A and B: Transthoracic echocardiography (TTE). (A) Parasternal long-axis view showing the bioprosthetic mitral valve with thickened calcified leaflets. (B) Parasternal 4-chamber view showing CW Doppler across the mitral inflow with a very high gradient (mean peak gradient = 28 mm Hg). (RV: Right ventricle; LV: Left ventricle; LA: Left atrium; AoV: Aortic valve).

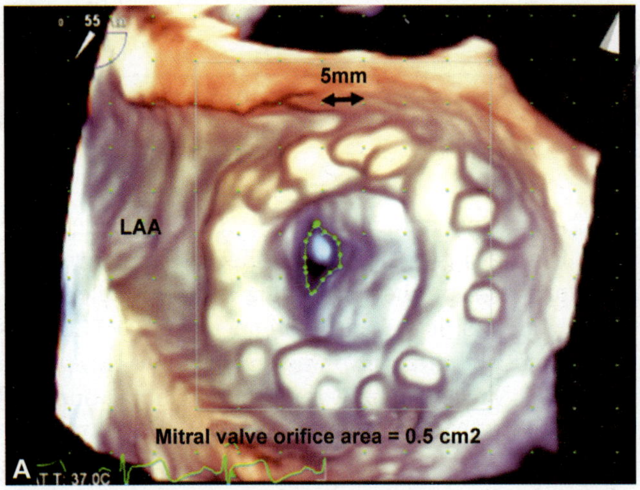

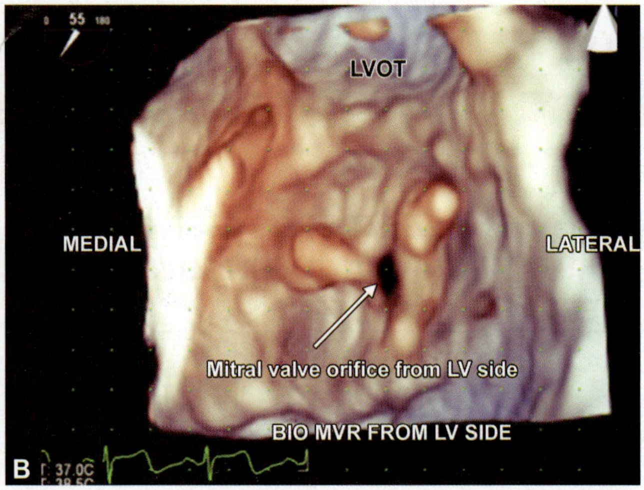

Figs. 57.2A and B: Preoperative 3D transesophageal echocardiography (3DTEE). (A) 3D zoom mode acquisition of the bioprosthetic mitral valve in surgical view (from left atrial side) shows a severely calcified, stenotic valve. Two leaflets are totally immobile and the third leaflet has only a limited opening. Using 3D grid calibration, planimetered mitral valve area was 0.5 cm^2 consistent with severely stenotic mitral valve. (B) Same acquisition of the mitral valve from left ventricular side shows a very stenotic orifice. (LAA: Left atrial appendage; LVOT: Left ventricular outflow tract).

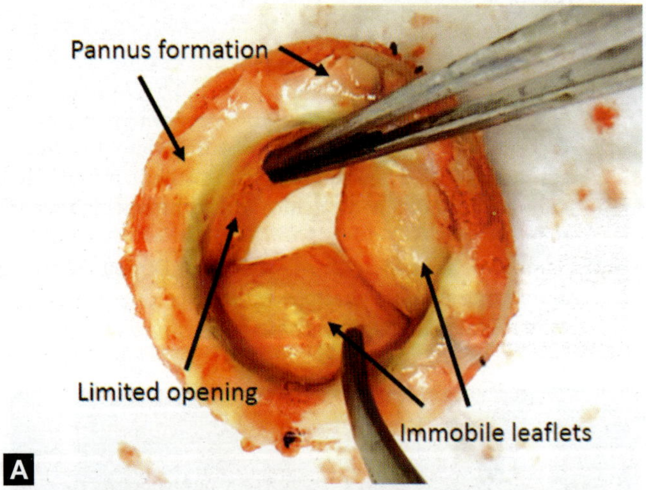

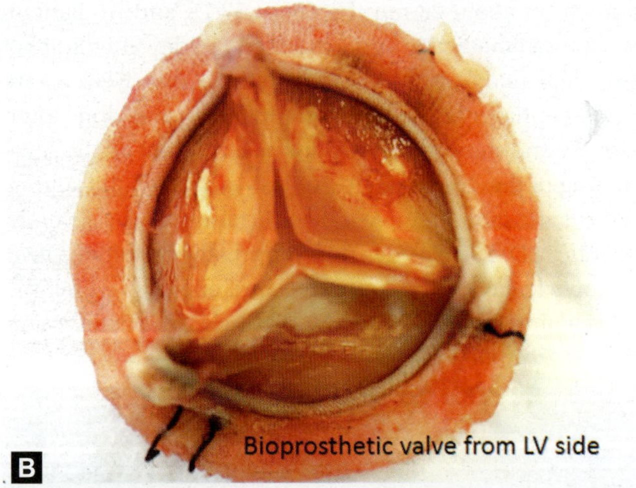

Figs. 57.3A and B: Surgical exploration of the bioprosthetic mitral valve. (A) Bioprosthetic mitral valve after extraction is shown from left atrial side. Whitish material is noted over the sewing ring consistent with pannus formation. Leaflets are rigid and calcified. Only one leaflet has limited opening and the other two leaflets are totally immobile. Mitral orifice opening is very similar to the preoperative 3D TEE image (Fig. 56.2A). (B) Bioprosthetic mitral valve from left ventricular (LV) aspect.

158: Preoperative 3D TEE zoom mode acquisition of the bioprosthetic mitral valve in surgical view shows limited opening of one leaflet and totally calcified and immobile the other two leaflets.
159: 3D TEE zoom mode of the mitral valve from left ventricular side showing a very narrow mitral orifice.
160: 3D TEE zoom mode of the mitral valve with triple display showing 3D surgical view and 2 other 2D reference views.
161: 3D TEE full volume color Doppler acquisition of the mitral valve showing severely stenotic mitral inflow and mild mitral regurgitation.

REFERENCES

1. Pibarot P, Dumesnil JG. Prosthetic heart valves. Selection of the optimal prosthesis and long-term management. Circulation 2009; 119: 1034-48.
2. Tsang W, Weinert L, Kronzon I, et al. Three-dimensional echocardiography in the assessment of prosthetic valves. Rev Esp Cardiol. 2011; 64: 1-7.

CASE 58

Chisato Izumi

A 76-year-old female. Post-MVR (St Jude prosthesis). Anticoagulant therapy was discontinued 1 week before eye surgery, and it was started again 2 days after surgery. Low-grade fever developed, thus 2D TTE was performed (Figs. 58.1 to 58.5) (162 and 163, MV = mitral valve replacement, arrow in 165 and 166 shows diastolic color Doppler flow signals in the LA) 10 days after surgery.

INR 1.18 (1 day prior to surgery)

INR 1.72 (10 days after surgery)

1. **What is an abnormal finding suggesting prosthetic valve dysfunction in this case?**
   (a) Abnormal leaflet motion in parasternal short axis view
   (b) Paravalvular mitral regurgitant flow signal
   (c) Abnormal diastolic color signal in the left atrium
   (d) Increased velocity of transmitral E wave.
   (e) None

Ans. (c)

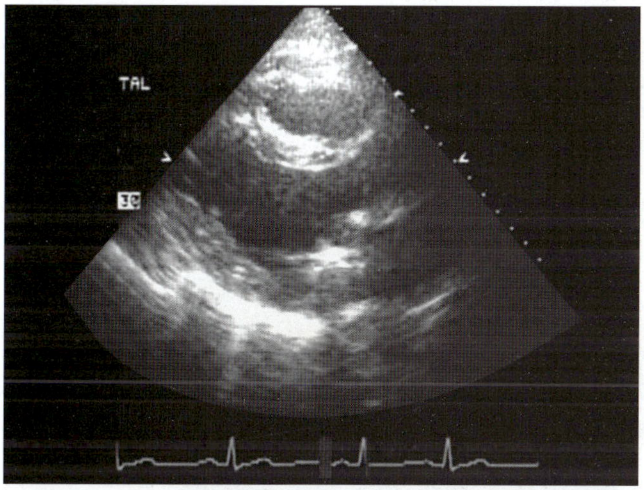

Fig. 58.1: Parasternal long-axis view.

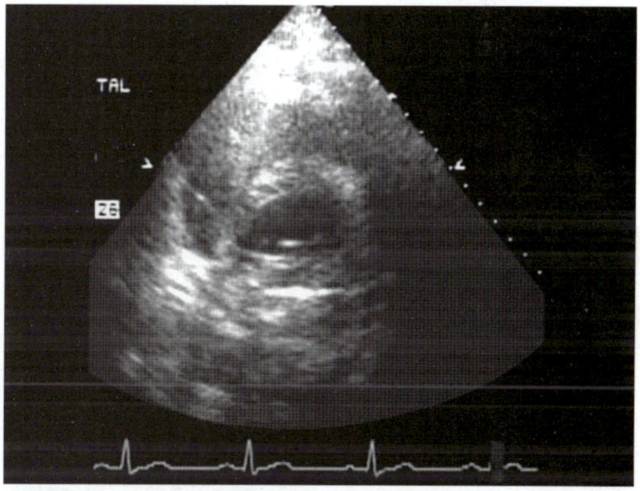

Fig. 58.2: Parasternal shot-axis view.

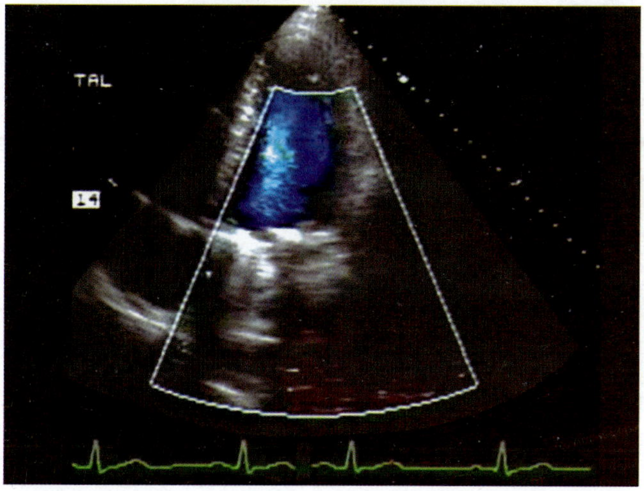

Fig. 58.3: Color Doppler image of apical 4-chamber view.

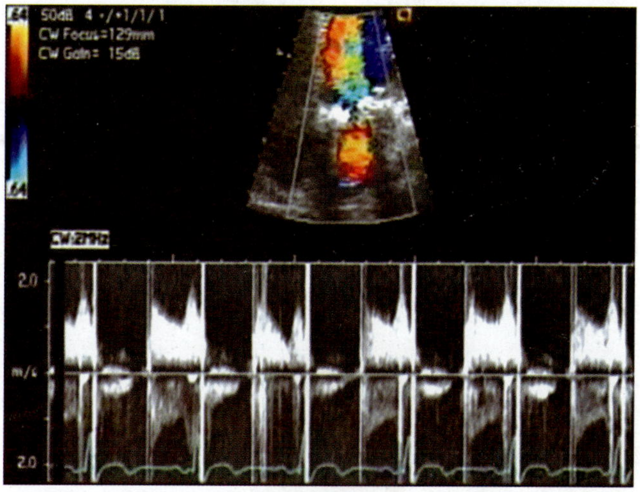

Fig. 58.4: Transmitral flow signal.

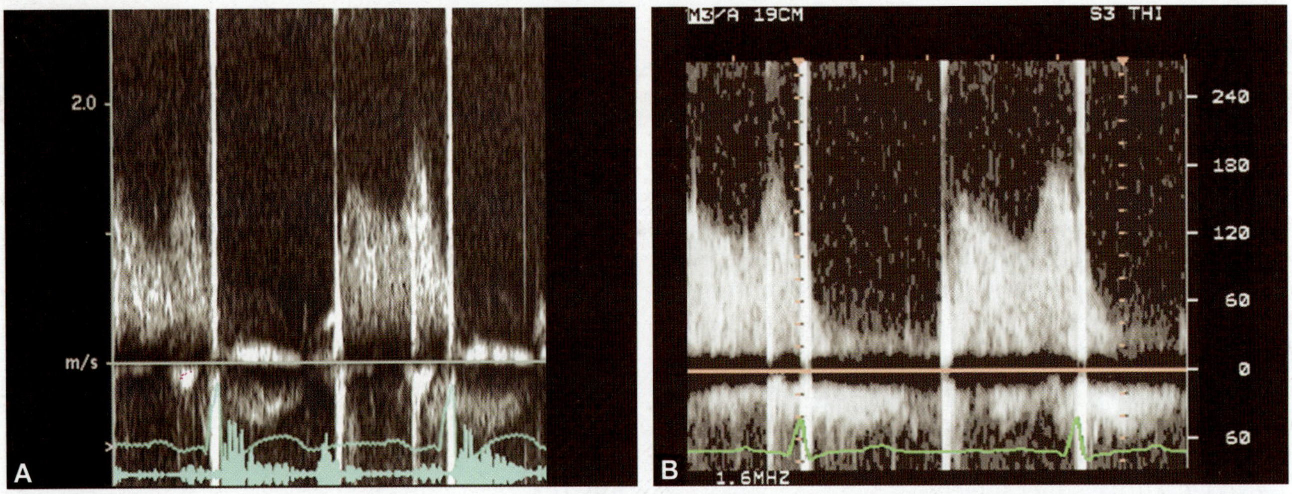

Figs. 58.5A and B: (A) Transmitral flow signal 1 month before admission. (B) Transmitral flow signal 10 days after eye surgery.

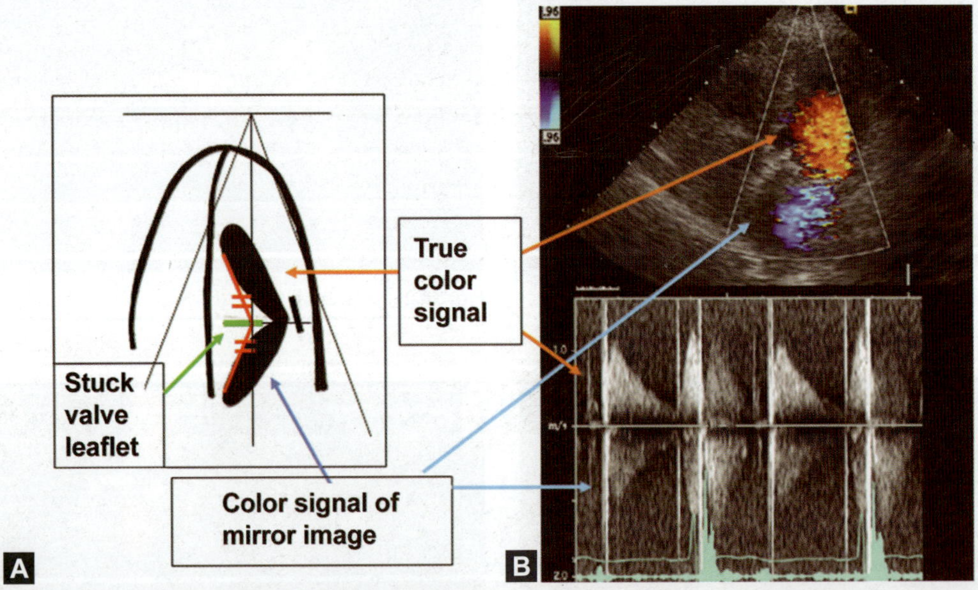

Figs. 58.6A and B: (A) A schematic drawing illustrating the mechanism of diastolic color signal in the LA. (B) Diastolic color signal in the LA.

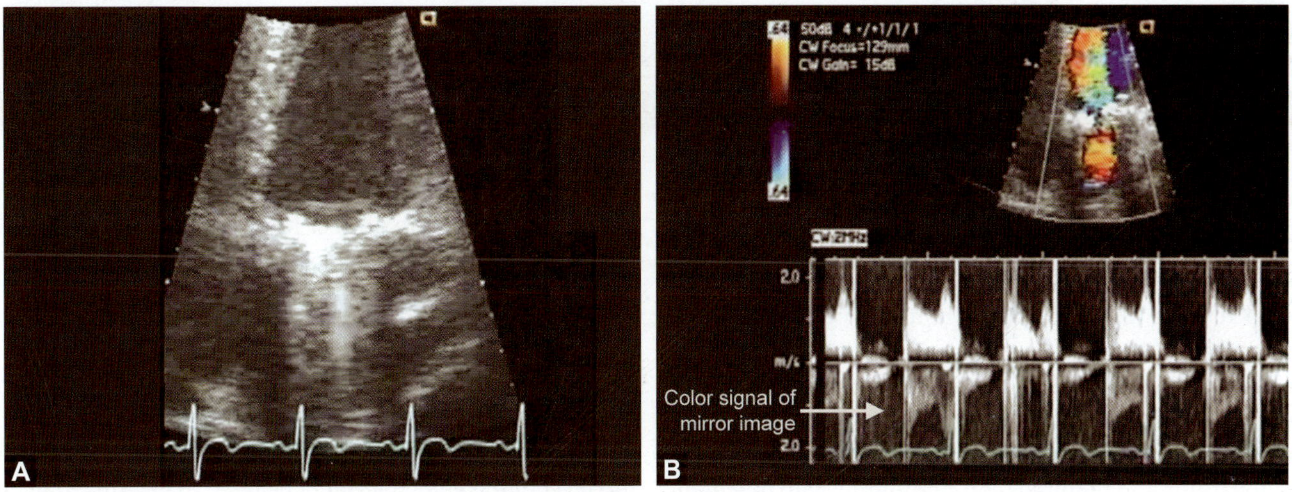

Figs. 58.7A and B: (A) Motion of the mitral prosthetic valve. (B) Flow signal record of transmitral flow and its mirror image.

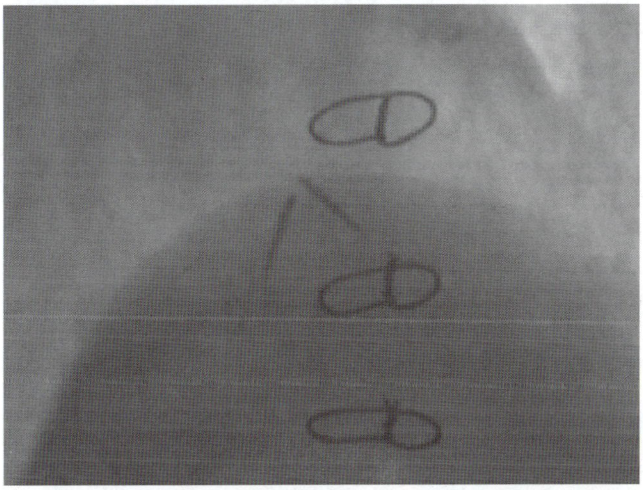

Fig. 58.8: Fluoroscopy of mitral prosthesis.

DISCUSSION

Peak velocity of transmitral flow did not increase compared to 1 month before admission (Fig. 58.5). Abnormal diastolic color signal in the LA was seen as a mirror image of transmitral flow which derived from a stuck leaflet (Figs. 58.6 and 58.7). Fluoroscopy of mitral prosthesis revealed that a leaflet was stuck (Fig. 58.8 and 🎥 164).

- There are many difficulties in echocardiographic diagnosis of prosthetic valve dysfunction due to various artifacts.
- However, "artifact" itself may be a clue to diagnosis of prosthetic valve dysfunction.
- Diastolic color signals in the LA are an abnormal finding suggesting mitral prosthetic valve dysfunction.

MOVIES 162 TO 166

CASE 59

Madeline Jankowski, Daniel R Schimmel, Vera H Rigolin

History

A 55-year-old male with sickle-cell anemia and end-stage renal disease presented with shortness of breath, lightheadedness, chest pressure, hypotension and bradycardia in April 2015. His cardiac history dates back to May 2014 when he underwent mitral valve (MV) repair for severe mitral regurgitation (MR). In January 2015, he developed endocarditis and required redo sternotomy with mechanical mitral valve replacement (31 mm mechanical On-X), tricuspid valve (TV) repair and MAZE procedure.

Transthoracic Echo (TTE) Findings

TTE was ordered with concern for recurrent endocarditis. Echo showed:

- Left ventricular ejection fraction of 40%, global hypokinesis
- Moderate right ventricular dilation and dysfunction
- Rocking of Mechanical MV
- Severe MR at the site of dehiscence at the posterolateral commissure (Fig. 59.1A and 167)
- Well-seated TV annuloplasty ring

Transesophageal Echo (TEE) Findings

TEE was done that same day to show a 1.6 cm × 0.3 cm crescent shaped defect along the 2 o'clock to 5 o'clock position of the mechanical MV, consistent with valve dehiscence with associated severe paravalvular MR. In the area of dehiscence, there was extensive necrotic tissue resulting in significant rocking of valve (arrow in 168 and 169).

Repeat TEE 3 weeks later showed an increase in size of the dehiscence that now extended from the 2 o'clock to 6 o'clock positions.

Patient Care

Because the patient was felt to be at high risk for redo valve surgery, he was evaluated for percutaneous closure of the paravalvular leak. Because of the large area of dehiscence and extensive necrotic tissue, the patient was felt to be at high risk for intraprocedural and late embolization of the percutaneous closure device. There was also concern that the patient's infection was not adequately controlled.

Discussion

Measuring and sizing paravalvular leaks is crucial in order to choose the correct percutaneous closure device. Quader et al.[1] suggest measuring the size of the defect at the level of the vena contracta using 3D TEE. This may be difficult when there is suboptimal image quality or when arrhythmia or patient movement result in stitch artifacts during full volume acquisitions. 2D and 3D TEE with color Doppler are also used during the procedure to evaluate any residual leaks post implantation. Kim et al.[2] uses the length and diameter of the defect from strut of the prosthesis to determine the maximum size (waist length and diameter) of a device (Figs. 59.1B and C, 170).

There are many devices that are used to plug paravalvular mitral valve leaks. Rihal et al[3] reviews some of the most common devices. At this time, there is not an FDA-approved device specifically made for plugging these leaks. As a result, other transcatheter devices such as an

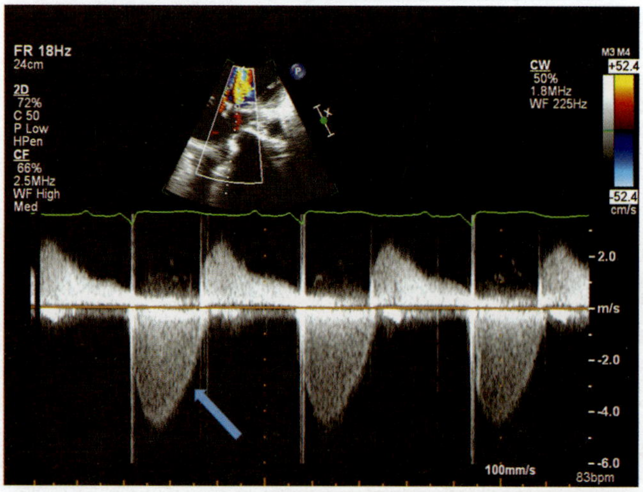

Fig. 59.1A: This image demonstrates the continuous wave Doppler through the MV on the TTE. The blue arrow shows the MR envelope. Note that the MR jet is almost as dense as the forward flow, revealing significant MR. The envelope is early peaking and triangular shaped indicating elevated left atrial pressures.

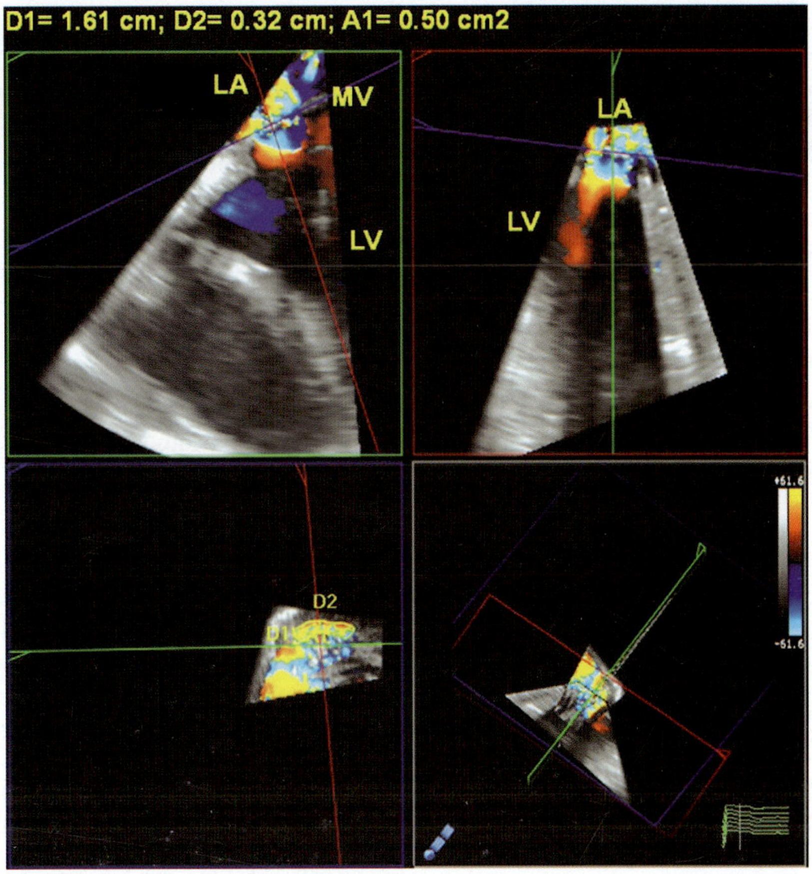

Fig. 59.1B: Accurate 3D measurement of the effective regurgitant orifice area of the perivalvular leak is best performed using multiplanar reconstruction. The 3D volume is divided into three orthogonal planes in order to locate and measure the effective regurgitant orifice area at the level of the vena contracta. The bottom left picture shows the en-face view of the defect found by aligning those planes.

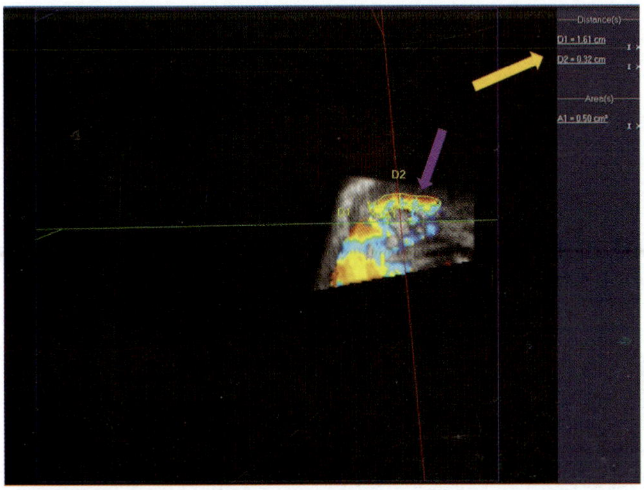

Fig. 59.1C: Accurate measurements can be made from the zoomed en-face view of the defect. The purple arrow shows the defect in systole with the color indicating the regurgitation. The yellow arrow shows the measurements of the width and length of the defect.

Amplatzer Septal occluder, muscular VSD occluder, duct occluder, vascular plug, or different vascular coils are used. Accurately sizing the defect assists in choosing the appropriate device. Shorter lesions may use the Amplatzer Septal occluder while longer lesions are plugged by Amplatzer muscular VSD or duct occluders. Caution is needed when using a larger closure device due to the risk of impairing prosthetic valve function. On the other hand, multiple smaller devices may increase the risk of embolization or recurrent infection.[4] Careful assessment of defect size and prosthetic valve function before choosing a device is necessary for a successful outcome.

The most common cause of prosthetic MV dehiscence is the presence of infection causing erosion of the surrounding area. Dehiscence of a prosthetic mitral valve is more common than that of the aortic valve. Ercan et al.[5] concluded that endocarditis is seen in 1–6% of patients with a prosthetic valve. Having a prior history of infective endocarditis increases the risk of recurrent endocarditis even after reoperation.

Classic echo features include a rocking motion of the prosthetic valve, but regurgitation may be hard to evaluate. This type of lesion can be easily missed on a TTE. The paravalvular leak in our patient was best seen in off axis views of the mitral valve. Turbulent flow is seen in these cases, but could be mistaken for forward flow through the valve. Also, regurgitation may be missed or underestimated due to shadowing artifact from the mechanical prosthesis. A TEE is helpful for evaluating severity of both valvular and paravalvular prosthetic valve regurgitation, particularly when the prosthesis is in the mitral position. When evaluating a patient for percutaneous closure of a paravalvular defect, the addition of 3D TEE is critical for localization and accurate sizing of the leak. The added information assists in choosing appropriate candidates for percutaneous closure and increases procedural success.

1. **Rocking motion of a mitral valve prosthesis on TTE may indicate:**
   (a) Well-seated prosthesis with normal gradients
   (b) Mitral valve dehiscence
   (c) Mitral valve prolapse
   (d) Severe aortic regurgitation

Ans. (b)

Mitral valve dehiscence. This "rocking motion" of the prosthesis indicates erosion of where the valve inserts into the annulus. This is a classical echocardiographic sign of dehiscence.

2. **In the spectral Doppler of continuous wave through a mitral valve with severe mitral regurgitation, what might you expect to see?**
   (a) Increased velocity of forward flow
   (b) Dense MR signal
   (c) Triangular shaped MR signal
   (d) MR velocities between 3 and 6 m/s
   (e) All of the above

Ans. (e)

All of the above. The forward flow through the valve will be increased because of the increase in regurgitant volume; the greater volume of flow that comes back through the valve has to go forward through the valve too. There will be a very dense MR signal because of the greater volume of RBCs being detected. The triangular shaped MR signal is caused by the faster equalization of pressure between the high pressure LA and the LV. The MR velocities depend on the systolic pressure difference between the LV and LA.

3. **TEE imaging is more helpful in assessing severity of prosthetic valve regurgitation because:**
   (a) Shadowing artifact by the valve may cause underestimation of the regurgitation on TTE
   (b) One cannot see the mitral valve on TTE
   (c) The esophagus sits behind the left atrium, making the mitral valve easy to see and evaluate
   (d) Accurate velocities of MR can only be obtained by TEE
   (e) (a) and (c)
   (f) All of the above

Ans. (e)

When looking at a TTE of a mechanical prosthesis, shadowing artifact can obscure the image to make it difficult to assess regurgitation. As seen in this case, MR could have been underestimated on TTE because we could not see the whole jet. TEE helps see the mitral valve in a different way because shadowing artifact is not present because of the view from behind the left atrium.

MOVIE LEGENDS

167: TTE 4 chamber view. Dual screen was used to see the 2D image alongside of the color Doppler. Significant rocking motion of the valve and thinning of the annulus can be seen. Severe paravalvular MR (arrow) is seen with color Doppler.

168: TEE image demonstrates the necrotic tissue of the thinned area (vertical arrow on the left) adjacent to the prosthetic mitral valve. Dual screen was used to demonstrate the location of the paravalvular MR (horizontal arrow on the right) across the necrotic tissue. Arrow shows rocking motion and MR.

169: 3D TEE image shows the prosthetic MV with defect along the 2 o'clock to 5 o'clock region (arrows).

170: 3D TEE image with color Doppler demonstrates the paravalvular MR jet (arrow). This image was used to measure the EROA seen in figures 1B and 1C using multiplanar reconstruction.

REFERENCES

1. Quader N, Davidson C, Rigolin V. Percutaneous Closure of Perivalvular Mitral Regurgitation: How Should the Interventionalists and the Echocardiographers Communicate? J Am Soc Echocardiogr 2015; 28(5):497-508.
2. Kim M, Casserly I, Garcia J, Klein A, Salcedo E, Carroll J. Percutaneous Transcatheter Closure of Prosthetic Mitral Paravalvular Leaks. J Am Coll Cardiol 2009;2(2):80-90.

3. Rihal C, Sorajja P, Booker J, Hagler D, Cabalka A. Principles of Percutaneous Paravalvular Leak Closure. JACC: Cardiovascular Interventions 2012; 5(2):121-130.
4. Gafoor S, Steinberg D, Franke J, Bertog S, Vaskelyte L, Hofmann I, Sievert H. Tools and Techniques—Clinical: Paravalvular leak closure. EuroIntervention, 2014;9:1359-1363.
5. Ercan S, Altunbas G, Deniz H, Gokaslan G, Bosnak V, Kaplan M, Davutoglu V. Recurrent Prosthetic Mitral Valve Dehiscence due to Infective Endocarditis: Discussion of Possible Causes. Korean J Thorac Cardiovasc Surg. 2013 Aug;46(4): 285–288.

CASE 60

Ahmad S Omran

MECHANICAL MITRAL VALVE DEHISCENCE, SEVERE PARAVALVULAR LEAK

This 34-year-old woman presented to our center with severe shortness of breath. She had a history of redo-mechanical mitral valve replacement (MVR) and tricuspid valve repair 13 years ago in another center. Initial transthoracic echocardiography (TTE) in our center showed normal left ventricular function. Doppler mitral inflow showed a very high E wave velocity with a normal pressure half-time and a suspected paravalvular leak in an off-axis short-axis view (Figs. 60.1A and B). There was severe tricuspid regurgitation (TR) with an estimated right ventricular systolic pressure (RVSP) of 60–70 mm Hg. Transesophageal echocardiography (TEE) was performed which showed two jets of severe paravalvular leak from two sides of the MVR (171). No obvious rocking motion of the MVR was noted. Exact location and extensions of the jets were not clear by 2D TEE, but 3D TEE en-face view in surgical orientation clearly showed the location of two broad jets. One jet was adjacent to the aorta around 12–2 o'clock (clock face orientation of MVR) and the second was posterior to the left atrial appendage (LAA) at 7–8 o'clock position (Figs. 60.2A and B, 172 and 173). Patient was discussed in our heart team meeting and a decision was made for surgical correction. Presence of multiple jets of MR and concomitant severe TR were not in favor of percutaneous closure of paravalvular leaks. In the cardiac operating room due to redo intervention for mitral valve, the surgeon decided to re-suture the area of the sewing ring dehiscence based on the map created by the 3D TEE surgical views (Figs. 60.3A and B). Tricuspid valve was also re-repaired. Intraoperative TEE showed a very good result with no residual paravalvular MR (174). Postoperative course was uneventful and patient was discharged home in good general condition. Follow-up echocardiography after one year showed a well-functioning MVR and only trace TR.

1. **In diagnosis and management of patients with mechanical mitral valve dehiscence, all of the following are correct *except*:**
   (a) Assessment of paravalvular leak in short-axis view is limited by acoustic shadowing of the posterior aspect of the valve-sewing ring.
   (b) Peak mitral E velocity of more than 1.9 m/s with normal pressure half-time has 90% sensitivity in the diagnosis of significant prosthetic MR.

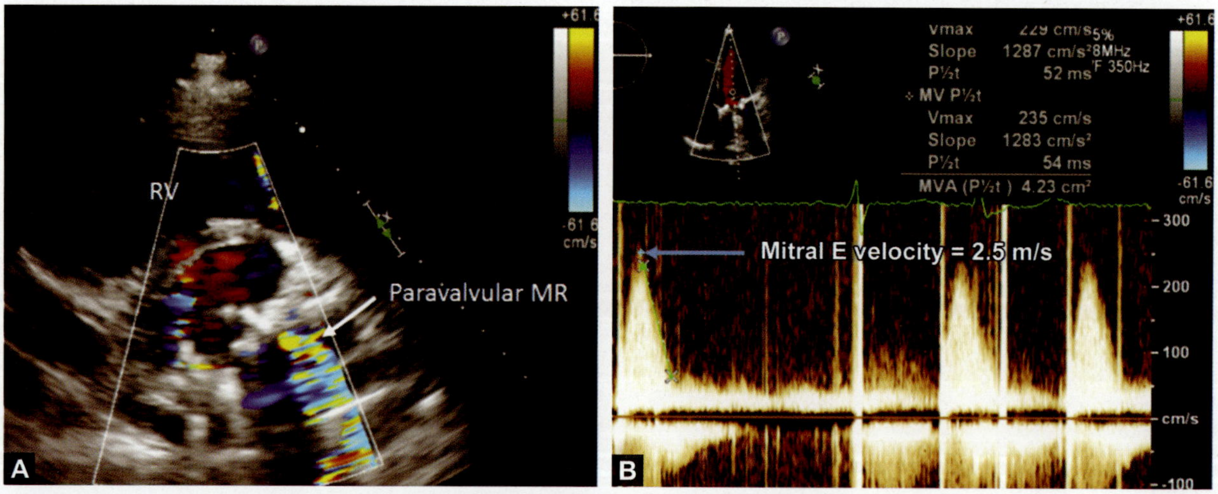

Figs. 60.1A and B: Transthoracic echocardiography (TTE). (A) Parasternal short-axis off-axis view showing paravalvular mitral regurgitation (MR). Mechanical mitral valve has a shadowing and masking effect on the degree of MR in this view. (B) CW Doppler of the mitral inflow shows a very high E wave velocity (2.5 m/s) consistent with significant transvalvular or paravalvular MR (RV: Right ventricle).

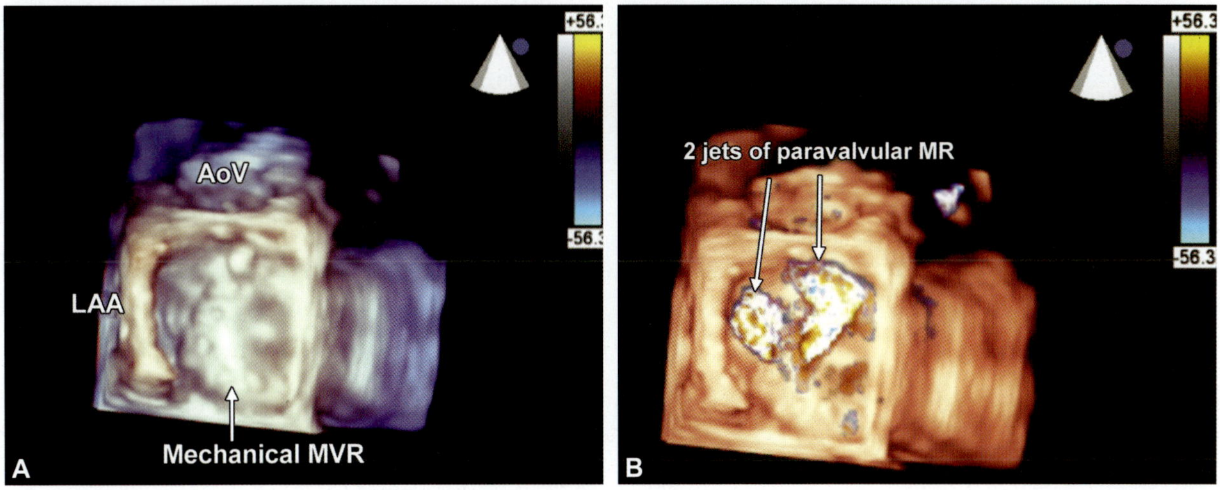

Figs. 60.2A and B: Preoperative 3D transesophageal echocardiography (3DTEE). (A) 3D zoom mode acquisition. Surgical view of the mechanical mitral valve (MVR) with color Doppler suppression shows MVR in clock face orientation. (B) Same view of the MVR with color Doppler shows two large jets of paravalvular leak, one adjacent to the aortic valve (AoV) at 12–2 o'clock and the second one posterior to the left atrial appendage (LAA) at 7–8 o'clock.

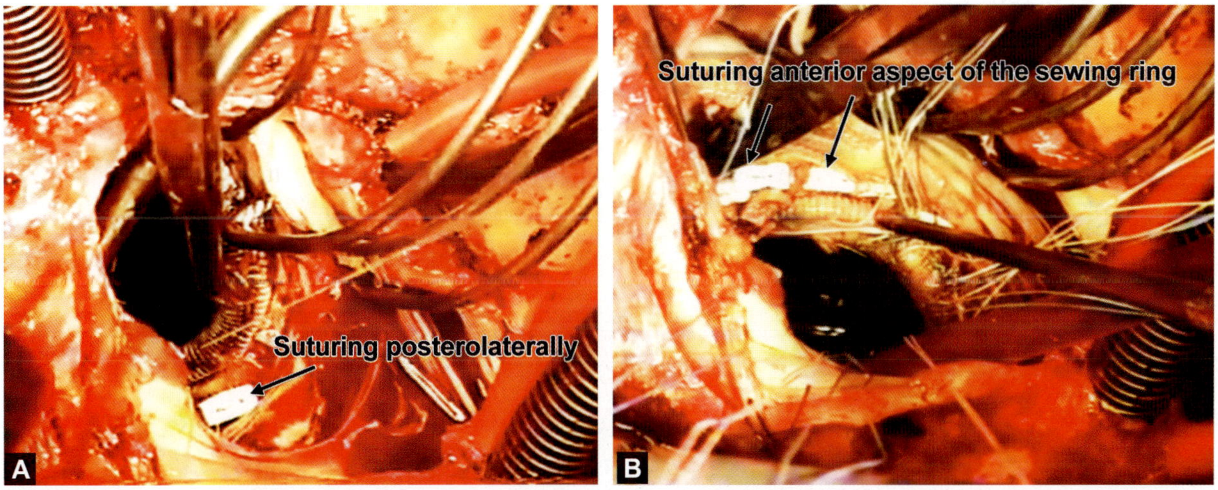

Figs. 60.3A and B: Surgical exploration of the mechanical mitral valve through the left atriotomy. (A) Re-suturing the posterolateral (7–8 o'clock) dehiscence of the sewing ring with two plegeted sutures. (B) More sutures were used to close the dehiscence at 12–2 o'clock.

(c) Real-time 3D TEE in cath lab can guide the cardiac interventionist in percutaneous closure of paravalvular leak in high-risk patients.
(d) Real-time 3D TEE with color Doppler underestimates the width of paravalvular leak compared to 2D TEE.

Ans. (d)

MOVIE LEGENDS

171: Preoperative 2D TEE 4-chamber view of the mechanical mitral valve showing two large jets of paravalvular leak from 2 sides.

172: Preoperative 3D TEE, surgical view of the mechanical MVR with full volume acquisition with suppressed color Doppler showing the clock face orientation of MVR.

173: Same view of previous movie with color Doppler showing two large jets of paravalvular leak at 7–8 o'clock and 12–2 o'clock.

174: Same view of previous movies immediately after re-suturing of the sewing ring showing no residual MR.

REFERENCES

1. Zoghbi WA, Chambers JB, Dumesnil JG, et al. Recommendations for evaluation of prosthetic valves with echocardiography and Doppler ultrasound. A report from the ASE/ACC/AHA/ EACVI and ESC. J Am Soc Echocardiogr 2009; 22:976-1008.
2. Franco E, Almeria C, de Agustin JA, et al. Three-dimensional color Doppler transesophageal echocardiography for mitral paravalvular leak quantification and evaluation of percutaneous closure success. J Am Soc Echocardiogr 2014; 27:1153-63.

CASE 61

John D Groarke, Judy R Mangion

TEE IN MITRAL VALVE REPAIR AND PERSISTENT MICROANGIOPATHIC HEMOLYTIC ANEMIA

A 79-year-old male presented for second opinion, with a 1-year prodrome of malaise, weight loss, progressive dyspnea and dark urine. Prior history was significant for mitral valve (MV) repair 9 years earlier for infective endocarditis.

Physical exam was notable for general pallor, anorexia, scleral icterus, and a pansystolic murmur, best heard at the apex. Laboratory data were consistent with a hemolytic anemia, with low hematocrit (24%) low haptoglobin (< 8 mg/dL), elevated LDH (2800 U/L), increased reticulocytes (10%), and increased total bilirubin (1.9 mg/dL). Peripheral blood smear confirmed a microangiopathic hemolytic anemia (Fig. 61.1). Endoscopy, computerized tomography of the thorax, abdomen and pelvis, and bone marrow biopsy did not identify a cause for the hemolytic anemia. Transthoracic echo showed a thickened mitral valve s/p repair with moderate to severe mitral regurgitation (MR) and no paravalvular leak. A transeosphageal echocardiogram (TEE) with live 3D imaging was performed for better mitral valve characterization (Figs. 61.2 and 61.3; and 175 and 176).

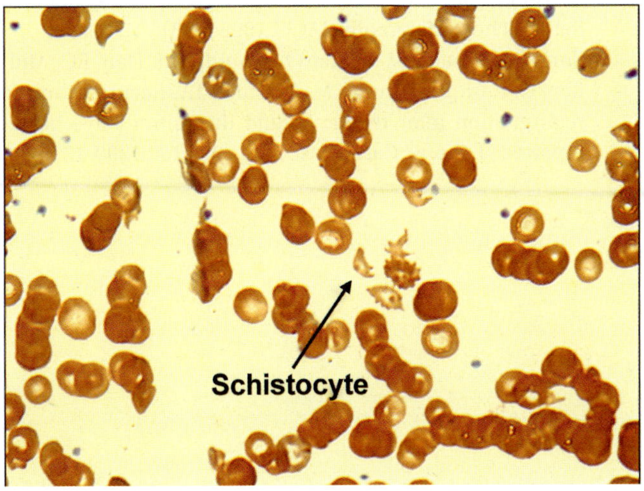

Fig. 61.1: Peripheral blood smear demonstrating evidence of intravascular hemolysis. Specifically, schistocytes (arrow) are present.

1. **Based on the TEE images, where does the mitral insufficiency originate in this patient?**
   (a) Valvular
   (b) Paravalvular
   (c) Both valvular and paravalvular
   (d) Unable to determine

Ans. (a)

TEE with color Doppler demonstrates three distinct high-velocity jets of mitral insufficiency, all located within the mitral valvular apparatus and within the annuloplasty ring.

2. **What is the likely etiology of this patient's hemolytic anemia?**
   (a) Hemolytic anemia of primary hematologic etiology
   (b) Hemolytic anemia caused by mitral leaflet perforation(s)
   (c) Hemolytic anemia caused by mitral paravalvular leak(s)
   (d) Age-related hemolytic anemia

Ans. (b)

TEE with 3D imaging demonstrates severe MR secondary to a focal perforation or cleft of the P3 scallop and a second focal perforation or cleft of the P1 scallop. A high-velocity MR jet originated from each defect.

Role of Echocardiography in Patient Care

TEE identified two focal MV perforations or clefts within the remotely repaired valve with resultant high-velocity MR as the cause of here-to-fore unexplained, chronic and persistent microangiopathic hemolytic anemia. This prompted surgical referral and subsequent MV replacement (MVR). Hemolysis resolved immediately following MVR and follow-up confirms sustained remission.

Summary and Discussion Points

TEE with live 3D imaging was the test of choice in identifying the etiology and guiding successful treatment of long-standing and persistent microangiopathic hemolytic anemia. Hemolysis is a rare mode of failure late s/p MV repair, and most commonly is associated with paravalvular

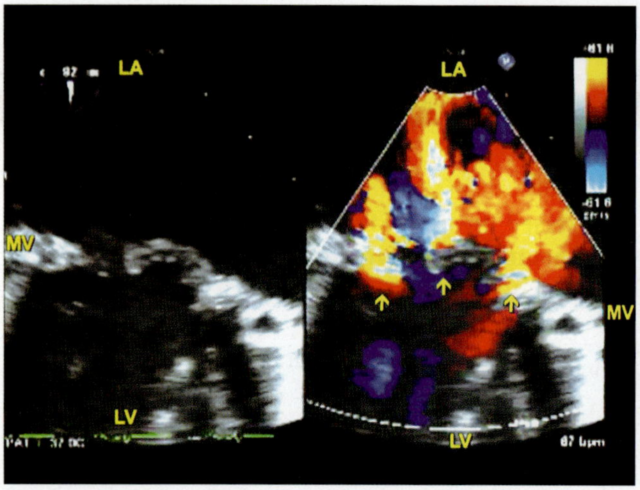

Fig. 61.2: Transesophageal echocardiography with color Doppler demonstrates severe mitral insufficiency with three distinct jets of valvular MR (arrows) originating from within the annuloplasty ring. Two of the mitral regurgitation jets emerge (arrows) from two separate perforations or clefts of the posterior leaflet, one involving the P3 scallop and the other involving the P1 scallop.

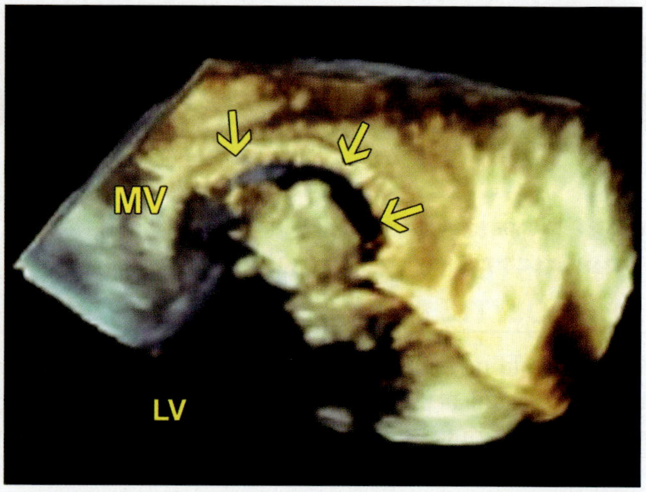

Fig. 61.3: Three-dimensional imaging confirms evidence of the leaflet perforations (arrows) which correlate with the high-velocity valvular regurgitant jets visualized on color Doppler.

leaks early following valve replacement. Microangiopathic hemolytic anemia in this case was late and secondary valvular defects that could only be identified with TEE. Our patient has continued to improve clinically s/p MVR.

MOVIE LEGENDS

175: Transesophageal echocardiography with color Doppler demonstrate severe mitral insufficiency with three distinct jets of valvular MR (arrows) originating from within the annuloplasty ring. Two of the mitral regurgitation jets emerge (arrows) from two separate perforations or clefts of the posterior leaflet, one involving the P3 scallop and the other involving the P1 scallop.

176: Three-dimensional imaging confirms evidence of the leaflet perforations (arrows) which correlate with the high velocity valvular regurgitant jets visualized on color Doppler.

REFERENCES

1. DeCesare W, Rath C, Hufnagel C. Hemolytic Anemic of Mechanical Origin with Aortic-Valve Prosthesis. N Engl J Med 1965;272:1045-1050.
2. Demirsoy E, Yilmaz O, Sirin G, Baran T, Tekin S, Sener D, Sonmez B. Hemolysis and mitral valve repair: A Report of Five Cases and Literature Review. J Heart Valve Dis 2008;17 (1):24-30.
3. Lam BK, Cosgrove DM, Bhudia SK, Gillinov AM. Hemolysis after mitral valve repair: Mechanisms and treatment. Ann Thorac Surg 2004;77:191-195
4. Yeo TV, Freeman WK, Schaff HV, Orszulak TA. Mechanisms of Hemolysis After Mitral Valve Repair: Assessment by Serial Echocardiography. JACC. 1998;32(3):717-723.
5. Suri RM, Schaff HV, Dearani JA, Sundt TM, Daly RC, Mullany C, Enriquez-Sarano M, Orszulak TA. Recurrent mitral regurgitation after repair: Should the mitral valve be re-repaired? J Thorac Cardiovasc Surg 2006;132:1390-1397.

MOVIE LEGENDS

185: Preoperative 3D TEE zoom mode acquisition of mitral and tricuspid valve in surgical view showing dehisced mitral ring and small size tricuspid annuloplasty ring.

186: Preoperative 3D TEE, same view as previous movie with slight rotation for better demonstration of the tricuspid annulus.

187: 3D TEE full volume color Doppler acquisition of the mitral valve showing severe MR, mostly originating from dehisced gap.

188: Immediate postoperative 3D TEE after mitral valve repair and implantation of a size 28 Physio ring.

REFERENCES

1. Koronzon I, Sugenge L, Perk G, et al. Real-time 3-dimensional echocardiography in the evaluation of post-operative mitral ring and prosthetic valve dehiscence. J Am Coll Cardiol 2009; 53:1543-7.
2. Hanson ID, Hanzel GS, Shannon FL. Mitral valve repair after annuloplasty ring dehiscence using MitraClip. Catheter Cardiovasc Inter. 2015 Oct 20.112.

CASE 65

Elsayed M, Alagic N, Uygur B, Turaga NSN, Chahwala JR, Adarna LG, Bulur S, Nanda NC

This is a 78-year-old male with MV prolapse and severe MR. He needed percutaneous placement of a second MV clip because residual MR was still significant after the first clip. 2D and 3D TEE were done in the cardiac catheterization laboratory. 189–191 are 2D TEE and 192–195 are 3D TEE.

1. **What is the severity of MR after placement of both MV clips (191)?**
   (a) Moderately severe
   (b) Moderate
   (c) Mild

Ans. (c)

MR is clearly mild. It was severe at baseline (189) before MV clip placement and remained eccentric and severe after the first clip (190). Nyquist limit was reasonable in 189 and 191, somewhat high in 190.

2. **What do the 3D TEE show? All statements below are correct *except*:**
   (a) 192 shows mainly A2 but also some A3 and P3 prolapse. These are easily identified when cropping the 3D data sets which show A3 and P3 placed more medially near TV. R, L and N represent right, left and noncoronary AV cusps, respectively
   (b) 193 shows deployment of the 2nd clip (arrowhead and #2, #1 represents the 1st clip).
   (c) 194 depicts cropping of the 3D data sets to identify both adjacently placed clips (#1 and #2).
   (d) 195 MPR mode. 2 orifices are well seen in the left lower panel, the 3rd orifice is not visualized in these images.
   (e) 192 also shows TV scallops.

Ans. (e)

Normally, there are no anatomic clefts in the TV but for the sake of convenience, each leaflet can be equally divided into 3 segments when describing prolapse.[1]

MOVIES 189 TO 195

REFERENCE

1. Pothineni KR, et al. Echocardiography. 2007;24(5)541-52.

CASE 66

Elsayed M, Alli O, Adarna LG, Alagic N, Uygur B, Chahwala JR, Bhagatwala K, Bulur S, Turaga NSN, Kattalan JJP, Nanda NC

This is a 74-year-old female with MVP and severe MR, who underwent MV clip repair. 2D and 3D TEE were done in the cath lab during the procedure.

1. **How many MV clips were placed in this patient? (Fig. 66.1 and 🎥 196–199)**
   (a) One clip
   (b) Two clips
   (c) Three clips

Ans. (b)

In this patient, two MV clips were placed because of significant residual MR following insertion of the first clip. The resulting 3 orifices (arrows) and the two clips (arrowheads) are well seen. Asterisk points to the delivering device (🎥 196–198). CW Doppler showed gradients from 2 orifices superimposed on each other, the gradient from one orifice being abnormally high (darker waveform). The gradients from the other two orifices were reasonable (Fig. 66.1). Only mild residual MR persisted after the procedure (🎥 199).

MOVIES 196 TO 199 🎥

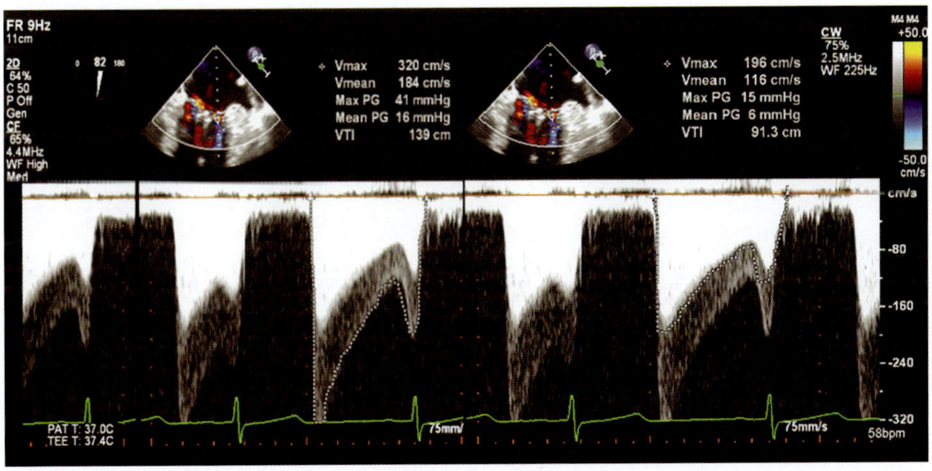

Fig. 66.1: Superimposed bright and dark waveforms from the two mitral orifices following mitral clip placement.

CASE 67

Bulur S, Nanda NC

The patient is an 81-year-old male, who recently underwent percutaneous MV clip repair for severe MR. 2DTTE was done.

1. **Arrow in 🎥 200 to 204 points to:**
   (a) MV clip with severe MR
   (b) MV clip, MV prolapse and moderate MR
   (c) Calcified MV apparatus with severe MR
   (d) MV clip, MV prolapse and mild MR

Ans. (d)

Both MV clip and MV prolapse are noted in 🎥 200. MR appears mild by color Doppler but it is eccentric and, therefore, most likely moderate. Also, the Nyquist limit is high at 61 cm/sec which will tend to underestimate MR severety. #1 and 2 in 🎥 202 point to a double orifice MV produced by insertion of the clip. Note that MR is mainly in the region of orifice #2.

2. **What does the arrow in 🎥 205 demonstrate:**
   (a) PFO with left to right shunt
   (b) Small ASD with left to right shunt
   (c) Congenital ASD with left to right shunt
   (d) Sinus venosus ASD with left to right shunt produced by MV clip

Ans. (b)

This small ASD was produced by transseptal puncture to enable the passage of the sheath and MV clip into the LA and MV. The puncture in the atrial septum was made superior to the PFO region (arrowhead in 🎥 206) to provide enough room in the LA to successfully maneuver placement of MV clip.

MOVIES 200 TO 206

CASE 68

Bulur S, Elsayed M, Nanda NC

This is a 67-year-old female with severe MR, who underwent percutaneous MV clip repair because she was not a surgical candidate due to co-existing morbidities. She came for an outpatient follow-up. Both 2D TTE and 3D TTE were done. The arrow in the movies points to the clip (207–210).

1. **What do the movies show?**
   (a) On 2DTTE, the clip appears to be attached to the posterior MV leaflet but not the anterior leaflet
   (b) There is significant residual MR
   (c) On 3D TTE, the clip appears attached to both MV leaflets with a resultant double orifice MV
   (d) All the above statements are correct
   (e) Only two of the above statements are correct, one statement is incorrect

Ans. (d)

3DTTE was superior to 2DTTE in this patient in displaying attachment of the clip to both anterior and posterior MV leaflets with a typical double orifice MV configuration (210). On 2DTTE, the clip is shown attached to the posterior leaflet but the anterior leaflet appears free with no evidence of clip (208). Despite the clip, the patient does have significant residual MR by color Doppler (209).

MOVIES 207 TO 210

CASE 69

Adarna LG, Elsayed M, Uygur B, Alagic N, Chahwala JR, Bhagatwala K, Bulur S, Turaga NSN, Kattalan JJP, Nanda NC

An 80-year-old male with a murmur of MR. 2D TTE was done (🎥 211).

1. **What does the movie show?**
   (a) Congenital double orifice MV
   (b) Acquired double orifice MV

Ans. (b)

The MV clip is clearly seen as an echogenic structure between the 2 MV inflow jets (#1 and #2). This patient underwent percutaneous MV clip placement for torrential MR due to MV A2 and P2 prolapse with chordae rupture. #3 and #4 represent residual MR from each of the two orifices.

MOVIE 211

CASE 70

Ahmad S Omran

MITRACLIP REPAIR IN DEGENERATIVE MITRAL VALVE DISEASE

This 76-year-old man presented to our center with acute pulmonary edema. Initial transthoracic echocardiography (TTE) showed a degenerative mitral valve with flail anterior leaflet (AMVL). Severe eccentric posteriorly directed jet of mitral regurgitation (MR) was noted. His left ventricular (LV) function was reduced with LV EF about 30%. After stabilization, the patient underwent coronary angiography which showed normal coronary arteries. Transesophageal echocardiography (TEE) was performed which confirmed the diagnosis of flail AMVL (at the A2 segment) with ruptured chordae (Figs. 70.1A and B, 212–214). During TEE, mitral valve (MV) was evaluated for possible MitraClip repair. Based on inclusion and exclusion criteria of EVEREST II Trial and EAE/ASE recommendations, this mitral valve was found to be suitable for percutaneous repair.

Patient was presented and discussed in our heart team. His overall assessment showed that he had a reasonable life expectancy, but a prohibitive surgical risk because of severe comorbidities. Decision by the heart team was to offer him percutaneous mitral valve repair (MitraClip repair).

Patient was transferred to the cath lab on the next day and the procedure was done under the guidance of 3D TEE, which was performed by an experienced echocardiographer. Because AMVL was flail and the mitral annulus dilated, multiple clip placement was planned by the operating team. Trans-septal puncture was performed at superior and posterior portion of the interatrial septum (IAS) guided by 3D TEE using the X-plane mode (Note: puncture site should be located about 4.5 cm above the level of the mitral valve closure and 2.5 cm posterior to the aortic root). As a technical rule, if multiple clip insertion is planned, the first clip should be inserted in the more medial portion of the mitral annulus to leave more space laterally for other clips. The first clip was successfully implanted. Clip stability and leaflet insertion were assessed by the 3D zoom mode and X-plane, and the degree of MR was evaluated as well (215–216). The degree of MR was only slightly reduced. The mean gradient across the mitral valve measured 2–3 mm Hg. The second clip was deployed by the same guiding catheter inside the left atrium in a more lateral position in relation to the first clip (220). Similar to the first clip,

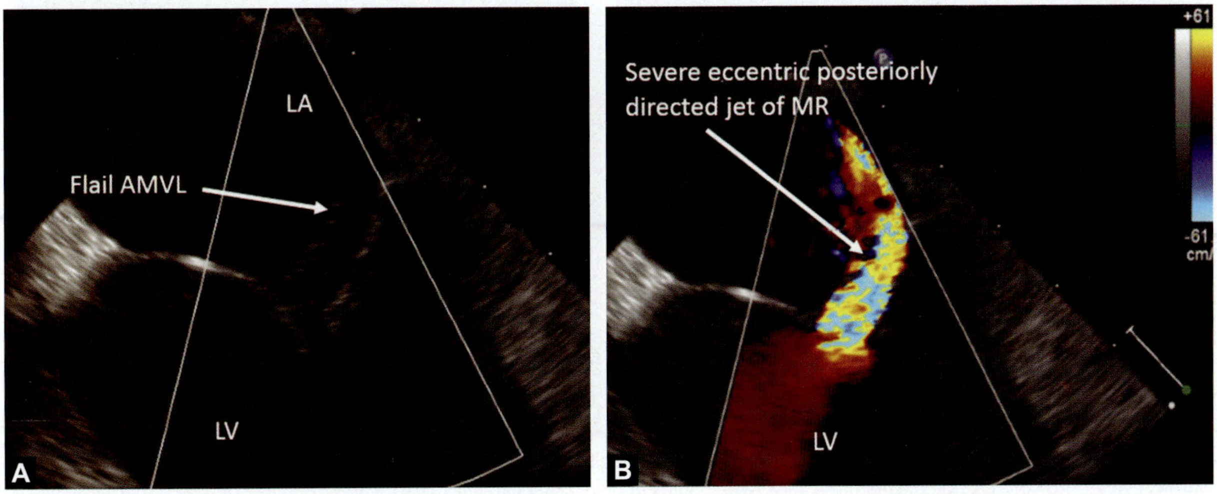

Figs. 70.1A and B: Pre-op TEE in the cath lab. (A) 2D TEE 4-chamber view showing degenerative mitral valve disease with a flail anterior mitral valve leaflet (AMVL) at middle segment (A2) and ruptured chordae. (B) Same view with color Doppler showing severe eccentric posteriorly directed jet of mitral regurgitation (MR). (LV: Left ventricle; LA: Left atrium).

the stability of the second clip was assessed carefully by 3D TEE in zoom and X-plane modes. More reduction of MR was noted but residual MR was still significant. Pulmonary venous inflow showed systolic blunting consistent with at least moderate MR. The mean gradient across the mitral valve was less than 4 mm Hg which encouraged the operating team to proceed with the third clip. After placement of the third clip, again lateral to the second one, only trivial MR remained. The mean gradient across the mitral valve was still less than 4 mm Hg at a heart rate of 80 beats per minutes, which ruled out any significant mitral stenosis. Pulmonary venous flow which had shown systolic reversal at pre-op echo, returned to an almost normal pattern. 3D TEE images of 3 clips in left atrial view and LV view as well as fluoroscopic are shown in this case (Figs. 70.2A and B, 3A and B, 217–219 and 221). Patient was extubated 2 hours later and discharged home the following day. At the 3-week follow-up, his general condition had significantly improved and TTE showed only mild residual MR and no significant mitral stenosis.

MitraClip repair received European CE Mark in 2008 and FDA approval for using in degenerative mitral valve disease in USA in 2013.[1] Currently more than 500 centers in the world are performing this procedure more than 27,000 patients have been treated by this method. In EVEREST II Trial, 184 patients were treated by MitraClip repair, about 73.4% of whom had degenerative mitral valve regurgitation and the rest had functional mitral valve disease. In the EVEREST group, 32% of patients had 2 clip insertion and the rest only one. In some European centers, insertion of 3 or 4 clips is becoming more popular in recent years. Currently, two large multicenter trials for MitraClip repair in functional MR are on the way: RESHAPE-HF in Europe and COAPT in North America.

Echocardiography plays a major role in appropriate selection of patients, monitoring the procedure in the cath lab, and in patients' follow-up.[2] It should be emphasized that, TEE, especially 3D TEE with live en-face view of the mitral valve during the procedure in cath lab, creates a common language between echo and interventional cardiologists. This common language plays a crucial role during the procedure.

1. In pre-op echocardiography for selection of the mitral valve for MitraClip repair, all of the followings are exclusion criteria *except*:

(a) Rheumatic mitral valve
(b) Degenerative mitral valve with flail posterior leaflet.
(c) Leaflet perforations.
(d) Mitral valve area less than 4 cm^2.

Ans. (b)

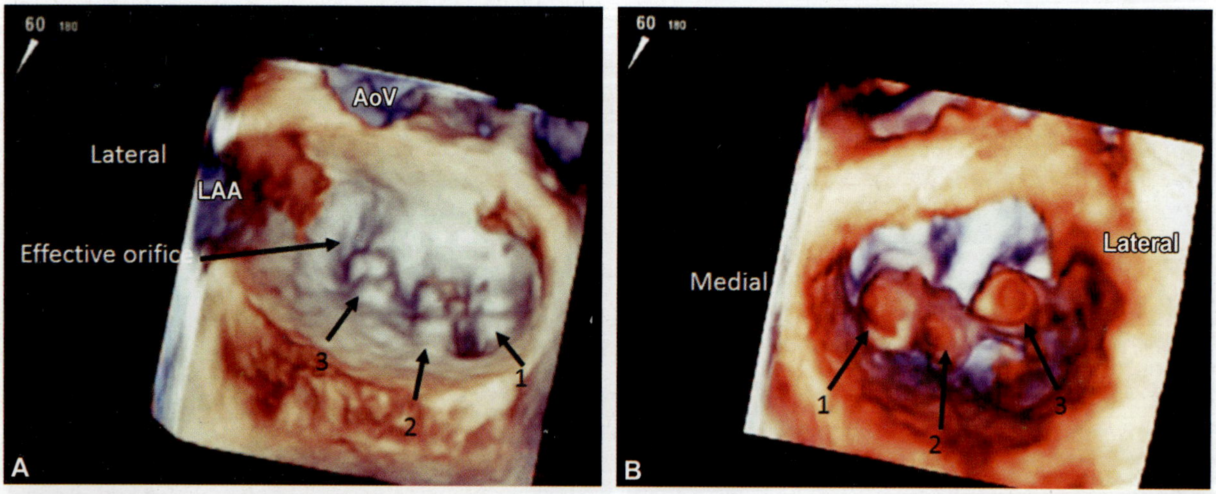

Figs. 70.2A and B: Post-op 3D TEE in the cath lab after insertion of 3 clips. (A) 3D TEE zoom mode acquisition of the mitral valve in en-face view (surgical view) showing LA side of the mitral valve with 3 clips in place. First clip (clip 1) is located medially between medial scallop of the posterior mitral leaflet (P3) and medial segment of the anterior mitral leaflet (A3). Other clips are located towards the lateral side of the mitral valve. New effective orifice of the mitral valve is located adjacent to the lateral commissure of the mitral valve and left atrial appendage (LAA). (B) 3D zoom mode of the mitral valve from left ventricular side. (AoV: Aortic valve).

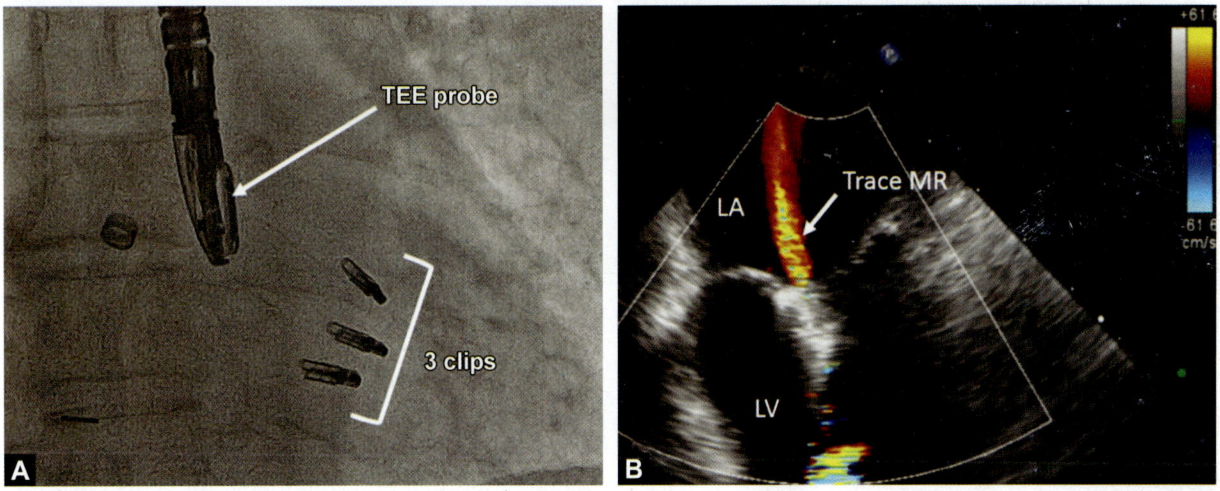

Figs. 70.3A and B: (A) Fluoroscopy view of the procedure showing side by side placement of 3 clips. TEE probe is seen in this image as well. (B) 2D TEE image with color Doppler performed toward the end of the procedure shows only trivial residual MR. (LA: Left atrium; LV: Left ventricle).

MOVIE LEGENDS

212: Preoperative TEE in the cath lab showing flail anterior mitral leaflet at the middle segment (A2).

213: Same view of previous movie with color Doppler showing severe eccentric posteriorly directed jet of MR.

214: 3D TEE zoom mode, surgical view showing flail A2 with ruptured chordae.

215: Same view of previous movie showing one clip insertion at the medial portion of the mitral closure line between A3 and P3.

216: Same view of previous movie with full volume acquisition showing significant residual MR after the first clip.

217: 2D TEE at commissural view after insertion of 3 clips showing trace residual MR.

218: 3D TEE zoom mode, surgical view of the mitral valve showing all 3 clips in place with good grasp of the leaflets and synchronized motion with heartbeats.

219: 3D TEE zoom mode, showing mitral valve from LV side with all 3 clips in place and good grasp of both mitral leaflets.

220: Fluoroscopic view after insertion of 2 clips. Clips are moving with each cardiac cycle in a synchronized manner with no jerk movement.

221: Fluoroscopic view after insertion of 3 clips showing normal motion.

REFERENCES

1. Mauri L, Foster E, Glower DD, et al. 4 year results of a randomized controlled trial of percutaneous repair versus surgery for mitral regurgitation. J Am Coll Cardiol 2013; 62:317-28.
2. Zamorano JL, Badano LP, Bruce C, et al. EAE/ASE recommendations for the use of echocardiography in new transcatheter interventions for valvular heart disease. J Am Soc Echocardiogr 2011;24:937-65.

CASE 71

Ahmad S Omran

MITRACLIP DETACHMENT

This 73-year-old man was admitted in our center with severe functional mitral regurgitation (MR). Transthoracic echocardiography (TTE) and transesophageal echocardiography (TEE) were performed to confirm the diagnosis and assess suitability for MitraClip repair. The patient was discussed in our heart team and was accepted for this procedure.

The next day, the patient was transferred to the cath lab and the procedure was performed by our MitraClip team including two interventional cardiologists and one echocardiographer. 3D TEE was used to guide and monitor the procedure. One clip was placed between the lateral scallop of the posterior mitral valve leaflet (P1) and the lateral segment of the anterior mitral valve leaflet (A1). 2D TEE showed a good reduction in the degree of MR (Figs. 71.1A and B, 222–223). 3D TEE zoom mode acquisition of the mitral valve (MV) from left ventricular side confirmed the stability of the device and adequate leaflet insertion (Fig. 71.2A, 224). Cardiac interventionists released the clip. Ten minutes after releasing, the degree of MR increased and became severe similar to the pre-op echo study (225). 3D TEE zoom mode from LV side showed the clip detached from the posterior mitral leaflet with attachment to only the anterior leaflet (Fig. 71.2B, 226 and 228). Fluoroscopy showed jerky movements of the clip during the cardiac cycle, which is one of the signs of partial detachment of the device (227). The procedure was stopped and the patient was transferred to CCU for further monitoring.

In CCU, the patient was awake and stable with no neurologic abnormality. Daily follow-up echoes were done, which showed no change compared to the post-op study in the cath lab. Six days after the procedure, TTE failed to show the presence of any clip in the region of the MV. The patient was still neurologically intact. TEE was performed immediately, which showed the clip was completely detached from the mitral leaflets, fallen into the LV cavity, and stuck between chordae and papillary muscles (229-231). Cardiac surgery team was consulted and a decision was made to transfer the patient to the operating room (OR) right away.

In the OR, the mitral valve was explored through the left atrium. The posterior mitral valve leaflet showed severe laceration of the middle and medial scallops (Figs. 71.3A and B). Two ruptured chordae were seen attached to the anterior mitral leaflet. These changes

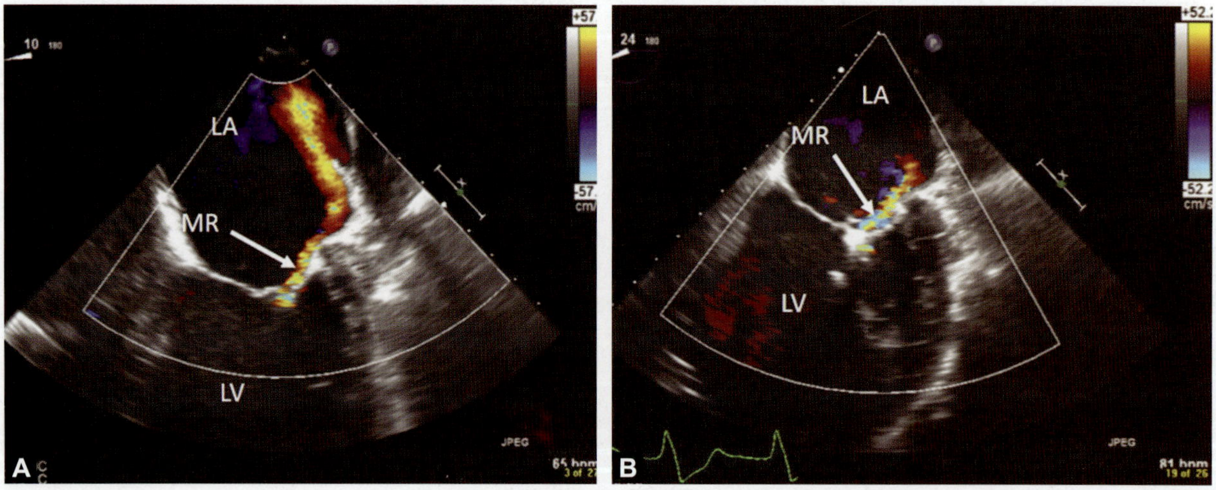

Figs. 71.1A and B: TEE in the cath lab. (A) Pre-op 2D TEE with color in 4-chamber view showing moderate to severe eccentric posteriorly directed jet of mitral regurgitation (MR). (B) Immediate post-op 2D TEE study shows mild residual MR after placement of one clip. (LV: Left ventricle; LA: Left atrium).

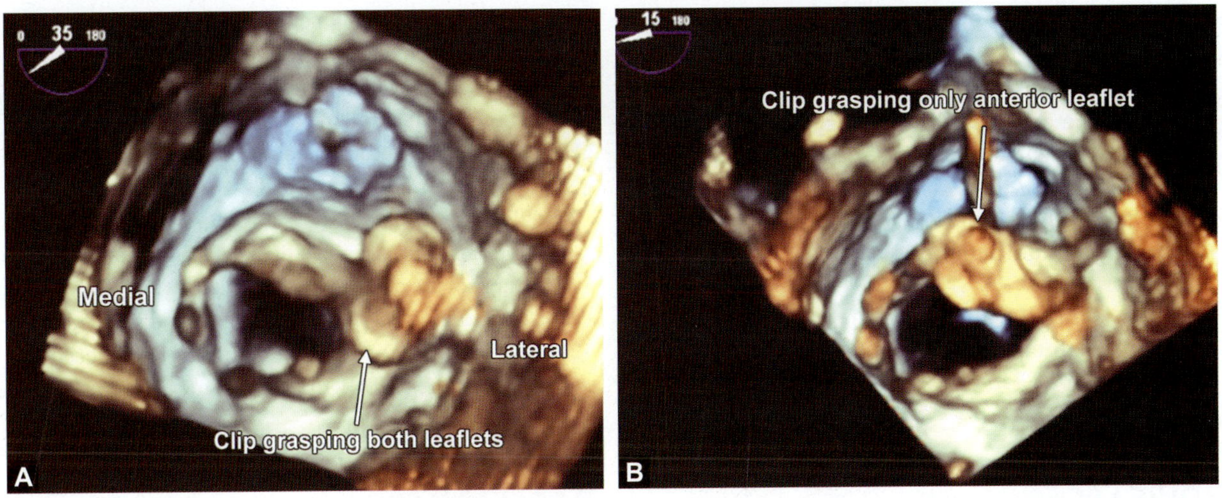

Figs. 71.2A and B: Post-op 3D TEE in the cath lab after insertion of one clip. (A) 3D TEE zoom mode acquisition of the mitral valve from LV perspective showing clip placed at lateral segments of the mitral valve. Clip appears grasping both leaflets equally. (B) Same view of the mitral valve 10 minutes after insertion of the clip showing attachment of the device only to the anterior leaflet.

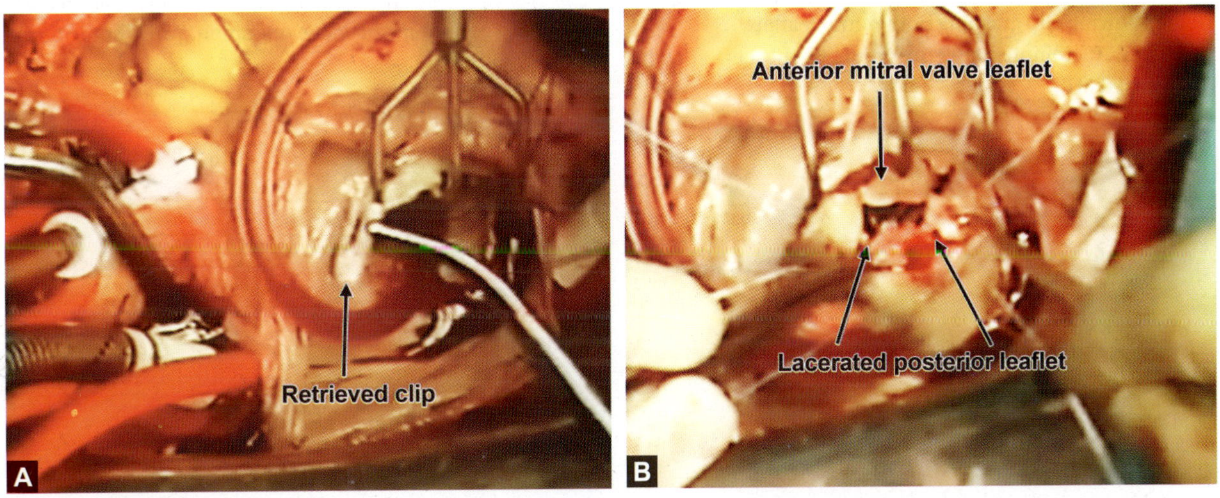

Figs. 71.3A and B: Surgical exploration through the left atrium. (A) Clip is shown retrieved from the left ventricular cavity. Clip was stuck between chordae. (B) Posterior mitral leaflet with damaged tissue. Two chordae of the anterior mitral leaflet were ruptured (not shown in this image).

on mitral valve had not been identified by pre-op TEE; therefore, they were attributed to iatrogenic tissue damage from multiple attempts during insertion of the clip. Mitral valve was repaired by replacing ruptured chordae and implanting an annuloplasty ring. Postoperative process was uneventful and the patient was discharged home in a good general condition a week later. Follow-up visit after 2 years showed the patient was still in good shape with NYHA class ll functional capacity. TTE at follow-up showed moderate residual MR.

Clip embolization is a rare complication of MitraClip repair. More commonly, the clip may partially become detached, which can usually be treated by surgery. Low rates of clip detachment have been reported in the literatures. As an example, in the EVEREST ll Trial, nine patients were noted in the first 12 months to have partial clip detachment; one additional patient developed partial clip detachment in the second year of trial.[1] In our cardiac center, this was the only case of clip detachment in the first year of our program. In the following 3 years, 50 cases of MitraClip repair were performed with no such a complication.

1. **In COAPT Trial (for treatment of patients with heart failure and functional mitral regurgitation), all of the followings are inclusion criteria *except*:**
   (a) Functional MR ≥ 3+ due to cardiomyopathy of either ischemic or nonischemic etiology.
   (b) Symptomatic patient (NYHA class ll, lll or ambulatory IV).
   (c) Decision of local heart team to decline the surgical treatment option due to prohibitive risk.
   (d) CABG or PCI in last 30 days.

Ans. (d)

MOVIE LEGENDS

222: Preoperative TEE in the cath lab showing moderate to severe eccentric posteriorly directed jet of mitral regurgitation.

223: Same view of previous movie after insertion of one clip. Only mild residual MR is noted.

224: 3D TEE zoom mode acquisition of the mitral valve from LV side showing clip grasping both mitral leaflets.

225: 2D TEE 10 minutes after insertion of the clip showing increased MR.

226: 3D TEE confirmation of partial detachment of the clip. Device is moving only with the anterior mitral leaflet.

227: Fluoroscopy view of the clip showing jerky movements of the clip with cardiac cycles.

228: 2D TEE in the cath lab showing attachment of the clip to only the anterior mitral leaflet.

229: 2D TEE on day 6 after procedure showing obvious flail anterior mitral leaflet (due to newly ruptured chordae). Ghost of the clip can be recognized within the chordae.

230: 2D TEE for better visualization of the dislodged clip.

231: 2D TEE in 4-chamber view showing severe eccentric posteriorly directed MR due to flail anterior mitral valve leaflet at A2.

REFERENCES

1. Whitlow PL, Feldman T, Pedersen WR, et al. Acute and 12-month results with catheter-based mitral valve repair. The EVEREST ll (Endovascular Valve Edge-to-Edge Repair) High Risk Study. J Am Coll Cardiol. 2012;59:130-9.
2. Giedel S, Schmoeckel M. Impact of failed mitral clipping in subsequent mitral valve operation. Ann Thorac Surg. 2014; 97:56-63.

CASE 72

Adarna LG, Nanda NC

Adult patient s/p metallic aortic prosthesis. 2D TTE was done.

1. **High gradients detected across an aortic prosthetic valve which shows completely normal leaflet motion by 2D echo (232, R = reverberation from prosthetic AV) may be due to all of the following *except*:**
   (a) Prosthesis patient mismatch
   (b) Severe prosthetic valve regurgitation
   (c) Pannus/thrombus formation
   (d) LVOT/supravalvar obstruction

Ans. (c)

Parasternal long axis view shows both leaflets of the metallic aortic prosthetic valve moving well consistent with no obstruction. Since metallic prosthetic valves normally show significant gradients, it is important to assess motion of individual leaflets and unrestricted motion helps rule out prosthetic obstruction. 3D echo may be helpful in assessing motion of both leaflets if only one leaflet or no leaflet is visualized on the 2D echo. Also, high gradients across normally functioning aortic prosthetic valves may be due to significant regurgitation or prosthesis patient mismatch.

MOVIE 232

CASE 73

Jaehoon Chung, Leon J Frazin

PREMATURE DEGENERATION OF BIOPROSTHETIC AORTIC VALVE

A 59-year-old male with past medical history of hypertension, type 2 diabetes and hyperlipidemia, who underwent aortic valve replacement with a 25-mm Freestyle stentless porcine valve for severe aortic stenosis due to bicuspid valve 7 years ago, presented to the emergency department complaining of worsening chest pain with exertion over the past 24 hours. On the physical exam, his blood pressure was 113/53 mm Hg. Heart rate was 74 beats per minute. Jugular venous pressure measures 8 cm H_2O. Cardiac auscultation revealed 3/6 systolic ejection murmur on the right upper sternal border. ECG did not show significant ST deviation. Troponin was 4.2 ng/mL. NT-pro BNP was 3450 pg/mL. Chest X-ray showed mildly increased pulmonary vascular congestion. Coronary angiography revealed no significant obstruction. Transthoracic echocardiography revealed normal left ventricular systolic function and a well seated bioprosthetic aortic valve with mean gradient of 26.4 mm Hg and peak velocity of 3.8 m/sec. Aortic valve area by the continuity equation was 1.5 cm^2. Further evaluation by transesophageal echocardiography was performed and the following clips were acquired (🎥 233–235).

1. **What is the diagnosis?**
   (a) Severe aortic stenosis
   (b) Severe aortic regurgitation
   (c) Normally functioning aortic valve
   (d) Paravalvular leak

Ans. (b)

2. **What is the underlying mechanism of Question 1?**
   (a) Premature degeneration of the prosthetic valve
   (b) Thrombus of the prosthetic valve
   (c) Pannus formation
   (d) Endocarditis

Ans. (a)

The transesophageal echocardiographic finding is consistent with severe aortic regurgitation secondary to premature degeneration of bioprosthetic aortic valve. Urgently, the patient was taken to the operating room. The aortic homograft was severely calcified. Left coronary cusp was completely degenerated and torn from the graft. There was severe inflammation on the coronary buttons. Histologic evaluation confirmed severe degeneration and calcification of the bioprosthesis (Figs. 73.1A and B). Subsequently, the whole aortic root was reconstructed with a 23 mm St. Jude valve conduit. The patient recovered without further complications.

Previous studies have shown that 25 to 40% of porcine heterograft prostheses have failed within 10 to 15 years of implantation.[1,2] The failure rate with porcine valves is higher with valves in the mitral position than in the aortic position.

A variety of factors can contribute to structural failure with bioprosthetic valves. Known risk factors are young age at the time of implantation, hyperparathyroidism, renal insufficiency.[3] Recently, Briand et al reported that metabolic syndrome is independently associated with accelerated degeneration of bioprosthetic valve.[4] In our case, the patient was relatively young at the time of the bioprosthetic valve implantation. In addition, our patient has had long standing metabolic syndrome and poorly controlled hypertension. Although the incidence is rare with the modern bioprosthetic aortic valve, premature degeneration should always be suspected in patients with high risk features.

MOVIE LEGENDS 🎥

233: 2 DTEE: Shows a flail bioprosthetic AVR with severe AR.
234 and 235: 2DTEE (left) and 3DTEE(right). Show a flail AVR with thickened leaflets.

REFERENCES

1. Hammermeister, K.E., et al., A comparison of outcomes in men 11 years after heart-valve replacement with a mechanical valve or bioprosthesis. Veterans Affairs Cooperative Study on Valvular Heart Disease. N Engl J Med, 1993. 328(18): p. 1289-96.

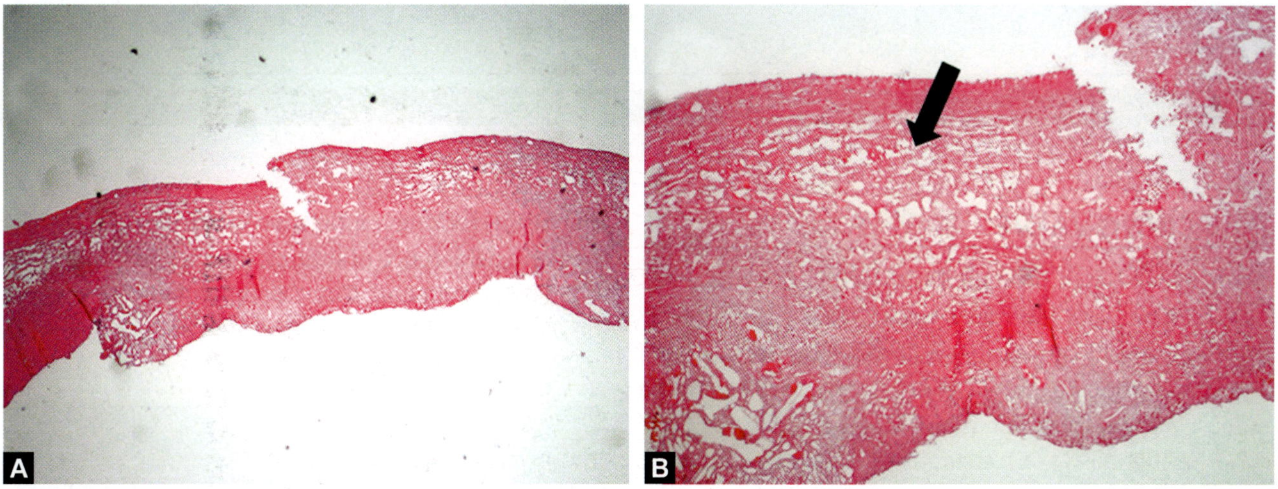

Figs. 73.1A and B: (A) Low power field of bioprosthetic valve leaflet. (B) High power field of the same slide. H & E staining of bioprosthetic valve leaflet demonstrates multiple vacuoles (indicated by a black arrow), consistent with severe degeneration and calcification.

2. Hammermeister, K., et al., Outcomes 15 years after valve replacement with a mechanical versus a bioprosthetic valve: final report of the Veterans Affairs randomized trial. J Am Coll Cardiol, 2000;36(4):1152-8.
3. Pibarot, P. and J.G. Dumesnil, Prosthetic heart valves: selection of the optimal prosthesis and long-term management. Circulation, 2009;119(7):1034-48.
4. Briand, M., et al., Metabolic syndrome is associated with faster degeneration of bioprosthetic valves. Circulation, 2006;114(1 Suppl):1512-7.

CASE 74

Armin Barekatain, Ahmed Abuzaid, Aiman Smer

ROCKING VALVE

A 49-year-old man presented with acute onset of shortness of breath and fever for 3 weeks. He has history of IV drug abuse and bioprosthetic aortic valve replacement 3 years ago. Blood cultures were drawn and he was started empirically on intravenous antibiotics. A transthoracic echocardiogram (TTE) demonstrated rocking motion (Figs. 74.1 and 74.2 and 236 and 237). In addition to the almost complete dehiscence of the aortic prosthesis, color Doppler shows significant paravalvular leak (Fig. 74.3 and 238). Unfortunately, the patient's clinical condition deteriorated dramatically and died a day later.

1. **In a patient with a rocking prosthetic valve, the most reliable technique for assessing paravalvular regurgitation severity is 2D echo rather than color Doppler.**
   (a) True
   (b) False

Ans. (a)

Significant rocking motion as in this patient signifies extensive dehiscence of sutures, indicative of severe paravalvular regurgitation. Color Doppler may underestimate the severity because of the dispersion of the jet by rocking

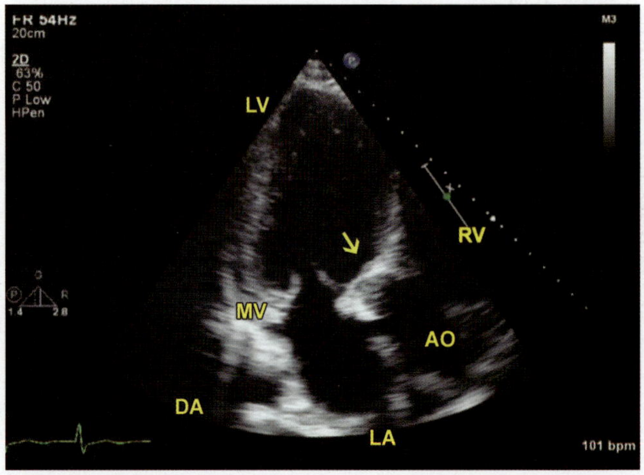

Fig. 74.2: TTE apical long axis view demonstrates same findings as above.

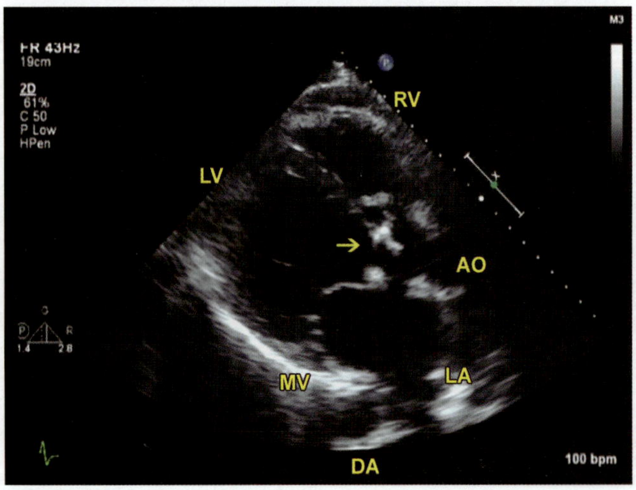

Fig. 74.1: TTE parasternal long axis view demonstrates rocking motion of the aortic bioprosthesis; this indicates significant dehiscence of the aortic bioprosthesis (arrow) and severe paravalvular AR. Note that the bioprosthesis leaflets are thickened and restricted.

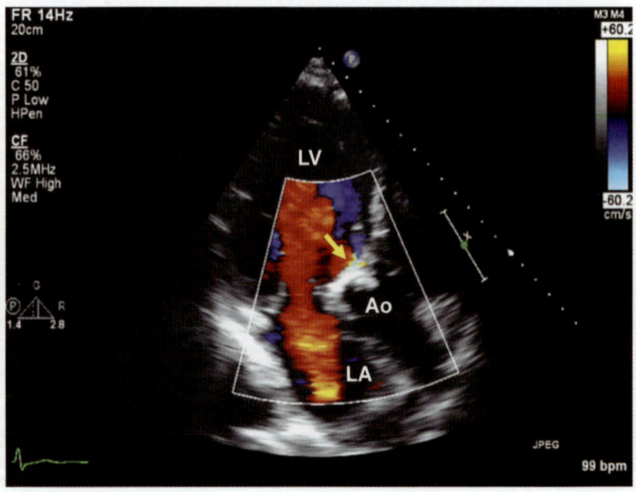

Fig. 74.3: TTE apical long axis view with color Doppler demonstrates para-valvular leak (arrow).

motion resulting in adequate color Doppler signals. In this patient also, paravalvular color Doppler signals are not as impressive as rocking motion.

MOVIE LEGENDS

236: TTE parasternal long axis view demonstrates rocking motion of the aortic bioprosthesis; this indicates significant dehiscence of the aortic bioprosthesis (arrow) and severe paravalvular AR. Note that the bioprosthesis leaflets are thickened and restricted.

237: TTE apical long axis view demonstrates same findings as above.

238: TTE apical long axis view with color Doppler demonstrates paravalvular leak (arrow).

CASE 75

Fabiola B Sozzi, Francois Bourlon

A 91-year-old man with severe symptomatic aortic stenosis underwent a transfemoral aortic valve (Edward Sapien XT23) implantation. One week later, the patient returned complaining of shortness of breath. This time severe aortic valve stenosis with migration of the prosthesis into the left ventricular outflow tract was found by TEE (arrow in Figs. 75.1 and 75.2, 🎥 239 and 240). Through the transgastric view, impingement of the protruding prosthetic valve on the anterior mitral leaflet was noted (arrow in Fig. 75.3 and 🎥 241). A successful subsequent urgent open heart surgery for device retrieval and prosthesis replacement with implantation of a bioprosthesis was performed.

This case highlights the importance of correctly sizing the annulus and evaluating the prosthetic valve for ensuring an accurate coaxial deployment.

1. **What is the structure visualized in the LVOT through the TEE midesophageal long-axis view (longitudinal view)?**
   (a) Discrete subvalvular aortic membrane (thin fibromuscular shelf located at the area of aorto-mitral continuity with extension toward the interventricular septum). It is frequently associated with congenital heart defects.
   (b) Endocardial vegetation in the LVOT
   (c) Caudal prosthetic valve migration into the LVOT
   (d) Calcified thrombus adherent to the LVOT

Ans. (c)

The calcificed native aortic valve, and the prosthetic valve displaced into the LVOT, are shown.

2. **What additional information does the color Doppler provide?**
   (a) Aortic stenosis
   (b) Aortic regurgitation
   (c) Aortic stenosis with the aliaising secondary to a subaortic membrane
   (d) None

Ans. (a)

Color Doppler TEE shows absence of significant aortic regurgitation.

3. **What is the structure visualized in the LVOT through the TEE deep transgastric long-axis view?**
   (a) Native calcified aortic valve
   (b) Prosthetic valve displaced into the LVOT
   (c) Discrete subvalvular aortic membrane

Ans. (b)

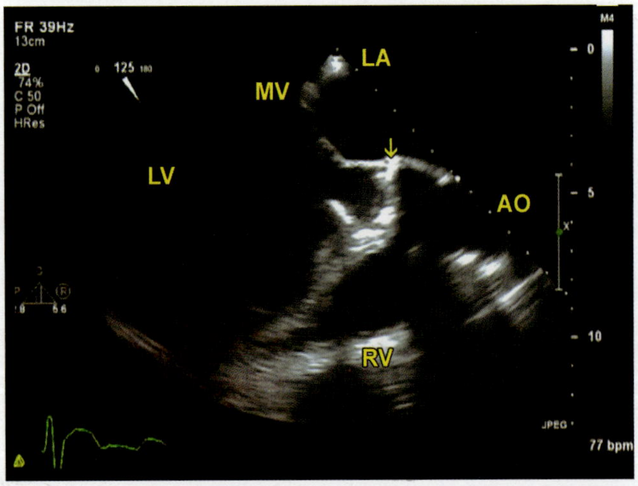

Fig. 75.1: TTE midesophageal long-axis view.

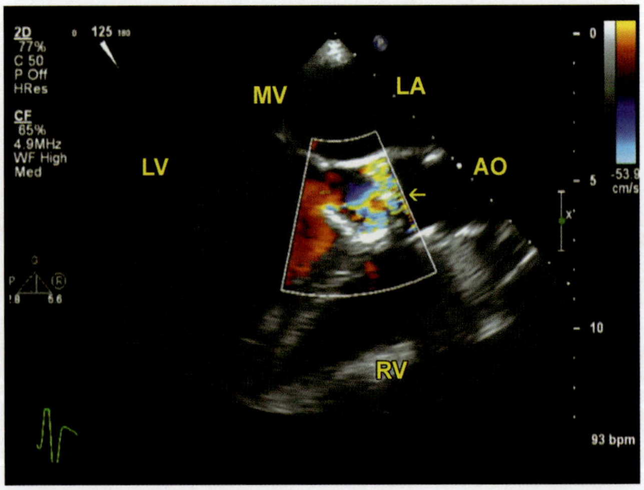

Fig. 75.2: TTE midesophageal long-axis view: Color Doppler.

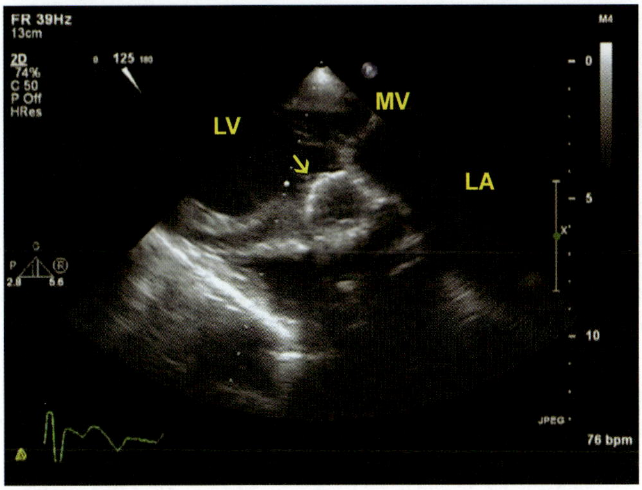

Fig. 75.3: TEE transgastric long-axis view (120°).

TEE transgastric long-axis view shows prominent prosthesis migration into the LVOT and impingement on the anterior mitral leaflet. This view is useful to show the aortic valve and the LVOT.

MOVIE LEGENDS

239: TEE midesophageal long-axis view.
240: TEE midesophageal long-axis view: Color Doppler.
241: TEE transgastric long-axis view (120°)

CASE 76

Ahmad S Omran

FAILED TRANSCATHETER AORTIC VALVE REPLACEMENT (TAVR)

This 74-year-old man was admitted in our center with a failed TAVR (TAVI). TAVR was performed in our center about a year ago because of severe aortic stenosis (AS) and mild aortic regurgitation (AR). His baseline left ventricular (LV) function was normal (LVEF about 55%). In the cath lab during TAVR, preoperative TEE showed trileaflet calcified aortic valve with aortic annulus size of 2.3 cm. He underwent TAVR with a CoreValve size 29. Postoperative TEE in the cath lab showed mild anteriorly located paravalvular AR. The position of the valve in the aortic root was normal by fluoroscopy (Figs. 76.1A and B, 242–244). He was followed in our center based on our TAVR protocol. Serial follow-up echo studies showed a gradual increase in the degree of paravalvular AR and a decrease in LV function.

His last transthoracic echocardiography done one year after the procedure showed moderate to severe AR (Figs. 76.2A and B) and LVEF of 25-35%. Decision was made by the heart team to balloon expand the TAVR. Patient was taken to the cath lab and several attempts for dilatatio were done using different sizes of balloons (245 and 246). The degree of paravalvular AR did not change. Patient was discharged for re-admission in a month and surgical intervention. In the cardiac surgery, the prosthesis was extracted from the aortic root with a great difficulty because of severe adhesion (Figs. 76.1A and B). The CoreValve which appeared intact was replaced by a conventional bioprosthetic aortic valve. The postoperative course was uneventful and the patient was discharged home after one week in a good general condition. Follow-up visit after 3 years showed the patient had a good functional capacity. TTE showed significant improvement of LV function to near normal, and a well-functioning bioprosthetic aortic valve.

1. **In echocardiographic assessment of transvalvular and paravalvular aortic regurgitation (AR) after TAVR, all of the following are correct *except*:**
   (a) Patients with mild or higher degree of AR have a worse outcome compared to patients with no or trivial AR.
   (b) Studies have shown that prosthesis undersizing, aortic annular calcification, and prosthesis long-axis malpositioning are the main causes for paravalvular AR.
   (c) Oversized prosthesis may cause central transvalvular AR.

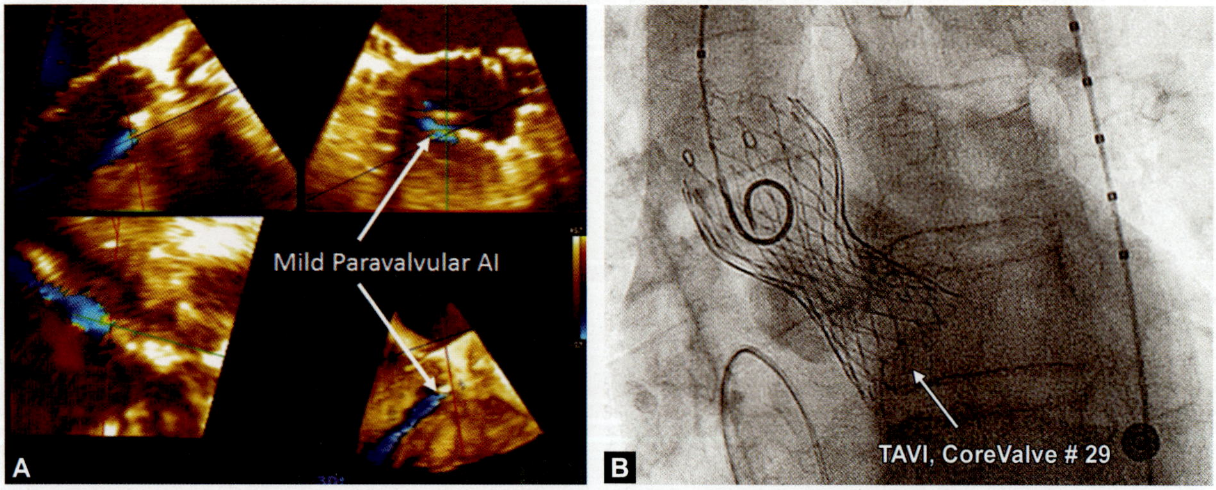

Figs. 76.1A and B: Intraoperative TEE and fluoroscopy in cath lab during TAVR procedure. (A) 3D TEE multiplanar reconstruction (MPR) mode acquisition showing mild paravalvular aortic regurgitation from anterior aspect of the aortic annulus. (B) Fluoroscopy view of CoreValve size 29 with acceptable position.

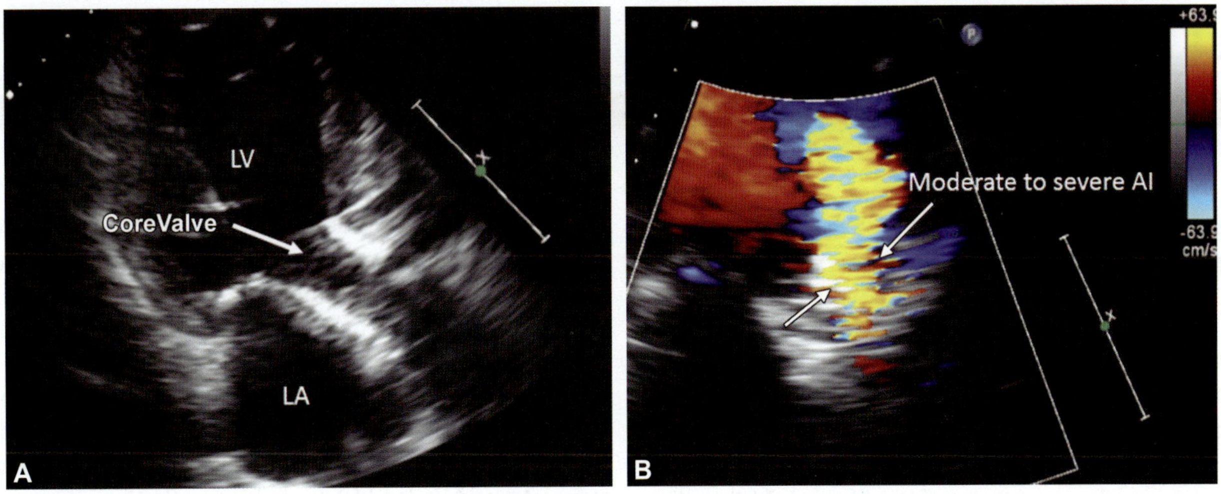

Figs. 76.2A and B: Follow-up transthoracic echocardiography (TTE) one year after TAVR. (A) Parasternal long-axis view showing CoreValve in normal position. (B) Moderate to severe aortic regurgitation, mostly paravalvular. (LA: Left atrium; LA: Left ventricle).

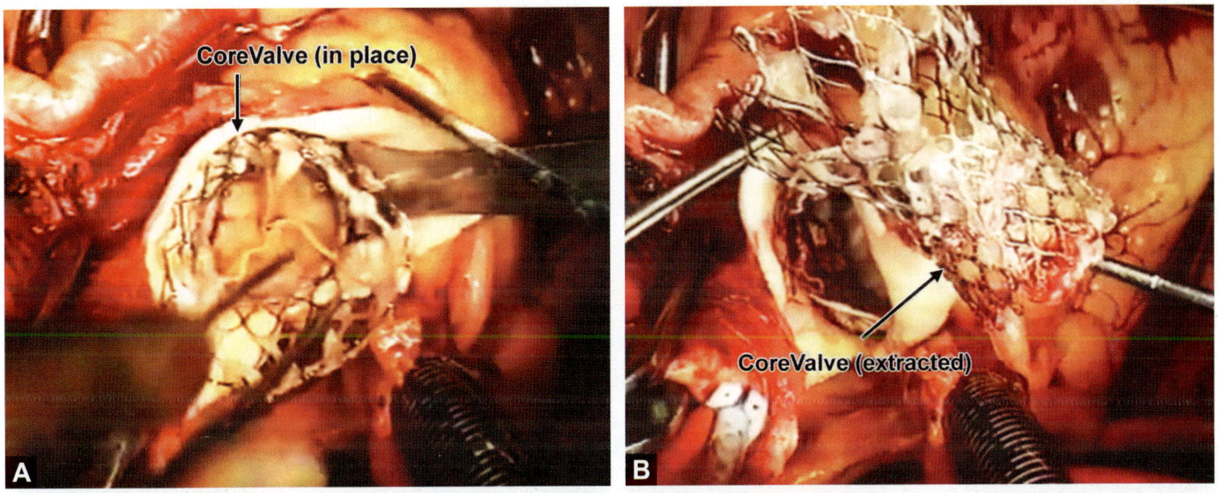

Figs. 76.3A and B: Surgical exploration of TAVR. (A) CoreValve is noted in place. Wire frame of TAVR was so deeply attached to the aortic wall that extraction of the valve was very challenging and time-consuming. (B) Extracting valve with intact frame and leaflets.

(d) Prevalence of moderate paravalvular AR is about 9% and moderate transvalvular AR 0.5% after TAVR.

Ans. (c)

MOVIE LEGENDS

242: Intraoperative 3D TEE in cath lab during TAVR showing mild paravalvular AR using X-plane.

243: 2D TEE in the cath lab in long-axis view showing mild paravalvular AR from the anterior aortic annulus.

244: 3D TEE zoom mode acquisition, showing the implanted valve from aortic perspective. TAVR is seated well.

245: 3D TEE in cath lab one year after TAVR when patient was taken for balloon expansion in an attempt to reduce paravalvular AR. Balloon inflation is demonstrated in the X-plane view.

246: Zoom mode live acquisition to demonstrate balloon inflation.

REFERENCES

1. Mihara H, Shibayama K, Jilaihawi H, et al. Assessment of postprocedural aortic regurgitation after TAVR. J Am Coll Cardiol Img. 2015;8(9):993-1003.
2. Shibayama K, Mihara H, Jilaihawi H, et al. 3-Dimensional assessment of features associated with transvalvular aortic regurgitation after TAVR: A real-time 3D TEE study. J Am Coll Cardiol Img. 2016;9(2):114-123.

CASE 77

Ahmad S Omran

BIOPROSTHETIC AORTIC VALVE ENDOCARDITIS

This 66-year-old man presented to our center with chronic history of fever, malaise, and weight loss. He was diagnosed with brucellosis six months previously and was being treated. He had a history of aortic valve replacement with a sutureless bioprosthetic valve (Edwards Intuity) 2 years ago due to aortic valve endocarditis. Recent blood cultures were positive for *Staph. aureus*. Initial transthoracic echocardiography (TTE) showed normal left ventricular function and mild bioprosthetic aortic valve regurgitation. There was haziness adjacent to the aortic root on the left atrial side with some color Doppler flow signals within (Figs. 77.1A and B). Transesophageal echocardiography (TEE) showed a honeycomb appearance around the aortic root, especially at the posterior aspect adjacent to the left atrium, and Doppler color flow signals within the cavities, consistent with aortic root abscess. A vegetation was noted and the abscess cavity extended to the aortic-mitral junction (Figs. 77.2A and B, 🎥 247 to 252). Patient was taken to the operating room (OR) after 3 days initial antibiotic therapy. Sutureless aortic valve which was infected at the posterior annulus was extracted. A large abscess cavity in the area of intervalvular fibrosa (aortic-mitral curtain) (Figs. 77.3A and B) was debrided and reconstructed using a bovine pericardial patch. Aortic and mitral valves were replaced by bioprosthetic valves. Immediate postoperative TEE showed a normally functioning bioprosthetic aortic valve, but there was a severe transvalvular MR from bioprosthetic mitral valve (MVR). More careful assessment of the MVR by 3D TEE in surgical view showed restriction of the movement of posterior two cusps as etiology for severe transvalvular MR (🎥 253 and 254). Findings were discussed with the surgical team in the OR and decision was made to place the patient back on pump. Surgical exploration found two sutures entrapping the two posterior cusps of the bioprosthetic mitral valve. Sutures were removed and patient came off the pump successfully. Re-assessment of the valve by 3D TEE (🎥 255 and 256) showed normal motion of the bioprosthetic mitral leaflets with no residual MR. Patient was discharged home one week later in a good general condition. Intraoperative 3D TEE played a crucial role in recognizing this intraoperative complication by

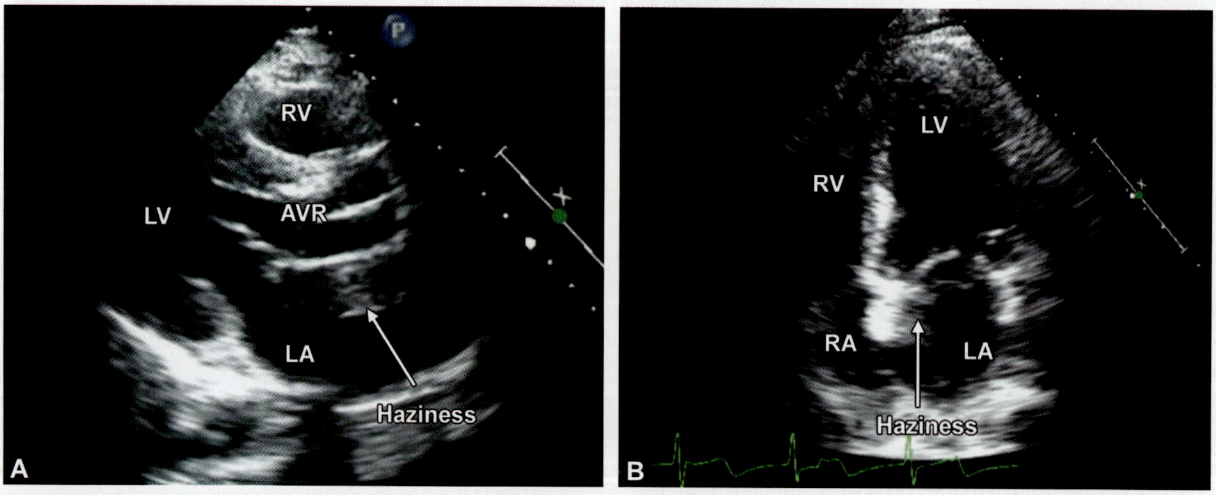

Figs. 77.1A and B: Transthoracic echocardiography (TTE). (A) Parasternal long-axis view showing bioprosthetic aortic valve (AVR) with haziness on the LA side. (B) Parasternal 4-chamber view showing same haziness inside the LA adjacent to the aortic root. Although this haziness could be an artifact, a periprosthetic abscess cavity should be considered in the differential diagnosis (RV: Right ventricle; LV: Left ventricle; RA: Right atrium; LA: Left atrium).

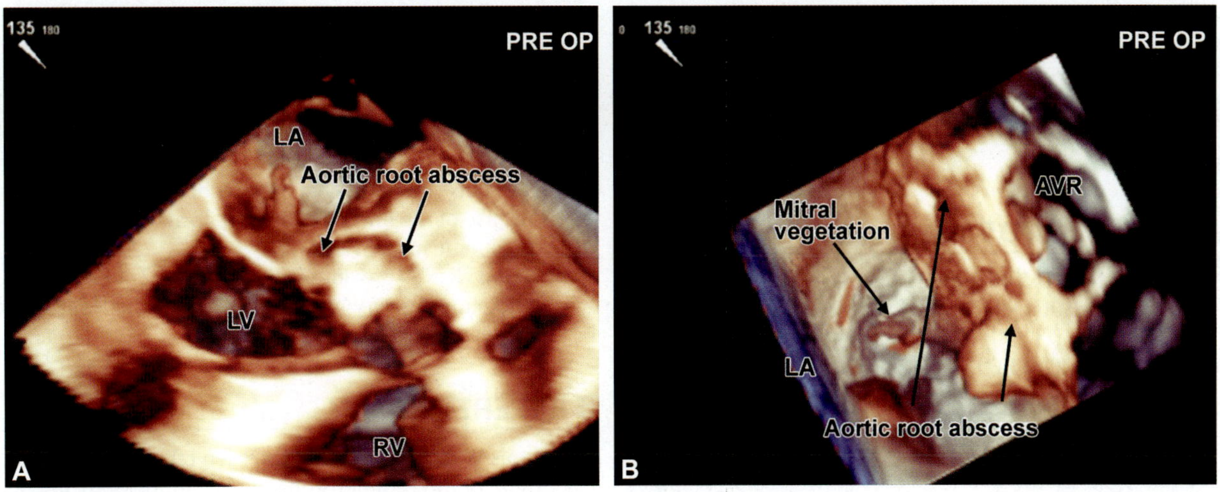

Figs. 77.2A and B: Preoperative 3D transesophageal echocardiography (3DTEE). (A) 3D zoom full-volume acquisition of the aortic root in long-axis view shows a large abscess cavity around the posterior aortic annulus with a multilobular (honeycomb) appearance. (B) 3D zoom mode acquisition of the aortic root shows the large abscess cavity between aortic root and LA involving the entire aortic-mitral curtain. Infection is extending to the base of the anterior mitral leaflet with a large mobile vegetation attached to the LA side of the anterior mitral leaflet. (RV: Right ventricle; LV: Left ventricle; LA: Left atrium; AVR: Aortic valve replacement).

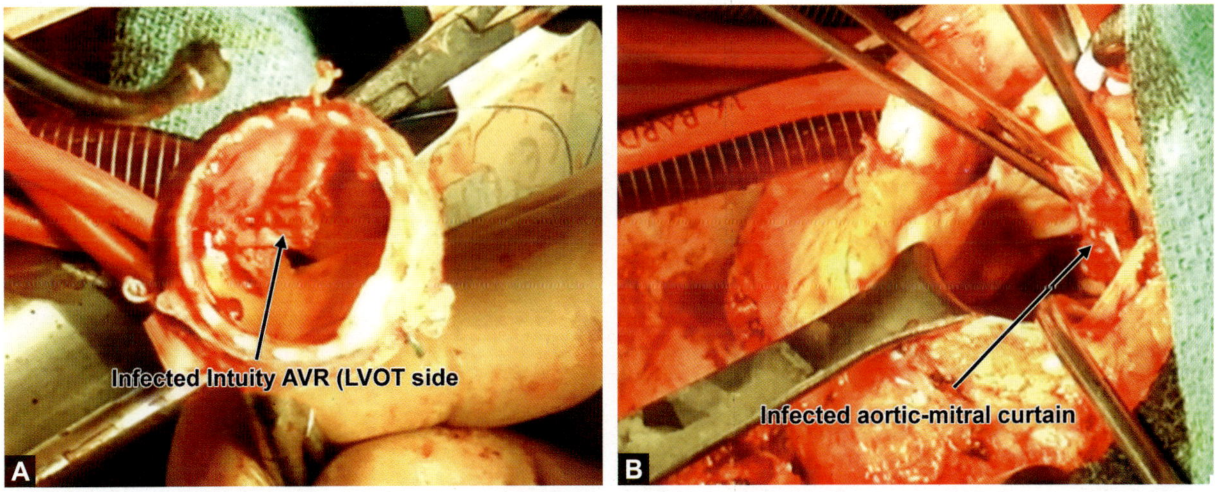

Figs. 77.3A and B: Surgical exploration of the aortic root. (A) Bioprosthetic aortic valve (Edwards Intuity valve) was extracted and is shown from LVOT side. Infection of the entire posterior annulus can be recognized. (B) Incision and debridement of the infected tissues of aortic-mitral curtain are shown. (LVOT: Left ventricular outflow tract).

diagnosing severe MR with associated restriction of two leaflets of the bioprosthetic mitral valve.

1. **In diagnosis and management of patients with prosthetic heart valve infective endocarditis (IE), all of the following are correct *except*:**
   (a) Based on 2014 ACC/AHA guidelines, TEE is indicated (class 1 recommendation) to diagnose IE of a prosthetic valve in the presence of persistent fever without bacteremia or a new murmur.
   (b) In periannular extension of prosthetic aortic valve endocarditis, 3D TEE may have additional value compared to 2D echocardiography.
   (c) Preoperative 3D TEE findings in prosthetic valve endocarditis have an excellent correlation with surgical findings.

(d) Based on 2014 ACC/AHA guidelines, early surgery is indicated in patients with IE complicated by heart block, annular or aortic abscess or destructive penetrating lesions.

Ans. (a)

MOVIE LEGENDS

247: Preoperative 2D TEE in long-axis view showing a large mobile vegetation attached to left atrial side of the anterior mitral leaflet.

248: Preoperative 2D TEE in long-axis view showing the bioprosthetic aortic valve (Edwards Intuity valve) with large multilobular abscess cavities (honeycomb appearance) at posterior aortic root.

249: Same view as the previous movie with color Doppler showing color flow signals inside the cavities and moderate paravalvular aortic regurgitation.

250: Preoperative 3D TEE in long-axis view showing perivalvular abscess cavities and rocking motion of the prosthetic aortic valve.

251: 3D TEE full volume acquisition of the aortic root in surgical view showing extension of the perivalvular abscess.

252: Rotation of previous view to visualize vegetation and extension of the infection to the aortic-mitral curtain.

253: 3D TEE immediately after aortic and mitral valve replacement showing restricted motion of two posterior cusps of the bioprosthetic mitral valve (stuck leaflets).

254: Same view as previous movie with full volume color Doppler acquisition showing severe transvalvular mitral regurgitation due to lack of leaflet coaptation.

255: 3D TEE immediately after second pump-run showing release of the mitral cusps with normally functioning bioprosthetic mitral valve.

256: Same view as previous movie with full volume color Doppler showing very good coaptation of the leaflets and no mitral regurgitation.

REFERENCES

1. Tanis W, Teske AJ, van Herwerden LA, et al. The additional value of three-dimensional etchocardiography in complex aortic prosthetic heart valve endocarditis. Echocardiography 2015;32(1):114-25.
2. Anwar AM, Nosir YF, Alasnag M, et al. Real time three-dimensional echocardiography: a novel approach for the assessment of prosthetic heart valves. Echocardiography 2014;31(2):188-96.
3. Nishimura RN, Otto CM, Bonow RO, et al. 2014 AHA/ACC Guideline for the management of patients with valvular heart disease. J Am Coll Cardiol. 2014;63(22): e57-185.

CASE 78

Roomi AU, Shah A, Siddiqui LI, Gupta N, Mohamed A, Nanda NC

The patient is a 73-year-old male, who had a mechanical AVR for degenerative AS 8 years ago. He is a known diabetic and hypertensive. He visited the Indian sub-continent from Middle East for vacation and received Ozone treatment for allergic rhinitis. Six weeks post treatment, he developed low-grade fever, night sweats and poor appetite.

CVS: Audible click in the aortic area with a grade IV/VI diastolic murmur.

Biochemistry: Hb: 8.5 mg/dl,WBC: 23,000, ESR: 109.
2D TTE done (257 and 258).

1. **What is the most likely diagnosis?**
   (a) Tuberculosis
   (b) Vasculitis
   (c) Infective endocarditis with aortic abscess
   (d) Sepsis.

Ans. (c)

This is a case of prosthetic valve endocarditis with aortic abscess rupture (arrow) into the LV cavity producing severe AR. The patient also has moderate MR. The patient subsequently had a successful redo AVR (bioprosthesis) and was discharged home without any complications.

MOVIES 257 AND 258

CASE 79

Ibrahim Osman, Robert Hartman, C Bogdan Marcu, Rajasekhar Nekkanti

ABSTRACT

Intracardiac fistulas are rarely seen and they are estimated to account for < 1% of all cases of infective endocarditis. Fistulization of paravalvular abscesses has been found in 6 to 9% of cases. Paravalvular aortic root abscess with intracardiac fistula formation is an exceedingly rare complication of infective endocarditis and even more rarely encountered in patients with bioprosthetic valve endocarditis. We report an unusual case of a 16-year-old African-American female with Turner's syndrome and aortic stenosis status post a bioprosthetic aortic valve replacement, who developed an aortic root abscess, complicated by an aortico-left atrial fistula. This case illustrates that a high index of suspicion, prompt diagnosis by echocardiography, proper antibiotic therapy and early surgical intervention are paramount to improve outcomes.

CASE PRESENTATION

A 16-year-old African-American female with past medical history of Turner's syndrome, aortic stenosis status post aortic valve replacement with replacement of ascending aorta and innominate artery due to post stenosis aneurysm and recently treated for a Methicillin-sensitive *Staphylococcus aureus* infective endocarditis with multiple subsequent negative transthoracic (TTE) and transesophageal echocardiography (TEE) studies who was admitted to our institution for acute respiratory distress, fever, hypotension and shortly after he became unresponsive with a brief CPR per protocol, intubated and started on vasopressors. There was evidence of significant volume overload on exam. Laboratory work-up revealed a leukocytosis, anemia, acute kidney and liver dysfunction, lactic acidosis and elevated BNP. ECG revealed sinus tachycardia. A transthoracic echocardiogram revealed a new aneurysm of the sinus of Valsalva, paravalvular leakage around the bioprosthetic aortic valve, suspecting an aortic root abscess. A small to moderate mobile mass beneath the aortic valve was noted likely representing a vegetation (259).

TEE revealed a perivalvular leak into a pseudoanuerysm draining to the left atrium, vegetation on the porcine aortic valve and normal left ventricular systolic function (Fig. 79.1 and 260). Cardiac CT was suggestive of vegetation near bioprosthetic aortic valve with pseudoaneurysm near left atrium (Figs. 79.2A to C).

The patient was taken urgently to the OR and underwent a redo sternotomy with a 20 mm Homograft aortic root replacement and closure of aortico-left atrial fistula with left atrial patch closure. Postoperative tissue samples from the excised aortic root and bioprosthetic valve also revealed growth of MSSA.

She achieved full recovery after prolonged and complicated post-operative course with severe acute kidney injury, acute liver injury, acute heart failure and profound anemia requiring transfusion. She was discharged home on long-term intravenous antibiotic therapy.

Role of Cardiovascular Imaging in the Diagnosis of Aortico-left Atrial Fistula

1. Which one of the following cardiovascular imaging modalities is the initial test of choice in the routine assessment of aortico-left atrial fistula?

(a) Transesophageal echocardiography
(b) Cardiac MRI
(c) Cardiac CT
(d) Transthoracic echocardiography
(e) Aortography

Ans. (d)

Since clinical diagnosis of aortico-atrial fistula (AAF) is difficult, definitive diagnosis is by a thorough echocardiographic evaluation. TTE is the initial test of choice in routine prosthetic aortic valve assessment and gradients estimation. Echocardiography plays an important role in the diagnosis of endocarditis and the identification of its complications. Aortography is the gold standard for diagnosis. However, noninvasive methods, such as contrast-enhanced CT, MRI, and echocardiography are currently preferred.

2. Transesophageal echocardiography can be used as an initial test of choice for assessing suspected endocarditis in which of the following clinical scenarios?

(a) Prosthetic heart valves
(b) Concomitant congenital heart diseases
(c) Previous endocarditis
(d) New murmur with acute heart failure
(e) All of the above

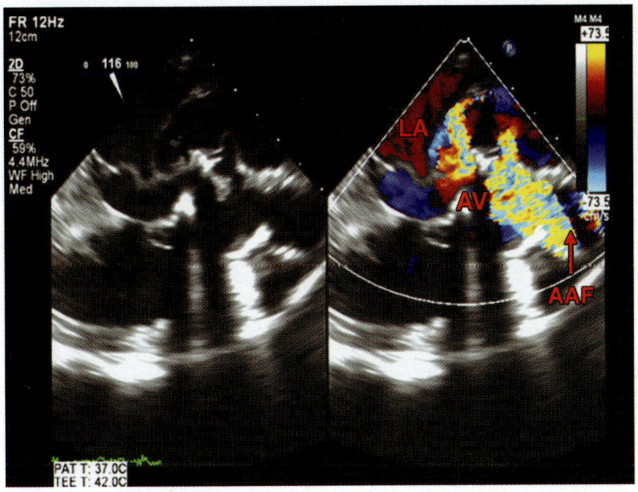

Fig. 79.1: TEE (long axis and short axis views) showed an aortic root abscess around a bioprosthetic aortic valve forming a fistulous communication to the left atrium. A color flow Doppler showing blood flow from the bioprosthetic aortic valve, into the aortic root abscess, which has ruptured into the left atrium, forming an aortico-left atrial fistula. There is a paravalvular aortic regurgitation.

Ans. (e)

TEE can be used as the initial test of choice in high-risk groups, such as patients with prosthetic heart valves, many congenital heart diseases, previous endocarditis and a new murmur with acute heart failure.

3. **Which of the following transthoracic echocardiography-limiting factors is true?**
   (a) The acoustic shadowing of the mechanical prostheses
   (b) Lack of optimal delineation of intracardiac pathology
   (c) Suboptimal signal to noise ratio and distance of transducer to the heart leading to lesser quality images with more attenuation
   (d) Turbulent flow through interchamber communication, small fistulous tracts and the coexistent complications with aortico-left atrial fistula
   (e) All of the above

Ans. (e)

Transthoracic echocardiography is limited by the acoustic shadowing of the mechanical prostheses, lack of optimal delineation of intracardiac pathology and suboptimal signal to noise ratio and distance of TTE transducer to the heart leading to lesser quality images with more attenuation. Turbulent flow of aortic to left atrium fistula can be mistaken on TTE particularly if near the prosthetic valve for prosthetic malfunction in the setting of endocarditis or heart failure. Inter-chamber communication and the fistulous tracts that are particularly small are less likely to be detected. The exact origin, chamber communications and even the size of the fistulous opening cannot be accurately assessed. Coexistent complications with AAF in the setting of aortic endocarditis, such as presence of annular abscess, extension to the upper interventricular septum or the subaortic area and pseudoaneurysm formation are not best seen by TTE.

4. **Which of the following statements makes TEE superior to TTE in real-time assessment of prosthetic valve function and morphology?**
   (a) TEE is crucial in detecting prosthetic valve malfunction, in assessing paravalvular leaks, and in detecting abscess or fistula formation.
   (b) Optimal delineation
   (c) Optimal signal-to-noise ratio
   (d) Superior images quality
   (e) (b) and (d)
   (f) All of the above

Ans. (f)

Multiple studies have compared TTE to TEE in the detection of both native and prosthetic valve septic complications and have showed that TEE is a far superior imaging modality. The proximity of the transducer and the higher signal-to-noise ratio are technical advantages of TEE over TTE. Furthermore, the posterior part of the aortic ring, which is in the far field in transthoracic imaging, is near field in the transesophageal approach, leads to better delineation. Detection of annular involvement and extension of the abscess cavity to the subaortic curtain or upper interventricular septum, all of which are crucial in planning surgical therapy, is also superior with TEE.

5. **Which one of the following TEE-limiting factors is true?**
   (a) Underestimation of cardiac involvement
   (b) Lack of optimal signal to noise ratio
   (c) The limitations of viewing a three dimensional structure such as the heart in a two dimensional fashion
   (d) Turbulent flow
   (e) (a) and (c)
   (f) All of the above

Ans. (e)

Cases of underestimation of cardiac involvement have also been reported with TEE. This reveals the limitations of viewing a three dimensional structure, such as the heart in a two dimensional fashion, a void which may be filled by 3-dimensional (3-D) echocardiography.

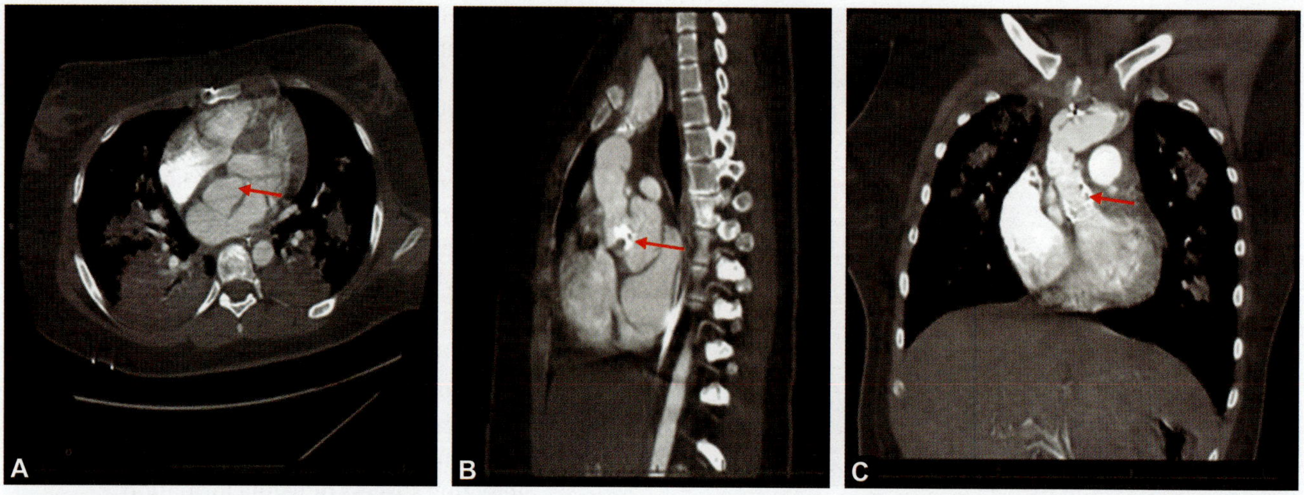

Figs. 79.2A to C: Cardiac CT with (A) coronal, (B) Sagittal and (C) Axial: revealed, "A large pseudoaneurysm (red arrow) measuring 4.7 x 4.7 x 4.3 cm in size that is located anterior and superior to the left atrium and medial to the right atrium, bilateral pulmonary consolidations. There was a small to moderate vegetation beneath the aortic valve".

6. Which of the following statements is true regarding cardiac CT advantages over cardiac MRI in the diagnosis of aortico-left atrial fistula?

(a) Higher spatial and temporal resolution
(b) Narrower field of view
(c) Nonionizing imaging modality
(d) Less renal complications

Ans. (a)

As prosthetic valve infectious endocarditis (IE) represents one of the most difficult situations for echocardiographic studies, cardiac CT seems to be especially useful in case of a negative or inconclusive echocardiographic study. However, contrast products should be used with caution in patients with renal failure or hemodynamic instability because of the risk of worsening renal impairment in combination with antibiotic nephrotoxicity. MRI offers the advantages of a non-ionizing imaging modality but is limited by its lower spatial resolution and availability in comparison with current CT scans.

MOVIE LEGENDS

259: Parasternal long and short axis views with Doppler color flow show a new aneurysm of the sinus of Valsalva, paravalvular leakage around the bioprosthetic aortic valve (aortic root abscess). Small to moderate mobile mass beneath aortic valve (vegetation). Turbulent flow (T) is also noted in LA.

260: Transesophageal echocardiogram in long and short axis views showing an aortic root abscess around a bioprosthetic aortic valve forming a fistulous communication to left atrium (arrowhead). A color flow Doppler shows blood flow from the bioprosthetic aortic valve, into the aortic root abscess, which has ruptured into the left atrium, forming an aortico-left atrial fistula. There is a paravalvular aortic regurgitation.

REFERENCES

1. Caruso A, Iarussi D, Materazzi C, Dialetto G, Covino F, Bossone E, Cotrufo M. Aortic Dissection with Fistula to Left Atrium: Diagnosis by Transesophageal Echocardiography with Successful Repair. J Am Soc Echocardiogr. 2000;13: 69–72. doi: 10.1067/mje.2000.102208. [PubMed] [Cross Ref]
2. Ananthasubramaniam K, Karthikeyan V. Aortic ring abscess with Aorto-atrial fistula complicating Fulminant Prosthetic Valve Endocarditis due to Proteus mirabilis. J Ultrasound Med. 2000;19:63–66. [PubMed]
3. Patsouras D, Argyri O, Siminilakis S, Michalis L, Sideris D. Aortic Dissection with Aorto-Left Atrial Fistula Formation Soon After Aortic Valve Replacement: A Lethal Complication Diagnosed By Transthoracic and Transesophageal Echcoardiography. J Am Soc Echocardiogr. 2002;15: 1409–11. [PubMed]
5. Shanewise JS, Martin RP. Assessment of endocarditis and associated complications with transesophageal echocardiography. Crit Care Clin. 1996;12:411–27. [PubMed]
6. Tamms MA, Guyssenhoven EJ, Bos E, de Jaegere P, Roelandt JR, Sutherland GR, Bom N. Enhanced morphological diagnosis in endocarditis by transesophageal echocardiography. Br Heart J. 1990;63:109. [PMC free article] [PubMed]
7. AHA scientific statement-Infective endocarditis: Diagnosis, Antimicrobial Therapy, and Management of Complications: A Statement for Healthcare Professionals From the

Committee on Rheumatic Fever, Endocarditis, and Kawasaki Disease, Council on Cardiovascular Disease in the Young, and the Councils on Clinical Cardiology, Stroke, and Cardiovascular Surgery and Anesthesia, American Heart Association: Endorsed by the Infectious Diseases Society of America Larry M. Baddour, MD, Chair; Walter R. Wilson, MD; Arnold S. Bayer, MD; Vance G. Fowler Jr, MD, MHS; Ann F. Bolger, MD; Matthew E. Levison, MD*; Patricia Ferrieri, MD; Michael A. Gerber, MD; Lloyd Y. Tani, MD; Michael H. Gewitz, MD; David C. Tong, MD; James M. Steckelberg, MD; Robert S. Baltimore, MD†; Stanford T. Shulman, MD; Jane C. Burns, MD; Donald A. Falace, DMD‡; Jane W. Newburger, MD, MPH; Thomas J. Pallasch, DDS, MS; Masato Takahashi, MD; Kathryn A. Taubert, PhD (Circulation. 2005; 111:e394-e433).

8. Imaging investigations in infective endocarditis: Current approach and perspectives. Franck Thunya,b,*, Jean-Yves Gaubertc,d, Alexis Jacquierc, Laetitia Tessonniere, Serge Cammillerie, Didier Raoultc, Gilbert Habiba, b. Archives of Cardiovascular Disease 2013:106;52-62.

SECTION 5

Endocarditis

CASE 80

Naveen Garg, Kanwal K Kapur

HEMODYNAMICS IN THE ICU

A 66-year-old male underwent tissue AVR. Postoperatively, he required high inotropic support and high antibiotic support, his heart rate was 120/min and blood pressure 90/60 mm Hg. Transesophageal echocardiography was done (261 to 263).

LVOT Diameter—2.1 cm, VTI 28 cm Vmax 209 cm/s

1. What do the above findings indicate?

(a) Stiff tissue AVR leaflets with high gradients.
(b) High LVOT velocity due to LVOT obstruction precipitated by inotropes.
(c) Significant MR due to unrecognized mitral valve pathology
(d) High antegrade transmitral velocity due to MR
(e) High cardiac output resulting from septicemia.

HEMODYNAMIC CALCULATIONS FROM TEE

1. Stroke Volume = LVOT AREA × LVOT VTI = 3.46 × 28 = 96.88 ml
2. Cardiac Output (CO) = HR × SV = 120 × 96.88 = 11.6L/min
3. Systemic Vascular Resistance (SVR) = 80 × (MAP-5)/CO = 448.3 dyne × s × cm^{-5}

Calculations

1. Stroke Volume SV = LVOT area × LVOT VTI (all measurements in 'cm' only)
   $= \pi d^2/4 \times$ LVOT VTI
   = 0.785 × d2 × LVOT VTI (in ml)
   In this example— d = 2.1 cm; LVOT VTI = 28 cm
   $= \pi d^2/4 = 0.785 \times 2.1 \times 2.1 = 3.46\ cm^2$
   SV = 3.46 × 28 = 96.88 ml
2. Cardiac Output (CO) = (SV × HR)/1000 (L/min)
   = (96.88 × 120)/1000
   = 11625.6/1000 = 11.6L (approx.)
3. SVR = 80 × (Mean Arterial Pressure – RA Pressure)/CO (For calculations RA pressures is assumed as 5 mm Hg)

$$MAP \simeq DP + \frac{1}{3}(SP - DP)$$

or equivalently

$$MAP \simeq \frac{2}{3}(DP) + \frac{1}{3}(SP)$$

or equivalently

$$MAP \simeq \frac{(2 \times DP) + SP}{3}$$

or equivalently

$$MAP \simeq DP + \frac{1}{3} PP$$

In this case— BP = 90/60 mm Hg
MAP = {(2 × 60) + 90}/3 = {120 + 90}/3 = 210/3 = 70 mm Hg
SVR = 80 × (70-5)/11.6 = 80 × 65/11.6 = 448.27 dyne × s/cm^{-5}

Note:
80 dyne × s × cm^{-5} = 1 mm Hg × min × L^{-1} = 1 Wu (Wood units)

DETAILS OF CALCULATIONS

Clue 1. Why so high a cardiac output ?
Clue 2. Why such a low SVR?

DILEMMA IN POSTOPERATIVE PERIOD

What is the most likely explanation of high CO with low SVR in the immediate postoperative period?

ANSWERS

1. Patient was not having transprosthetic obstruction because LVOT VTI/AO VTI = 28/54.6= 0.51. Significant transprosthetic obstruction is likely only if this VTI ratio is < 0.30 (Figs. 80.3 and 80.4).
2. Significant mitral pathology (either regurgitation or obstructive) is unlikely since high flow velocities are observed across both mitral and aortic valves. These findings can be explained by a high cardiac output state (Figs. 80.1 and 80.2).

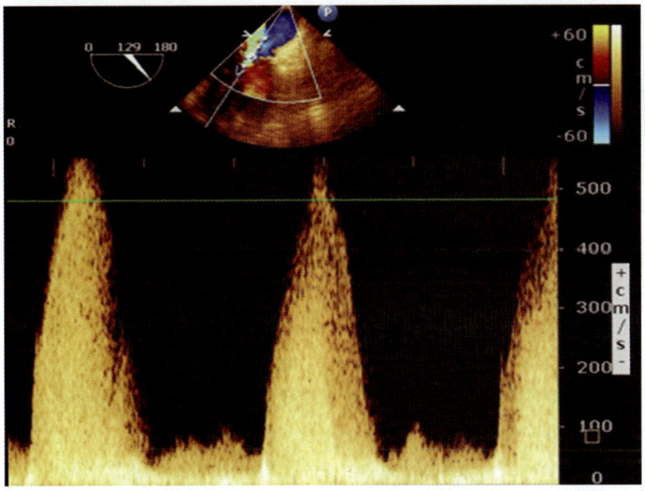

Fig. 80.1: TEE Continuous wave Doppler. Shows mitral regurgitation.

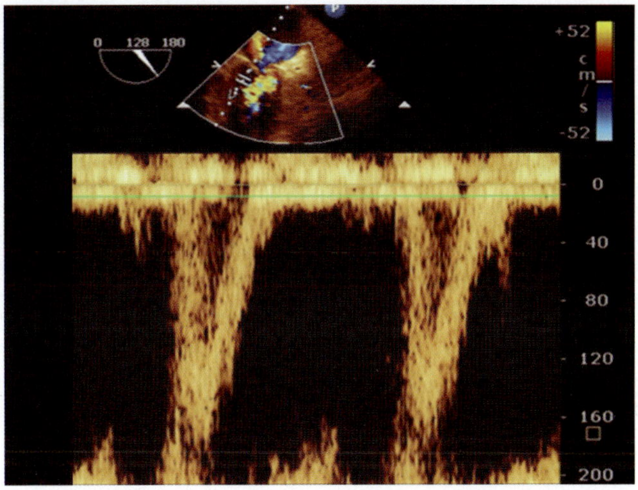

Fig. 80.2: TEE Pulse wave Doppler. Shows mitral in flow pattern.

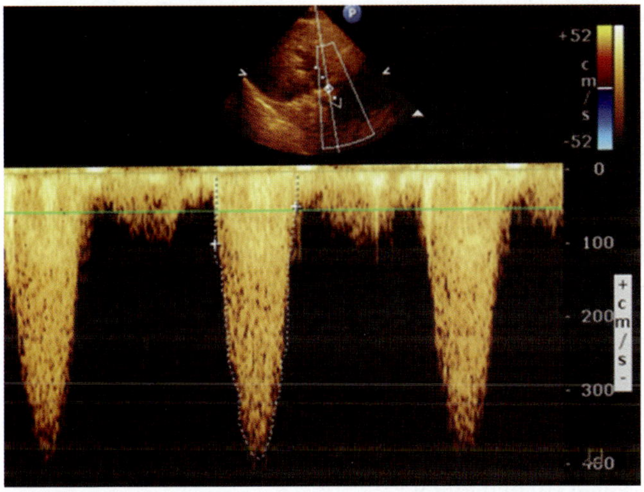

Fig. 80.3: TEE Continuous wave Doppler. Also shows high gradients across the tissue AVR (Transgastric view). V_{max} (maximum peak velocity) = 390 cm/s, VTI (Velocity time integral) = 54.6 cm, maximum peak gradient (PG) = 61 mm Hg, Mean PG = 35.9 mm Hg.

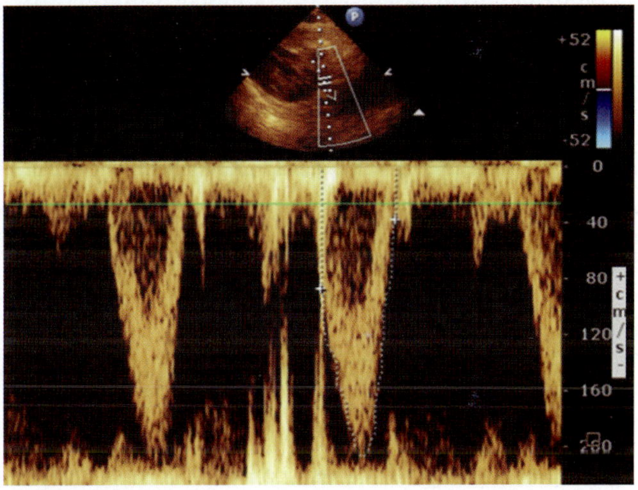

Fig. 80.4: TEE Pulse wave Doppler. Shows LVOT gradients by pulsed Doppler obtained in the transgastric view.

3. As depicted in Figure 80.5, the LVOT appears wide open; thus significant LVOT narrowing can be excluded.
4. Therefore, the most logical explanation is that the patient has SEPSIS, which could be due to exacerbation of pre-existing and unrecognized infection or acquired intraoperatively.

The classical hemodynamics of septicemia are high cardiac output with low SVR and failure to maintain adequate arterial pressure without the use of inotropes.

Colistin 2 million units were added to the existing antibiotic regimen (Meropenam and Targocid) and the patient responded well. See TTE-263A and 263B.

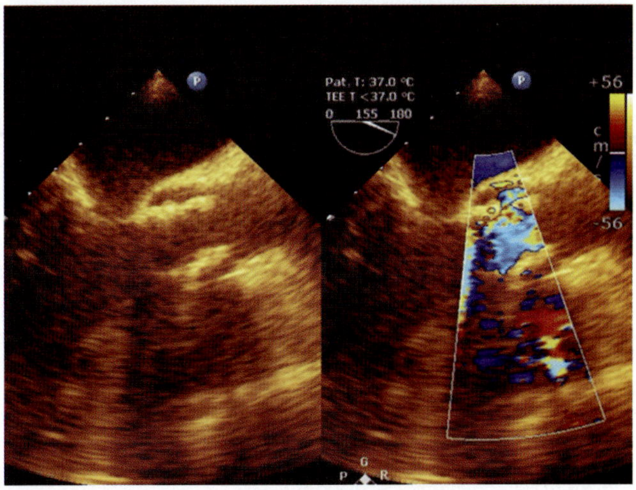

Fig. 80.5: TEE. Long axis view showing AVR.

POSTOPERATIVELY

His blood reports later showed:

HIGH total WBC count 18000/dL (which later increased to 25000)

N-86 L-12 E- 2

HIGH ESR—60 mm/h

Blood Cultures—Sterile

(Probably due to the preoperative use of antibiotics)

Patient was discharged after 2 weeks of hospital stay with normal pressure gradients across the tissue AVR and normal velocities across all cardiac valves.

CONCLUSION

Thus, proper interpretation of non-invasively derived hemodynamics from TEE studies could be extremely useful in the appropriate diagnosis and management of critically ill patients.

CARDIAC OUTPUT AND CARDIAC INDEX

Cardiac output = Stroke Volume × HR
(CO) (SV)

SV = CSA of valve or vessel × VTI (velocity time integral)

CSA = $\pi D^2/4$ where D = Annular diameter

- CO = SV × HR
- SV = CSA × Velocity x time

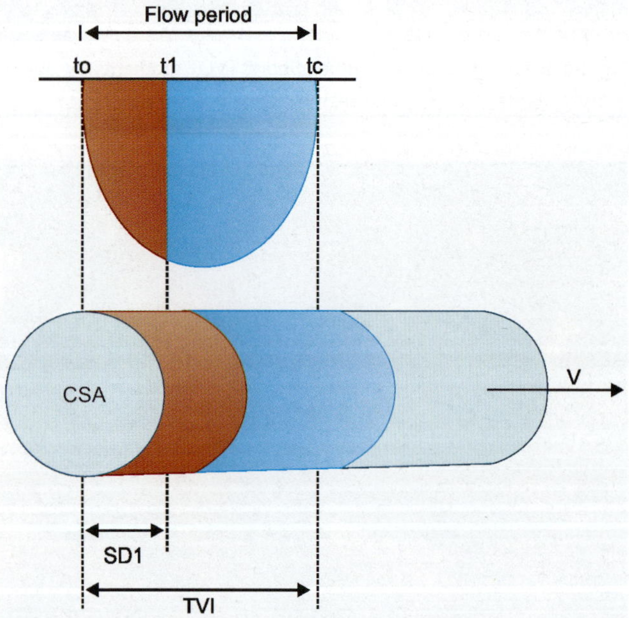

Fig. 80.6: Hemodynamic calculations.

- SV = CSA × VTI
- CSA = $\pi D^2/4 = 3.142 \times D \times D/4$; CSA = $0.785D^2$
- CO = $0.785D^2 \times$ VTI × HR

SYSTEMIC VASCULAR RESISTANCE (SVR)

It is the resistance offered by the systemic arterioles and capillaries to the flow of blood across the systemic circuit. It is the ratio of the pressure drop across the systemic vascular bed to the systemic blood flow. The arterial end of the circuit is the ascending aorta while the venous end is the IVC/ RA. Owing to the pulsatile nature of blood flow the pressure drop across the systemic circuit is the difference in mean pressures between the aorta and the RA.

Mean Ao pressure = DP + 1/3 PP assuming that Diastole duration is 2/3 of cardiac cycle

Mean IVC/RA pressure is the CVP which is estimated by the IVC size

Correlation Between RA Pressure (CVP) and IVC Appearance

CVP 0–5 mm Hg: IVC totally collapses on inspiration and is <1.5 cm in diameter

CVP 5–10 mm Hg: IVC collapses >50% on inspiration and is 1.5 to 2.5 cm in diameter

CVP 11–15 mm Hg: IVC collapses <50% on inspiration and is 1.5 to 2.5 cm in diameter

CVP 16–20 mm Hg: IVC collapses <50% on inspiration and is >2.5 cm in diameter

CVP >20 mm Hg: No change in IVC on inspiration and is >2.5 cm in diameter

SVR = (Mean Ao pressure – Mean RA pressure) (mm Hg)/cardiac output (L/min) = Wood Units (Wu)

1 Wu = dyne x sec x cm^{-5}

Normal SVR = 10-20 Wu = 800 – 1600 dyne x sec x cm^{-5}

Causes of Low SVR with high CO...

- Septicemia
- Chronic liver disease
- Renal failure with fluid overload
- Chronic anemia
- AV fistula

Causes of High SVR with low CO.....

- Accelerated hypertension
- Dehydration

- Congestive cardiac failure
- Renal failure with hypertension

The importance of SVR computation is that it could indicate the etiology of the Shock syndrome in patients admitted in the Emergency Room or the ICU. For example, in Septic Shock due to peripheral vasodilation there is increased CO and thus the computed SVR is low (less than 800 dynes) ; on the other hand in cardiogenic shock owing to low cardiac CO, the SVR is high (more than 1600 dynes).

MOVIES 261 TO 263

CASE 81

Arnav Kumar, Masood Ahmad

TRANSESOPHAGEAL THREE DIMENSIONAL ECHOCARDIOGRAPHY IN MITRAL VALVE ENDOCARDITIS

The following case was originally published by us in Circulation 2013;128:e204-e206.

A 66-year-old man with history of mitral valve prolapse is admitted to the emergency room with four day history of progressive dyspnea, cough and hemoptysis. Patient develops hypotension (blood pressure, 96/61 mm Hg), tachycardia (heart rate, 122 beats per minute), and respiratory distress (36 breaths per minute with oxygen saturation of 86% on room air) with a fever of 38.7°C (101.7°F). Physical examination is remarkable for grade 5 of 6 holosystolic murmur along the left sternal border and bibasilar rales. Numerous palpable petechial lesions are noticed on the foot. Patient is admitted to the coronary care unit and intubated. Blood cultures are drawn and broad-spectrum antibiotics are started. Two dimensional transthoracic echocardiography is done and suggests a mobile mass attached to the mitral valve. Two sets of blood cultures, 48 hours apart, grew coagulase negative *Staphylococcus lugdunensis*. Skin biopsy done on admission confirms leukocytoclastic vasculitis. Movie 264 is a real time three-dimensional transesophageal echocardiogram. Surgeon's view of the mitral valve is shown with segments of the anterior leaflet (A1, A2, and A3) and scallops of the posterior leaflet (P1, P2, and P3). Patient is taken to the operating room and a 33-mm Epic tissue bioprosthesis is placed in the mitral position. Microscopic examination of valve tissue reveals severe acute inflammation with fibrinous exudates and bacterial colonies consistent with acute bacterial endocarditis. Tissue culture also grows *Staphylococcus lugdunensis*. The patient has an uneventful postoperative course and is discharged on a 4-week regimen of intravenous vancomycin and oral rifampicin.

1. **The movie clip 264 shows all of the following *except*:**
   (a) Mitral valve vegetation on P2 scallop
   (b) Mitral valve vegetations on P1 and P3 scallops
   (c) No vegetation on anterior leaflet
   (d) Flail segment of the posterior leaflet
   (e) Perforation in anterior mitral leaflet

Ans. (b)

The echocardiographic features of typical of infective endocarditis are: (1) an oscillating intracardiac mass on a valve or supporting structure or in the path of a regurgitation jet or on an iatrogenic device, (2) abscess, (3) new partial dehiscence of a prosthetic valve, or (4) new valvular regurgitation. The attachment site of the vegetation to the mitral and tricuspid valves is usually on the atrial side. A vegetation appears as an echogenic and mobile mass attached to the endocardial surface of the valve or to the prosthetic material in the heart. The sensitivity of detecting a vegetation with two-dimensional transthoracic echocardiography (TTE) is 65 to 80% and with TEE, 95%.

2. **In left-sided valve endocarditis, the embolic complications are increased with the following echo characteristics of the vegetation:**
   (a) Greater mobility
   (b) Extent and size (Greater than 11 mm in size)
   (c) Vegetation on the mitral valve
   (d) Consistency (less calcific)
   (e) All of the above

Ans. (e)

In left-sided valve endocarditis, the frequency of embolic complications increase with the greater mobility, extent, consistency (less calcific), and size of the vegetation.[2] When vegetations are larger than 11 mm, 50% or more of patients develop at least one complication of infective endocarditis. In patients with tricuspid valve endocarditis, pulmonary embolism is the most common complication (69%). Patients with a large (>10 mm) vegetation involving the mitral valve are at increased risk for embolic events, but vegetation size does not correlate with the degree of heart failure and patient survival.[3]

3. **In the setting of infective endocarditis, the following are indications for surgery *except*:**
   (a) Severe CHF
   (b) Recurrent emboli
   (c) Valve abscess
   (d) Large fungal vegetations
   (e) Repeat blood cultures positive in 48 hours

Ans. (e)

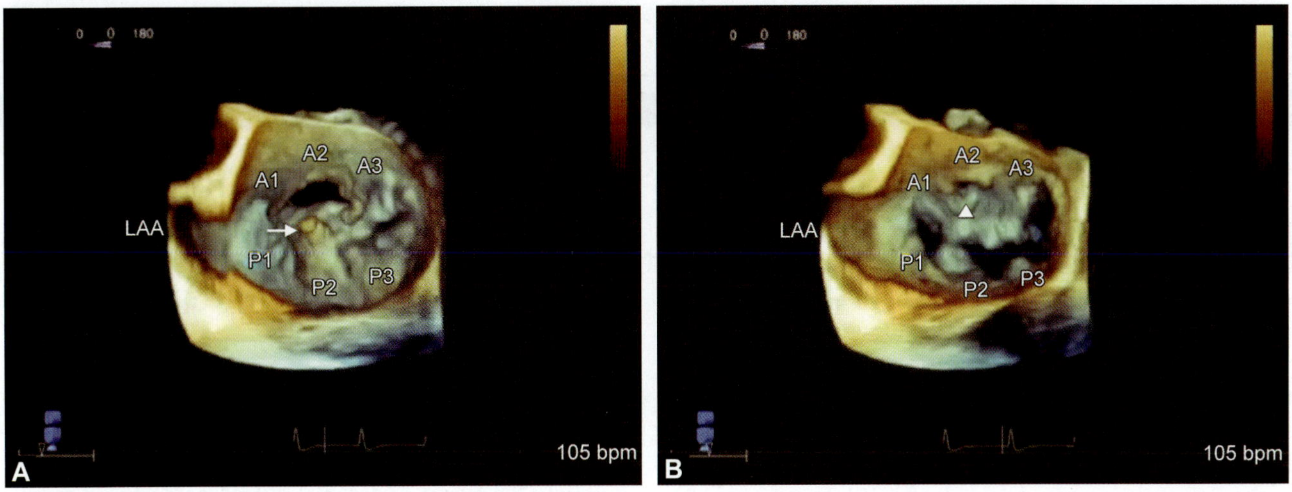

Figs. 81.1A and B: 3D TEE surgeon's view of the mitral valve with anterior (A1, A2 and A3) and posterior (P1, P2 and P3) scallops. Vegetation attached to P2 (arrow) and perforation in A2 (arrowhead).

If blood cultures are positive in 48 hours, continue antibiotics. If patient received correct antibiotics for six days and still blood cultures are positive, then proceed with surgery (persistent bacteremia).

4. **In patients with complicated, left sided native valve endocarditis, the greatest reduction in mortality with valve surgery has been noted in:**
   (a) Patients who had moderate to severe congestive heart failure
   (b) Immunocompromised state
   (c) Staphylococcus aureus bacteremia
   (d) Refractory infection
   (e) Pericardial effusion

Ans. (a)

A review of 513 adults with left-sided native valve endocarditis showed that valve surgery was associated with reduced mortality (16% vs. 33%) at 6 months. The greatest reduction in mortality with valve surgery was noted in patients who had moderate to severe congestive heart failure (14% vs. 51%).[4]

5. **All of the following incremental information helpful to surgeons was provided by real time three-dimensional transesophageal echocardiography in the above case *except*:**
   (a) Partially flail P2 segment
   (b) Perforation in the anterior leaflet
   (c) A clear view of all individual mitral valve scallops
   (d) Precise location of the vegetation
   (e) Mitral annular abscess

Ans. (e)

Real time three-dimensional trans-esophageal echocardiography helped to accurately visualize the partially flail P2 segment and perforation in the anterior leaflet (264 and Figs. 81.1A and 1B). However, mitral annular abscess is not seen. These findings are confirmed intraoperatively. Real time three-dimensional Transesophageal echocardiography is an important tool to accurately visualize valvular structural abnormalities that can help surgeons plan procedures in advance.

MOVIE LEGEND

264: Three-dimensional transesophageal echocardiogram, surgeon's view of the mitral valve showing a partially flail P2 scallop with a vegetation (arrow in Fig. 81.1A) and a perforation at the base of the A2 segment of anterior mitral leaflet (arrowhead in Fig. 81.1B).[1]

REFERENCES

1. Arain FA, Williams BD, Lick SD, Boroumand N, Ahmad M. Echocardiographic, histopathologic, and surgical findings in Staphylococcus lugdunensis mitral valve endocarditis after prostate biopsy. Circulation. 2013;128:e204-6.
2. Sanfilippo AJ, Picard MH, Newell JB, et al. Echocardiographic assessment of patients with infectious endocarditis: prediction of risk for complications. J Am Coll Cardiol. 1991;18:1191-9.
3. Mugge A, Daniel WG, Frank G, Lichtlen PR. Echocardiography in infective endocarditis: reassessment of prognostic implications of vegetation size determined by the transthoracic and the transesophageal approach. J Am Coll Cardiol. 1989;14:631-8.
4. Vikram HR, Buenconsejo J, Hasbun R, Quagliarello VJ. Impact of valve surgery on 6-month mortality in adults with complicated, left-sided native valve endocarditis: a propensity analysis. JAMA. 2003;290:3207-14.

CASE 82

Ahmad S Omran

INFECTIVE ENDOCARDITIS OF MITRAL VALVE

This 54-year-old man presented to our center with severe shortness of breath. He had a history of culture negative infective endocarditis six months previously which was treated medically in our hospital. Transthoracic echocardiography (TTE) showed severe mitral regurgitation (MR) due to flail anterior mitral valve leaflet (Figs. 82.1A and B). There were no vegetations or other signs of active endocarditis. Transesophageal echocardiography (TEE) was performed which showed a large perforation in the middle of the AMVL. Multiple jets of severe MR were noted (Figs. 82.2A and B, 🎥 265-267). Patient was taken to the operating room for surgical intervention. Because of history of gastric disease, mitral valve repair was a preferred option compared to mitral valve replacement. During surgery, the mitral valve was inspected from a left atriotomy approach. A large perforation was noted in the middle of the AMVL which was patched by autologous fresh pericardium (Figs 82.3A and B). A size 32 Physio ring was used for mitral annuloplasty (🎥 268 and 269). Immediate postoperative TEE showed no residual MR. Patient was discharged home in a good condition. Follow-up echocardiography showed an excellent result with no MR and no significant gradient across the mitral valve.

1. In echocardiographic assessment and management of patients with infective endocarditis (IE) all of the following are correct *except*:

(a) Based on ACC/AHA guidelines, TEE is recommended in all patients with known IE when complications have developed or are clinically suspected.

(b) Intraoperative TEE is class 1 indication for patients undergoing valve surgery for IE

(c) In surgical cases of IE in the setting of active infection of the mitral valve, mitral valve replacement is preferable to valve repair.

(d) In patients undergoing mitral valve replacement after six weeks of antibiotic therapy, the 30-day mortality is about 10%.

Ans. (c)

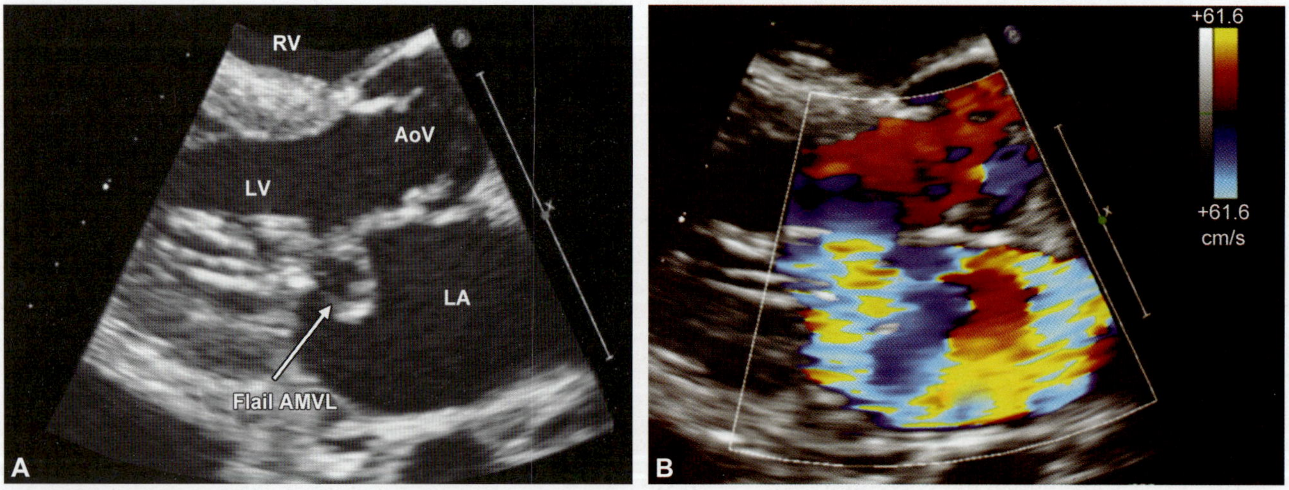

Figs. 82.1A and B: Transthoracic echocardiography (TTE). (A) Parasternal long-axis view shows a large flail anterior mitral valve leaflet (AMVL). (B) Several multiple jets of mitral regurgitation (MR) due to flail and fenestrated AMVL. (LA: Left atrium; LV: Left ventricle; RV: Right ventricle; AoV: Aortic valve).

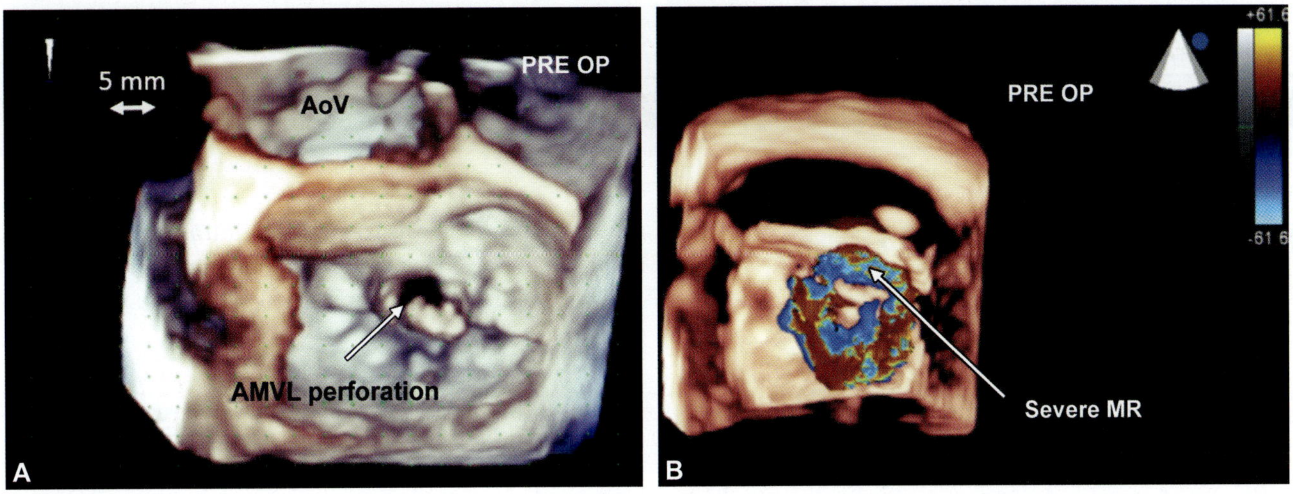

Figs. 82.2A and B: Preoperative 3D transesophageal echocardiography (3DTEE). (A) 3D zoom mode acquisition in surgical view of the mitral valve shows a large perforation in the middle of the anterior mitral valve leaflet (AMVL). Perforation site appears healed with regular margin. (B) Same view of the mitral valve showing multiple jets of severe MR, mostly originating from the perforation site. (AoV: Aortic valve).

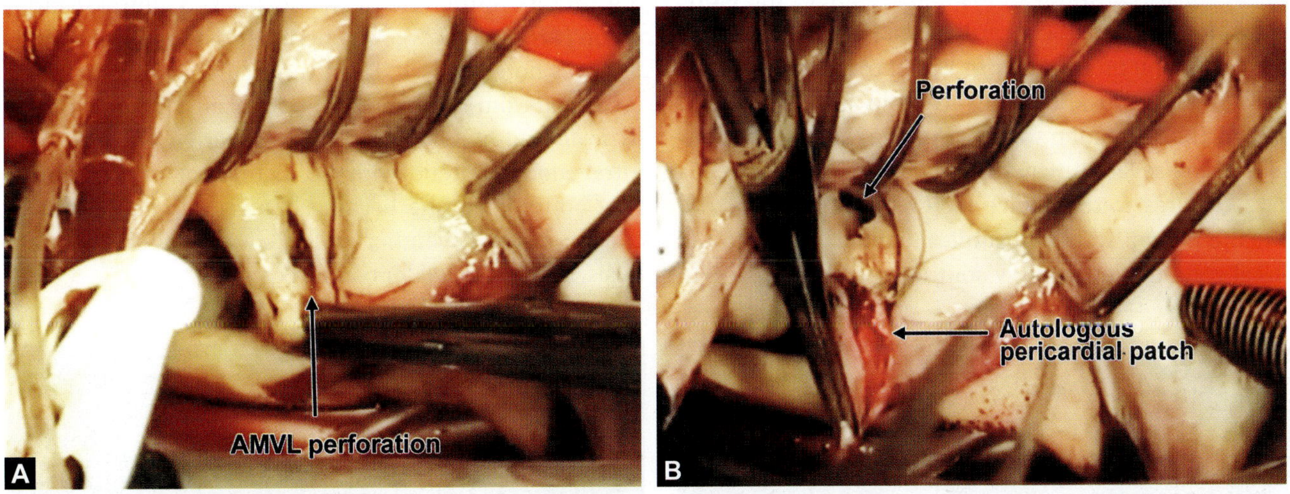

Figs. 82.3A and B: Surgical exploration of the mitral valve via left atriotomy. (A) Perfect correlation is seen with preoperative 3D TEE finding. Large perforation is seen with clean margins. (B) A patch of fresh autologous pericardium was used to repair the perforation. A size 32 Physio ring was implanted for annuloplasty.

MOVIE LEGENDS

265: Preoperative 3D TEE, surgical view of the mitral valve, showing a large perforation in the middle of the anterior mitral valve leaflet.

266: Preoperative 3D TEE in mitral commissural view showing several multiple jets of MR.

267: 3D TEE same view as movie 265 showing origin of MR mostly from the perforation of the anterior leaflet.

268: Intraoperative 3D TEE showing mitral valve after repair. Anterior leaflet appears bulky due to insertion of a large pericardial patch.

269: Same view as previous movie showing no residual mitral regurgitation.

CASE 83

Aiman Smer, Muhammad Soubhi Azzouz

INFECTIVE ENDOCARDITIS COMPLICATED WITH ACUTE PULMONARY EDEMA

A 50-year-old woman with a history of poorly controlled diabetes mellitus, hypertension and end stage kidney disease on hemodialysis presented with altered mental status. No fever, chills, chest pain or shortness of breath. Vitals stable. Pertinent laboratory studies revealed elevated white blood count at 26 × 10^3 cells/microL, hemoglobin 8.1 g/dL, and very low platelet count at 17,000/microL. Creatinine of 10.8 mg/dL and blood urea nitrogen of 107 mg/dL. Brain magnetic resonance imaging revealed numerous acute infarcts consistent with cardioembolic source. Therefore, she had transthoracic echocardiogram (TTE) that showed large vegetation on the anterior leaflet of the mitral valve, measuring 33 mm × 20 mm (arrow in Figure 83.1 and 270). The vegetation was obstructing the mitral inflow and causing severe functional mitral stenosis (Fig. 83.2). Blood cultures were positive for *Corynebacterium striatum*. The patient was poor surgical candidate due to her critical condition and poorly controlled comorbidities. In the same time, she was treated with intravenous antibiotics per infectious disease recommendation.

One month later, she presented with acute pulmonary edema and septic shock.

1. What's your diagnosis?

(a) Embolization of the mitral valve vegetation
(b) Mitral valve perforation with severe mitral regurgitation
(c) Large pericardial effusion with tamponade
(d) Worsening mitral stenosis

Ans. (b)

Repeat TTE revealed hyperdynamic left ventricle with severe left ventricular hypertrophy. There is perforation of the anterior mitral valve leaflet with severe mitral regurgitation (271 to 273). A component of the mitral vegetation was noted as well. Right ventricular systolic pressure increased from 30 to 85 mm Hg. Clinically, the patient was hypoxic and hypotensive. She was started on CPAP and intravenous diuretic with no significant improvement. Few hours later, she became bradycardic and had PEA cardiac arrest. Given her critical status and dismal prognosis, family elected for comfort care.

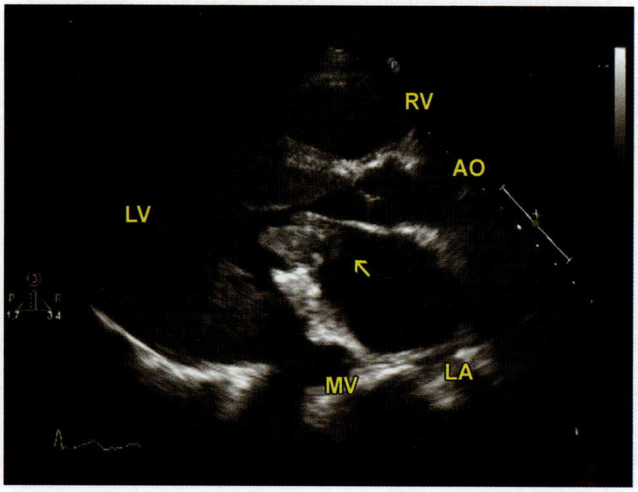

Fig. 83.1: TTE parasternal long axis view showing a large mobile echo density mass (arrow) attached to the anterior leaflet of the mitral valve on the atrial side, measuring 33 mm x 20 mm). Also, note the severe left ventricular hypertrophy due to long-standing uncontrolled hypertension and end stage kidney disease.

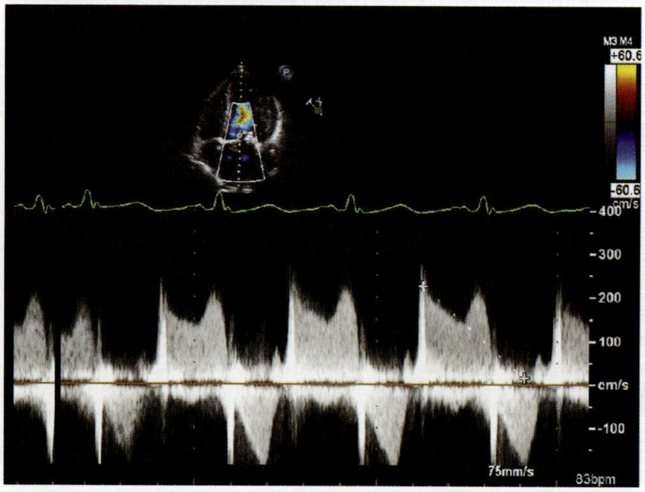

Fig. 83.2: TTE apical four chamber view with tissue Doppler of the mitral valve inflow demonstrating severe function mitral stenosis. Estimated mitral valve area via pressure half time is 1.2 cm^2, peak mitral inflow velocity 2.3 m/sec and mean pressure gradient 14 mm Hg.

MOVIE LEGENDS

270: TTE parasternal long axis view revealed a large mobile echo density mass (arrow) attached to the atrial side of the anterior leaflet of the mitral valve, measuring 33 mm × 20 mm). Note that there is also a very mobile component of the vegetation protruding into the left atrium during systole.

271: TTE parasternal long axis view and color Doppler revealed a perforation/rupture of the anterior leaflet of the mitral valve with torrential mitral regurgitation. There is flail segment in the same area of the previously noted vegetation (arrow).

272: TTE apical four chamber view zoomed at the mitral valve in panning motion revealing that the perforation is affecting the same area of previously noted vegetation (arrow) on the anterior leaflet.

273: TTE apical five chamber view showing a perforation of the anterior mitral leaflet in the mid segment with flail A2 segment. The anterior leaflet is still thickened and a component of the vegetation (arrow) is attached to it .

CASE 84

Dinesh Gautam, Rahul Choudhary, Gaurav Singhal, Kotti K, Aashish Agarwal, Elsayed M, Nanda NC

This is a 30-year-old female with a past history of prolonged fever of unknown origin. She presented with a murmur of MR. 2D and 3D TTE were done.

1. **What may be the cause of perforation (arrow) in the anterior mitral valve leaflet (Figs. 84.1 to 84.8 and 274-279)?**
   (a) Rheumatic mitral valve disease
   (b) Autoimmune mitral valve disease
   (c) Barlow's disease
   (d) Congenital anterior mitral valve cleft/perforation
   (e) Bacterial endocarditis

Ans. (e) Bacterial endocarditis

Because of past history of prolonged fever, the perforation (arrow) with severe MR is possibly due to endocarditis involving the MV. MV is mildly thickened and shows

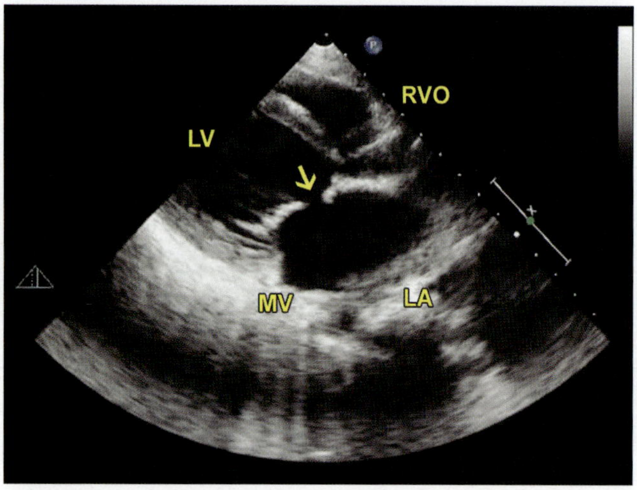

Fig. 84.1: Parasternal long axis view. Arrow points to a perforation in the anterior MV leaflet. LA is dilated.

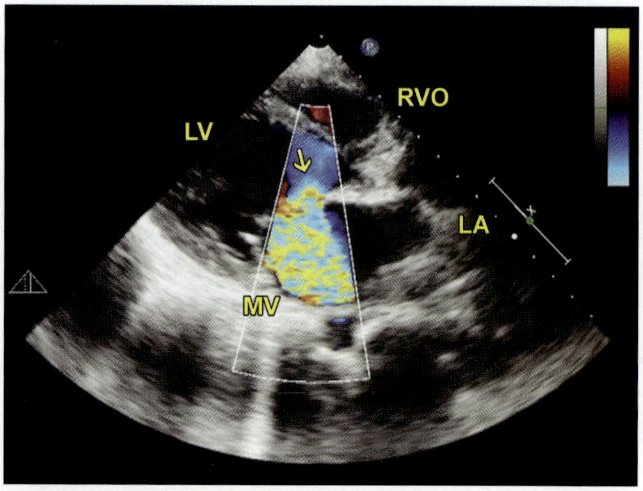

Fig. 84.2: Color Doppler examination showing severe MR through the perforation (arrow) in the anterior MV leaflet.

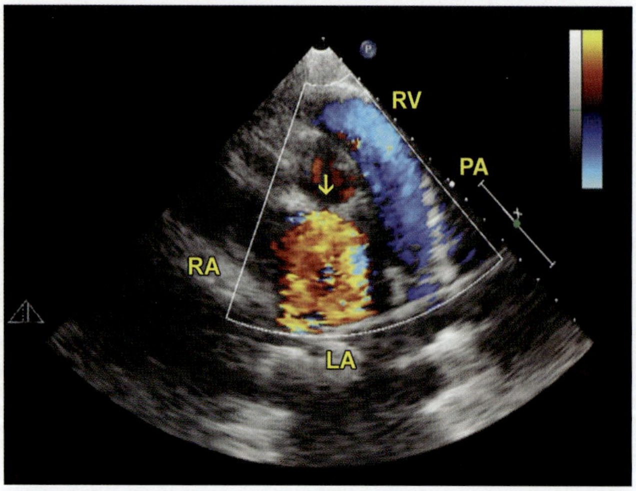

Fig. 84.3: Color Doppler examination. Short axis view showing severe MR through the perforation (arrow) in the anterior MV leaflet.

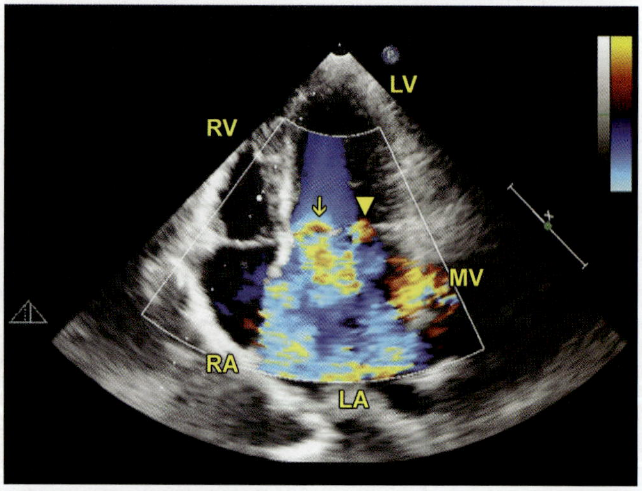

Fig. 84.4: Color Doppler examination. Apical four chamber view demonstrating severe MR through the perforation (arrow) in the anterior MV leaflet.

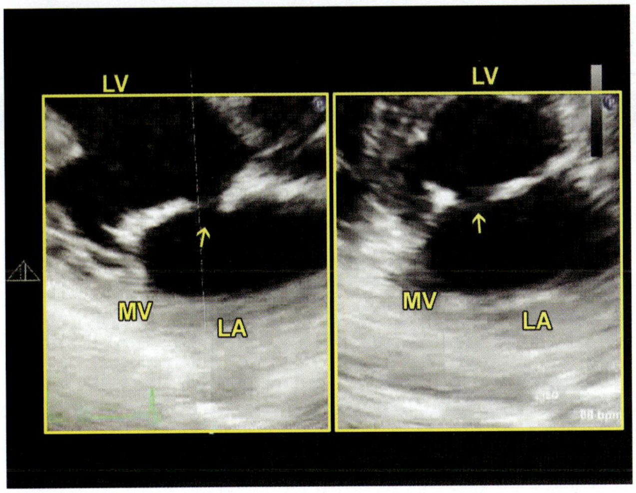

Fig. 84.5: Arrow points to a perforation in the anterior MV leaflet.

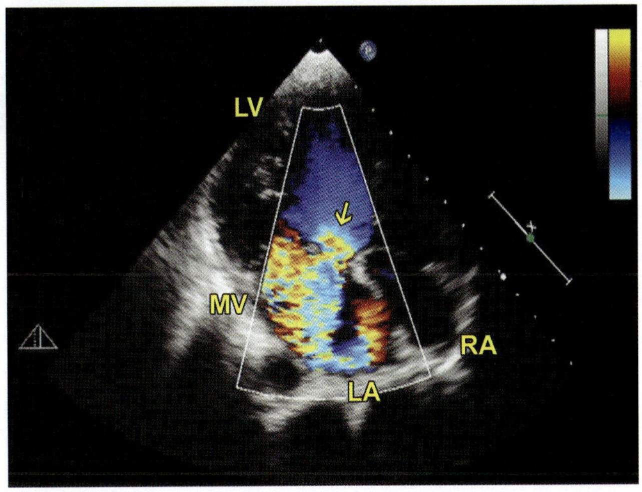

Fig. 84.6: Color Doppler study demonstrating severe MR through the perforation (arrow) in the anterior MV leaflet.

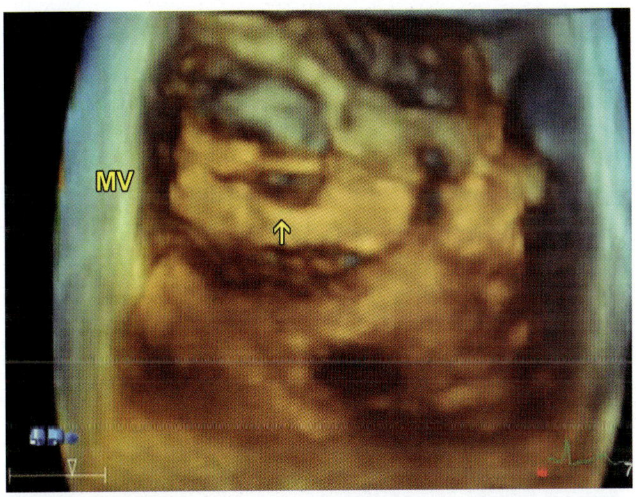

Fig. 84.7: 3D TTE. Anterior MV leaflet perforation (arrow) viewed en face in short axis.

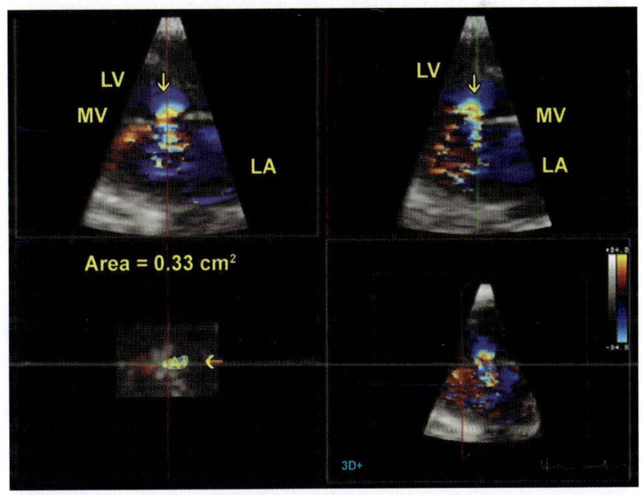

Fig. 84.8: 3DTTE. Measurement of the area of vena contracta (arrow in the left lower panel) of MR occurring through the perforation (arrow in upper panels) in the anterior MV leaflet.

prolapse of posterior leaflet (arrowhead in 274). Arrowhead in 277 shows a second jet of MR through the coaptation point. A congenital cleft does not usually occur in the basal portion. The other conditions listed do not per se result in a perforation.

2. **MR in this patient is very severe by 2D color Doppler with 2 jets, one through the perforation (arrow) and the other centrally at the coaptation point (arrowhead in 277). However, by 3D color Doppler, the vena contracta (VC) area is 0.33 cm^2 which is consistent with moderate MR. Severe MR should have a VC area > 0.4 cm^2. What may be the reason for this finding?**
   (a) The VC of the central jet was measured and not MR from perforation.
   (b) The Nyquist limit is very high at ovcr 85 cm/s.
   (c) Color Doppler 3D TTE is unreliable in cases of MV perforations.

Ans. (b) The Nyquist limit is very high at over 85 cm/s.

The Nyquist limit should have been lower around 61 cm/s or less when using 3D color Doppler for assessing VC size. High Nyquist limits may affect the size of VC.

Figures 84.7 and 84.8 and 280 and 281 are 3D TTE.

MOVIES 274 TO 281

CASE 85

Moneal Shah, Robert WW Biederman

MULTIMODALITY IMAGING FOR A MITRAL VALVE MASS

A 41-year-old female with a history of antiphospholipid antibody (APL) syndrome presented with acute vision loss and found to have a retinal artery occlusion. She subsequently was referred for a transesophageal echocardiogram to rule out cardiac embolism. A four chamber view revealed an echo density attached to the tip of the posterior leaflet of the mitral valve involving both the atrial and ventricular sides of the valve (282A). Color Doppler showed an eccentric, anteriorly-directed jet of mitral regurgitation (282B). Blood cultures were drawn which were negative. In order to obtain tissue characterization, she was referred for a cardiac MRI. T2-weighted dark-blood imaging showed increased signal from the mitral valve mass indicating active inflammation (Fig. 85.1). In addition, post-gadolinium contrast imaging revealed patchy myocardial enhancement consistent with myocarditis (Fig. 85.2).

1. **The modality best-suited for mitral valve mass imaging is:**
   (a) TTE
   (b) TEE
   (c) Cardiac MRI
   (d) Cardiac CTA

Ans. (b)

Transesophageal echo provides the best combination of structural and functional assessment of the mitral valve. While cardiac MRI can provide tissue characterization of masses, the highly mobile nature of valvular masses can prove challenging for visualization by MRI. Cardiac CTA can be used for mitral valve imaging; however, given the radiation and contrast needed, it is not a preferred option.

2. **Etiology of this valvular mass is most likely:**
   (a) Bacterial endocarditis
   (b) Thrombus
   (c) Papillary fibroelastoma
   (d) Libman-Sacks endocarditis

Ans. (d)

The patient had no prior viral prodrome to suspect viral myocarditis; rather, it was felt this was lupus myocarditis. Given that finding and the history of APL, the etiology of the valvular mass was most likely marantic (Libman-Sacks) endocarditis.

Libman-Sacks endocarditis is a nonbacterial manifestation of valvular heart disease associated with systemic lupus erythematosus (SLE). Libman-Sacks lesions affect

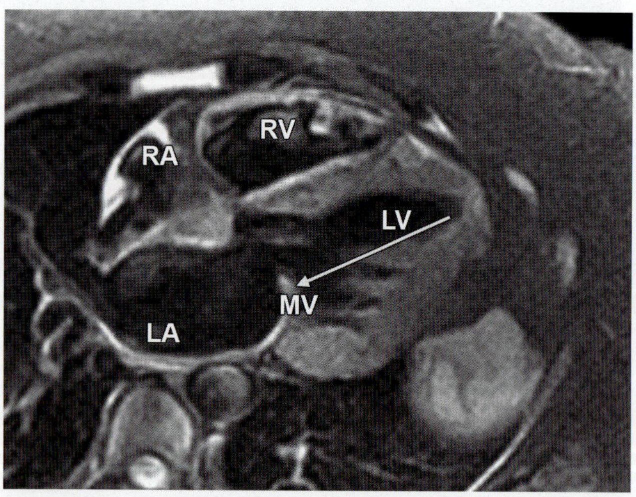

Fig. 85.1: T2-weighted 4-chamber image showing increase signal (arrow) of the mitral valve mass indicating inflammation.

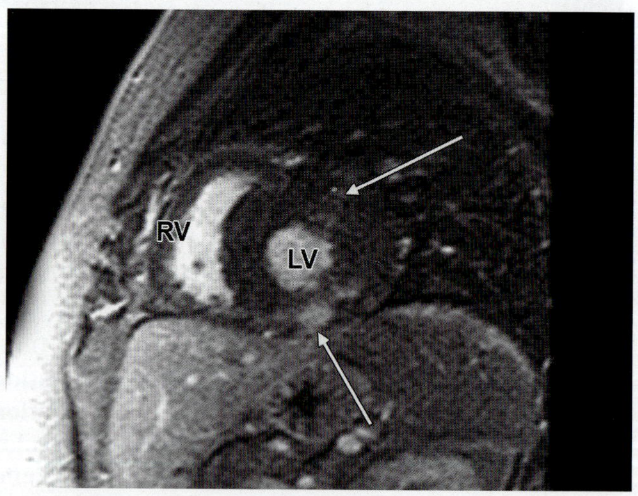

Fig. 85.2: Post-gadolinium contrast short axis image showing patchy enhancement of the inferior and anterior walls (arrows) consistent with myocarditis.

the valve either by generalized thickening or focal vegetations most commonly on the ventricular side of the left-sided valves. Histologically, these lesions are due to fibrin deposition with an inflammatory mononuclear infiltration. As in this patient, these lesions cause regurgitation typically, rather than stenosis. A higher prevalence of Libman-Sacks endocarditis was found in SLE patients with APL than in patients without APL. The lesions are benign, however, embolic phenomenon have been reported typically as a cerebrovascular ischemic event. As was done in this patient, antiocoagulation is typically the treatment for secondary prevention for embolic events.[1]

MOVIES 282A AND B

REFERENCE

1. Hojnik M, George J, Ziporen L, Shenfeld, Y. "Heart Valve Involvement (Libman-Sacks Endocarditis) in the Antiphospholipid Syndrome." Circulation. 1996;93:1579-87.

CASE 86

José Carlos Armendariz Ferrari, Yudy Miluska Roldan Concha, Alfredo Sotomayor Estrada

SEVERE CARDIAC COMPROMISE DUE TO SKIN INFECTION (PEDIATRIC PATIENT)

The patient is a 6-year-old child from Peru. Two months before being admitted to the hospital, he presented with a complicated Varicella cutaneous bacterial infection. He later developed impetigo, pyodermatitis and cellulitis. A month later, he developed fever with progressive respiratory difficulties, orthopnea, edemas and abdominal pain. He was transferred to our hospital because he was found to have cardiomegaly.

The patient was admitted in a really bad shape (BP: 70/50 mm Hg, HR 128 pm, RR 20 pm). He was pale with multiple cutaneous lesions. He showed distal necrotic areas on both feet and hand fingers (Figs. 86.1A and B). He had multiple petechias and rales were heard over the lower two-thirds of his lungs. He had gallop rhythm but no murmurs . The liver was enlarged and tender with ascites.

The laboratory exams showed severe systemic compromise.

Hematological Findings

- Anemia, leukocytosis with left deviation
- Nitrogen retention

Urine Analysis

- Hematuria
- Altered hepatic profile
- Raised transaminases (AST-ALT and GGTP)
- Abnormal albumin/globulin ratio, CK/CK MB were normal.

EKG (Fig. 86.2)

Sinus tachycardia, anterior and lateral myocardial injury and infarction.

Chest X-ray (Fig. 86.3), Cardiomegaly and right pleural effusion.

Echocardiogram

Figures 86.4A to C. 283: Parasternal long axis (A). 284: Basal short axis (B). 285 LV short axis (C). Show important pericardial effusion with presence of abundant fibrin and a mobile mass in the LV cavity protruding into the LVOT and aorta.

Figures 86.5A to C and 286. Apical 5 chamber (A), 287 apical 4 chamber (B), and 288 apical 2 chamber (C) views show mid apical akinesis of the LV. Also, a mobile mass with attachment at the level of the mitral subvalvular

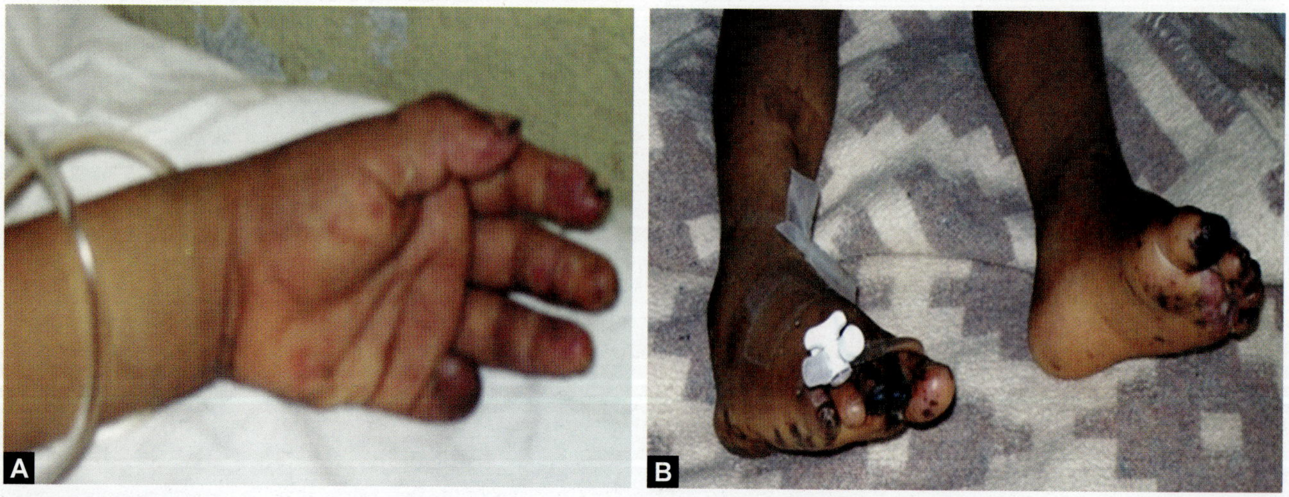

Figs. 86.1A and B: Distal necrotic lesions in hands and feet.

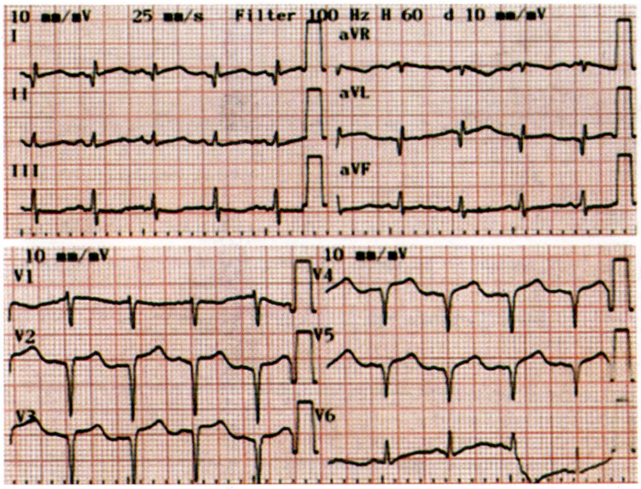

Fig. 86.2: Echocardiography.

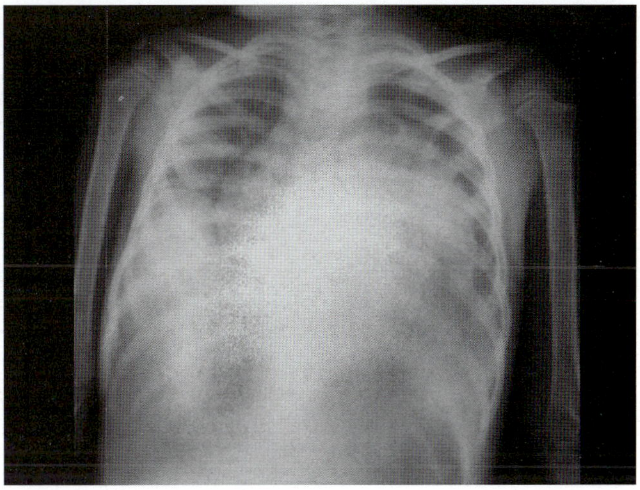

Fig. 86.3: Chest X-ray.

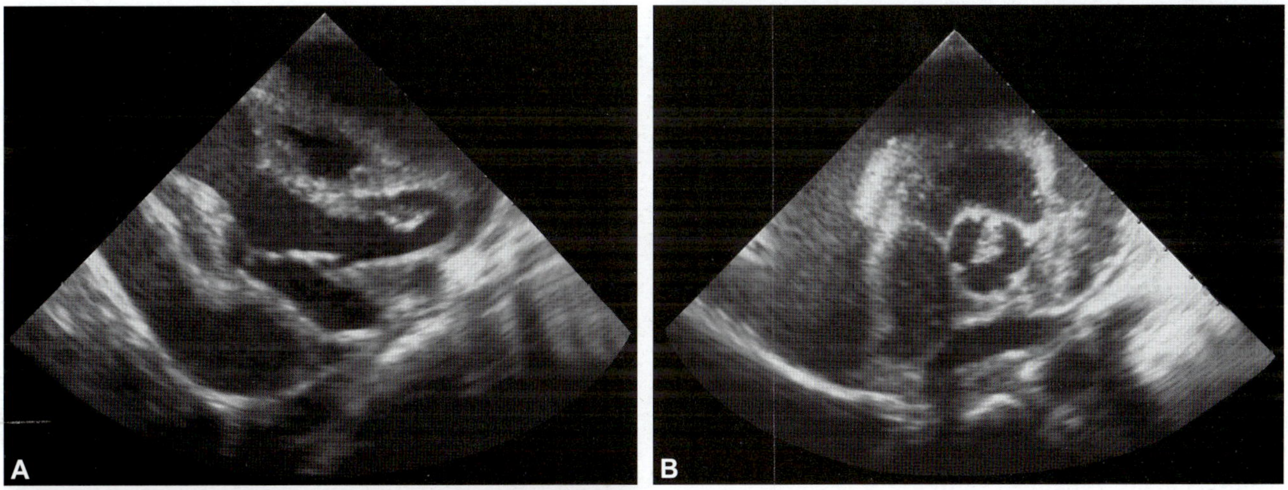

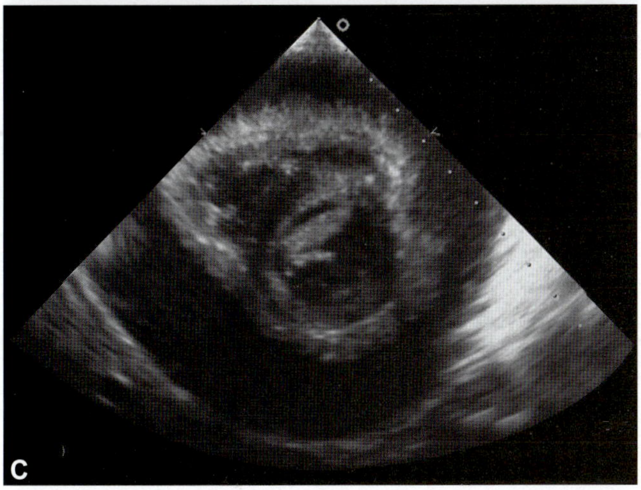

Figs. 86.4A to C: 2D Echocardiography. (A) Parasternal long axis 283; (B) Parasternal basal short axis 284; (C) Parasternal short axis at LV level 285.

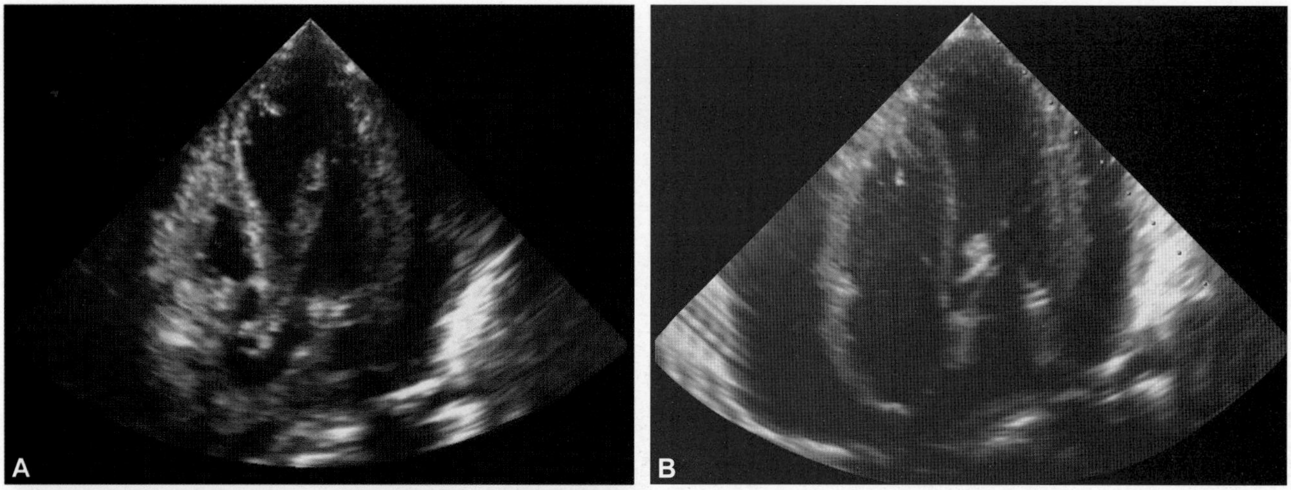

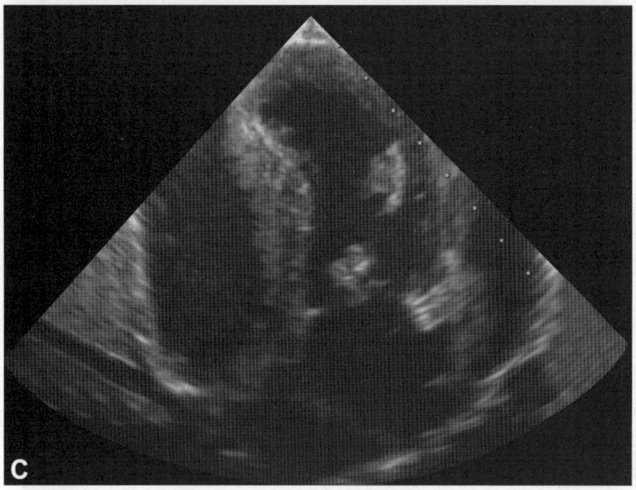

Figs. 86.5A to C: 2D Echocardiography apical views. (A) 5 chamber view (286); (B) 4 chamber view (287); (C) 2 chamber view (288).

apparatus protruding into the LVOT and aorta. Note the proximity of the mass to the ostium of the left main coronary artery in the 5 chamber view.

Figure 86.6 (287). The apical 4 chamber view and pulsed Doppler study show abnormal ventricular coupling suggesting increased intrapericardial pressure plus akinesis of the medial apical region of the LV.

The patient was rushed into surgery with the goal of excising the vegetation due to the high risk of new embolic events. The surgical findings were pyogenic pericarditis, multiple vegetations attached to the mitral subvalvular apparatus including the chordae tendineae and papillary muscles and extensive scarring in the apical region of the left ventricle. The patient unfortunately died during surgery.

The anatomy-pathology study showed vegetations (fibrin, inflammatory cells and bacteria colonies) and myocyte necrosis (Figs. 86.7A to C).

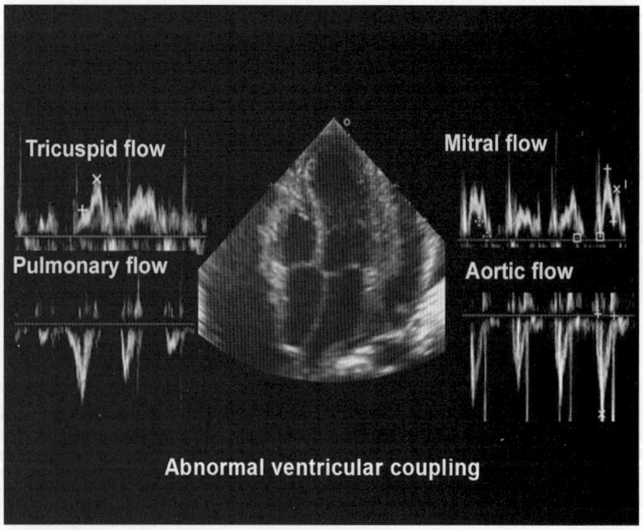

Fig. 86.6: Pulsed wave Doppler study.

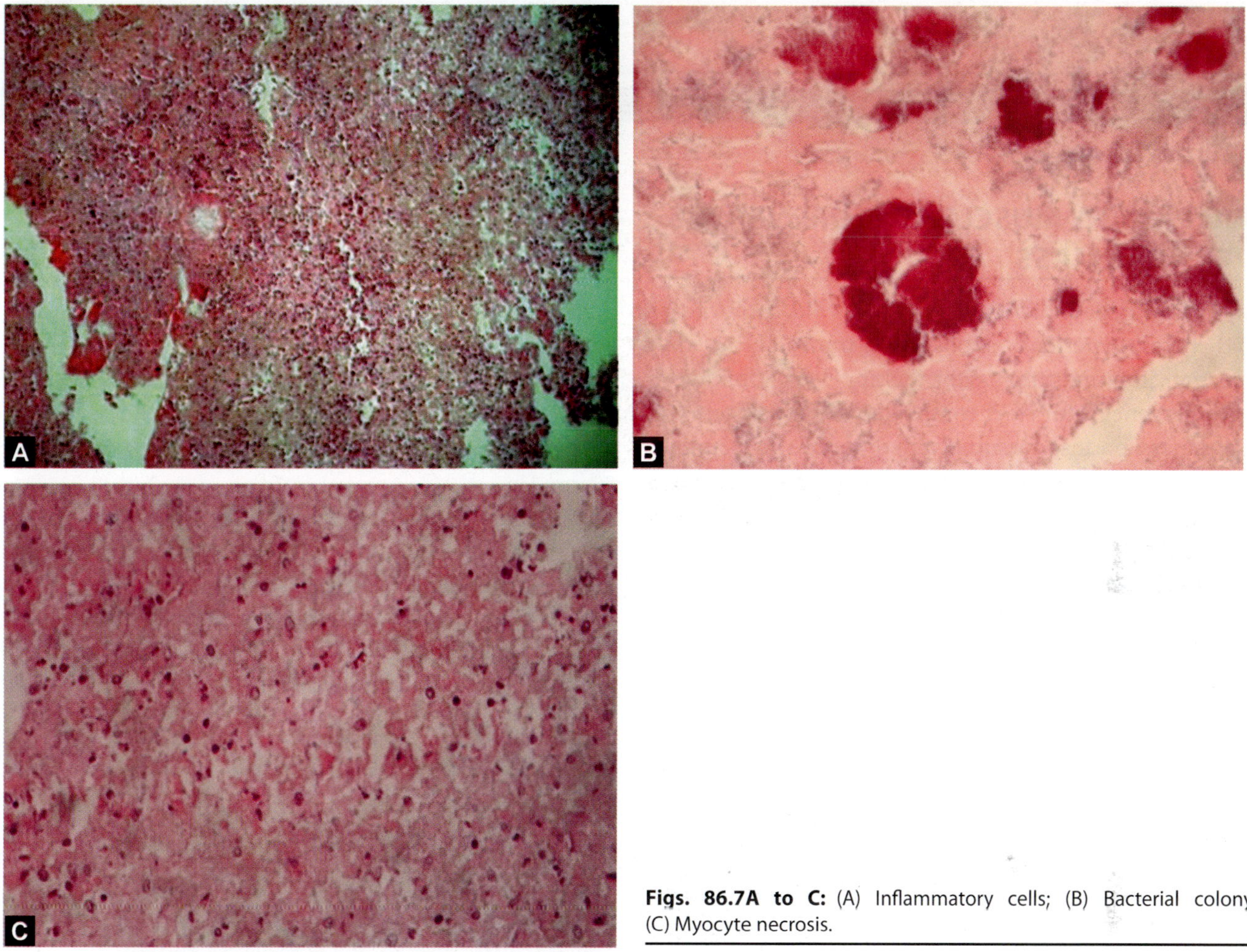

Figs. 86.7A to C: (A) Inflammatory cells; (B) Bacterial colony; (C) Myocyte necrosis.

Final Diagnosis

- Bacterial endocarditis
- Systemic pyogenic embolism
- Myocardial infarction due to septic coronary embolism
- Pyogenic pericarditis

This case shows an unusual complication of Varicella. This is the first case we have ever observed in our facility. It is likely that the poor nutritional status of the patient due to economic issues had an important bearing on the final tragic outcome.

Two -dimensional echocardiography with Doppler was of great utility in the diagnosis of all the structural and functional complications in our patient.

MOVIES 283 TO 288

CASE 87

Naveen Garg, Kanwal K Kapur

PAPILLARY MUSCLE RUPTURE VERSUS FUNGAL MASS

An African male patient about 58 years old, known case of diabetes, hypertension, post renal transplant on anti-rejection immunosuppressant therapy, was admitted in the emergency with chief complaints of sudden onset of drowsiness, perfuse sweating, and dyspnea. On examination, his pulse rate was irregular and blood pressure was 110/70 mm Hg. On examination he had bilateral chest crepitations and muffled heart sounds. His laboratory investigations revealed hypoglycemia with random blood sugar (RBS) 32 mg/dL, Hb-10 gm%, TLC-6.8 × 10^3/microL, N-82, L-10, M-7, E-1, Trop-T-positive, Anti-CMV-positive, blood urea 108 mg/dL, and serum creatinine 1.3 mg/dL.

His ECG reveals atrial fibrillation and chest X-ray shows bilateral pulmonary edema with cardiomegaly. CECT of brain showed multiple infarcts (Figs. 87.1A to C).

Transthoracic echocardiography was performed that shows a fluttering mass in LA with severe MR and pericardial effusion (289A to D). 2DTTE reveals a distended inferior vena cava with no respiratory variation and TR jet velocity of 47.1 mm Hg. His calculated PASP was 65 mm Hg.

2DTEE was done for further assessment of the mass. TEE showed the mass was a torn papillary muscle, which had led to his acute condition (290A to F and Fig. 87.2).

Live/real time 3D images were also acquired during TEE and analysed offline. The 3D images provided more insight and identified the torn muscle as the anterolateral

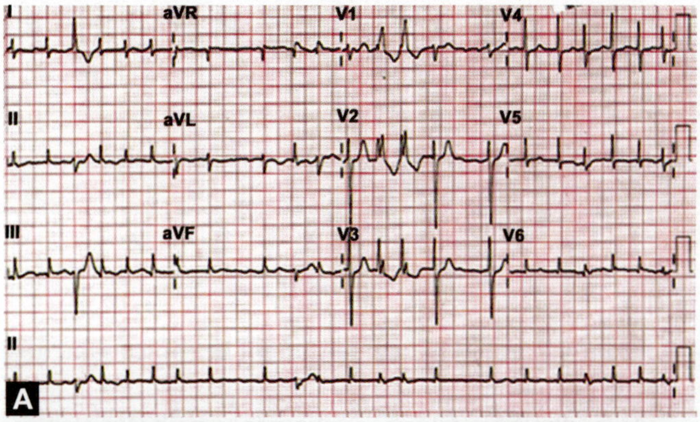

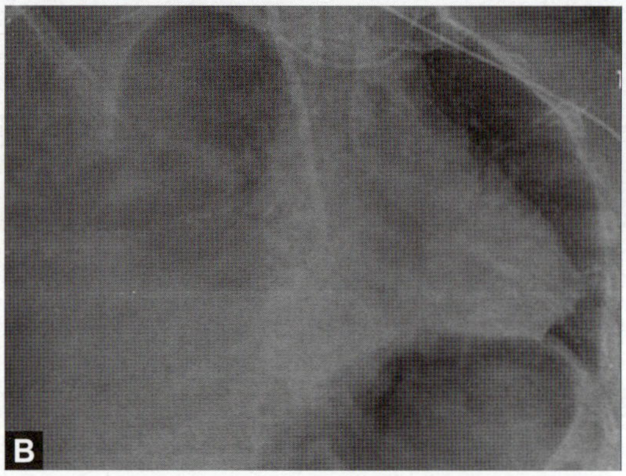

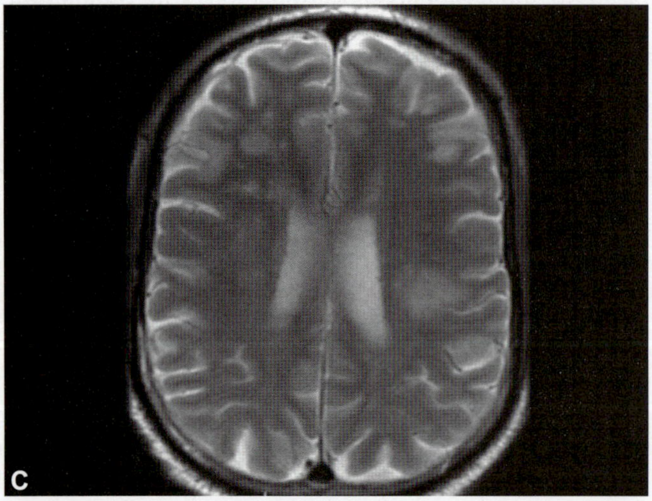

Figs. 87.1A to C: (A) ECG showing AF; (B) X-ray shows pulmonary edema; (C) CT-HEAD – Multiple infarcts.

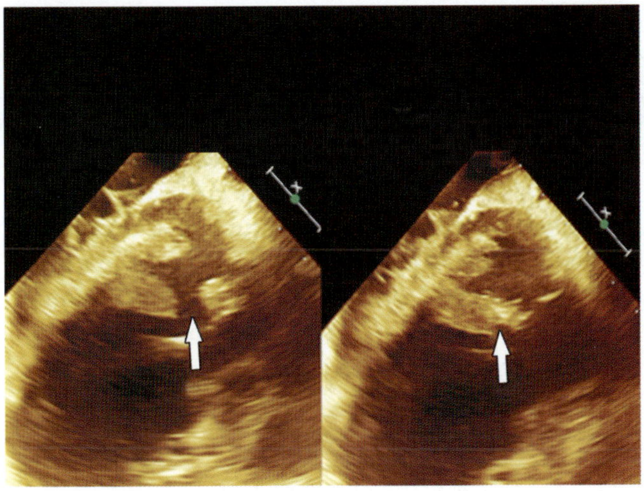

Fig. 87.2: TEE shows torn papillary muscle (arrows).

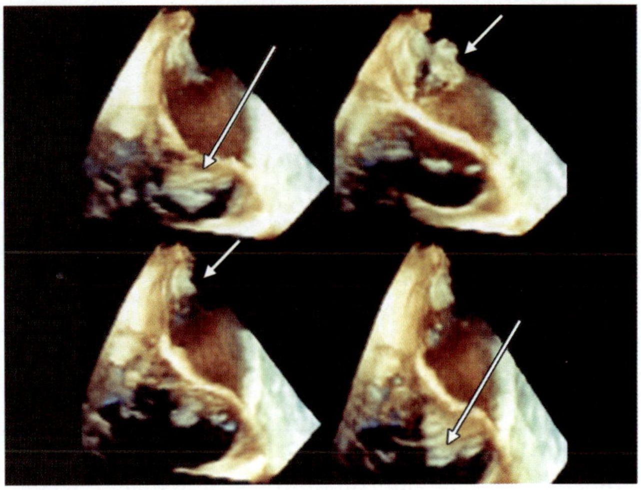

Fig. 87.3: 3D echo reveals fluttering mass (arrows) in LA.

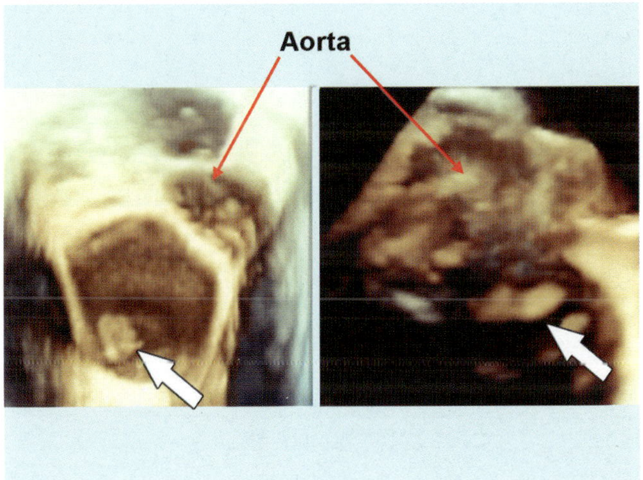

Fig. 87.4: 3D echo shows anterolateral papillary muscle involvement (white arrows).

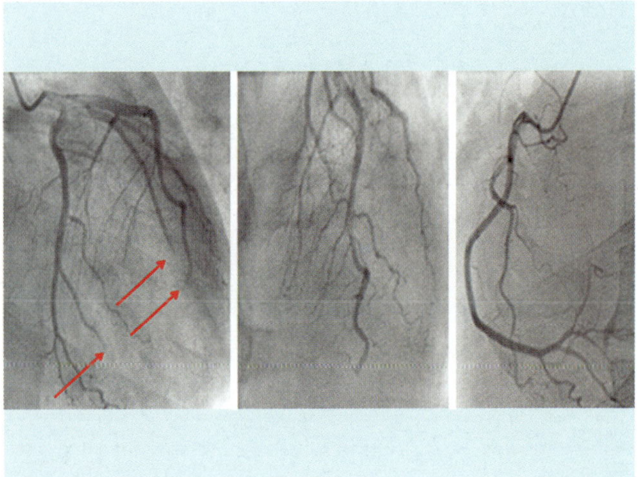

Fig. 87.5: Coronary angiogram (CAG) shows abrupt blockage of LAD, RAMUS and OM1 (red arrows).

papillary muscle (291A to F and Figs. 87.3 and 87.4). Coronary angiogram revealed abrupt blockage of mid LAD, ramus and OM1 (Fig. 87.5).

The patient was taken up for mitral valve replacement. At surgery the ruptured mass in LA was excised and was diagnosed as anterior papillary muscle rupture. The post-operative period was complicated by septicemia to which the patient eventually succumbed. The histology report of the excised mass showed infiltration of Aspergillosis fungal infection (Fig. 87.6).

DISCUSSION

Papillary muscle rupture is more common in inferior wall myocardial infarction. Of all the papillary muscle ruptures, the posteromedial papillary muscle rupture is 3–4 times more common than the anterolateral. It is probably due to the single artery perfusion of posteromedial and dual supply of anterolateral papillary muscle. Single artery supply by RCA in case of inferior infarcts results in more devastating infarction and rupture of posteromedial papillary muscle. The dual supply by LAD and LCx reduces the

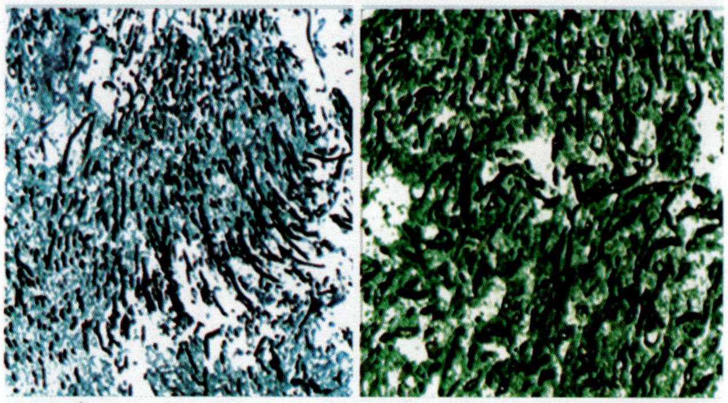

Fig. 87.6: Histopathology of the LA mass showing Aspergillosis fungal hyphae.

probability of infarction/rupture of the anterolateral papillary muscle. Causes of rupture of papillary muscle include myocardial infarction, infective endocarditis, trauma, cardiomyopathies or iatrogenic. Papillary muscle infection due to fungus is rare.

This Case—The angiographic appearance of coronary arteries in our patient (abrupt cut-off) suggests embolic occlusion of arteries (distal LAD, ramus and OM1) rather than atherosclerotic obstruction. The interesting feature in our patient is 3D TEE diagnosis of rupture of anterolateral papillary muscle as a result of embolization from a fungal vegetation. A combination of 3D TEE along with histological confirmation of fungal etiology helped in identifying the pathophysiological process.

MOVIE LEGENDS

289A to D: Transthoracic echocardiography
290A to F: Transesophageal echocardiography
291A to F: 3D echocardiography

CASE 88

Pizzano Nelson

A 20-year-old male presented with fever, chills, coughing and dyspnea, which started 3 days before, rapidly progressive, associated with weakness. Personal history included in hospital treatment due to a lower respiratory tract infection at the age of six months which required intravenous antibiotic administration. Physical examination revealed regular tachycardia, rales at lower 1/3 of left hemi thorax. Laboratory work showed a remarkable high white cells count. A chest X-ray was taken which showed an image consistent with pneumonia. Therefore, antibiotic treatment was begun. After a few days of treatment slight general improvement was noted but from the second day on fever and coughing were reinstalled, dyspnea increased, peripheral O2 desaturation was confirmed, and hematic sputum appeared.

Blood cultures were ordered and an echocardiogram was performed.

TTE revealed a mass related to tricuspid valve. A TEE was performed then which clearly showed a mobile mass on the tricuspid valve consistent with a vegetation, a prominent Eustachian valve and a catheter-like structure coming into the right atrium from the superior vena cava with a small highly mobile mass at its tip (🎥 292 to 294 and Figs. 88.1 to 88.3).

A CT scan was ordered which confirmed the catheter-like image in the location described as well as dense areas in both lungs. (Fig. 88.4).

A second round of blood cultures grew *Candida albicans*.

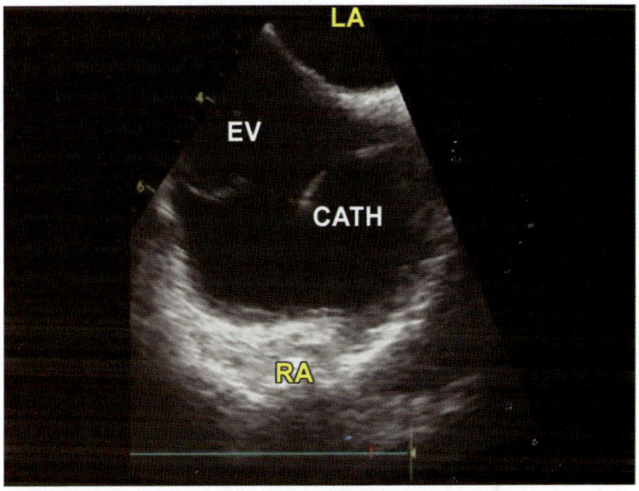

Fig. 88.2: TEE view of right atrium (RA) showing an Eustachian valve (EV) and a catheter-like image (CATH) coming from the superior vena cavae.

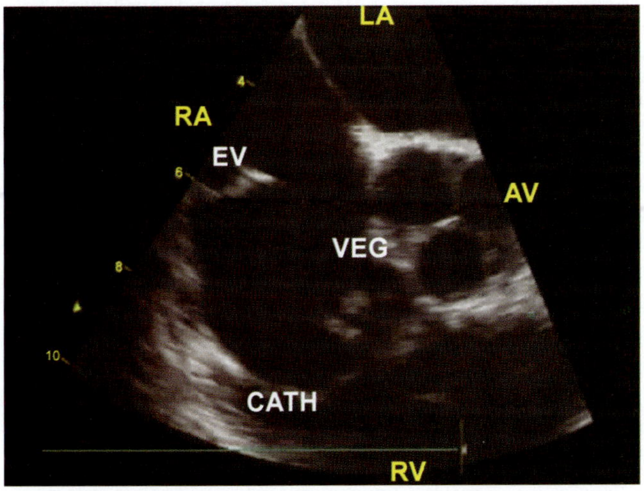

Fig. 88.1: TEE view of right atrium (RA), left atrium (LA), aortic valve (AV), right ventricle (RV), showing Eustachian valve (EV), vegetation (VEG) attached to tricuspid valve (TV), and catheter-like image (CATH).

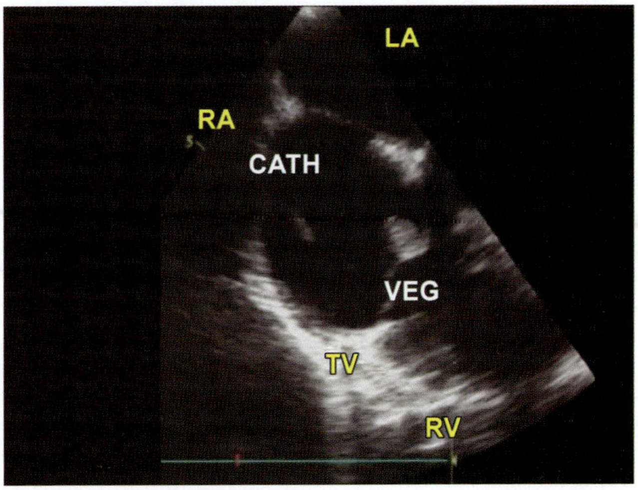

Fig. 88.3: TEE view showing catheter-like image (CATH) in the right atrium (RA) and a vegetation (VEG) on the tricuspid valve (TV).

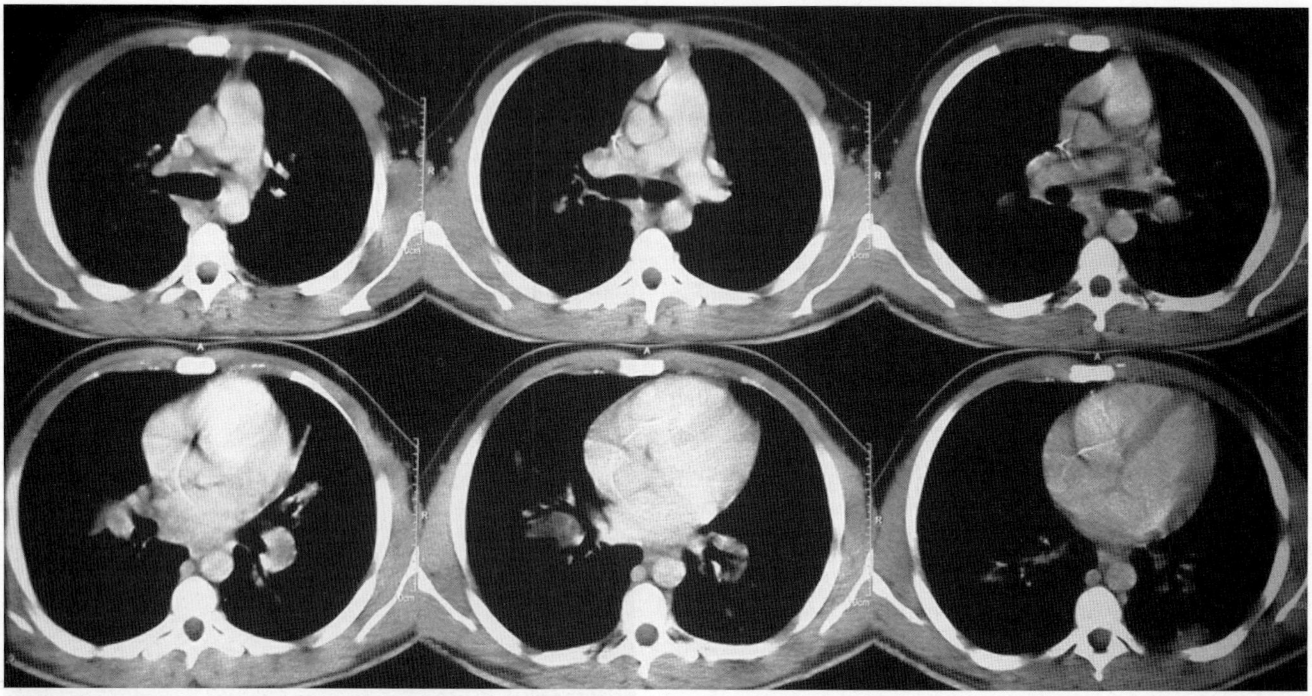

Fig. 88.4: CT scan showing a catheter-like image in the right heart coming from the superior vena cavae.

Discussion

This patient was interpreted as suffering from an acute pneumonia. After having a bad evolution, tests were ordered to clarify diagnosis. Infectious endocarditis and subsequent septic pulmonary infarction was then diagnosed, caused by a fungus probably favored by an I/V line left in the right heart when in hospital for treatment 20 years ago.

Fluconazole was then administered and surgical extraction of remaining catheter was done.

Patient did well and was discharged after a few days.

It must be highlighted the concomitant viewing by TEE of three different structures (292 to 294). One is a normal but rather large filamentous structure which corresponds to Eustachian valve. A mass on tricuspid valve, which is an acquired structure consistent with a vegetation. And last but not least, a very uncommon image consistent with a "forgotten" intravenous line which shows a small mass on the tip, also consistent with infectious endocarditis.

MOVIES 292 TO 294

CASE 89

Uygur B, Bulur S, Nanda NC

The patient was a 59-year-old male with ICD implantation in 2009 who was referred because of TV/ICD vegetations. Blood cultures detected methicillin sensitive coagulase negative Staphylococcus and he was placed on antibiotic therapy. Because of his deteriorating clinical condition, it was decided to send him for urgent surgery. However, this was delayed because of a low platelet count. His platelet count was subsequently brought up above 100,000/mL but 1 day before surgery he had respiratory and cardiac arrest and died. 2D and 3D TTE movies are shown.

1. **What does the arrow show (🎥 295 to 298)?**
   (a) Large clots involving the TV and ICD lead (L)
   (b) Large vegetations involving the TV and ICD lead (L)
   (c) Infected thrombi cannot be excluded

Ans. (c)

The ICD lead is clearly seen embedded in the masses. The TV is not fully visualized; hence it also appears to be involved. Because the masses are very large, they are more likely to be thrombi. Positive blood cultures and the patient's rapidly deteriorating clinical condition suggest the presence of infection and therefore these masses could be infected thrombi or a combination of thrombi and vegetations. 🎥 298 is 3D subcostal examination. Arrowhead points to the ICD lead.

MOVIES 295 TO 298 🎥

CASE 90

Bulur S, Elsayed M, Nanda NC

This is a 26-year-old patient bed ridden with spina bifida and neurogenic bladder. He developed pericardial effusion which was drained. He had lines placed in the right heart and subsequently developed fever. Several 2D TTEs and TEEs were done.

This patient illustrates the value of follow up echocardiograms. He began with no liver congestion, normal LV and RV function and no obvious TV vegetations. He was noted to have a bicuspid AV with mild thickening. Then he developed a large pericardial effusion of unknown etiology with poor RV function. This improved following fluid drainage but later developed a large pericardial hematoma. Around this time, lines were placed in the right heart for monitoring pressures. He subsequently developed TV vegetations and LV-RA and then LV-RV shunts (acquired Gerbode defect) 🎥 299-311 and Figures 90.1 to 90.5. Dates and timings of movies are given.

1. **How are LV – RV and LV – RA shunts differentiated from AO–RV shunt?**
   (a) AO–RV shunt would show high velocity flows in both systole and diastole.
   (b) LV–RV and LV–RA shunts would show high velocity flows only in diastole
   (c) AO–RV shunt shows high velocity flow in systole but not diastole
   (d) It is difficult to differentiate the two unless one does a careful 2D color Doppler examination to show the shunt origin from either the AO or LV.

Ans. (a)

Because the pressure in the AO is high in both systole and diastole and the pressures in RV and RA are normally much lower, AO–RV shunt (as well as AO-RA shunt) will occur throughout the cardiac cycle (continuous murmur on auscultation). On the other hand, the difference between LV and RV/RA diastolic pressures is very low and hence there is no high velocity shunting in diastole in the case of LV–RV/RA shunt.

2. **This patient has a bicuspid AV. What other important 2D echocardiographic parameters should one assess?**
   (a) Aortic valve area
   (b) Presence and severity of AR
   (c) Size of the aortic root up to the mid ascending aorta
   (d) All of the above

Ans. (d)

3. **What is the most common congenital cardiac anomaly which affects 1–2% of the population?**
   (a) Ventricular septal defect

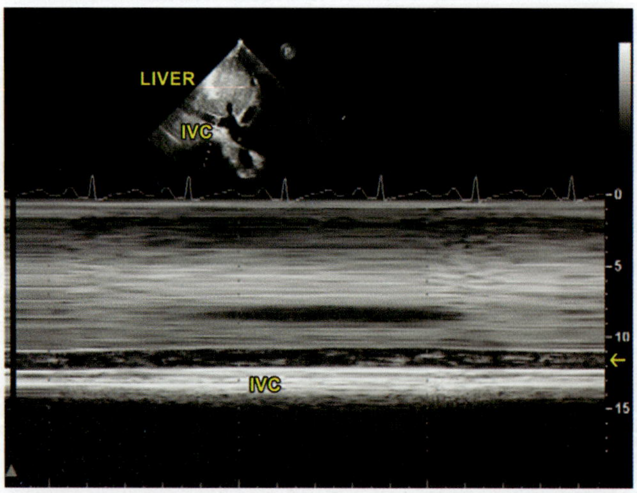

Fig. 90.1: M-mode image. Subcostal examination. Spontaneous echo contrast signals indicative of low flow state are noted in the IVC.

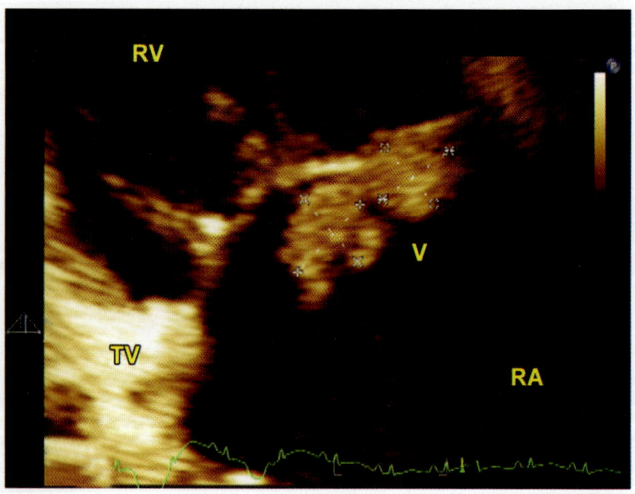

Fig. 90.2: Vegetations (V) on both atrial and ventricular aspects of TV.

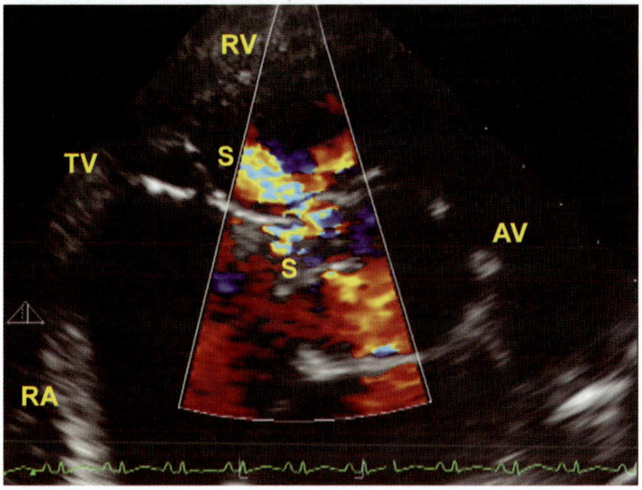

Fig. 90.3: LV-RV and LV-RA shunts(S). Gerbode defects.

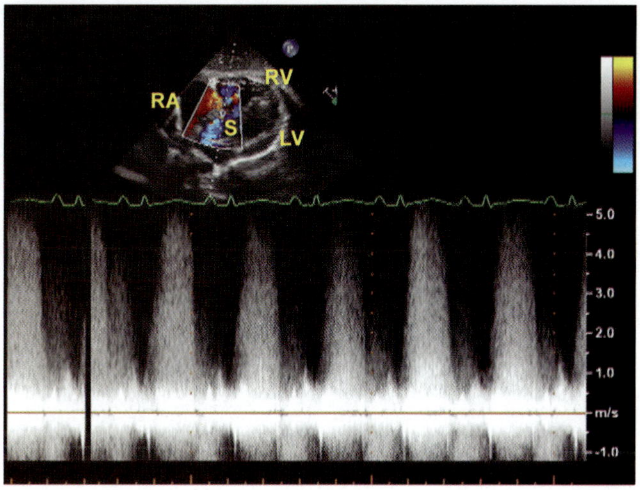

Fig. 90.4: LV-RA/RV shunt (Gerbode shunt) visualized subcostally. CW Doppler shows a very high velocity over 5 m/s indicating a restrictive defect with no significant elevation of RV systolic pressure.

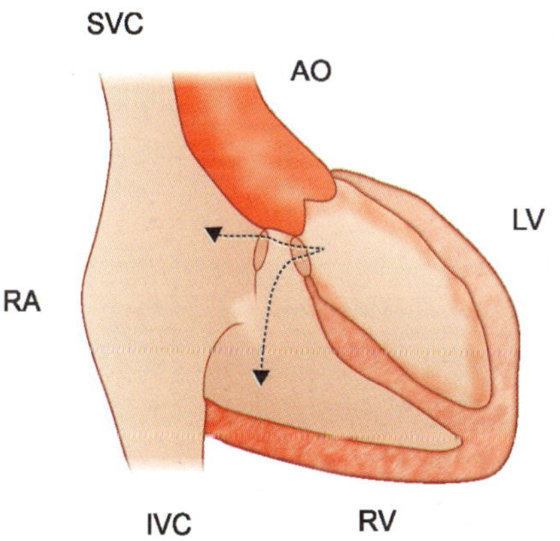

Fig. 90.5: Schematic diagram showing both LV-RA and LV-RA-RV shunts (Gerbode defects).

(b) Coronary artery fistula
(c) Patent ductus arteriosus
(d) Bicuspid aortic valve

Ans. (d)

4. **What are the usual complications of bicuspid aortic valve?**
   (a) Aortic stenosis
   (b) Aortic regurgitation
   (c) Endocarditis
   (d) A and B
   (e) All of the above

Ans. (e)

MOVIE LEGENDS

299: Subcostal view showing normal liver texture.
300: Bicuspid AV with mild thickening (asterisk)
301: PE. Thickened TV, no vegetations.
302: Large PE. Poor RV function. RV free wall shows no thickening in systole.
303: Large PE. Mild TR and no TV vegetations.
304: Arrow shows spontaneous contrast in IVC indicating low blood flow state.
305: Arrow shows a large pericardial thrombus following PE drainage. (C = catheter in the right heart).
306: Line/catheter (C) in the right heart. Mild TR.
307: LVO-RA shunt (S) just beneath the TV (Gerbode shunt).
308 & 309: Vegetations (V) on both atrial and ventricular aspects of TV. Some vegetations are adjacent to AV.
310: Shows LV-RV and LV-RA shunts (Gerbode shunt).
311: LV-RA/RV shunt (Gerbode shunt) visualized subcostally. The texture of liver has changed. It shows small multiple echo densities giving a typical "starry sky appearance". These result from accentuation of portal venule walls because of diminished liver parenchymal echogenicity from edema of hepatocytes. This occurs with hepatic congestion due to right sided heart failure. It is also noted in other conditions such as acute hepatitis and toxic shock syndrome.[1]

REFERENCES

1. Abu-Judeh HH. The "starry sky" liver with right-sided heart failure. AJR Am J Roentgenol. 2002 Jan;178(1):78. PubMed PMID: 11756091.

2. Nanda NC, Gramiak R, Manning JA. Echocardiography of the tricuspid valve in congenital left ventricular-right atrial communication. Circulation. 1975 Feb;51(2):268-72. PubMed PMID: 1112006.

3. Gerbode F, Hultgren H, Melrose D, Osborn J. Syndrome of left ventricular-right atrial shunt; successful surgical repair of defect in five cases, with observation of bradycardia on closure. Ann Surg. 1958 Sep;148(3):433-46. PubMed PMID: 13571920; PubMed Central PMCID: PMC1450812.

CASE 91*

Gulotta JC, Gaba S, Bulur S, Joson M, Sungur A, Nanda NC

The patient is a 26-year-old male with tetralogy of Fallot and pulmonary atresia who was admitted with one week history of fever, dyspnea and pulmonary edema. Previously he had surgical VSD closure, a shunt placement with homograft between RV and PA, a stent placement in proximal LPA with subsequent redilation and a valved conduit between RV and PA.

On examination the patient was febrile, hypotensive and tachypneic. He had a loud precordial systolic murmur, a diastolic murmur, bilateral basal rales and bilateral lower limb edema.

2D TTE, 2D TEE and subsequently 3D TTE were performed. Figures 91.1-91.3 and 91.4A-C. 🎥 312A-D, 313, 314 A and B and 315 A-H.

1. **When performing an echocardiographic examination what windows should be used?**

   (a) Standard left parasternal, apical, subcostal and suprasternal windows

   (b) An attempt should be made to additionally examine all available windows including right parasternal approach, bilateral supra- and infraclavicular examination and examination from the back

Ans. (b)

In this patient conduit vegetations by 2D TTE were demonstrated only when an acoustic window underneath the left clavicle was utilized. The patient developed cardiogenic and septic shock, hypoxic respiratory failure and acute renal shut down. He was begun on multiple antibiotics and supportive measures and survived despite a long and complicated course. The plan is for future PV conduit and AV replacement.

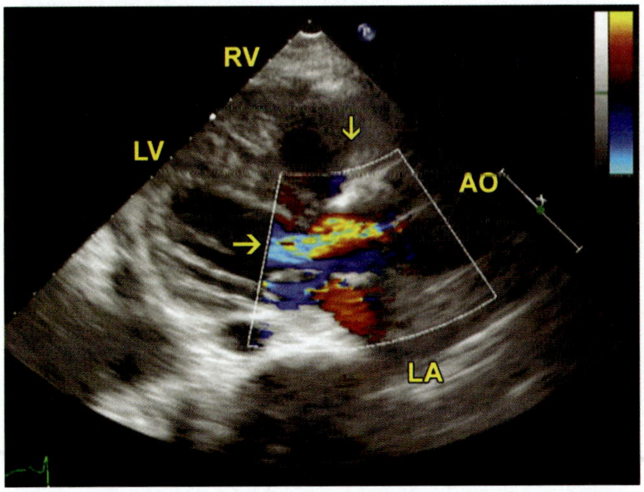

Fig. 91.1: Two-dimensional transthoracic echocardiography in tetralogy of Fallot postrepair. Top arrow shows a thickened patch suspicious for vegetation. The lower arrow shows moderate aortic regurgitation. 🎥 312A–D. Movie 312D shows peak and mean gradients across the tricuspid valve (TV) of 77 and 40 mm Hg, respectively. AO = aorta; LA = left atrium; LV = left ventricle; RA = right atrium; RV = right ventricle; TR = tricuspid regurgitation.

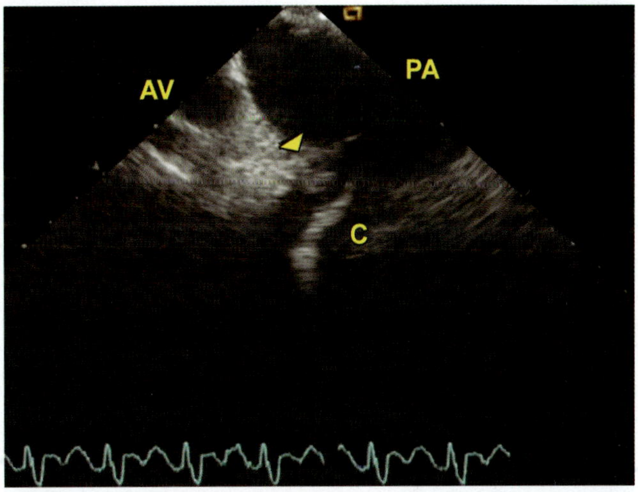

Fig. 91.2: Multiplane two-dimensional transesophageal echocardiography in tetralogy of Fallot postrepair. Arrowhead shows a large mass like vegetation in the conduit (C) which is seen connected to the pulmonary artery (PA). 🎥 313. AV = aortic valve; AA = ascending aorta.

*This case is reproduced with permission from: Gulotta JC, Gaba S, Bulur S, Joson M, Sungur A, Nanda NC. Echocardiography. 2015 Feb;32(2):361-4.

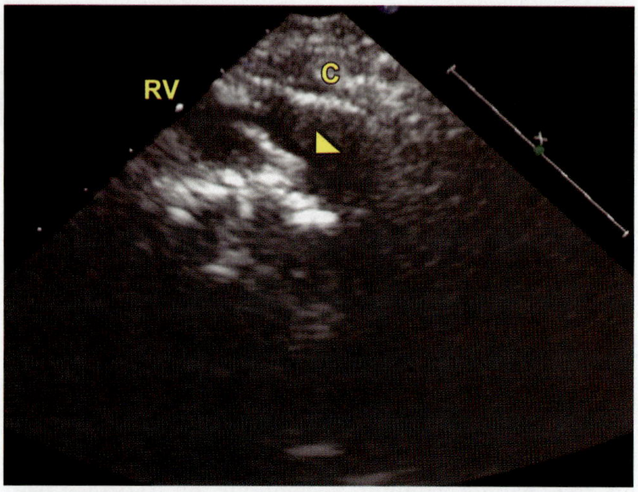

Fig. 91.3: Two-dimensional transthoracic echocardiography in tetralogy of Fallot postrepair. Examination was repeated with the transducer placed below the left clavicle. Arrowhead shows a large mobile vegetation in the conduit (C). 314A and B. Arrow in 314B shows torrential conduit valve regurgitation. Abbreviations as in Figure 91.1.

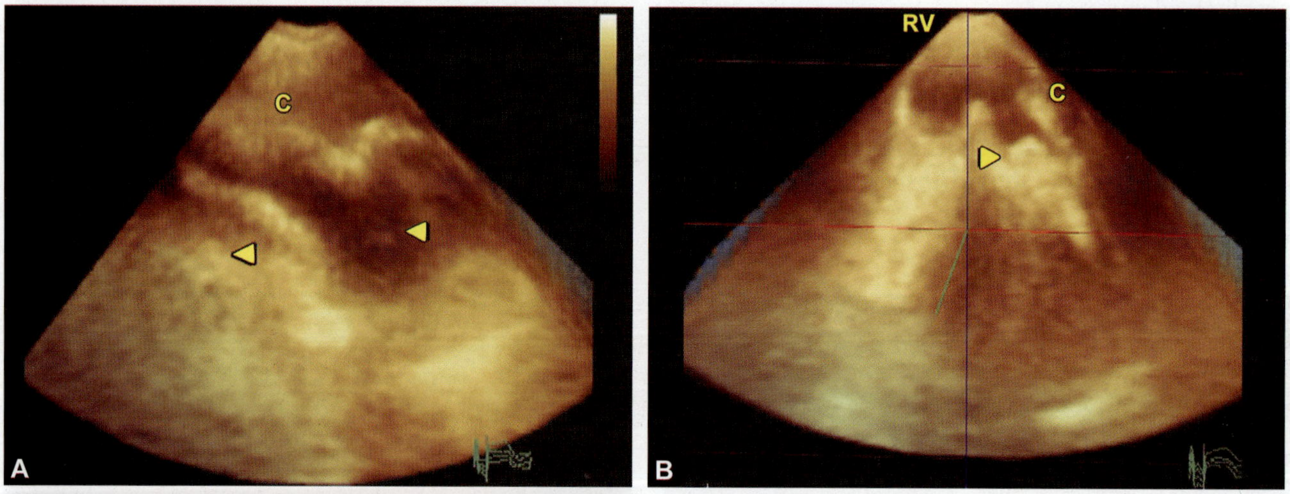

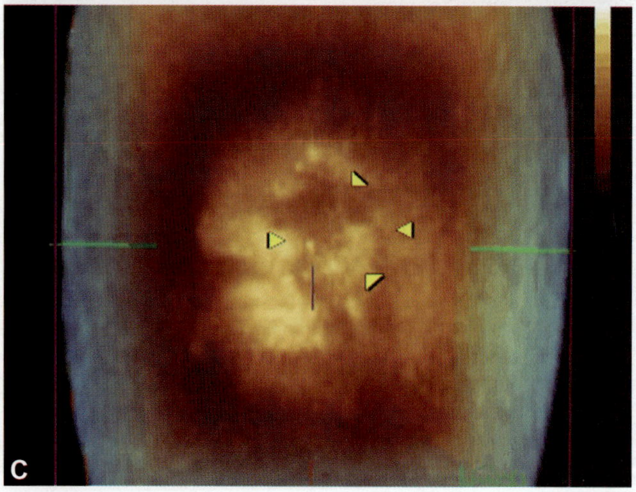

Figs. 91.4A to C: Live/real time three-dimensional transthoracic echocardiography in tetralogy of Fallot postrepair. A–C. Arrowheads point to vegetations involving the prosthetic valve and the conduit (C). The large vegetation seen on the two-dimensional study is noted in A. The junction of the C with the RV is well seen in B. Panel C depicts multiple vegetations viewed from the top. 315A–H. P in 315D indicates prosthetic valve. R points to reverberatory artifacts in 315E. 315G represents multiplanar mode used for making measurements. 315H shows the volume (V1) of the largest vegetation (0.38 mL), two smaller vegetations (V2 and V3, 0.04 and 0.02 mL, respectively) and composite volume (V4) of the 5 smallest vegetations (0.12 mL).

MOVIES 312A TO D, 313, 314A AND B AND 315A TO H

SECTION 6

Coronary Artery Disease

CASE 92

Guler EC, Nanda NC

This 50-year-old female with known systemic hypertension sought attention because of intermittent chest pains. 2D TTE was performed (🎥 316). Apical 4-chamber view is shown.

1. **How would you assess LV wall motion in this patient?**
   (a) Assess LV epicardial motion
   (b) Assess LV endocardial motion
   (c) Assess LV myocardial motion
   (d) Assess motion of all the above

Ans. (b)

Motion of the endocardium (the innermost layer, arrows) which moves more than the other two layers should be considered when evaluating LV function. Evaluation of only the epicardium (outer layer) specially if the endocardium and the myocardium (middle layer) are not well visualized or not visualized at all could incorrectly suggest hypokinesis because the epicardium generally moves less than the endocardium as can be noted in this patient. In such cases, it is important to adjust the transducer position and angulation to try to optimally image the endocardium. Contrast echo is also very useful to delineate the endocardial border. Care needs to be taken also to maximize the distance between the base and apex of the LV to avoid foreshortening. Motion of the RV is also evaluated similar to LV.

MOVIE 316 🎥

CASE 93

Elkaryoni A, Arisha MJ, Barssoum K, Mohamed A, Nanda NC

This is a 53-year-old male with non-ST elevation myocardial infarction. His body surface area is 2.2 m^2. 2D TTE was done (317A and B).

1. **Parasternal long axis view (317A) shows the following:**
   (a) Markedly hypokinetic anterior septum
   (b) Normal motion of inferolateral wall
   (c) Hyperkinesis of inferolateral wall
   (d) (a) and (b) are correct
   (e) (a) and (c) are correct

Ans. (e)

The inferolateral wall shows compensatory hyperkinesis because of the markedly hypokinetic septum.

2. **The arrow in the parasternal short axis view (317B) points to:**
   (a) Epicardial fat pat
   (b) Organized pericardial effusion with fibrin
   (c) Organized pericardial effusion following partial rupture of LV wall
   (d) Only (b) and (c) are correct
   (e) All of the above are correct

Ans. (d)

Epicardial fat pad is noted anterior to the organized pericardial effusion (arrow). It is not clear whether this patient developed pericardial effusion due to heart failure which subsequently organized or whether there was a small rupture due to myocardial infarction which was sealed with fibrin. Since the effusion is localized anteriorly with no fluid posteriorly, a sealed rupture is more likely. In the short axis view, the anterior septum and both anterior and anterolateral walls are hypokintetic.

MOVIES 317A AND B

CASE 94

Taher A, Elsayed M, Alagic N, Uygur B, Turaga NSN, Chahwala JR, Adarna LG, Bulur S, Nanda NC

A 59-year-old male referred for echocardiogram before CABG.

Apical 4 chamber views show thin and hypokinetic apical inferoseptum (arrow in 318) and apical RV free wall hypokinesis (arrow in 319).

1. **Name the LV walls in parasternal long-axis and apical 4 chamber views?**
   (a) Inferolateral and anteroseptal; inferoseptal and anterolateral
   (b) Posterior and septal; inferoseptal and anterolateral
   (c) Posterior and anteroseptal; septal and lateral
   (d) Posterolateral and anteroseptal; inferoseptal and free wall

Ans. (a)

In the parasternal long-axis view the walls are named inferolateral and anteroseptal.

In the 4 chamber view they are denoted as inferoseptal and anterolateral.

In the 2 chamber view the walls are designated as inferior (next to liver) and anterior.

2. **Which coronary arteries you suspect are significantly stenosed in this patient?**
   (a) LAD and RCA
   (b) LAD only
   (c) LAD and RCA/CX
   (d) RCA and CX

Ans. (a)

The distal septum is supplied by LAD and the RV free wall by the RCA. However the distal portion of RV free wall is often supplied by LAD. Thus (b) may also the correct answer.

320 is from another patient showing RV apical dyskinesis (arrow).

MOVIES 318 TO 320

CASE 95

Bulur S, Elsayed M, Alagic N, Uygur B, Turaga NSN, Chahwala JR, Adarna LG, Nanda NC

This male patient is 81-year-old and has a history of coronary artery disease. 2D TTE was done.

1. **What does the arrow in the parasternal long-axis view show (🎥 321)?**
   (a) Hypokinesis of LV inferolateral wall and RV free wall
   (b) Hypokinesis of LV inferior wall and RV free wall
   (c) Hypokinesis of LV inferolateral wall and RV free wall plus trivial pericardial effusion located posteriorly
   (d) Hypokinesis of LV inferior wall and RV free wall plus trivial pericardial effusion located posteriorly

Ans. (c)

Hypokinesis of LV inferolateral wall (posterior wall) is easily recognized by comparing it with the ventricular septum which shows normal motion and thickening in systole. The visualized RV wall is hypokinetic. There is trivial pericardial effusion but the relatively echolucent space in front of the pericardium represents normal myocardium. This appearance is due to the homogenous nature of myocardium without any significant interfaces in this area. In most instances, the normal myocardium is more echogenic than in this patient because it has several interfaces which result in the production of echo signals.

2. **Which coronary artery is likely involved in this patient?**
   (a) LAD
   (b) LAD
   (c) RCA or LCX
   (d) Only RCA
   (e) Only LCX

Ans. (d)

LV inferolateral wall is generally supplied by RCA or LCX. RV free wall is supplied by RCA. Since both walls are involved, significant RCA stenosis would be expected in this patient.

🎥 322 is from another patient demonstrating LV inferolateral wall dyskinesis (arrow).

MOVIES 321 AND 322

CASE 96

Alagic N, Adarna LG, Elsayed M, Uygur B, Turaga NSN, Chahwala JR, Bulur S, Nanda NC

The patient is a 53-year-old male with history of previous myocardial infarction. 2DTTE was done.

1. **Which view is shown (🎥 323)?**
   (a) Apical 4 chamber view
   (b) Apical 2 chamber view
   (c) Apical long-axis view
   (d) Para-apical view

Ans. (b)

Neither RV nor RA is visualized in the movie clip, only the LV and LA. Hence, it is apical 2 chamber view.

2. **What does the arrow in the movie clip point to?**
   (a) Hypokinesis and dyskinesis of proximal LV inferoposterior wall
   (b) Dyskinesis of proximal LV inferoposterior wall
   (c) Dyskinesis of proximal LV inferior wall
   (d) Both hypokinesis and dyskinesis may be normally seen in this view

Ans. (c)

In the apical 2 chamber view, LV inferior and anterior walls are imaged. The proximal inferior wall is clearly seen bulging outward in systole (dyskinesis) from previous myocardial infarction involving this area.

3. **Which coronary artery is most likely involved?**
   (a) RCA or LCA
   (b) Only RCA
   (c) Only LCA
   (d) RCA plus LAD
   (e) LCA plus LAD

Ans. (b)

LV inferior wall is generally supplied by the RCA.

🎥 324 is from another patient showing aneurysmal proximal LV inferior wall (arrow) delineated by contrast echocardiography.

🎥 325 is from a different patient showing LV apical aneurysm (arrows) predominantly involving the apical inferior wall (left arrow).

MOVIES 323 TO 325

CASE 97

Adarna LG, Bulur S, Elsayed M, Alagic N, Uygur B, Turaga NSN, Chahwala JR, Nanda NC

The patient is a 67-year-old male in heart failure. He has history of myocardial infarction in the past. 2DTTE movies are shown (🎥 326 to 328).

1. **All of the following statements are true *except*:**
   (a) The arrow points to a thrombus in the LV apex which is aneurysmal (AN)
   (b) Mild aortic regurgitation (AR) is noted
   (c) The arrow shows an artifact in the LV apex
   (d) The echo findings are consistent with past myocardial infarction

Ans. (a)

Contrast echocardiography done with a commercially available agent clearly shows complete filling of the LV apex with no evidence of thrombus. The echo density visualized is therefore most likely an artifact. Contrast echocardiography is most useful in excluding a thrombus or another space occupying lesion in the LV apex.

🎥 329 to 331 are from another patient showing a large echo density (arrow) in the LV apex. Contrast echo shows absence of any mass and therefore the echo density is an artifact.

MOVIES 326 TO 331 🎥

CASE 98

Kul Aggarwal, Archana Vasudevan, Sudarshan Balla

Why is this patient short of breath?

A 76-year-old male presented with one month history of shortness of breath on exertion. Had a previous history of sick sinus syndrome and permanent pacemaker implant. His echocardiogram is shown here (Fig. 98.1 and 332):

The echocardiogram is most consistent with:

1. LV aneurysm
2. LV pseudoaneurysm
3. RV akinesis
4. LV diverticulum

Discussion

Patient underwent a cardiac catheterization study with coronary angiography and LV angiography. Found to have a totally occluded right coronary artery and nonobstructive left coronary system. His TEE (Fig. 98.2 and 333) and LV angiography (Fig. 98.3 and 334) are shown here.

This case illustrates the presence of a large true LV aneurysm following an inferior infarct. The occluded RCA is consistent with the territory of this aneurysm. A true aneurysm typically has a large "neck" and a smooth wall whereas a false aneurysm has a narrow neck and irregular track. A diverticulum is generally very small in size. LV aneurysms are more common at the apex following an anterior myocardial infarction. Complications include heart failure, ventricular arrhythmias and LV thrombus with potential for systemic embolization.

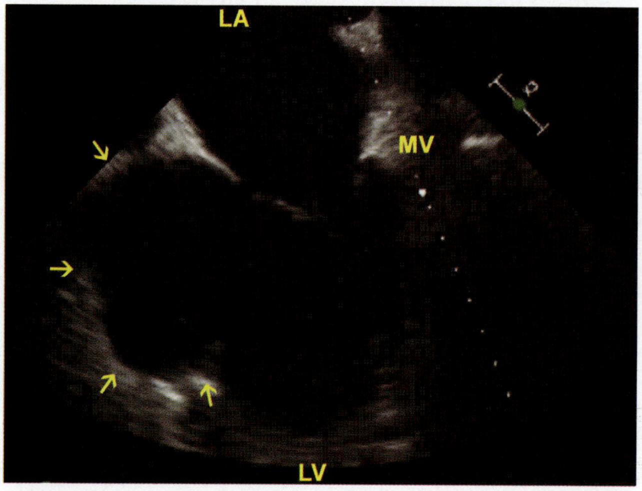

Fig. 98.2: Transesophageal echocardiography. Shows same findings as above.

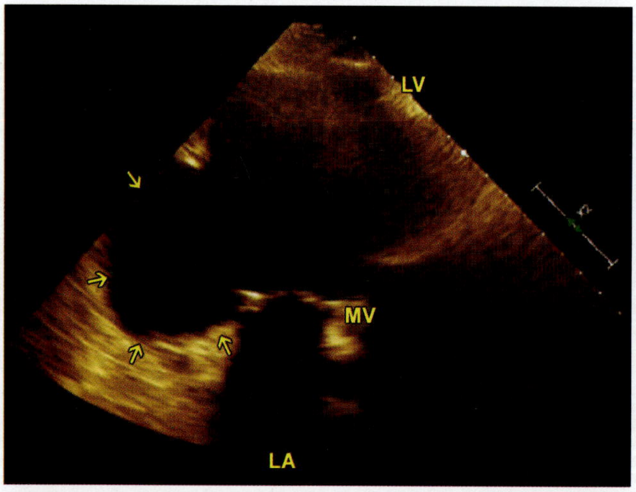

Fig. 98.1: Transthoracic apical view showing a very large true LV aneurysm (arrows) with a wide opening.

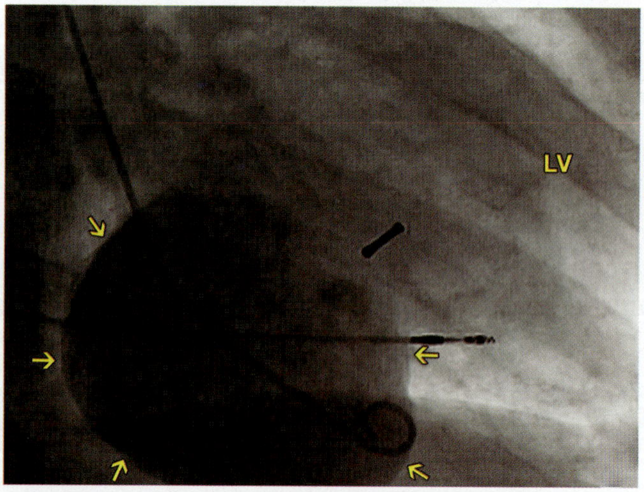

Fig. 98.3: LV angiogram also showing the same findings.

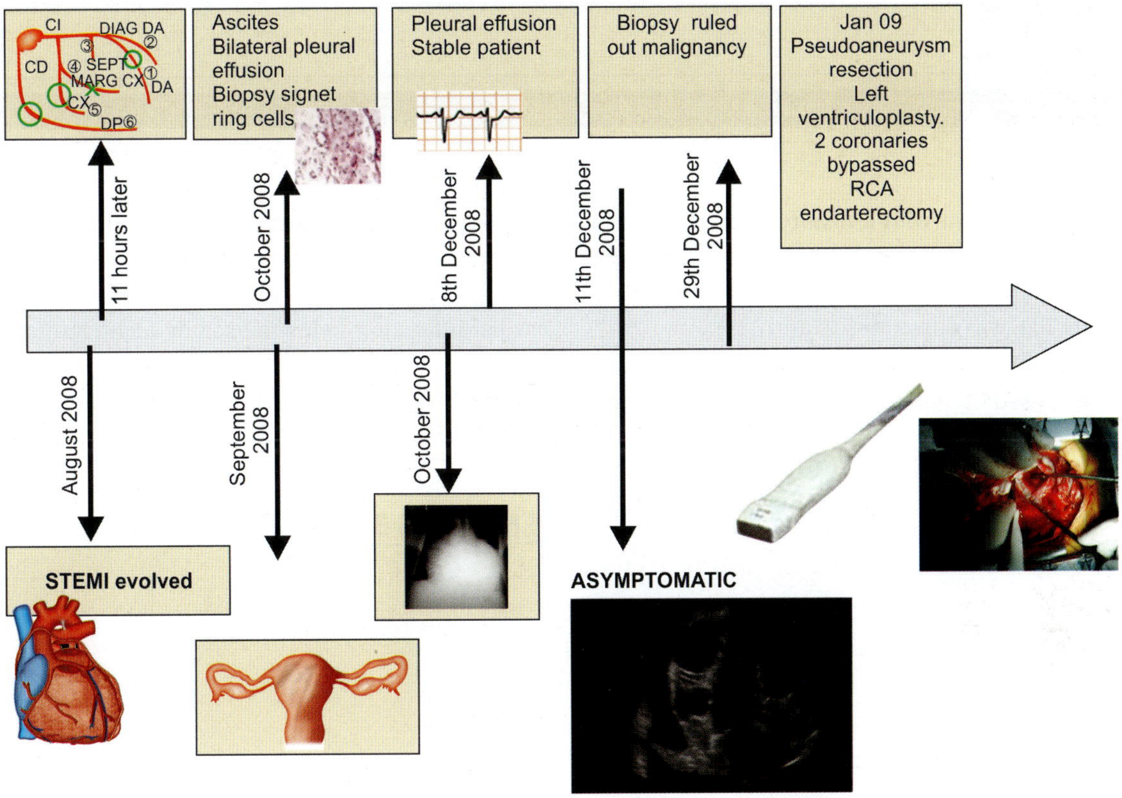

Fig. 101.5: Timeline of medical history, evolution.

MOVIE LEGENDS

337 to 339: 2D TTE. Arrows show multiple pseudoaneurysms and the arrowhead points to pleural effusion.

CASE 102

Adarna LG, Elsayed M, Taher A, Alagic N, Uygur B, Turaga NSN, Chahwala JR, Bulur S, Nanda NC

This is an elderly patient with a history of previous myocardial infarction who developed a harsh systolic precordial murmur. No murmur was noted prior to myocardial infarction. 2D TTE was done (340 and 341).

1. **What are the findings on the echo?**
   (a) Decreased LV function
   (b) Decreased RV function
   (c) Ventricular septal rupture with left to right shunt
   (d) Ventricular septal rupture with right to left shunt

Ans. (c)

The large rupture in the mid portion of the septum (arrow) is clearly seen with flow signals moving from LV to RV through the defect. No history of murmur prior to myocardial infarction helps to exclude a congenital ventricular septal defect. Both LV and RV function appear normal. Poor RV function heralds adverse prognosis in patients with ventricular septal rupture.

MOVIES 340 AND 341

CASE 103

Ahmad S Omran

POST-MYOCARDIAL INFARCTION SEPTAL RUPTURE (POST MI VSD)

This 71-year-old man was transferred to our center on day 2 post-myocardial infarction (MI). He had developed a new harsh holosystolic murmur best heard at the left lower sternal border. He was originally admitted to an outside hospital with an anterolateral MI. On transfer to our hospital, he was clinically not in cardiogenic shock. Initial transthoracic echocardiography (TTE) showed a large serpiginous septal rupture involving the distal anterior septum. It also showed a large left to right ventricular shunt with a peak gradient (PIG) of about 85 mm Hg (Figs. 103.1A and B). Left ventricular ejection fraction (LV EF) was about 30–35%. Right ventricular systolic pressure (RSVP) estimated by tricuspid regurgitation velocity was about 50–60 mm Hg. Right ventricular (RV) function was normal. Patient was discussed in our heart team meeting and a decision was made for surgical repair.[1] He was taken to the cardiac operating room the next day. Preoperative 3D TEE confirmed the diagnosis made by TTE. The exact location and extension of the defect were identified in a surgical view (Fig. 103.2A, 342 to 344). The ventricular septal defect (VSD) was measured as 1.7 × 2.5 cm. Surgical exploration showed a totally infarcted anterolateral wall. VSD was explored through an incision in the anterior wall. Bovine pericardial patch was used to exclude the VSD from the left ventricle (Figs. 103.3A and B). LV incision was then closed using double Teflon sheets. Postoperative TEE immediately after repair showed a well-seated patch with no residual VSD shunt. Apical part of the left ventricle (dead space) which was excluded became part of the right ventricle and has communication with RV through the VSD (Fig. 103.2B and 345). Patient had CABG as well in target coronary arteries.[2] He was discharged home in good general condition. Follow-up visit after 5 years showed the patient was in good functional capacity. TTE at follow-up showed no residual VSD and LVEF of about 35–40%.

1. **In diagnosis and management of post-MI VSD, all of the followings are correct *except*:**
   (a) Surgical repair of post-MI VSD should be done immediately after diagnosis even if the patient is not in cardiogenic shock
   (b) Septal perforation develops on the average 2–3 days after myocardial infarction
   (c) Right ventricular failure is a relative contraindication for surgical repair

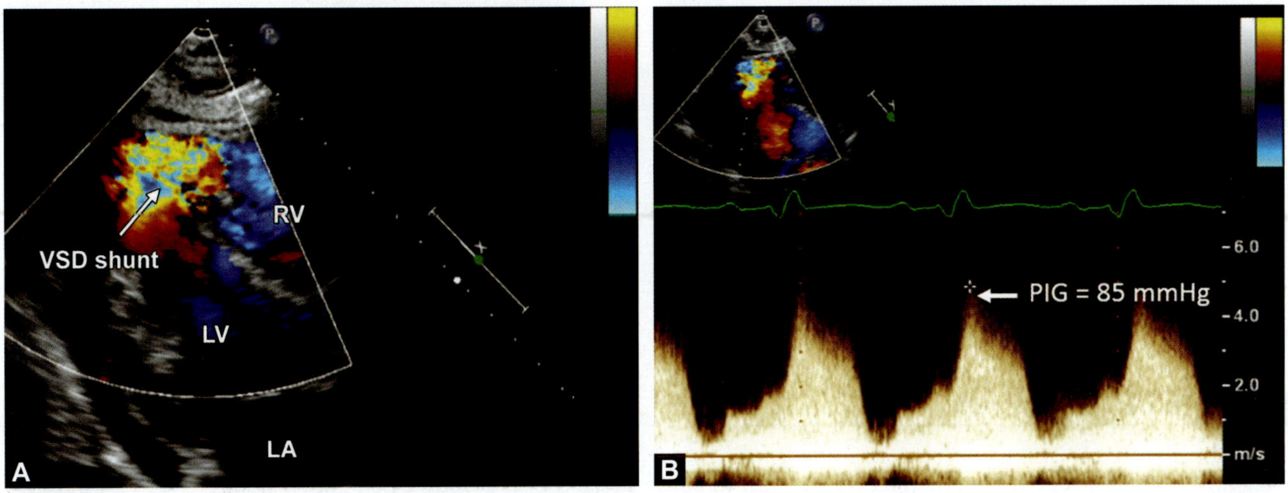

Figs. 103.1A and B: Transthoracic echocardiography (TTE). (A) Low parasternal long-axis view showing a large distal anterior septal rupture with LV to RV shunt. (B) Parasternal 4-chamber view with CW Doppler across the VSD showing peak gradient of 85 mm Hg. This high gradient is against the presence of significant pulmonary hypertension. (RV: Right ventricle; LV: Left ventricle; LA: Left atrium).

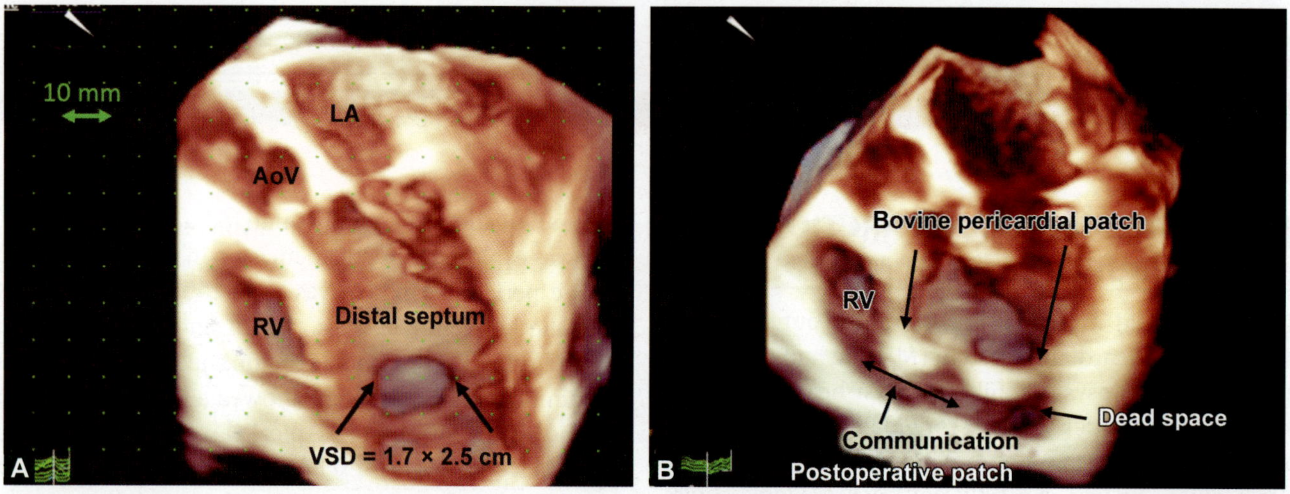

Figs. 103.2A and B: Pre- and postoperative 3D transesophageal echocardiography (3DTEE). (A) 3D TEE full volume acquisition of left ventricle showing en-face view of the distal ventricular septum. (B) Surgical view after repair with exclusion of the VSD. In this view VSD is part of the RV and communicates with the dead space of LV apex which is already excluded from the LV. (LA: Left atrium; AoV: Aortic valve; RV: Right ventricle).

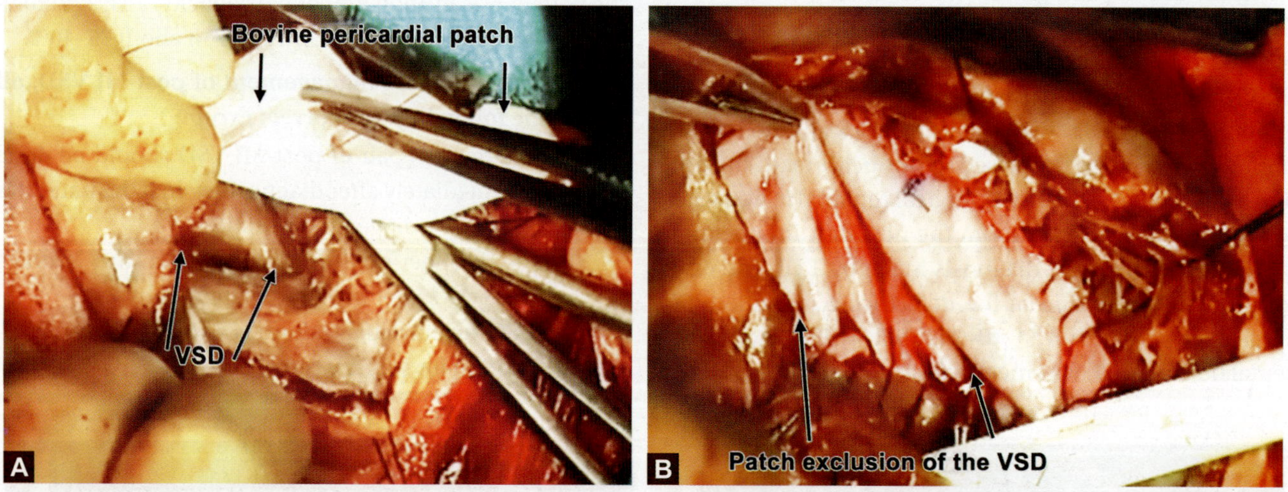

Figs. 103.3A and B: Surgical repair of the VSD. (A) Exploration of the VSD and preparation of the bovine pericardial patch for repair. (B) Large bovine patch is sutured in left ventricle (LV) above the VSD to the healthy margins of the defect. LV apex is excluded. At the end, LV apex, and VSD are part of the right ventricle.

(d) In-hospital mortality of surgical repair is about 30% and chance of recurrence after repair is 10–40%

Ans. (a)

MOVIE LEGENDS

342: Preoperative 3D TEE full volume acquisition with triple display showing en-face view of the VSD and corresponding 2D TEE views.
343: Same view as previous movie with more focus on VSD.
344: Same view as previous movies with more rotation showing the defect as the surgeon views it.
345: Same views as previous movies after surgical repair. Bovine pericardium seen excluding the left ventricle from the apex. VSD has become part of the right ventricle.

REFERENCES

1. Coskun KO, Coskun ST, Popov AF, et al. Experiences with surgical treatment of ventricle septal defect as a post infarction complication. J Cardiotho Surg 2009; 4:3.
2. Arnaoutakis GJ, Zhao Y, George TJ, et al. Surgical repair of ventricular septal defect after myocardial infarction: outcomes from the Society of Thoracic Surgeons National Database. Ann Thorac Surg 2012;94(2):436-43.

CASE 104

Marina Leitman, Boris Orlov, Eli Peleg, Zvi Vered

RUPTURE OF PAPILLARY MUSCLE FOLLOWING REPERFUSION

Introduction

In the era of primary percutaneous intervention in acute ST elevation myocardial infarction, mechanical complications of myocardial infarction have become infrequent. Nevertheless, rupture of papillary muscle occurs, and is related usually to late arrival and lack or insufficient coronary intervention. On the other hand, rapid restoration of blood supply to the coronary artery during angioplasty may lead to reperfusion injury and do continuous damage to the myocardium. We describe a patient with acute myocardial infarction complicated with partial rupture of papillary muscle 4 days after stenting of the left circumflex coronary artery.

Case Description

A 67-year-old male with history of coronary artery bypass surgery 20 years previously, was admitted into the intensive coronary care unit due to pulmonary cdcma, that required mechanical ventilation. The electrocardiogram showed ST segment depression in precordial leads and troponin level of 1.84 ng/ml was consistent with non ST elevation myocardial infarction. Urgent transesophageal echocardiography detected severe left ventricular dysfunction with infero-postero-lateral akinesis and moderate mitral regurgitation secondary to restricted posterior mitral valve leaflet motion (Figs. 104.1, 104.2, 346 and 347). The angle between the posterior leaflet and the mitral annulus plane was 52.7°, consistent with ischemic angle. Coronary angiography showed occluded left circumflex coronary artery that was successfully opened and covered with stent; internal mammary graft to the left anterior descending artery was patent. Intra-aortic balloon pump was inserted and patient's condition appeared to improve. Despite the successful reperfusion and initial stabilization, on the 4th day the patient's condition deteriorated, blood pressure fell and noradrenalin was administered. Chest X-ray showed worsening of pulmonary edema, and blood gases analysis showed hypoxia.

A second transesophageal echocardiography showed better contraction of the posterolateral wall, less ischemic restriction of the posterior leaflet—ischemic angle was

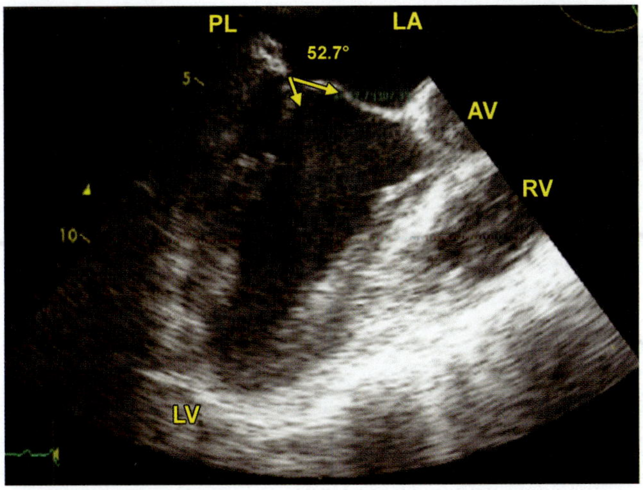

Fig. 104.1: 1st TEE. Ischemic mitral valve with restricted posterior leaflet (PL) characteristic of ischemic mitral valve. Angle between mitral annulus plane and posterior leaflet is 52.7° (between the arrow). Posterior wall of the left ventricle is akinetic.

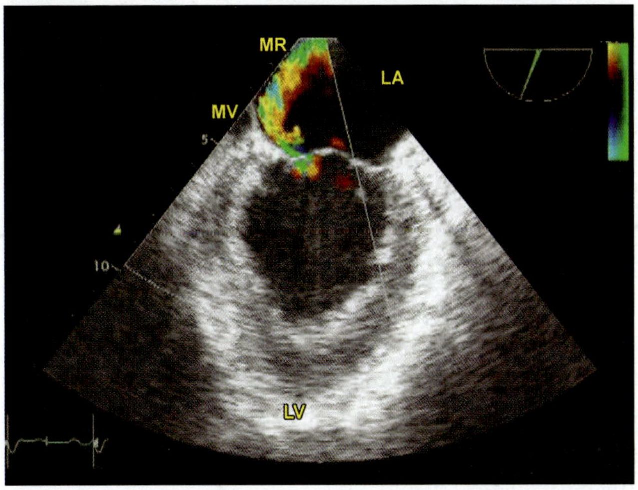

Fig. 104.2: 1st TEE. Posterior direction of mitral regurgitation (MR) jet consistent with ischemic mitral regurgitation which is moderate in severity.

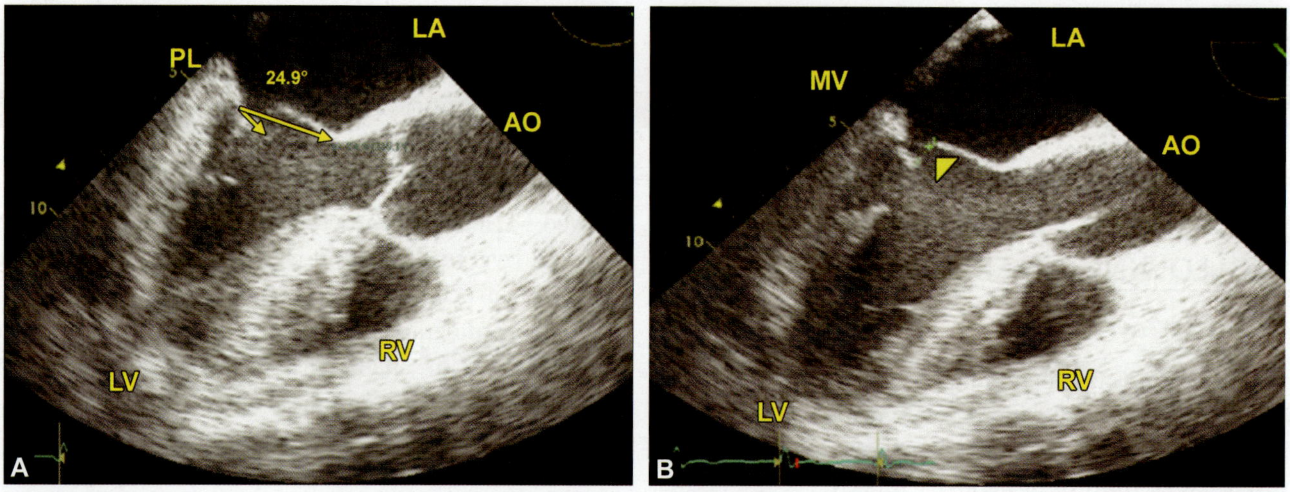

Figs. 104.3A and B: 2nd TEE. (A) Posterior leaflet of mitral valve shows better motion—angle between mitral annulus and posterior leaflet is 24.9° (between the arrow). (B) A lack of coaptation of mitral valve (arrowhead) with flail noncoapting anterior mitral valve leaflet. Posterior wall of the left ventricle contracts well, posterior leaflet movement is less restricted.

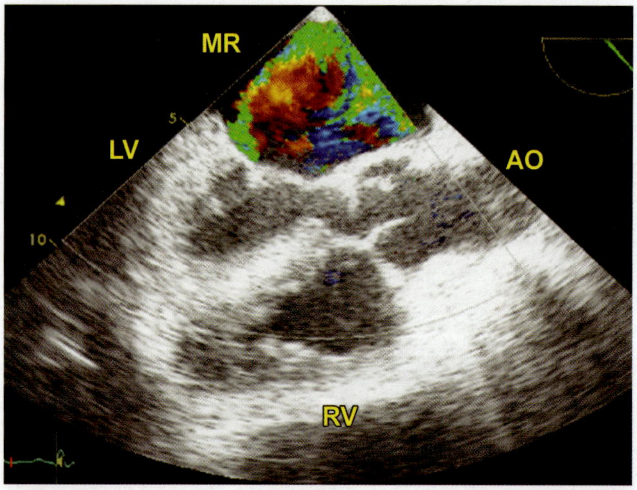

Fig. 104.4: 2nd TEE. Posteriorly directed jet of severe mitral regurgitation.

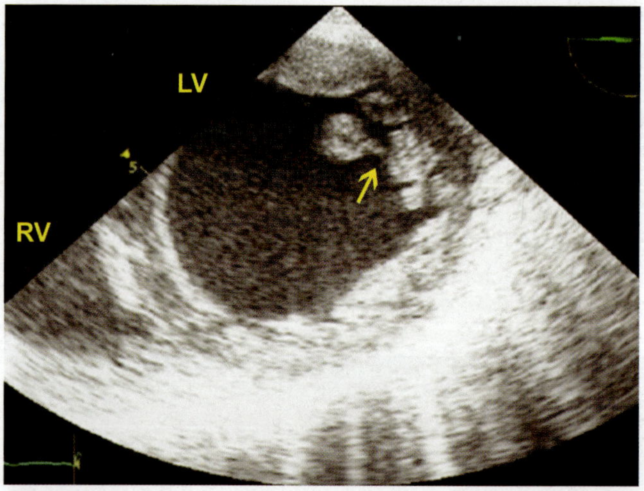

Fig. 104.5: 2nd TEE. Transgastric view. Posterior papillary muscle (arrow) is almost ruptured.

24.9°, excessive motion of the flail anterior leaflet with loss of coaptation and severe mitral regurgitation (Figs. 104.3A and B, 104.4, 348 and 349). The anterior head of the posterior papillary muscle was partially ruptured (Figs. 104.5, 104.6, 350 and 351).

Urgent surgery revealed partial rupture of necrotic papillary muscle that was removed, (Fig. 104.7) and the mitral valve was replaced successfully by a biological valve.

Comment

Rupture of papillary muscle is a serious mechanical complication of ST elevation[1] and non-ST elevation myocardial infarction,[2] more often occurring 2–7 days after myocardial infarction,[3] but may occur as late as 28 days after MI.[4] Its occurrence is rare—0.26% of patients with acute myocardial infarction.[5] Posteromedial papillary

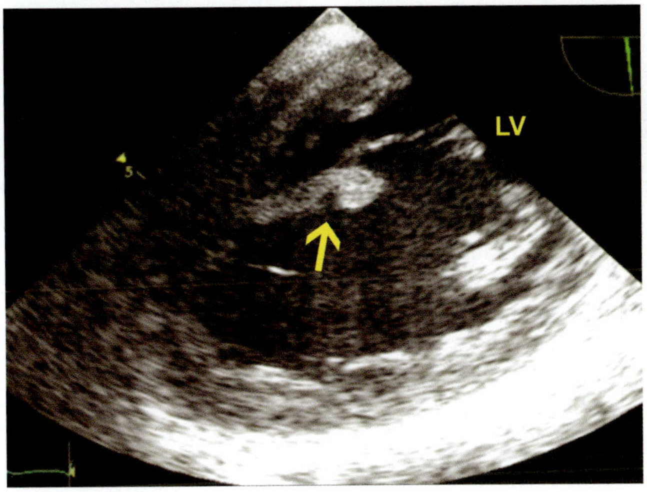

Fig. 104.6: 2nd TEE. Transgastric view. Anterior head of posterior papillary muscle (arrow) is almost ruptured.

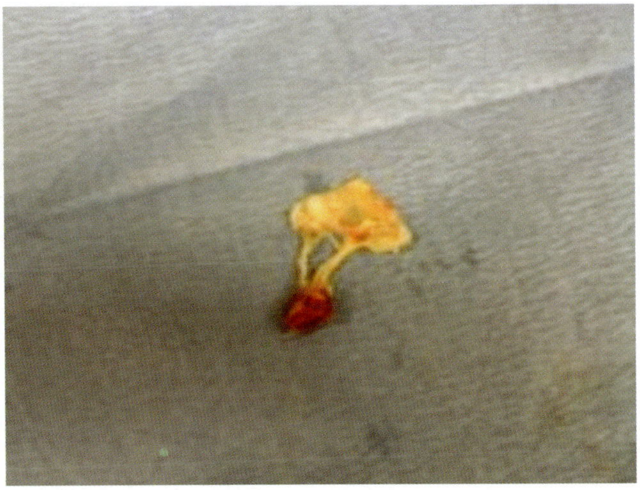

Fig. 104.7: Excised necrotic ruptured posterior papillary muscle.

muscle rupture is almost three times more frequent than the anterolateral—73 vs. 27% respectively,[7] due to non-uniform blood supply. The posterior papillary muscle has single vessel, while the anterior papillary muscle has dual vessel blood supply, that was confirmed with sonicated albumin microbubbles injection.[6] Overlap exists between electrocardiographic and pathological definition of myocardial infarction—ST elevation myocardial infarction is presumed to be transmural, while non-ST elevation myocardial infarction is thought to be subendocardial. Rupture of papillary muscle may complicate both: ST elevation and non-ST elevation myocardial infarction. In a classical pathological series of 17 consecutive patients complete rupture of papillary muscle occurred in 3, 8 had partial rupture, 6 patients had rupture of 1 of 2 or 2 of 5 heads of papillary muscle, 9 of 17 had subendocardial and 8 transmural myocardial infarction.[4]

Rupture of papillary muscle, similarly to other mechanical complications of myocardial infarction is usually associated with first acute myocardial infarction and the left ventricular cavity is usually of normal size.[7] Myocardial infarction that causes a rupture of posterior papillary muscle is often of small- to moderate- size. The left ventricle has enough systolic function to exert shear forces on the papillary muscle that lead to its rupture.[8] When patients with ischemic cardiomyopathy have acute myocardial infarction the heart is "too weak" to rupture and mechanical complications of myocardial infarction are rare.[7] This was not the case in our patient who had severe left ventricular dysfunction. Why after reperfusion, despite of better contraction of posterior wall our patient experienced incomplete rupture of papillary muscle?

In this case, before revascularization typical ischemic mitral valve appearance was seen, ischemic angle was more that 45°—a cutoff of successful restrictive annuloplasty.[9]

After reperfusion, the posterior leaflet of the mitral valve moved better, the "ischemic angle" of the posterior leaflet, relatively to the plane of the mitral annulus diminished (24.9°), but mitral regurgitation worsened. In the context of excessive motion of the anterior leaflet with loss of coaptation and acute flail configuration, organic mitral regurgitation due to papillary muscle pathology was suspected, and was confirmed on the transesophageal transgastric view and on surgery.

An additional important point: posterior orientation of mitral regurgitation jet is unusual in rupture of the posterior papillary muscle but may happen due to rupture of the anterior head.

In this case, rupture of the papillary muscle occurred 4 days after reperfusion, again highly unusual. We managed to find only one report of rupture of papillary muscle that occurred immediately after late reperfusion.[10]

Reperfusion may cause endothelial cells dysfunction with production of the potent vasoconstrictor endothelin-1 and oxygen free radicals that induce coronary vasoconstriction; activation of platelets and leucocytes with prothrombotic phenotype, production of oxidants, increased fluid and extravasation of protein alongwith re-entry of calcium can induce massive myofibril contraction and contraction band necrosis.[11]

Although rupture of papillary muscle is rare, papillary muscle infarction occurs quite often—among 738 patients with reperfused ST elevation myocardial infarction papillary muscle infarction was found by cardiac magnetic resonance in 104 patients (14%) and was associated with larger infarction, more pronounced reperfusion injury and higher mortality. In 53% the papillary muscle was completely infarcted.[12]

We believe that in this patient the leading cause for papillary muscle rupture was reperfusion injury.

Conclusion

Rupture of papillary muscle may occur after reperfusion. If rupture of papillary muscle occurs after revascularization, reperfusion injury should be considered.

Ischemic angle of the posterior leaflet of mitral valve can be measured routinely in functional-ischemic mitral regurgitation, and this measurement can provide an objective parameter regarding mitral valve motion and pathology.

MOVIE LEGENDS

346: 1st TEE. Ischemic mitral valve with restricted posterior leaflet (PL) characteristic of ischemic mitral valve. Angle between mitral annulus plane and posterior leaflet is 52.7°. Posterior wall of the left ventricle is akinetic.

347: 1st TEE. Posterior direction of mitral regurgitation (MR) jet consistent with ischemic mitral regurgitation which is moderate in severity.

348: 2nd TEE. A. Posterior leaflet (PL) of mitral valve shows better motion - angle between mitral annulus and posterior leaflet is 24.9°. B. A lack of coaptation of mitral valve with flail noncoapting anterior mitral valve leaflet. Posterior wall of the left ventricle contracts well, posterior leaflet movement is less restricted.

349: 2nd TEE. Posteriorly directed jet of severe mitral regurgitation.

350: 2nd TEE. Transgastric view. Posterior papillary muscle (arrow) is almost ruptured.

351: 2nd TEE. Transgastric view. Anterior head of posterior papillary muscle (arrow) is almost ruptured.

REFERENCES

1. O'Gara PT, Kushner FG, Ascheim DD, et al.; American College of Cardiology Foundation/American Heart Association Task Force on Practice Guidelines. 2013 ACCF/AHA Guideline for the Management of ST-Elevation Myocardial Infarction A Report of the American College of Cardiology Foundation/American Heart Association Task Force on Practice Guidelines Circulation. 2013;127:e362-e425.
2. Amsterdam EA, Wenger NK, Brindis RG, et al. 2014 AHA/ACC Guideline for the Management of Patients with Non-ST-Elevation Acute Coronary Syndromes: a report of the American College of Cardiology/American Heart Association Task Force on Practice Guidelines. J Am Coll Cardiol. 2014;64(24):e139-228.
3. Wei JY, Hutchins GM, Bulkley BH. Papillary muscle rupture in fatal acute myocardial infarction: a potentially treatable form of cardiogenic shock. Ann Intern Med. 1979;90(2):149-52.
4. Nishimura RA, Schaff HV, Shub C, et al. Papillary muscle rupture complicating acute myocardial infarction: analysis of 17 patients. Am J Cardiol. 1983;51(3):373-7.
5. French JK, Hellkamp AS, Armstrong PW, et al. Mechanical complications after percutaneous coronary intervention in ST-elevation myocardial infarction (from APEX-AMI). Am J Cardiol. 2010;105(1):59-63.
6. Voci P, Bilotta F, Caretta Q, et al. Papillary muscle perfusion pattern. A hypothesis for ischemic papillary muscle dysfunction. Circulation. 1995;91(6):1714-8.
7. Barbour DJ, Roberts WC. Rupture of a left ventricular papillary muscle during acute myocardial infarction: analysis of 22 necropsy patients. J Am Coll Cardiol. 1986;8(3):558-65.
8. Jolly S, Hutchison S. Papillary muscle rupture post-myocardial infarction. Cardiology rounds. 2003;8(4).
9. Magne J, Pibarot P, Dagenais F, et al. Preoperative posterior leaflet angle accurately predicts outcome after restrictive mitral valve annuloplasty for ischemic mitral regurgitation. Circulation. 2007;115(6):782-91
10. Kamohara K, Yoshikai M, Murayama J. Complete rupture of the posterior papillary muscle caused by late reperfusion for acute myocardial infarction. Jpn J Thorac Cardiovasc Surg. 2006;54(3):124-7.
11. Verma S, Fedak PW, Weisel RD, et al. Fundamentals of reperfusion injury for the clinical cardiologist. Circulation. 2002;105(20):2332-6.
12. Eitel I, Gehmlich D, Amer O, et al. Prognostic relevance of papillary muscle infarction in reperfused infarction as visualized by cardiovascular magnetic resonance. Circ Cardiovasc Imaging. 2013;6(6):890-8.

CASE 105

Roomi AU, Shah A, Siddiqui LI, Elsayed M, Bulur S, Nanda NC

A 47-year-old male with anterior wall STEMI, received thrombolytic therapy. Next day, he became hemodynamically unstable. Chest X-ray showed acute pulmonary edema. Bedside TEE was done (Figs. 105.1 to 105.3 and 352 to 354).

1. **What is your diagnosis?**
   (a) Papillary muscle rupture with severe MR
   (b) LV tumor with severe MR
   (c) MV vegetation with severe MR

Ans. (a)

History of myocardial infarction with an LV mass protruding into LA is typical of papillary muscle rupture (arrows in 352 and 353). The patient did not have any clinical stigmata of endocarditis.

2. **What is the percentage of patients in whom the ruptured papillary muscle does not prolapse and is not seen in the LA?**
   (a) About 5%
   (b) About 10%
   (c) About 20%
   (d) About 25%
   (e) About 30%

Ans. (d)

In these patients, it is important to carefully examine the LV for the ruptured papillary muscle which will appear as a mobile echodensity.

3. **What are the causes for absence of prolapse of ruptured papillary muscle into the LA?**
   (a) Ruptured papillary muscle is trapped by the chordae in the LV

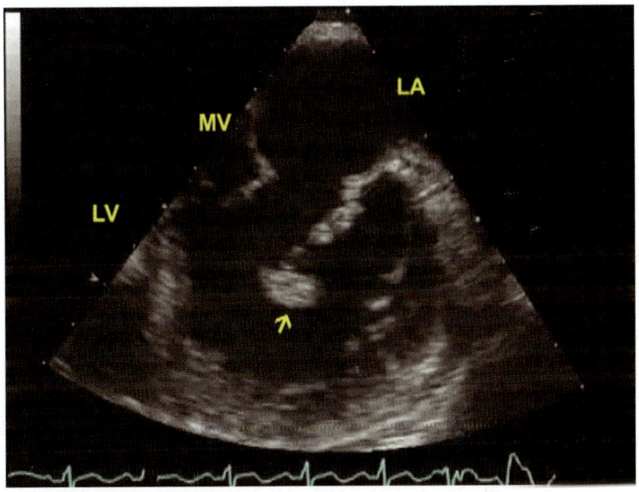

Fig. 105.2: Arrow points to the ruptured papillary muscle.

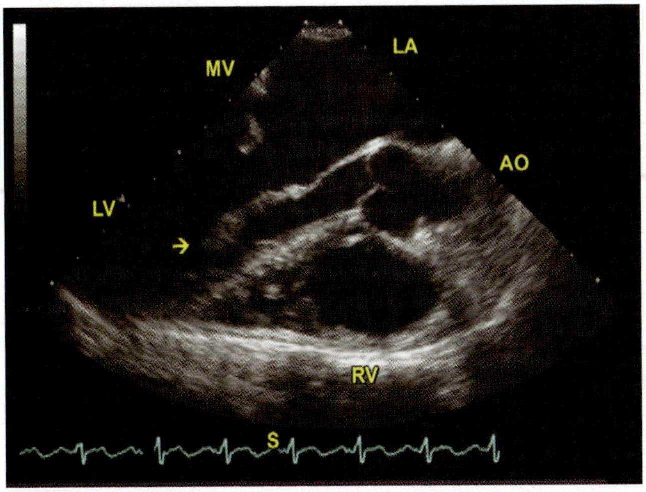

Fig. 105.1: Arrow points to the ruptured papillary muscle.

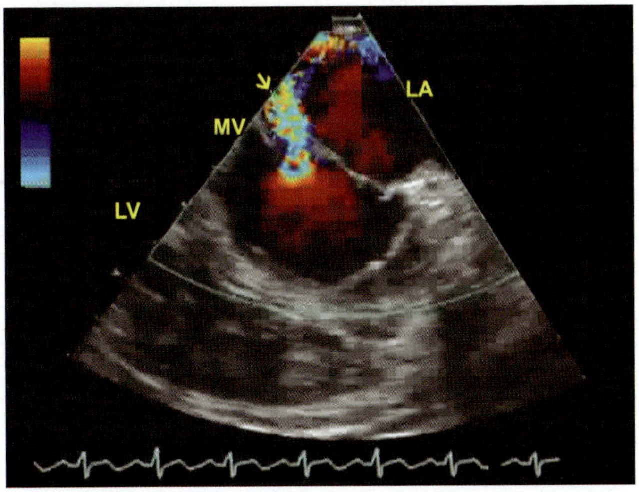

Fig. 105.3: Arrow points to significant MR which is also shown in Movie 354.

(b) Rupture is partial, not complete
(c) Only (a) is correct
(d) Only (b) is correct
(e) Both (a) and (b) are correct

Ans. (e)

Surgical findings: Confirmed rupture of anterior papillary muscle which was managed by St. Jude mechanical mitral valve prosthesis (#27).

Arrow in Figure 105.3 and 354 points to MR.

MOVIES 352 TO 354

CASE 106

Elsayed M, Alagic N, Uygur B, Turaga NSN, Chahwala JR, Adarna LG, Bulur S, Nanda NC

This is a 62-year-old male with chest pain and arthritis. Resting echocardiogram was normal except for a very small pericardial (P) effusion. He was referred for dobutamine stress echocardiogram. As soon as dobutamine IV dose was increased from 30 to 40 mcg/kg/minute with hand grip, his systolic blood pressure dropped to 92 mm Hg from 150 mm Hg. He did not complain of chest pain but felt jittery. There were no wall motion abnormalities (355 to 357).

1. **What would you do?**
   (a) Stop dobutamine
   (b) Stop hand grip
   (c) Continue both dobutamine and hand grip till target heart rate is reached
   (d) Check LVOT gradient

Ans. (d)

In this patient LVOT gradient increased from 6 mm Hg (Fig. 106.1) at rest to > 64 mm Hg (Fig. 106.2). SAMs of MV did not develop but LV cavity obliteration in systole was noted (357). Dobutamine was stopped, the high gradient reverted to normal, the BP normalized and the patient did well.

2. **How would you exclude hypertrophic cardiomyopathy (HCM) in this patient given that his LVOT was narrow at 17 mm and the LV walls were at the upper limit of normal in thickness or borderline hypertrophied?**
   (a) Perform a follow-up echocardiogram at 3 months to recheck for HCM
   (b) Check LVOT gradient with Valsalva during recovery at the same visit

Ans. (b)

There was no evidence of LVOT obstruction by CW Doppler during Valsalva which was performed in the recovery phase. LVOT obstruction may develop with dobutamine which resolves with discontinuation of the drug in patients with no evidence of HCM.

MOVIES 355 TO 357

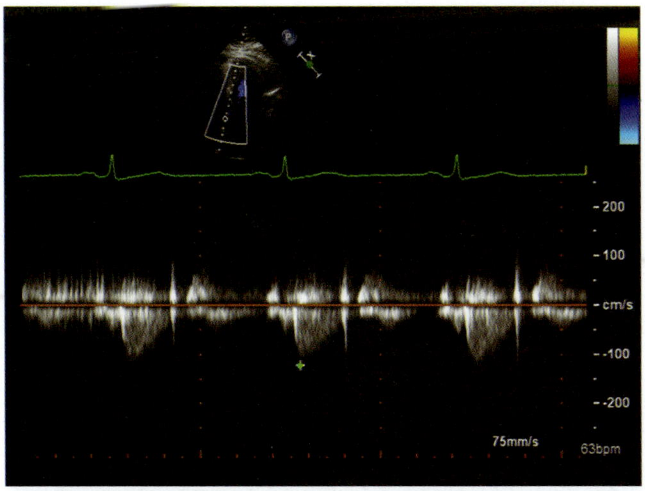

Fig. 106.1: Resting LVOT velocity showing no significant obstruction.

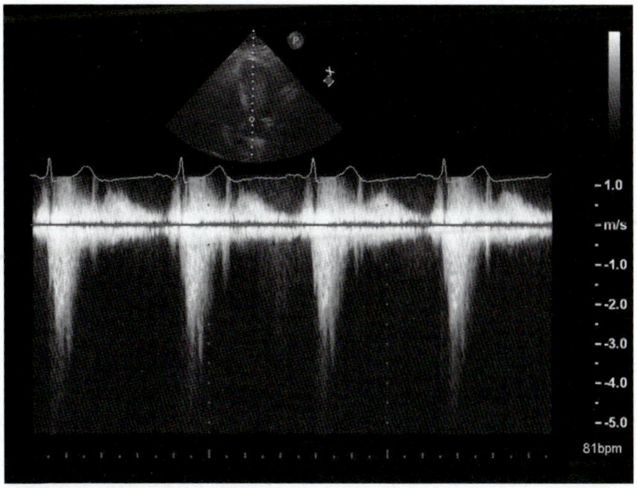

Fig. 106.2: LVOT interrogation using CW Doppler demonstrating a peak gradient of more than 64 mm Hg.

CASE 107

Elsayed M, Alagic N, Uygur B, Turaga NSN, Chahwala JR, Adarna LG, Bulur S, Nanda NC

Dobutamine stress echo studies from another 53-year-old female status post-cardiac transplantation with mild LV hypertrophy, narrow LVOT width of 13 mm and no resting obstruction are shown. Clinically there was concern regarding development of ischemic heart disease. At a Dobutamine dose of 20 mcg/kg/minute, patient developed typical MV SAMs and a peak gradient of 123 mm Hg across the LVOT. Dobutamine was stopped.

1. **Does this patient have HCM?**
   (a) Yes
   (b) No

Ans. (a)

With a relatively small dose of Dobutamine, the patient developed SAMs typical of HCM (Fig. 107.1 and 358) as well as a very high LVOT gradient (Fig. 107.2). 359 and 360 show apical 4 and 2 chamber views.

2. **What are the typical echo features of MV SAMs in HCM?**
   (a) SAMs begin a short interval after MV closure and revert to baseline sometime before the next MV opening.
   (b) SAMs begin immediately after MV closure and do not revert to baseline till the MV opens.

Ans. (a)

Typical SAMs will begin only during LV ejection (short interval after MV closure) when the Venturi phenomenon or "drag" effect occurs. They will revert to baseline as soon as LV ejection ceases with discontinuation of the above phenomenon. MV opening will occur a short time after cessation of LV ejection.

3. **There are several possible mechanisms which causes hypotension during Dobutamine stress echo. Which of the following does not cause hypotension?**
   (a) Excessive stimulation of cardiac mechanical receptors leading to vasodepressor response with peripheral dilatation and hypotension.
   (b) Isolated increase in systemic vascular resistance
   (c) Decrease in cardiac output (CO) due to LV cavity obliteration and reflex bradycardia
   (d) LVOT/mid LV cavity obstruction

Ans. (b)

4. **Which of the following statements is not true regarding Dobutamine?**
   (a) It is a sympathomimetic drug.
   (b) It stimulates alpha1 receptors

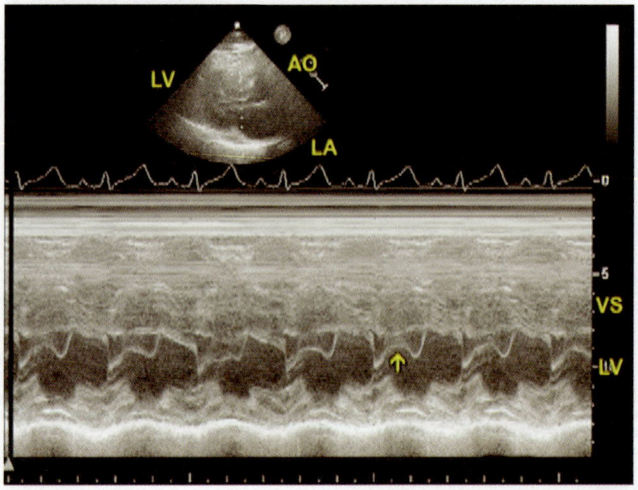

Fig. 107.1: Arrow points to a typical SAM well seen on the 2D directed M-mode.

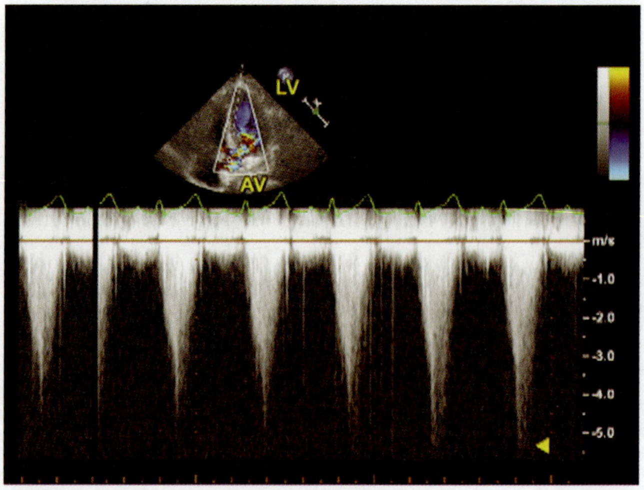

Fig. 107.2: LVOT interrogation by CW Doppler demonstrates a very high gradient of 123 mm Hg.

(c) It stimulates beta 1 and 2 receptors
(d) In peripheral vasculature, alpha 1 mediated vasoconstriction is offset by beta 2 mediated vasodilation.
(e) None of the above.

Ans. (e)

5. Regarding arrhythmias which may occur during Dobutamine stress echo, which of the following statements is incorrect?

(a) Six or more PVCs/minute (about 15%)
(b) Non sustained ventricular tachycardia (3.5%)
(c) Supraventricular tachycardia (3.4%)
(d) Second degree AV block (0.6%)
(e) Atrial flutter/fibrillation (0.1–0.6%)
(f) If done properly, no arrhythmia should ever occur

Ans. (f) *Source*: Martes H, Sawada SG, Ryan T, et al. Circulation 1993;88:15-19.

6. Most common side effects of Dobutamine stress echo are all of the following *except*:

(a) Nausea (8%)
(b) Anxiety (6%)
(c) Headach (4%)
(d) Tremor (3.7%)
(e) Urgency (1%)
(f) Pedal edema (unknown incidence)

Ans. (f) *Source*: Martes H, Sawada SG, Ryan T, et al. Circulation 1993;88:15-19.

MOVIES 358 TO 360

CASE 108

Adarna LG, Elsayed M, Alagic N, Uygur B, Turaga NSN, Chahwala JR, Bulur S, Nanda NC

This is a middle aged patient complaining of vague chest pains. LV and RV function were normal and no wall motion abnormalities were noted. An attempt was made to image the proximal left main (LMCA) and right (RCA) coronary arteries by 2D TTE.

1. **Which statement is correct?**
   (a) Proximal LMCA and RCA are normal
   (b) LMCA shows nonstenotic atherosclerotic plaques

Ans. (a)

The top arrow points to proximal RCA and bottom arrow to LMCA. Both are clear in 361. 2D gain is high in 362 producing artifacts mimicking small plaques in LMCA.

MOVIES 361 AND 362

CASE 109

Alok Saurav, Aiman Smer

LARGE MASS COMPRESSING THE RIGHT VENTRICULAR OUTFLOW TRACT

A 91-year-old woman with a history of three vessel CABG in 1990 found to have an incidental mediastinal mass on chest X-ray (Fig. 109.1), after a ground level fall. Precordial exam revealed grade III/VI continuous murmur at the right sternal border. Transthoracic echocardiogram (TTE) showed a large 8 × 7 cm mass compressing the right ventricular outflow tract (Fig. 109.2) with evidence of continuous flow into it on color Doppler (363) and contrast administration (364).

1. **Which of the following describes your diagnosis?**
   (a) Pericardial mesothelioma
   (b) Pericardial cyst
   (c) Saphenous venous graft pseudoaneurysm
   (d) Primary cardiac lymphoma

Ans. (c)

CT chest showed a large pseudoaneurysm originating from the diagonal coronary artery bypass graft (Fig. 109.3). Review of operative records revealed surgical course complicated by hemothorax requiring re-exploration of the chest. Intraoperatively oozing around the proximal anastomosis of SVG to diagonal branch was repaired. She

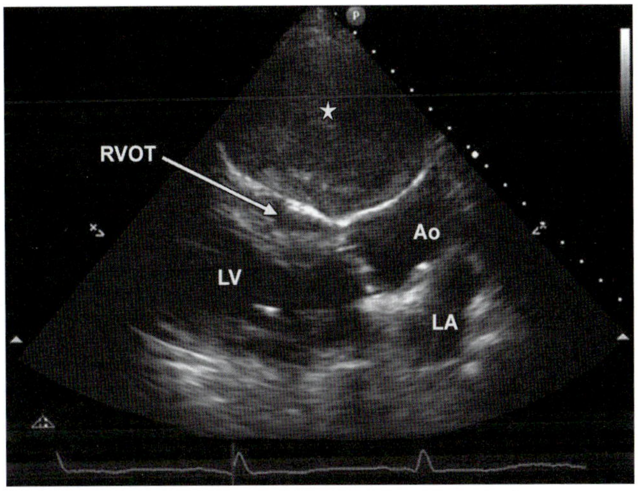

Fig. 109.2: 2D TTE. Parasternal long-axis view showing a large pseudoaneurysm (star) compressing the right ventricular outflow tract (RVOT). (LV: Left ventricle; LA: Left atrium; Ao: Aorta).

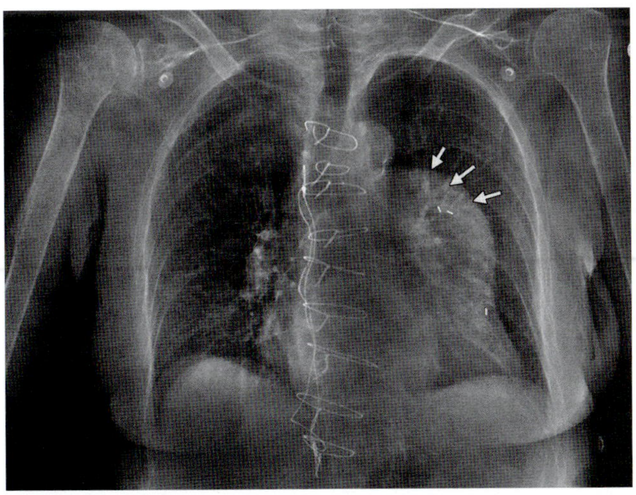

Fig. 109.1: Chest X-ray anteroposterior supine view demonstrating a large mediastinal mass (arrows).

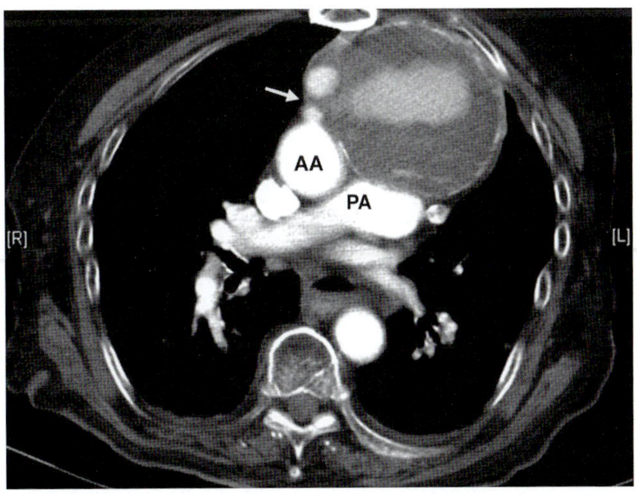

Fig. 109.3: Computed tomography (CT) of the chest showing the pseudoaneurysm originating from the diagonal coronary artery bypass graft (arrow). (AA: Ascending aorta; PA: Pulmonary artery).

remained asymptomatic until this admission. Options of surgical and endovascular repair were discussed. However, considering her asymptomatic status, advanced age, and high risk for operative complications family elected for conservative approach.

MOVIE LEGENDS

363: 2D TTE. Parasternal long-axis view with color flow (arrow) imaging showing the continuous flow into the pseudoaneurysm (star).

364: 2D TTE. Parasternal long-axis view with definity contrast showing the contrast filling the pseudoaneurysm (arrow).

CASE 110

Roomi AU, Shah A, Siddiqui LI, Gupta N, Mohamed A, Nanda NC

A 41-year-old male, known case of diabetes mellitus, hypertension and dyslipidemia, sustained anterior wall myocardial infarction and underwent percutaneous coronary angioplasty with stenting. Subsequently, he remained asymptomatic with unremarkable physical examination. A routine follow-up 2D TTE was done (🎥 365 and 366).

1. **What is the abnormal finding?**
   - (a) LAD infarction
   - (b) Dilated LV
   - (c) Mild PR
   - (d) Foreign body
   - (e) All of the above

Ans. (e)

A stent (arrow in 🎥 365 and 366) is clearly seen protruding into the aortic root. This stent had been placed in the left main coronary artery. CT scan (Fig. 110.1, arrow = stent) was done and showed no evidence of dissection or any other pathology. Since the patient was completely asymptomatic, no intervention was planned.

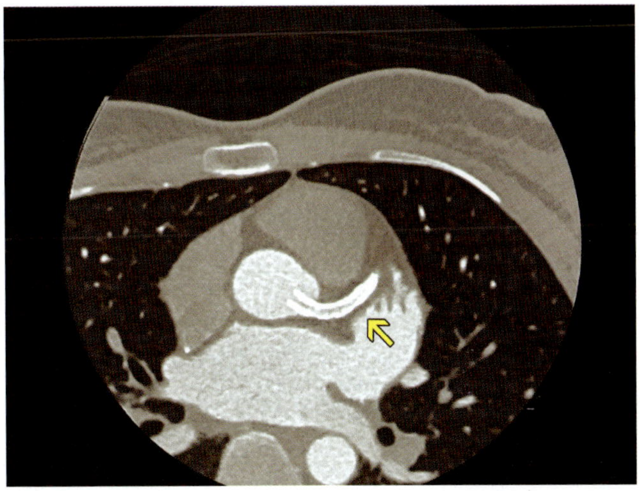

Fig. 110.1: CT scan. Arrow points to the stent protruding into the AO.

MOVIES 365 AND 366 🎥

CASE 111

Mohamed A, Gupta N, Elsayed M, Nanda NC

The patient is a 64-year-old female with COPD and past history of pulmonary embolism. She is morbidly obese weighing 300 Lb (136 kg). Her height was 74 inches and body surface area (BSA) 2.6 M2.

1. **What does the arrow show (367 to 369)?**
   (a) Mediastinal tumor
   (b) Thick chest wall with rib abnormalities
   (c) Breast implant
   (d) Pericardial/epicardial fat pad

Ans. (d)

The echo densities in the very large fat pad (3 cm in thickness) represent areas of fibrosis. Generally, fat deposition around the heart is in the form of fibrofatty tissue. Its size has been shown to be related to various risk factors for atherosclerosis and coronary artery disease.

MOVIES 367 TO 369

SECTION 7

Left Ventricle, Right Ventricle and Cardiomyopathy

CASE 112

Ramdas G Pai

SHORT OF BREATH

1. **What is the cause of these (Figs. 112.1 and 112.2) observations?**
   (a) Pericardial constriction
   (b) Restrictive cardiomyopathy
   (c) Deep breathing
   (d) Severe left and right ventricular dysfunction

Ans. (d)

- Severe left and right ventricular dysfunction. There is pulsus alternans of both RV and LV. There is alternating decrease in both amplitude and duration of both TR velocity and LV outflow. Figures 112.3 to 112.6 illustrate the various components of pulsus alternans.

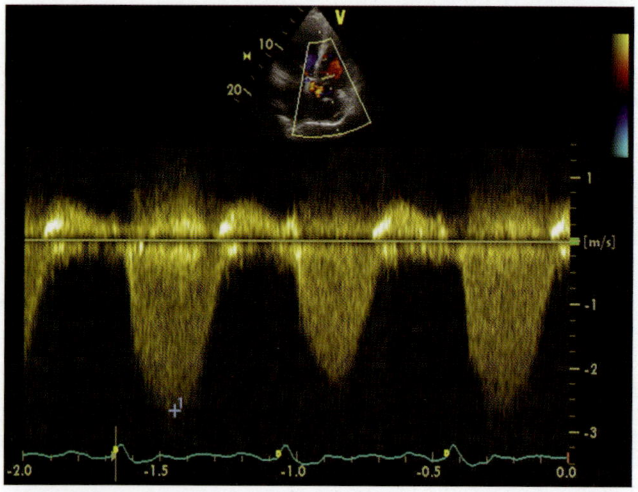

Fig. 112.1: TR velocity.

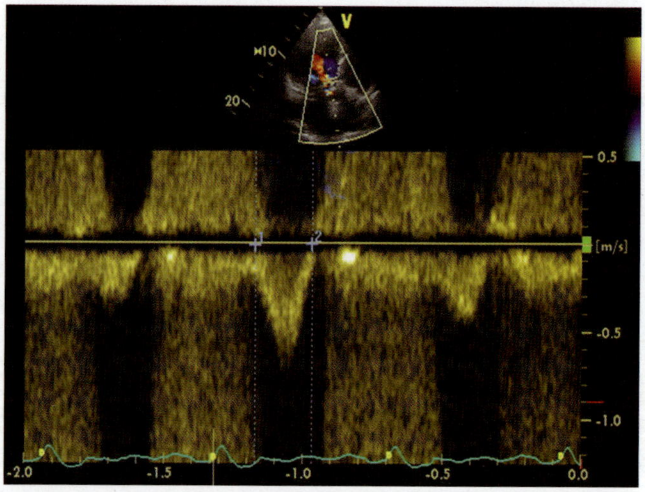

Fig. 112.2: Left ventricular outflow tract (LVOT).

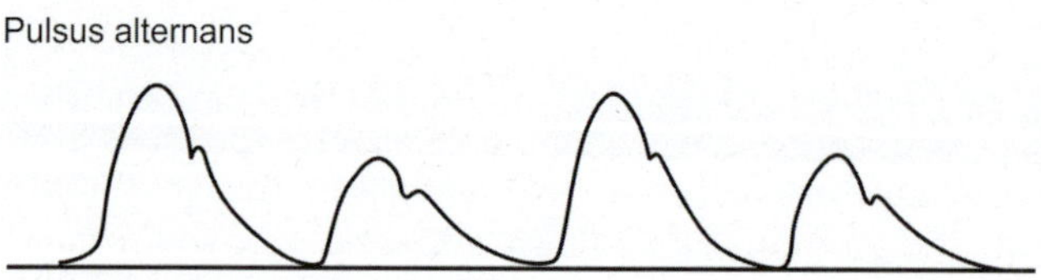

Fig. 112.3: Pulse wave tracing in pulsus alternans: Note the lower pulse volume with every other beat.

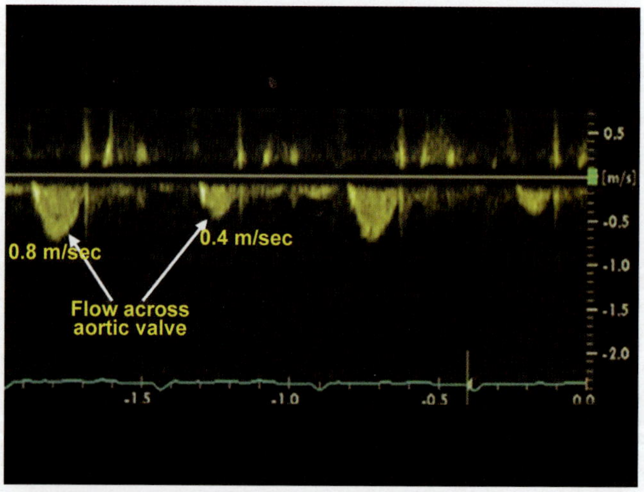

Fig. 112.4: Flow across aortic valve: Note lower velocity and duration of flow with every other beat resulting in lower stroke volume with those beats.

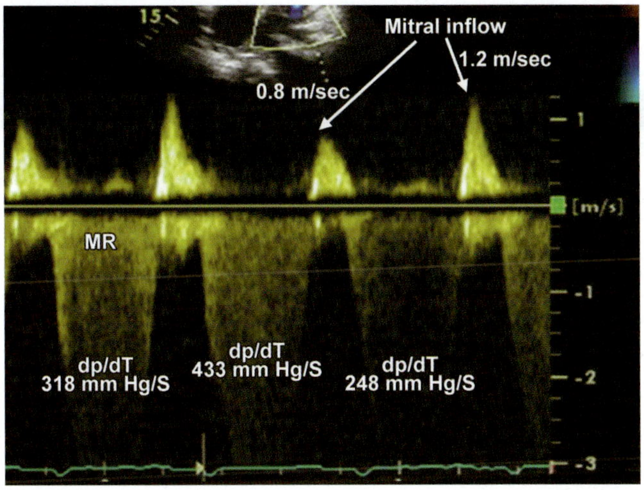

Fig. 112.5: Transmitral flow: Note reduced transmitral flow with every other beat. When the left ventricle receives higher filling, the left ventricular dP/dt is higher as calculated from the associated mitral regurgitation signal.

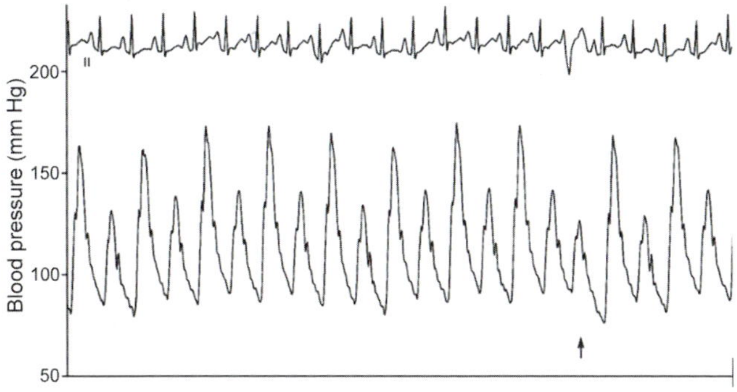

Fig. 112.6: Arterial pulse tracing in a patient with pulsus alternans.

DISCUSSIONS: PULSUS ALTERNANS

Causes of Pulsus Alternans

- Severe LV or RV dysfunction
- Severe increase in afterload
- May be precipitated by tachycardia

Possible Mechanisms of Pulsus Alternans

- Increased preload sensitivity and beat to beat change in EDV
- Altered Ca^{2+} handling by sarcoplasmic reticulum

CASE 113

Alagic N, Adarna LG, Chahwala JR, Elsayed M, Uygur B, Turaga NSN, Bulur S, Bhagatwala K, Elkaryoni A, Arisha MJ, Nanda NC

The IVCs imaged from the subcostal view in four different adult patients are shown (370 to 373).

1. (370):

(a) The RA pressure is normal
(b) The RA pressure is mildly elevated
(c) The RA pressure is very low
(d) The RA pressure is moderately elevated

Ans. (a)

The maximal inner dimension of the IVC measures 20 mm which is normal (21 mm is upper limit of normal) and it collapses more than 50% during respiration or with sniff. Findings are consistent with normal RA pressure (0–5 mm Hg, average 3 mm Hg).

2. (371 and 372A and B):

(a) The RA pressure is normal
(b) The RA pressure is mildly elevated
(c) The RA pressure is moderately elevated
(d) The RA pressure is markedly elevated

Ans. (d)

The IVC is enlarged to more than 21 mm and shows minimal (<50%, 371) or no collapse (372A and B). Therefore, the RA pressure is markedly elevated more than 15 mm Hg. In these cases often the TV inflow shows restrictive filling, tricuspid E/E′ >6 and the diastolic flow is predominant in hepatic veins (systolic filling fraction less than 55%). The IVC would also be enlarged with minimal or no collapse in patients with pericardial tamponade, constrictive pericarditis and moderately severe to severe TR. If the IVC is normal in size or is dilated but shows >50% collapse then the RA pressure is 5–10 mm Hg, average 8 mm Hg.

3. (373):

(a) The RA pressure is normal
(b) The RA pressure is mildly elevated
(c) The RA pressure is very low
(d) The RA pressure is moderately elevated

Ans. (c)

In these cases, the IVC is very small with normal or no collapse. This is seen in patients with hypovolemia and usually the ventricles are hyperdynamic in order to maintain normal stroke volumes.

MOVIES 370 TO 373

CASE 114

Chahwala JR, Elsayed M, Alagic N, Adarna LG, Bhagatwala K, Bulur S, Turaga NSN, Nanda NC

1. What does the arrow in the color M-mode examination of an adult patient show (🎥 374)?

(a) Slope of mitral inflow propagation velocity in the apical 4-chamber view

(b) MR

Ans. (a)

Normal values are greater than 50 cm/sec. Lower values are seen in patients with LV diastolic dysfunction.

MOVIE 374

CASE 115

Chahwala JR, Elsayed M, Alagic N, Uygur B, Turaga NSN, Adarna LG, Mohamed A, Gupta N, Bulur S, Nanda NC

Mitral valve inflow and Doppler tissue imaging (DTI) tracings in a middle-aged patient with diabetes mellitus are shown (Figs. 115.1 to 115.3).

1. **Does this patient have increased left-sided filling pressures?**
   (a) Yes
   (b) No

Ans. (a)

The ratio of mitral inflow velocity to average of maximum early diastolic (E') lateral and medial mitral annulus velocities by DTI is high at 18.14 (normal ratio ≤ 14). Also the ratio of mitral E to A on the mitral inflow is high at 3 (restrictive physiology, normal ratio ≤ 2). MV deceleration time is also reduced at 116 ms and normal is 160–240 ms. High mitral E to E' ratio, high mitral E to A ratio and reduced MV deceleration time (DT) are all indicative of increased left sided filling pressure (diastolic dysfunction). Caveats for these ratios are significant MR and significant MV annular calcification (MAC) which will increase mitral inflow velocity (E) resulting in a falsely elevated ratio.

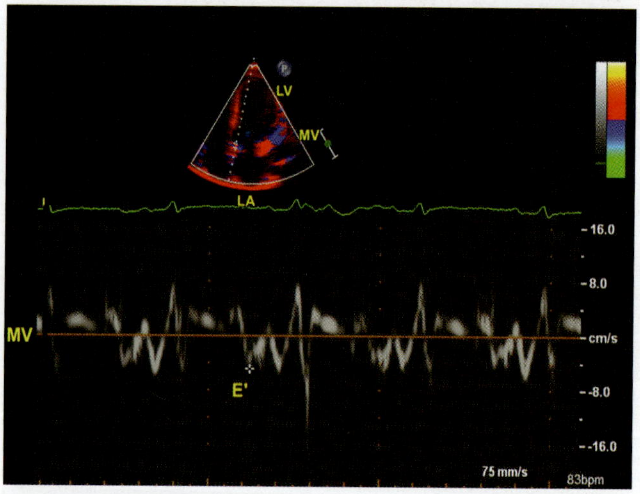

Fig. 115.1: Maximum early diastolic medial mitral annulus velocity (E') is shown.

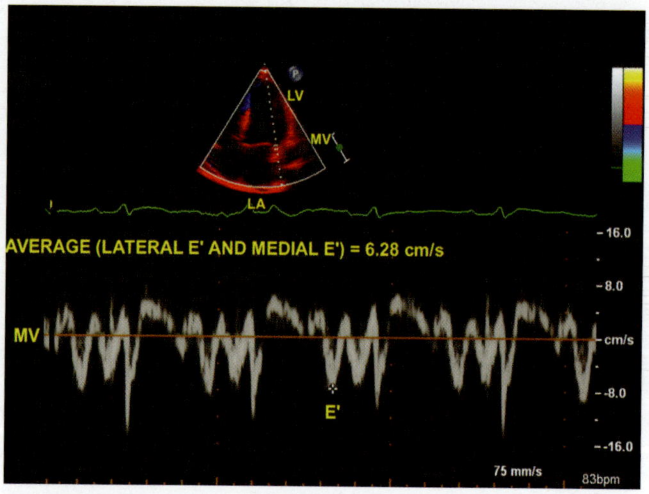

Fig. 115.2: Maximum early diastolic (E') lateral mitral annulus velocity is shown.

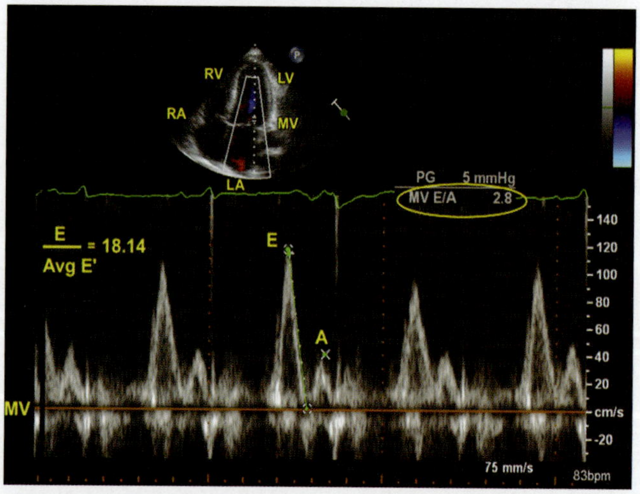

Fig. 115.3: Maximum early diastolic (E) and atrial systolic (A) mitral inflow velocities are shown.

CASE 116

Chahwala JR, Elsayed M, Alagic N, Uygur B, Turaga NSN, Adarna LG, Bulur S, Nanda NC

Mitral inflow tracing in an adult patient with heart failure (Fig. 116.1).

1. **All statements are correct regarding L-wave *except*:**
   (a) It is not often noticed.
   (b) L-wave represents continued pulmonary vein mid-diastolic LA flow into the LV through the MV.
   (c) It may be seen in patients with clinical heart failure with both normal and reduced systolic function. It may be an indicator of advanced LV diastolic dysfunction.
   (d) Computer models suggest that L-wave may be related to reduced active relaxation of the LV together with high LV stiffness resulting in prominent oscillatory movement of the diastolic LV-LA pressure gradient.
   (e) Practically all patients with LV diastolic dysfunction will have L-waves.
   (f) It may be normally seen in patients with slow heart rates (bradycardia).
   (g) It has a prognostic value and these patients more often require hospitalization with heart failure.
   (h) L-wave may also be recorded by M-mode.

Ans. (e)

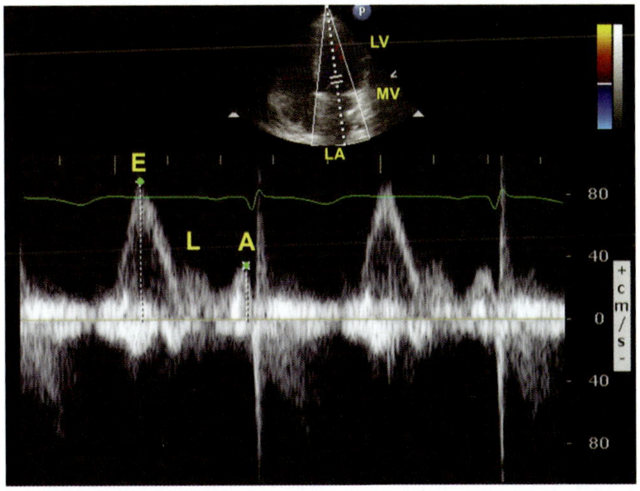

Fig. 116.1: Mitral inflow tracing showing a prominent L wave measuring more than 20 cm/s.

REFERENCE

1. Kerut EK. The mitral L-wave: a relatively common but ignored useful finding. Echocardiography. 2008 May;25(5): 548-50. doi: 10.1111/j.1540-8175.2007.00626.x. Epub 2008 Feb 12. PubMed PMID: 18279403.

CASE 117

Anastasia Vamvakidou, Roxy Senior

A 27-year-old man presented to the emergency department with right-sided weakness, facial droop and progressive dysphasia. He had a CT head which revealed a left sided middle cerebral artery infarct. He was found to be in atrial fibrillation (AF). As part of the investigation for a cardiac source of embolic stroke, he had an echocardiogram both with and without an echo contrast agent(🎥 375 to 380).

1. **What is the striking feature in the right ventricle (RV)?**
   (a) RV apical aneurysm
   (b) RV moderator band
   (c) RV pressure and volume overload
   (d) RV dilatation

Ans. (a)

There is left ventricular (LV) pressure and volume overload as it is obvious from the bulging of the inter-atrial and inter-ventricular septum toward the RV in both systole and diastole. RV is dilated with impaired radial and longitudinal function; however the striking feature is the RV apical aneurysm which hugs around the LV apex.

2. **What is the LV structural abnormality?**
   (a) LV apical aneurysms
   (b) Non-compaction
   (c) LV thrombus
   (d) Apical hypertrophic obstructive cardiomyopathy (HOCM) (advanced)

Ans. (a)

In the apical 4-chamber views there are obvious LV apical aneurysms mainly seen in the contrast-enhanced images. There is no LV thrombus or non-compaction present.

3. **What is the likely cause of LV systolic dysfunction in this man?**
   (a) Arrhythmogenic right ventricular cardiomyopathy (ARVC)
   (b) Dilated cardiomyopathy
   (c) Atrial septal defect (ASD)
   (d) AF induced tachycardiomyopathy

Ans. (b)

According to the revised criteria for the diagnosis of ARVC, the presence of RV apical aneurysms together with severe right ventricular outflow tract (RVOT) dilatation in parasternal long axis (PLAX)/parasternal short axis (PSAX) views are required to make the diagnosis echocardiographically (RVOT PSAX 39 mm, RVOT PLAX 39 mm translate to severe dilatation in this case). However, LV has to be normal or mildly impaired which is not the case here.[1] An ASD would primarily be associated with grossly globally dilated RV (especially compared to the LV), which is not present here. AF induced tachycardiomyopathy primarily affects the LV. A cardiac MRI during his admission confirmed the presence of dilated cardiomyopathy with multiple LV aneurysmal areas and only limited subendocardial LV apical scarring.

MOVIES 375 TO 380 🎥

REFERENCE

1. Marcus F, McKenna W, Sherrill D, et al. Diagnosis of arrhythmogenic right ventricular cardiomyopathy/dysplasia. Proposed modification of task force criteria. Circulation. 2010;121:1533-41.

CASE 118

Bhagatwala K, Elsayed M, Alagic N, Uygur B, Turaga NSN, Chahwala JR, Adarna LG, Mohamed A, Gupta N, Bulur S, Nanda NC

This is an adult patient presenting with severe shortness of breath and heart failure. 2D Transthoracic Echocardiogram (TTE) was done (381 to 386).

1. **What is the estimated left ventricular ejection fraction (LV EF) in this patient?**
   (a) 10–15%
   (b) 25%
   (c) 26–30%
   (d) 31–35%

Ans. (a)

The LV shows extremely poor function. 381 and 382 represent parasternal long and short axis views. There is no thrombus but a few trabeculations in the LV apex (apical four 383, and apical five 384 chamber views). Calcification is noted at the tip of a papillary muscle (384, apical 5-chamber view). An ICD lead (P) is also seen in 383 and 384. Left atrial appendage (LAA) is clear without a clot in 385 (apical 2-chamber view). 386 is apical long axis view. RV function is also extremely poor in this patient.

MOVIES 381 TO 386

CASE 119

Bulur S, Elsayed M, Nanda NC

A 39-year-old patient with heart failure (Fig. 119.1 and 387 and 388).

1. **In ischemic cardiomyopathy with significant MR which of the following echocardiographic parameters are related to recurrent MR and poor prognosis after MV annuloplasty?**
   (a) MV coaptation distance > 10 mm.
   (b) Systolic tenting area >2.5 cm^2.
   (c) Posterior MV leaflet angle > 45 degrees.
   (d) Distal anterior MV leaflet angle >25 degrees.
   (e) End-systolic inter-papillary muscle distance >20 mm.
   (f) Posterior papillary muscle intervalvular fibrosa distance >40 mm.
   (g) Systolic sphericity index >0.7
   (h) LV end diastolic dimension > 65 mm, left ventricular (LV) end systolic dimension >51 mm.
   (i) All of the above.
   (j) Some of the above but not all.

Ans. (i)

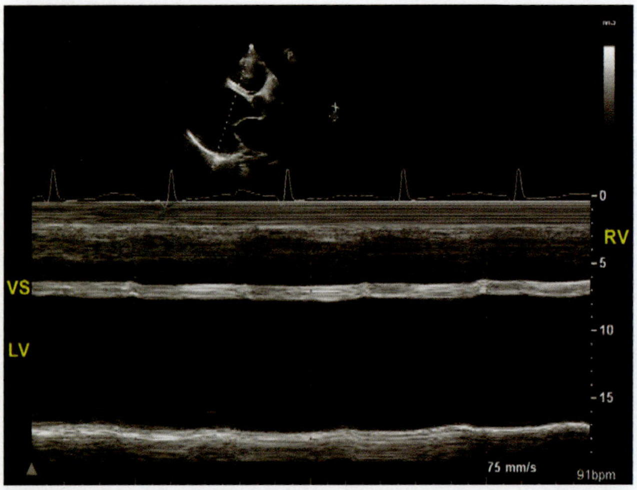

Fig. 119.1: M-mode showing marked LV dialatation with poor function.

The above parameters have been linked to poor outcome and recurrent MR after MV annuloplasty. They need to be further validated using larger number of patients.

2. **Regarding LAA in 388 which of the following statements are correct?**
   (a) LAA thrombus can be confidently excluded.
   (b) LAA thrombus cannot be excluded and multiplane 2D TEE would need to be performed if clinically indicated.
   (c) Since the 2D images are of good quality, 3D TTE can be performed and that should more confidently exclude LAA thrombus if clinically indicated.
   (d) 3D TEE would be superior to 3D TTE if the 2D TTE image quality was sub-optimum.

Ans. (c and d)

The apical 2-chamber view shown, represents only a thin slice of LAA and the thrombus may still be present in other areas and lobes of LAA. With 3D modality the entire extent of LAA is included in the acquired data set facilitating systematic cropping (sectioning) of the appendage and thrombus can be more confidently excluded. In this patient the 2D image quality is good and hence 3D TTE—which is based on 2D TEE images—would be expected to provide a more confident assessment of LAA precluding-use of the more invasive 2D TEE and 3D TEE.

MOVIE LEGENDS

387: Parasternal long axis view. There is a clear separation between RV (arrowhead) and LV (arrow) sides of VS. The LV portion of VS is thin and echogenic consistent with fibrosis. MV coaptation (C) point is centrally displaced into LV with restriction of motion of both leaflets resulting from remodeling of LV. This is consistent with dilated cardiomyopathy as opposed to ischemic cardiomyopathy where the coaptation point may be eccentrically displaced with more restricted motion of the posterior mitral leaflet.

388: Apical 2-chamber view showing LAA without any obvious thrombus.

CASE 120

Bulur S, Nanda NC

This is a 21-year-old male with muscular dystrophy. 2D TEE had to be done while the patient was sitting in a chair. Because of poor quality examination, an echo contrast agent was intravenously administered to optimally define the LV endocardial border (389 to 391).

1. **Which is the correct statement?**
   (a) LV is globally dilated with poor function (LVEF <25%) and thinning of walls. RV function is normal.
   (b) LV is globally dilated with poor function (LVEF <25%) and thinning of walls. RV function cannot be evaluated adequately since only a small portion of the RV is imaged.

Ans. (b)

Contrast echo is very useful to delineate LV and RV endocardial borders in patients with poor acoustic windows. Dilated cardiomyopathy may be associated with muscular dystrophy.

MOVIES 389 TO 391

CASE 121

Alagic N, Nanda NC

This is a middle-aged male complaining of shortness of breath on mild exertion who was noted to be in heart failure. 2D TTE was done (392 and 393) and repeated one month later after he was placed on Coumadin (394 and 395).

1. **What do the initial apical 4-chamber views (392 and 393) show?**
   (a) A large mobile thrombus in the LV apex
   (b) A huge trabeculation in the LV apex
   (c) A mobile tumor such as a myxoma in the LV apex
   (d) An echo artifact in LV apex needs to be ruled out
   (e) The diagnosis cannot be made unless a contrast echo or 3D is done

Ans. (a)

The mass is most likely a large thrombus (oblique arrow) because it is associated with poor LV function which results in blood flow stasis thereby providing a good milieu for thrombus formation. The multiple small echolucencies seen within the thrombus probably represent areas of lysis or liquefaction resulting from natural lytic factors normally present in blood which tend to dissolve the clot. Giving Coumadin further facilitates dissolution of the thrombus that is evident in 394 (apical 2-chamber view) and 395 (apical 4-chamber view) which show significant reduction in the size of the thrombus. The horizontal arrow in 395 points to small associated trabeculations which are not mobile. In this patient the highly mobile thrombus can be differentiated from a trabeculation which would generally be much smaller, less mobile and often multiple. LV myxoma or other type of tumor would be less likely as the LV function would be expected to be normal. An echo artifact is generally much less echogenic and may extend beyond the borders of the LV which clinches the diagnosis.

MOVIES 392 TO 395

CASE 122

Bulur S, Nanda NC

This patient is a 58-year-old male presenting with heart failure. 2D Transthoracic Echocardiogram (TTE) was done (396A to D).

1. **What would you estimate the LVEF in this patient?**
   (a) < 25%
   (b) 25–30%
   (c) 30%
   (d) 30–35%
   (e) 35%

Ans. (a)

LV function is very poor in this patient with hardly any motion of LV walls.

Normal LV function	= LVEF 52–72% (male)
	LVEF 54–74% (female)
Mild LV dysfunction	= LVEF 41–51% (male)
	LVEF 41–53% (female)
Moderate LV dysfunction	= LVEF 30–40%
Severe LV dysfunction	= LVEF <30%

2. **How would you categorize RV function in this patient?**
   (a) Moderate dysfunction
   (b) Normal function
   (c) Cannot evaluate accurately because RV free wall is not well seen
   (d) Poor function

Ans. (d)

RV wall in the apical 4 chamber and parasternal long axis views show poor motion. This patient also has a pacemaker lead (L) in the RV and severe TR which may have been accentuated by the pacemaker lead crossing the TV. Closed arrows point to spontaneous contrast echoes in the LV resulting from low cardiac output and open arrows show apical trabeculations.

3. **LV end-diastolic internal dimension in this patient measured 5.4 cm. Does this mean LV enlargement?**
   (a) Yes
   (b) No

Ans. (b)

Upper limit of normal for males is 5.8 cm and for females 5.2 cm. This internal dimension is also measured at the level of MV tips at the beginning of QRS complex of the ECG.

MOVIES 396A TO D

REFERENCE

1. Lang RM, Badano LP, Mor-Avi V, et al. Recommendations for cardiac chamber quantification by echocardiography in adults: an update from the American Society of Echocardiography and the European Association of Cardiovascular Imaging. J Am Soc Echocardiogr. 2015 Jan;28(1):1-39.e14.

CASE 123

Chahwala JR, Bhagatwala K, Elsayed M, Alagic N, Uygur B, Turaga NSN, Adarna LG, Bulur S, Nanda NC

The patient is a 54-year-old male who was first seen 5 months ago complaining of shortness of breath and found to be in heart failure. Subsequently, his symptoms improved on standard medical regimen. He is 70 inches tall and weighs 196 lb. His blood pressure is 96/52 mm Hg and heart rate 67/minute. Both initial and current 2D TTE movie clips are shown side by side (397 to 401).

1. **Comparison of the movie clips shows a definite improvement in both LV and RV function as compared to 5 months ago. This statement is:**
   (a) True
   (b) False

Ans. (a)

The overall function of both ventricles is still diminished but there is definite improvement in wall motion compared to the initial study. Placing the movies side by side is helpful in assessing this. A contrast agent was administered because the endocardium of more than 2 adjoining segments was not visualized in the apical 4-chamber view on standard 2D TTE.

2. **All the following statements are true *except*:**
   (a) He may have suffered from some sort of myocarditis which has improved over time.
   (b) He may have dilated cardiomyopathy of unknown origin and the improvement in function is due to optimal medical therapy given to treat his heart failure. His heart rate has also come down.
   (c) Given his age, he most likely has ischemic cardiomyopathy and the improvement in function is due to PTCA which he may have undergone after the initial echocardiogram.
   (d) Segmental wall motion abnormalities may occur in dilated cardiomyopathy although they are more common in ischemic heart disease.

Ans. (c)

Generally, RV wall motion is normal in ischemic cardiomyopathy unless there is severe involvement of RCA or the patient has suffered from myocardial infarction involving the RV also. Even so, the RV would be expected to show segmental and not generalized hypokinesis/akinesis.

MOVIES 397 TO 401

CASE 124

Arisha MJ, Elkaryoni A, Nanda NC

The patient is a 53-year-old male with dilated cardiomyopathy and congestive heart failure who has had several follow-up 2D TTEs. His LV is markedly dilated to 92 mm with severe generalized hypokinesis (🎥 402 to 406). Initial and repeat 2D TTE five months later following optimal medical management are shown (🎥 402 and 403 without an echo contrast agent, 🎥 404 to 406 with contrast).

1. **Is the nomenclature of LV walls correct in all movies?**
   (a) Yes
   (b) No, needs some corrections

Ans. (a)

🎥 402 to 406 represent parasternal long axis, parasternal short axis, apical 4-chamber, apical 2-chamber and apical 5-chamber views.

A: Anterior wall; AL: Anterolateral wall; AS: Anterior septum; I: Inferior wall; IL: Inferolateral wall; IS: Inferior septum; P: Pacemaker.

MOVIES 402 TO 406 🎥

CASE 125

Bulur S, Nanda NC

This is a 70-year-old male with dilated cardiomyopathy and left bundle branch block who underwent cardiac resynchronization therapy (CRT). 2D echoes before (407, left panel) and after (407, right panel) CRT are shown.

1. **What do the movies show?**
   (a) There is significant improvement in motion of both VS and PW (inferolateral wall) as well as RV wall following CRT
   (b) There is significant improvement in motion of both VS and PW (inferolateral wall) but RV wall motion is unchanged following CRT
   (c) There is no significant change in LV wall motion following CRT

Ans. (b)

There is a clear improvement in LV wall motion. However, the quality of the study is suboptimal and injection of an echo contrast agents would have been helpful in more clearly defining the LV endocardial borders. RV wall motion was normal at baseline and did not show any changes following CRT.

MOVIE 407

CASE 126

Ghazwan Elias, Mohammed Hasoon, Christian S Breburda

ECHO GUIDED VERSUS ADAPTIVE CRT OPTIMIZATION

Introduction

Cardiac resynchronization therapy (CRT) has become a new, effective treatment modality in patients with drug-resistant advanced congestive heart failure. Despite careful selection, as many as 30 to 40% of patients do not respond to CRT.[1] Echocardiographic (echo) optimization of atrioventricular delay (AVD) was studied in several randomized trials of CRT; however, biventricular (BIV) pacemaker optimization is often underutilized and instead, the default device settings for adaptive (P and QRS automated) CRT are used. We first described grey scale 2D strain,[5] recently 3D strain imaging has been introduced for optimization in device therapy in heart failure. We are reporting a case of non-ischemic DCM in whom we used a new biventricular pacer that automatically adjusts atrioventricular (AV) times, called adaptive CRT.

A 52-year-old African-American female with past medical history of hypertension, thalassemia and non-ischemic dilated cardiomyopathy diagnosed in July 2014 presented with 2-block dyspnea on exertion after 3 months on Guideline Directed Medical Therapy (GDMT).

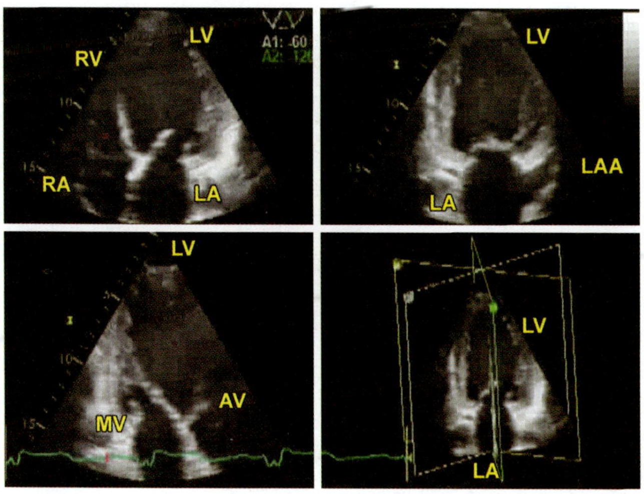

Fig. 126.1: 3D Echo. Apical triplane view. Dilated cardiomyopathy (DCM).

Physical exam showed blood pressure of 100/62 mm Hg, pulse 88 bpm, height 172 cm and weight 102 kg. Cardiac exam showed regular heart rate, sinus rhythm, normal S1, S2 and no murmurs. Lungs were clear to auscultation bilaterally. Transthoracic echo showed left atrial and left ventricular enlargement, ejection fraction (EF) of 15% (408), restrictive left ventricular filling, and E/e' of 24 (Figs. 126.2A and B, 409). He was categorized as New York Heart Association (NYHA) class II, C. The patient was referred for device therapy—cardiac resynchronization device (CRD).

1. **What further diagnostic workup should be done at this point?**
   (a) 3D strain echo
   (b) Cardiac MRI
   (c) Contrast echo
   (d) Stress echo
   (e) Cardiac computed tomography (CCT)

Ans. (a)

With 3D strain echo we can measure global longitudinal strain (GLS) (Figs. 126.1 and 126.3). GLS is a measure of LV longitudinal systolic function and may be superior to EF in dilated cardiomyopathy. The normal value of GLS is less than –18%. It is negative because it measures the degree of systolic myocardial deformation during contraction. In this case, GLS was significantly abnormal < –10% (410).

2. **In addition to optimized GDMT what is the best therapeutic approach for this patient?**
   (a) Place an implantable cardioverter defibrillator (ICD)
   (b) Place a cardiac resynchronization device (CRD)
   (c) Place CRD-ICD
   (d) Place a quadripolar lead CRD
   (e) Place a dual chamber pacemaker

Ans. (d) See comments for question 3

3. **After device implantation, patient should undergo which of the following studies?**
   (a) Repeat transthoracic echo
   (b) 3D strain echo for lead pacing site optimization
   (c) 3D strain echo
   (d) Contrast echo
   (e) Stress echo

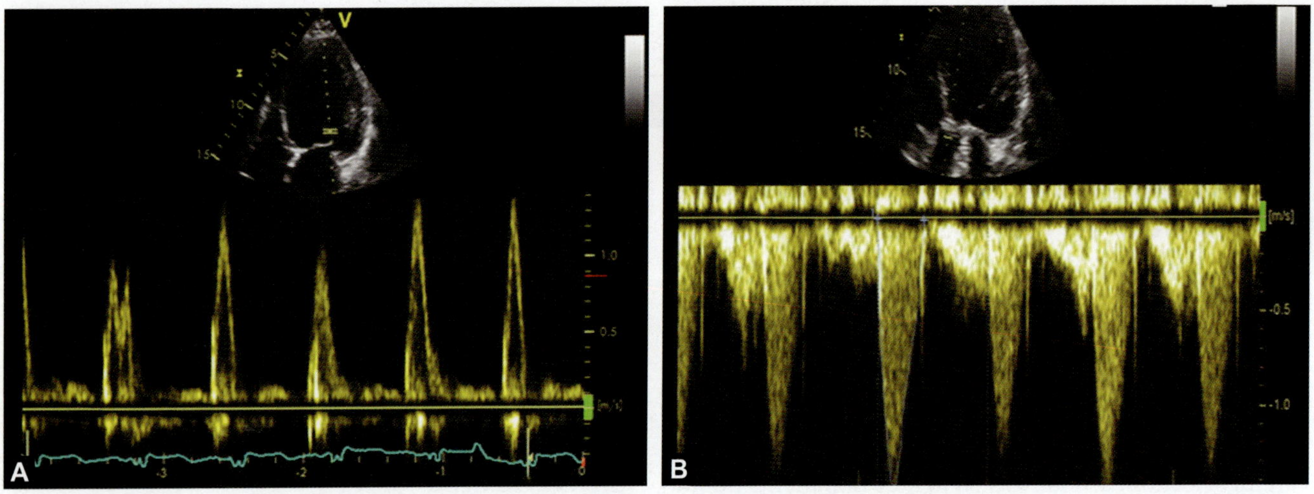

Figs. 126.2A and B: Shows MV inflow (A) and AV outflow (B) Doppler tracings.

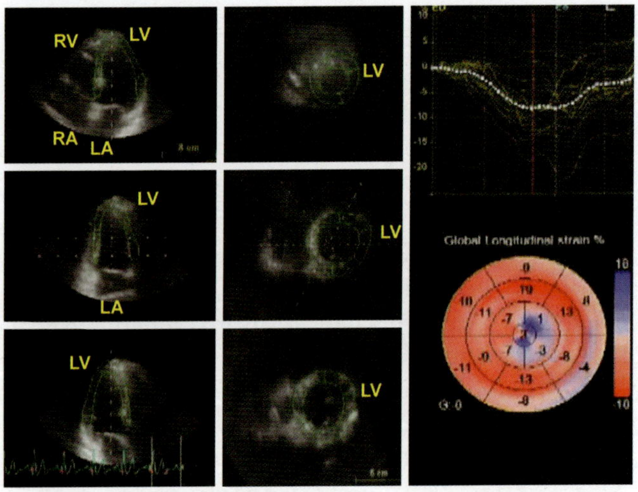

Fig. 126.3: Global longitudinal Strain (Bulls Eye) by 3D echo.

Ans. (b)

There are new devices available (Medtronic adaptive CRT) that automatically optimize the AV delay.[2,4] By promoting intrinsic RV conduction, Adaptive CRT reduces RV pacing and increases device longevity for patients with normal AV conduction. In addition to that a new Quardipolar LV lead was introduced that allows to optimize the pacing sequence in the LV, from four different pacing sites. This allows for various pacing vector directions from the tip of the LV lead close to the LV apex or a midventricular level in the vicinity of the diaphragm[3] or at the base of the heart or even originating from the tip of the right ventricle (RV) lead to any of the lead position in the LV and with reverse directions. In our case we optimized the LV pacing sequence by studying 3D strain imaging and tissue synchronous imaging (TSI) with each combination of pacing vectors [Figs. 126.5(TSI), 412].

4. Which of the following 3D strain bulls eye represent the optimized Quadripolar lead setting resulting in maximum global longitudinal strain?

(a) 70 L1-RV

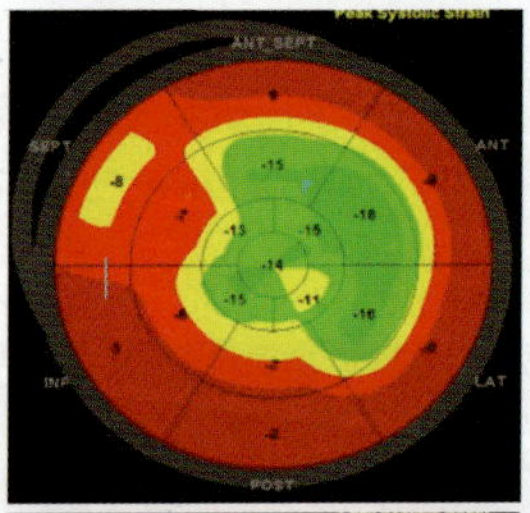

(b) 90 L4-RV

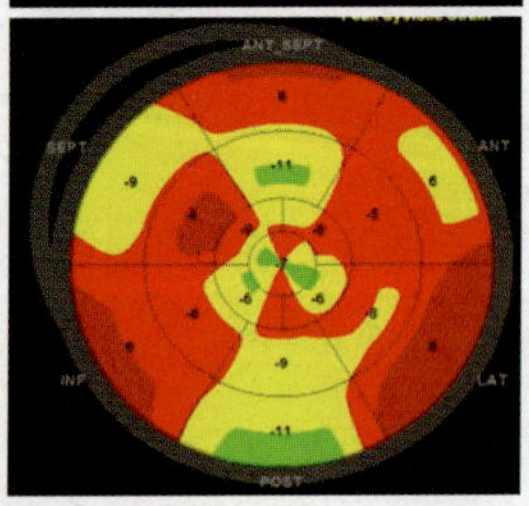

(c) 90 L1-RV

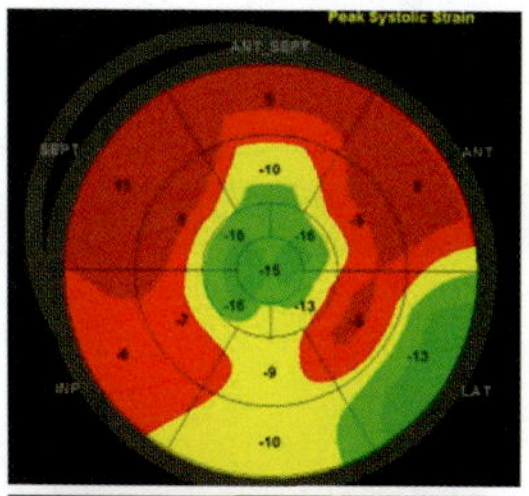

(d) 100 L1-L4

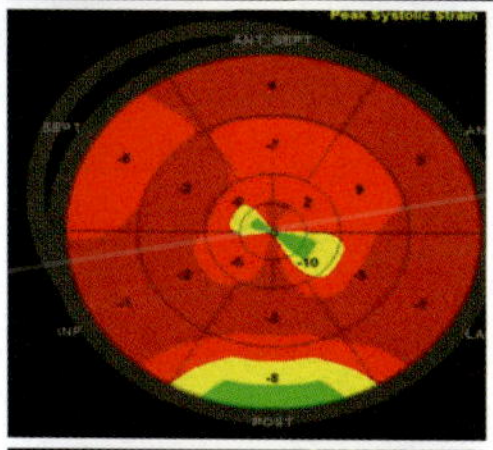

(e) 100 L4-L1

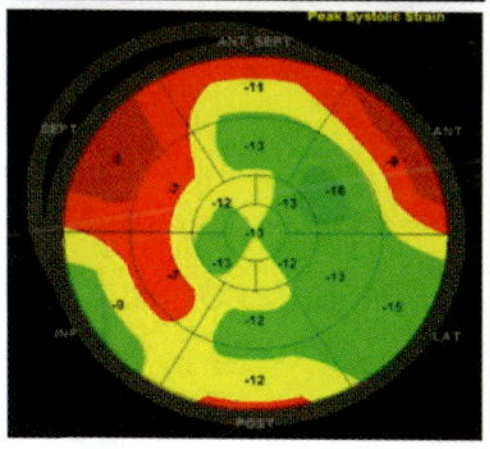

Ans. (e)

Choice E shows the largest area (green) of the normal GLS (U-shaped). The best result was with AV delay of 100 msec with pacing from the base of the left ventricular (LV) lead L4 to the Apex LV lead L1 (Fig. 126.4 and 411).

DISCUSSION

We demonstrate the feasibility of 3D strain imaging in the assessment of the Quadripolar lead CRD. With each pacing setting we were able to obtain different 3D strain patterns, mitral Doppler inflow and aortic outflow. We were able to optimize the pacing settings guided by the 3D strain patterns. Echo guidance may have a future role for LV Quadripolar adaptive CRD.

MOVIES 408 TO 412

REFERENCES

1. Abraham WT, Fisher WG, Smith AL, et al. Cardiac resynchronization in chronic heart failure. N Engl J Med. June 13, 2002;346(24):1845-53.
2. Biffi M, Zanon F, Bertaglia E, et al. Short-spaced dipole for managing phrenic nerve stimulation in patients with CRT: the "phrenic nerve mapping and stimulation EP" catheter study. Heart Rhythm. January 2013;10(1):39-45.
3. Biffi M, Foerster L, Eastman W, et al. Effect of bipolar electrode spacing on phrenic nerve stimulation and left ven-

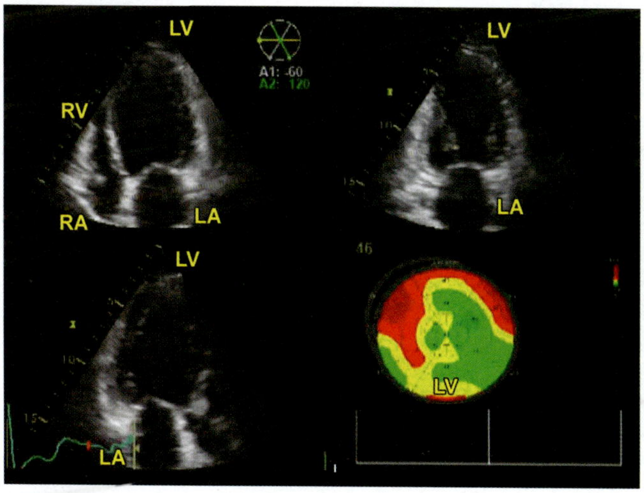

Fig. 126.4: LV quadripolar lead optimized 100 msec L4-L1. L represents pacing sites on the Quadripolar AV lead, L1 Apex pacing site, L2-L3 midventricular pacing site and L4 LV base pacing site.

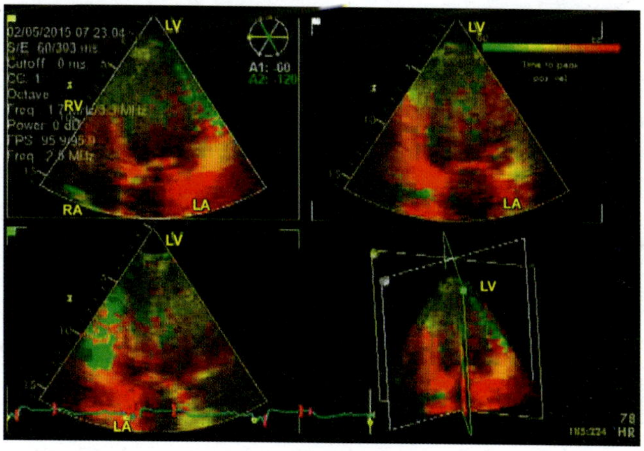

Fig. 126.5: Tissue synchronous imaging (TSI).

CASE 127

Sridhar Venkatachalam, Masood Ahmad

A 33-year-old male with known non-ischemic cardiomyopathy presented with New York Heart Association (NYHA) class IV symptoms. His clinical picture was consistent with cardiogenic shock. After initiation of inotropic support with Milrinone, he remained hypotensive and oliguric. A percutaneous left ventricular assist device (Impella 2.5 L) was inserted via right common femoral artery access. At the time of placement in the cardiac catheterization laboratory, two-dimensional transthoracic echocardiography (2D-TTE) was used to confirm the position of the blood-inlet tip in the left ventricular cavity. However, when the patient arrived in the cardiac care unit, suction alarms were noted with lower than expected flows. Bedside 2D-TTE demonstrated Impella catheter in the left ventricle, although the blood-inlet tip could not be visualized satisfactorily in the parasternal long axis view (Figs. 127.1A and B). Real time three-dimensional transthoracic echocardiography (3D-TTE) was performed subsequently. With 3D-TTE, the blood inlet tip was seen embedded into the papillary muscle in the parasternal long axis view (Fig. 127.1C and 413). The short axis cropped 3D caudal view on 3D-TTE demonstrated the tip abutting the posterior wall of the left ventricle (Fig. 127.1D). The Impella catheter was pulled back and the tip was repositioned to a depth of 3.5 cm below the level of aortic valve in the left ventricular cavity (Figs. 127.1E and F, 414).

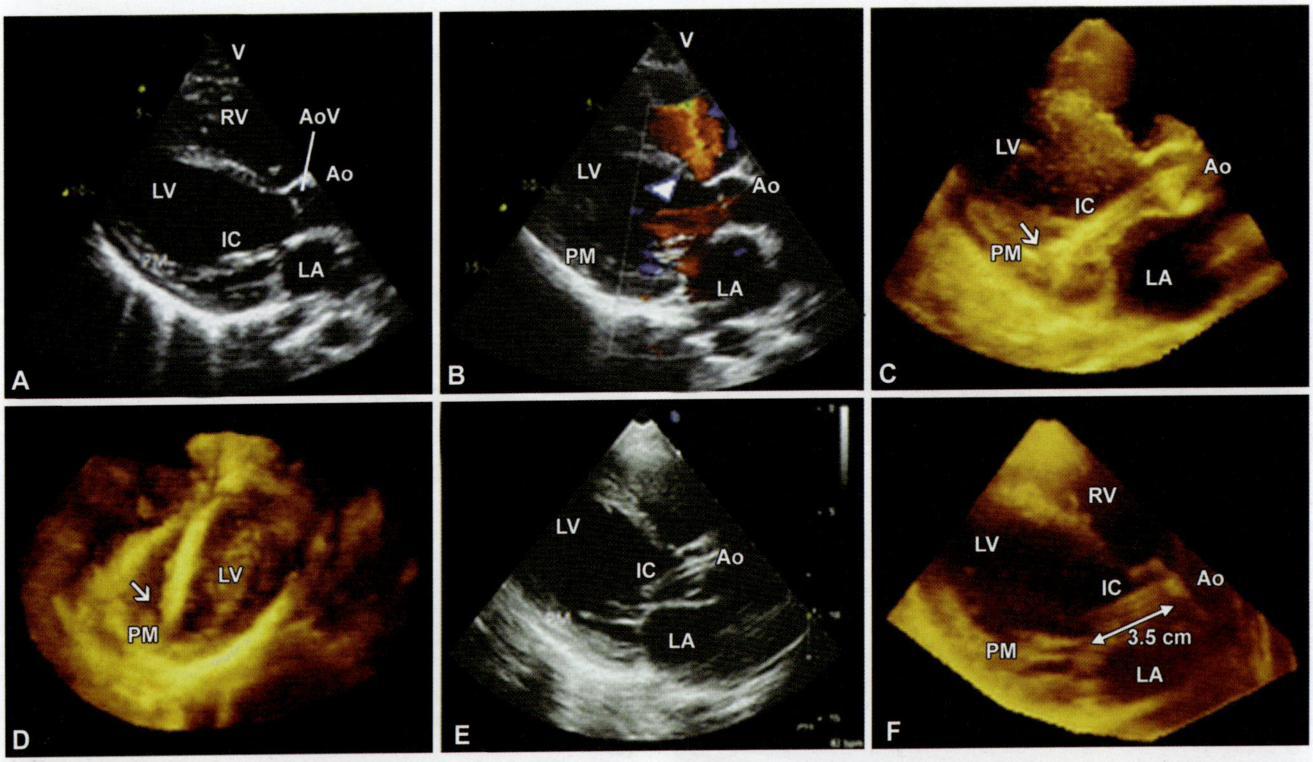

Figs. 127.1A to F: Two-dimensional transthoracic echocardiography (2D-TTE) parasternal long-axis view showing the transvalvular position of Impella catheter with poor visualization of the blood-inlet tip (Panel A). 2D-TTE with color Doppler imaging demonstrates flow at the outlet area below the aortic valve (arrowhead, Panel B). Three-dimensional transthoracic echocardiogram (3D-TTE) shows the blood-inlet distal tip of the Impella catheter imbedded into the papillary muscle (arrow, Panel C, Movie clip 1). Cropped 3D caudal short-axis view from the left ventricular side shows inflow tip touching the posterior left ventricle wall (arrow, Panel D). 2D-TTE parasternal long axis view after Impella catheter pull back reveals the inflow tip below aortic valve in the left ventricular cavity (Panel E). 3D-TTE clearly shows the inflow catheter tip distance at approximately 3.5 cm below the aortic valve plane (double-headed arrow, Panel F, Movie clip 2). (Ao: Aorta; AoV: Aortic valve; IC: Inflow catheter; LA: Left atrium; LV: Left ventricle; PM: Papillary muscle; RV: Right ventricle).

1. The following findings if present on 2D-TTE would be considered a potential contraindication for placement of Impella pump:

(a) Mechanical aortic valve
(b) Aortic valve stenosis with valve area $<1.5\ cm^2$
(c) Moderate to severe aortic insufficiency
(d) All of the above

Ans. (d)

Choices (a), (b) and (c) are listed as contraindications by the manufacturer.

2. Echocardiographic findings with optimal Impella catheter inlet positioning include all *except*:

(a) Color Doppler showing a dense mosaic pattern of turbulence near the outlet area below the aortic valve
(b) Catheter inlet 4 to 4.5 cm below the aortic valve in the left ventricular cavity
(c) Catheter pointing towards the left ventricular apex
(d) Catheter outlet area above the aortic valve

Ans. (a)

When correctly positioned, color Doppler would show a dense mosaic pattern of turbulence above the aortic valve at the outlet of the Impella catheter. A catheter that is too far into the ventricle would result in the mosaic pattern beneath the aortic valve. Choice (b), (c) and (d) indicate correct positioning.

3. With regard to placement of Impella, the incorrect statement is:

(a) Fluoroscopic guidance is not always required at the time of insertion
(b) Catheter repositioning can be performed safely at the bedside with 2D TTE in most cases
(c) Suction alarms, low flow or hemolysis may all be indicative of catheter migration
(d) When using transesophageal echocardiography, the mid-esophageal long axis view is preferred

Ans. (a)

The Impella pump should be inserted under fluoroscopic guidance in the catheterization laboratory to allow visualization of the entire catheter and remove slack. A portable C-Arm fluoroscopy may be used for subsequent confirmation of position. Minor catheter repositioning can be performed safely at the bedside with 2D-TTE imaging. Choice (c) and (d) are correct.

4. The next best bedside test in the assessment of Impella pump blood-inlet tip when 2D-TTE views are suboptimal is:

(a) Chest X-ray
(b) Transesophageal echocardiogram
(c) 3D-TTE
(d) Fluoroscopy

Ans. (c)

Although transesophageal echocardiogram may be used in this situation, the next best step would be to perform 3D-TTE. In addition to being less invasive, cropped images from 3D-TTE provide sufficient detail to assist in localizing Impella catheter position.[1] Chest X-ray and fluoroscopy are generally not helpful for optimal positioning of the catheter tip after insertion.

MOVIES 413 AND 414

REFERENCE

1. Abusaid GH, Ahmad M. Transthoracic real time three-dimensional echocardiography in Impella placement. Echocardiography. 2012;29:E105-E106.

CASE 128

Adarna LG, Elsayed M, Alagic N, Uygur B, Turaga NSN, Chahwala JR, Mohamed A, Gupta N, Bulur S, Nanda NC

This is a 48-year-old male who presented with severe LV global hypokinesis with an estimated EF of 10–15%. He underwent left ventricular assist device (LVAD) implantation. 2D TTE was done (415 to 421).

1. **Which of the following statements is incorrect?**
   (a) Arrow in 415 (parasternal long axis view) points to a cannula in LV apex which is pumping blood from LV into the proximal ascending aorta. The arrowhead points to the rightward shift of the interventricular septum.
   (b) Hollow arrow in 415 shows the AV practically closed throughout the cardiac cycle.
   (c) 416 (parasternal long axis view) shows mild AR. Severe AR would have compromised systemic perfusion since a significant proportion of blood pumped into the ascending aorta would have regurgitated back into the LV.
   (d) 417 (M-mode) shows occasional partial opening and closing of the AV (arrow).
   (e) P in 418 (AV short axis view) represents an implantable cardioverter defibrillator (ICD). Note the closed position of the AV throughout.
   (f) Arrow in 419 (LV short axis view at the level of the papillary muscle) shows rightward shift of ventricular septum.
   (g) 420 is a short axis view near the level of LV apex showing the cannula (arrow).
   (h) Arrow in 421 shows red flow signals representing LV blood being directed into the pump.
   (i) Pulsatile LVADs are synchronized with EKG.

Ans. (i)

Pulsatile LVADs are not synchronized with EKG. Rightward shift of the ventricular septum may result from high LV diastolic pressures because of improper LVAD speed setting, device dysfunction, inlet obstruction and severe AR. Leftward shift may signal excessive LV decompression due to excessive pump speed, significant TR and RV systolic dysfunction. A patent foramen ovale (PFO) needs to be closed at the time of device implantation due to the increased risk of hypoxemia and paradoxical embolization. The arrow in 422 shows a color Doppler artifact from the LV cannula.

423 is an M-mode taken from another patient with LVAD showing minimal opening movement of the AV (arrow).

MOVIES 415 TO 423

CASE 129

Adarna LG, Bulur S, Alagic N, Uygur B, Nanda NC

Adult patient who underwent mitral valve replacement (MVR) and left ventricular assist device (LVAD). 2D TTE was done (🎥 424, R = reverberation from MVR).

1. **Do you think this patient needs a LVAD on the basis of 🎥 424.**
   (a) Yes
   (b) No

Ans. (b)

Left ventricular assist device is needed to pump the blood out of the LV into the ascending aorta (AO) to maintain perfusion. In this patient, LV function appears to have normalized and LVAD may not be necessary. MVR is also moving well. AV motion is markedly reduced because most of LV blood is drawn by the cannula (arrow) and very little moves through the AV. RV function also appears reasonable.

MOVIE 424 🎥

CASE 130

Gupta N, Mohamed A, Elsayed M, Nanda NC

Color Doppler flow signals in the aortic arch (ACH) and descending aorta (DA) are shown in an adult patient (🎥 425 and 426).

1. **What is the etiology of these flow signals?**
   (a) These flow signals are occasionally seen normally
   (b) Severe AR
   (c) Flow signals from collaterals entering the DA in a patient with aortic coarctation
   (d) Could be related to LVAD which this patient may have

Ans. (d)

This patient does have a left ventricular assist device (LVAD). It is possible that the aortic cannula is inserted somewhat higher up in the ascending AO resulting in these prominent flow signals. Continuous flow signals (arrow) are also noted on PW Doppler examination in 🎥 426.

MOVIES 425 AND 426

CASE 131

Andre Dias, Nikoloz Koshkelashvili, Aman Amanullah

An 80-year-old man with past medical history significant for seizure disorder, hypertension and hyperlipidemia presented to emergency department (ED) with witnessed generalized tonic-clonic seizure that lasted for 30 minutes. On admission his blood pressure was 214/92 mm/Hg, with heart rate of 39 beats per minute, a respiratory rate of 12 and oxygen saturation of 97% on room air. The respiratory and cardiovascular examination results were unremarkable except for bradycardia. The electrocardiogram (EKG) in the ED revealed complete heart block shown in Figure 131.1. Laboratory results were remarkable for an initial elevated troponin I of 1.2 ng/mL. Patient underwent transvenous pacemaker placement and coronary angiography the same day (Figs. 131.2 and 131.3). Echocardiogram shortly after the procedure is shown in Figure 131.4 and 427 and 428.

1. **Based on the information provided what is the most likely diagnosis?**
   (a) Extensive myocardial infarction in the LAD territory
   (b) Stress induced cardiomyopathy with apical clot
   (c) Large scar from prior significant LAD infarct
   (d) Severe hypokinesis of anterior wall secondary to infiltrative process

Ans. (b)

Takotsubo cardiomyopathy (TCM) also known as apical ballooning syndrome or stress-induced cardiomyopathy is a peculiar reversible condition often affecting postmenopausal women after a stressful event. The underlying mechanisms have not been completely elucidated but several hypotheses, such as catecholamine cardiotoxicity, microvascular dysfunction and coronary artery spasm, have been implicated.[1-3] The diagnosis of TCM was made based on the Modified Mayo Clinic Criteria:[4] absence of pheochromocytoma or myocarditis, presence of modest elevation in cardiac troponin accompanied by transient hypokinesis of the left ventricular distal segments sparing the base. Normal coronary anatomy excluded myocardial infarction as the culprit factor.

Our case also emphasizes the importance of recognizing potential complications associated with TCM such as cardiac thrombus formation (arrow in 427 and 428).

2. **How would you manage this patient?**
   (a) Percutaneous coronary intervention
   (b) Refer to CT surgery for revascularization
   (c) Start systolic heart failure regimen consisting of beta blocker, ACE inhibitor with anticoagulation
   (d) Emergent thrombolytic therapy

Ans. (c)

There is no obstructive coronary artery disease and therefore no indication for percutaneous coronary intervention or revascularization. Patient should be treated for systolic

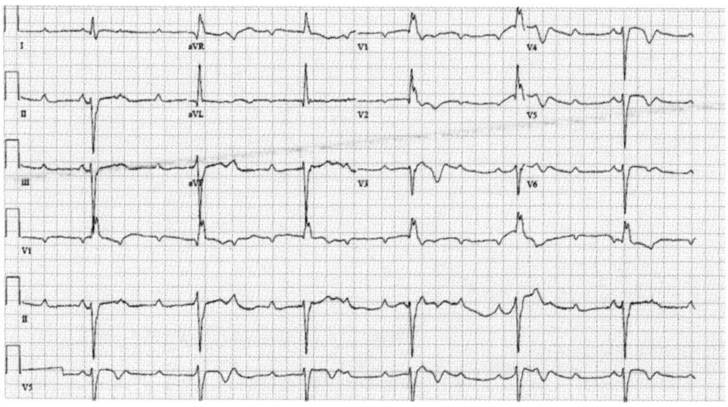

Fig. 131.1: ER EKG.

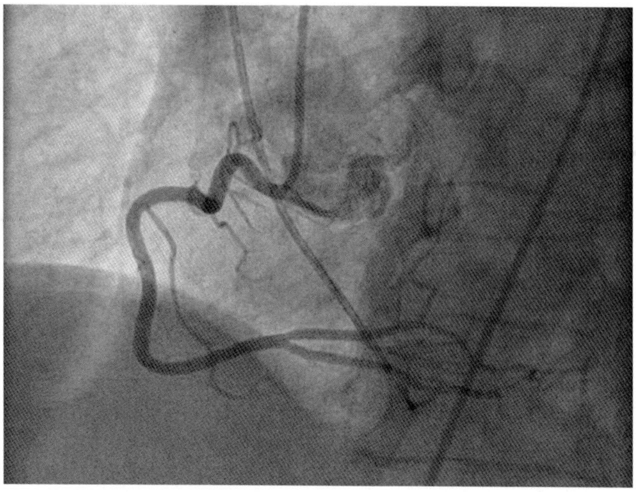

Fig. 131.2: Right coronary artery.

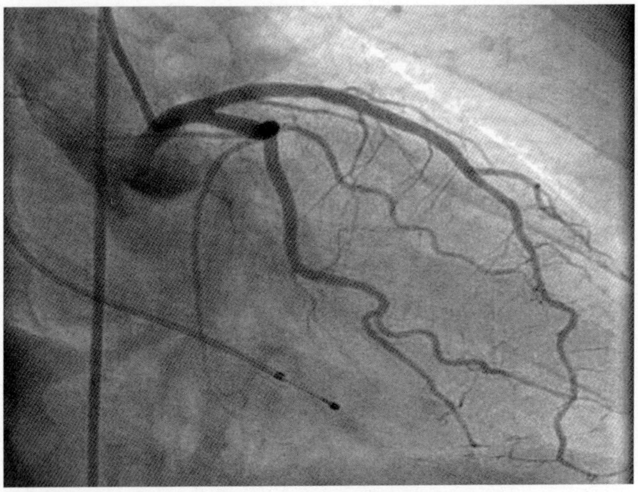

Fig. 131.3: Left coronary system with pacemaker lead.

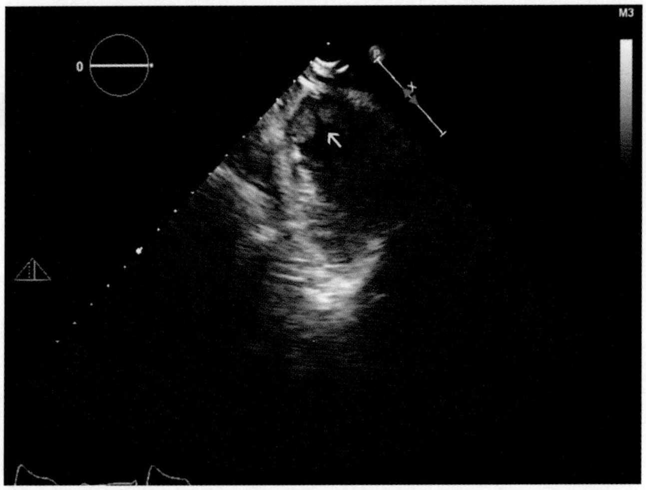

Fig. 131.4: Apical thrombus (arrow) on echocardiogram.

left ventricular dysfunction and anticoagulation given the presence of LV thrombus.

MOVIES 427 AND 428

REFERENCES

1. Gianni M, Dentali F, Grandi AM, et al. Apical ballooning syndrome or takotsubo cardiomyopathy: a systematic review. Eur Heart J. 2006;27(13):1523-9.
2. Kurowski V, Kaiser A, von Hof K, et al. Apical and midventricular transient left ventricular dysfunction syndrome (tako-tsubo cardiomyopathy): frequency, mechanisms, and prognosis. Chest. 2007;132(3):809-16.
3. Prasad A, Lerman A, Rihal CS. Apical ballooning syndrome (tako-tsubo or stress cardiomyopathy): a mimic of acute myocardial infarction. Am Heart J. 2008;155(3):408-17.
4. Bybee KA, Kara T, Prasad A, et al. Systematic review: transient left ventricular apical ballooning: a syndrome that mimics ST-segment elevation myocardial infarction. Ann Intern Med. 2004;141(11):858-65.

CASE 132

Hanumanth K Reddy, Raghuveer Kura, Rakesh Sharma, Ravi Komatireddy, Nishchayjit Basra

CHEST PAIN AND SHORTNESS OF BREATH IN A PHYSICIAN

A 70-year-old physician was admitted with chest pain, diffuse T inversions on EKG and positive cardiac enzymes. The patient is on valsartan for hypertension. Rest of the medical history is unremarkable. Personal history revealed overwhelming professional stress associated with medicare regulations. Physical examination was unremarkable except for tachycardia with a heart rate of 110 beats/minute, S3 gallop and sparse rales over lung bases. Cardiac enzymes were mildly elevated and chest X-ray showed mild pulmonary edema (refer to 429 and 430 before answering the following questions).

1. **The cause of symptoms in this patient is:**
   (a) Dilated cardiomyopathy
   (b) Ischemic cardiomyopathy
   (c) Takotsubo cardiomyopathy
   (d) Sarcoidosis

Ans. (c)

2. **The treatment for this condition includes:**
   (a) Supportive and symptomatic therapy
   (b) Steroids and methotrexate
   (c) ACE inhibitors and beta blockers
   (d) Diuretics and digoxin

Ans. (a)

3. **Clinical course and prognosis of this condition is generally:**
   (a) Downhill and fatal
   (b) Favorable and may recover completely
   (c) Chronic with a propensity for refractory heart failure
   (d) None of the above

Ans. (b)

The patient's condition improved with supportive and symptomatic therapy (see 431). Treatment included diuretics, beta-blockers, ARB, heparin and aspirin. Lipid profile was within normal limits.

One year later, the patient's long-term wife passed away and the patient was severely stressed out. He was readmitted to the hospital with a similar presentation as before with complete eventual recovery.

DEFINITION OF TAKOTSUBO CARDIOMYOPATHY

Left ventricle assumes an appearance of a Japanese octopus fishing pot called a takotsubo. Stress cardiomyopathy with transient apical ballooning and left ventricular systolic dysfunction, which usually recovers within a few weeks.

EPIDEMIOLOGY OF TAKOTSUBO CARDIOMYOPATHY

This condition probably accounts for ≈1% to 2% of all cases of suspected acute myocardial infarction. It is more common in post-menopausal women after exposure to sudden, unexpected emotional or physical stress.[1]

MAYO CLINIC DIAGNOSTIC CRITERIA[1]

1. Transient hypokinesis, akinesis, or dyskinesis in the left ventricular mid-segments with or without apical involvement
2. Frequently, but not always, a stressful trigger
3. Absence of obstructive coronary disease or a plaque rupture
4. New ECG abnormalities (ST-segment elevation and/or T-wave inversion)
5. Modest elevation in cardiac troponin; and
6. Absence of pheochromocytoma and myocarditis.

DIFFERENTIAL DIAGNOSIS OF TAKOTSUBO CARDIOMYOPATHY

Since patients with Takotsubo cardiomyopathy present with chest pain, ST, T changes and positive cardiac enzymes, they frequently undergo catheterization which eliminates the apical wall motion abnormalities from critical coronary artery disease.

As shown in Figure 132.1A, echocardiographic 429 and angiographic 430, apical ballooning characterizes

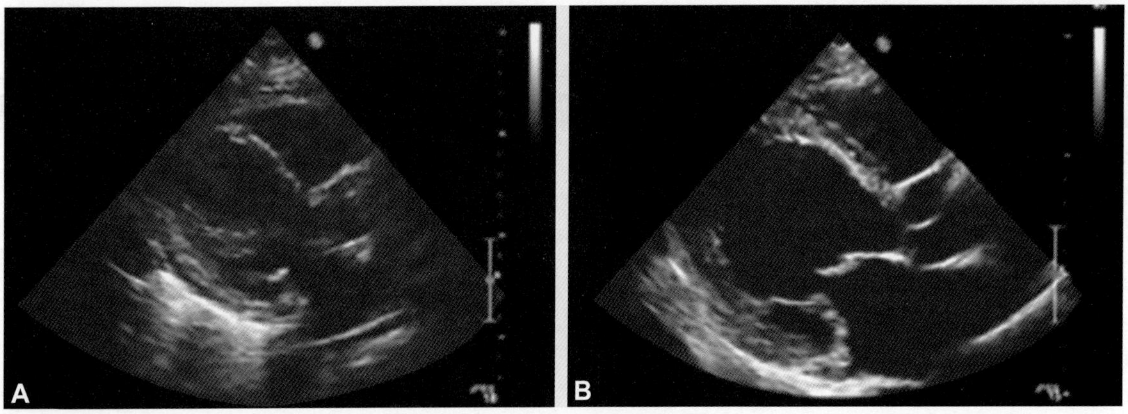

Figs. 132.1A and B: Differential contractile patterns. (A) Takotsubo cardiomyopathy; (B) Dilated cardiomyopathy.

Takotsubo cardiomyopathy in contrast to the global hypokinesis typical of dilated cardiomyopathy shown in Figure 132.1B.

431 is an echocardiogram showing normalized LV systolic function of a Takotsubo patient.

TAKOTSUBO CARDIOMYOPATHY: DISCUSSION

Patients with Takotsubo cardiomyopathy have high levels of serum catecholamines and plasma brain natriuretic peptide (BNP). Myocardial biopsy has shown interstitial infiltrates consisting primarily of mononuclear lymphocytes, leukocytes, and macrophages; myocardial fibrosis; and contraction bands with or without overt myocyte necrosis. The inflammatory changes and contraction bands distinguish Takotsubo cardiomyopathy from coagulation necrosis seen in myocardial infarction resulting from coronary artery occlusion.

Wittstein et al.[3] compared admission plasma catecholamine concentrations between a group of 13 patients with stress cardiomyopathy who had transient apical ballooning and a group of 7 patients hospitalized for acute myocardial infarction (Killip class III). The plasma levels of both epinephrine and norepinephrine were remarkably increased in the stress cardiopathy patients.[2]

The authors suggested that the elevated catecholamine levels might be responsible for the systolic dysfunction, however, elevated catecholamine levels are not uniformly found in patients with this syndrome. High plasma catecholamine levels in patients with pheochromocytoma are well known to induce reversible cardiomyopathy. The myocardial histological changes in Takotsubo cardiomyopathy are quite similar to those of catecholamine cardiotoxicity in both animals and humans. These changes, which differ from those in ischemic cardiac necrosis, include contraction band necrosis, neutrophil infiltration, and fibrosis pattern. These histological changes are usually noted in Ca^{2+} overload states. Therefore, it has been proposed that Ca^{2+} overload in myocardial cells produces ventricular dysfunction in catecholamine cardiotoxicity. Lyon et al.[4] have proposed that the high circulating epinephrine levels might trigger a switch in cardiomyocyte intracellular signaling changing Bar-Gs protein coupling to Bar-Gi coupling. Bar-Gi protein activation was shown to cause negative inotropic effect on human myocardium.

In summary, the apical ballooning that characterizes Takotsubo cardiomyopathy reflects toxic high local concentrations of catecholamines, not coronary artery or microvascular disease. The pattern of left ventricular dysfunction may result from both myocardial cellular rupture and withdrawal of β-adrenoceptors.

MOVIE LEGENDS

429: Transthoracic echocardiogram (TTE) 2-chamber showing apical ballooning with good LV contraction.
430: Left ventricle (LV) angiogram during cardiac catheterization.
431: TTE apical 4-chamber showing improved LV function.

REFERENCES

1. Akashi YJ, Goldstein DS, Barbaro G, et al. Takotsubo cardiomyopathy: a new form of acute, reversible heart failure. Circulation. 2008;118:2754-62.
2. Nef HM, Mollmann H, Weber M, et al. Release pattern of cardiac biomarkers in left ventricular apical ballooning. Int J Cardiol. 2007;115:128-9.
3. Wittstein IS, Thiemann DR, Lima JA, et al. Neurohormonal features of myocardial stunning due to sudden emotional stress. N Engl J Med 2005;352:539-48.
4. Lyon AR, Rees P SC, Prasad P, et al. Nature Clinical Practice Cardiovascular Medicine 2008;5:22-29.

CASE 133

Claudia Carolina Cajas-Morales, Nilda Espinola-Zavaleta, Jose Antonio Arias-Godinez, Juan Francisco Fritche-Salazar, Nydia Avila-Vanzzini, Maria Eugenia Ruiz-Esparza, Angel Romero-Cardenas, Maria Del Sol Ordaz

A 21-year-old male was seen one year ago with moderate-effort dyspnea and lower extremity edema. He sought our attention recently because of increasing dyspnea, paroxysmal nocturnal dyspnea and increased waist circumference. On physical examination, the apex was in the 6th left intercostal space outside the midclavicular line. He also had lower left parasternal lift, gallop rhythm, murmur of mitral and tricuspid insufficiency, ascites and edema of lower limbs. Transthoracic echocardiography and magnetic resonance imaging (MRI) were performed and the images are shown below.

1. **What is the diagnosis (Figs. 133.1, 133.2, 432 and 433)?**
   (a) Left ventricular hypertrophy
   (b) Myocarditis
   (c) Dilated cardiomyopathy with left ventricular non-compaction
   (d) Severe mitral regurgitation

Ans. (c)

Left ventricular non-compaction is a rare entity with the prevalence of 0.1–3% in the general population. It is characterized by abnormal trabeculations particularly

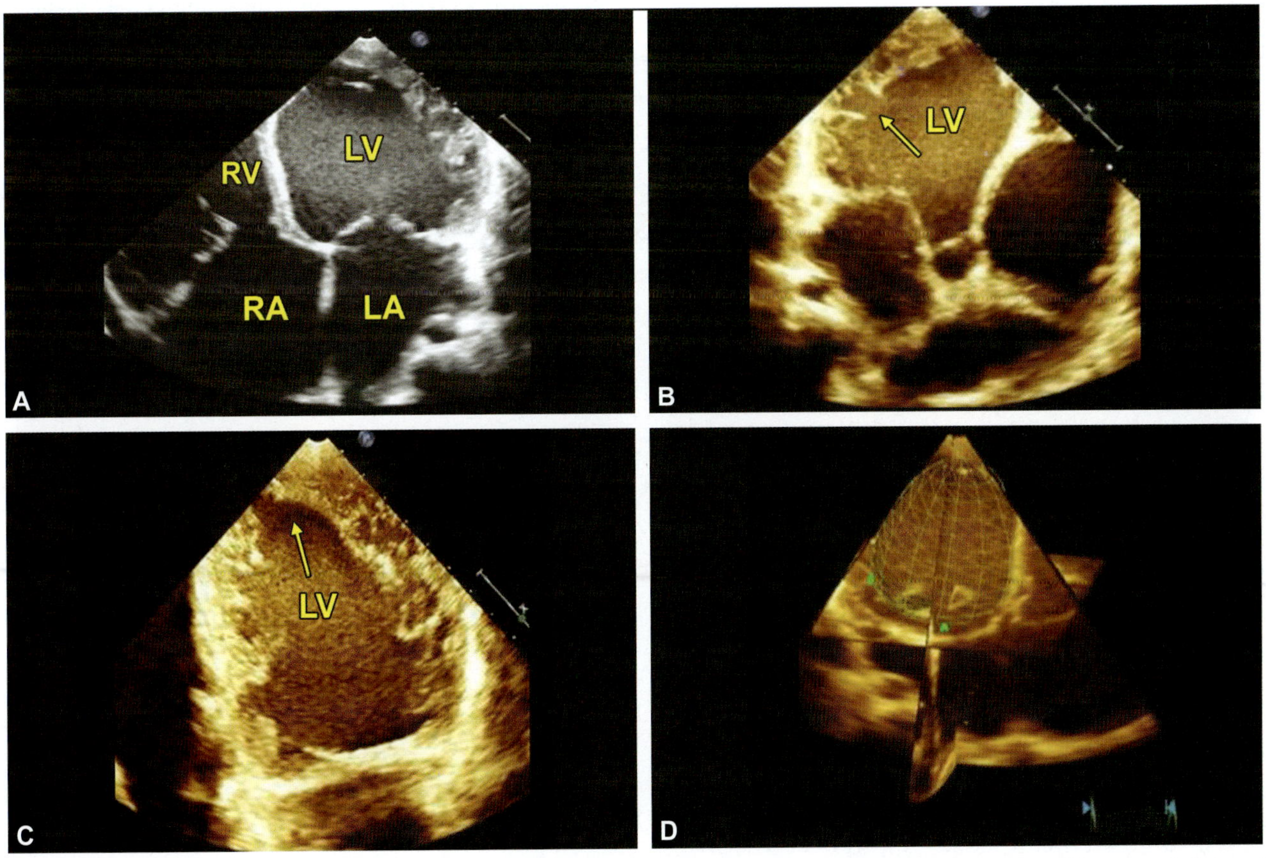

Figs. 133.1A to D: Two-dimensional images in the apical four (A), five (B) and two (C) chambers views showing dilatation of all 4 cardiac cavities and hypertrabeculation (arrows in all figures and movies) in the anterolateral and apical walls of LV. (D) LV systolic function by 3D echocardiography. (RV: Right ventricle; RA: Right atrium; LV: Left ventricle; LA: Left atrium).

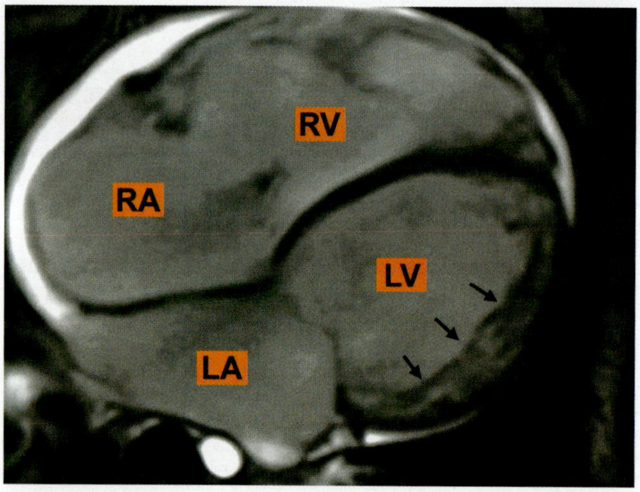

Fig. 133.2: MRI. Cine gradient echo 4-chamber, showing significant dilatation of the four cardiac chambers with hypertrabeculation of LV anterolateral and apical walls. Arrows point to multiple trabeculations consistent with LV non-compaction. Also pericardial effusion is observed. (RV: Right ventricle; RA: Right atrium; LV: Left ventricle; LA: Left atrium).

at the apex, but hypertrabeculations can occur in other left ventricular (LV) regions. The most common clinical presentation is heart failure, arrhythmias or thromboembolism.[1,2] Echocardiography and MRI have been crucial in addressing this cardiomyopathy. The most used diagnostic criteria in both echocardiography and MRI is the ratio of non-compacted to compacted myocardium of > 2: 1 and > 2.3: 1, respectively. Another approach used in MRI is the percentage of trabecular mass > 20%. There are different types, but non-compaction associated with dilated LV has a worse prognosis. Treatment is symptomatic, defibrillator, cardiac resynchronization therapy and cardiac transplantation.

MOVIE LEGENDS

432 and 433: 2D TTE five-chamber views with color Doppler showing mitral and tricuspid regurgitation.

REFERENCES

1. Towbin JA, Lorts A, Jefferies JL. Left ventricular non-compaction cardiomyopathy. Lancet. 2015;386:813-25.
2. Espinola-Zavaleta N, Soto ME, Muñoz-Castellanos L, et al. Non-compacted Cardiomyopathy: clinical-echocardiographic study. Cardiovas Ultrasound. 2006;4:35.

CASE 134

Bulur S, Adarna LG, Elsayed M, Alagic N, Uygur B, Turaga NSN, Chahwala JR, Nanda NC

The patient is a 60-year-old female who presented with heart failure. She underwent MV replacement for severe MR a few years ago. At that time LV function was noted to be poor. 2D (434) and 3D TTE (435 and 436) were done.

1. **What do the arrows point to (434 to 436)?**
    (a) Multiple clots in a poorly functioning LV
    (b) Tumor in LV apex
    (c) Multiple trabeculations in a poorly functioning LV
    (d) Both multiple trabeculations and clots in a poorly functioning LV
    (e) In my experience, artifacts in LV apex look exactly like this

Ans. (c)

This patient has multiple trabeculations visualized by both 2D and 3D TTE consistent with LV noncompaction. Trabeculations appear more numerous by 3D TTE than 2D TTE which has also been shown in the past. It is best to consider diagnosing this rare entity only if numerous trabeculations are noted in the LV and other criteria are present. 3D can also calculate the trabecular volume by subtracting the compacted volume from the total LV volume. Multiplying the trabecular volume by 1.05 which is the specific gravity of cardiac muscle will give the trabecular mass. In this patient, LV end-systolic volume (ESV) with trabeculations included measured 150 mL by 3D TTE and 78 mL excluding trabeculations. Therefore, the trabecular volume was 72 mL which is 48% of LV volume (72/150 = 48%). The trabecular mass would be 75.6 g (72 × 1.05).

437 is 2D TTE from another adult patient. Arrows in the apical long axis view show multiple trabeculations consistent with LV noncompaction.

MOVIES 434 TO 437

REFERENCE

1. Rajdev S, Singh A, Nanda NC, et al. Comparison of two- and three-dimensional transthoracic echocardiography in the assessment of trabeculations and trabecular mass in left ventricular noncompaction. Echocardiography. 2007 Aug;24(7):760-7.

CASE 135

Mohamed A, Gupta N, Elsayed M, Taher A, Nanda NC

This is a 56-year-old male being evaluated for a renal transplant. 2D TTE was done (438 to 440, 438 is an echo contrast study).

1. **What are the echo findings (438 to 440)??**
   (a) Large LV with diminished function and bilateral pleural effusion (arrows in 439 and 440).
   (b) Large LV with diminished function, multiple trabeculations (arrows in 438) raising the possibility of non-compaction and bilateral pleural effusion (arrows in 439 and 440).

Ans. (b)

MOVIES 438 TO 440

CASE 136

Supawat Ratanapo, Gyanendra K Sharma

NON-COMPACTION CARDIOMYOPATHY WITH LV THROMBUS

A 35-year-old man with no known cardiac history presented with acute right hemiparesis and was found to have acute left middle cerebral artery stroke. Transthoracic echocardiogram was performed as a part of stroke work up. Short axis view was obtained (Figs. 136.1, 136.2, 441 and 442). A focused 4-chamber view with contrast echocardiogram showed thrombus is left ventricle (Fig. 136.3 and 443).

1. **Which statement is true regarding his cardiac condition?**
   (a) Ratio of non-compacted to compacted layers are more than 2 from the end-systolic image of the left ventricle is a common diagnostic criteria.
   (b) Left ventricular thrombus is the most common presentation of this cardiac condition
   (c) Prominent trabeculations of the myocardium are always due to congenital abnormality occurring since childhood and not seen in any other cardiac abnormalities.
   (d) This condition does not increase risk of sudden cardiac death in the future.
   (e) Most of genetic-associated case is X-linked abnormalities.

Ans. (a)

a. The Commonly used echocardiographic criteria is based on Jenni criteria[1] which is the series of 34 patients with non-compaction cardiomyopathy.
   1. Absence of coexisting cardiac abnormalities.
   2. Left ventricular wall has 2 distinctly identifiable layers; thin compacted myocardium and a thicker non-compacted endocardial layer of trabecular meshwork with deep endomyocardial spaces/recesses. An end systolic ratio of non-compacted to compacted layers of > 2 is considered diagnostic.
   3. The predominant localization of the pathology is to mid-lateral, apical, and mid-inferior segments.
   4. Color Doppler evidence of flow into the inter-trabecular recesses.

b. Most common manifestation of non-compaction cardiomyopathy is dyspnea and heart failure.

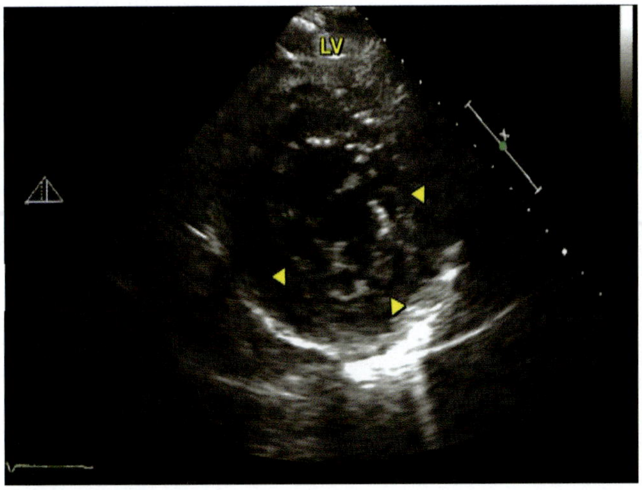

Fig. 136.1: Short-axis image of non-compaction cardiomyopathy showed hypetrabecular endocardium (arrowheads).

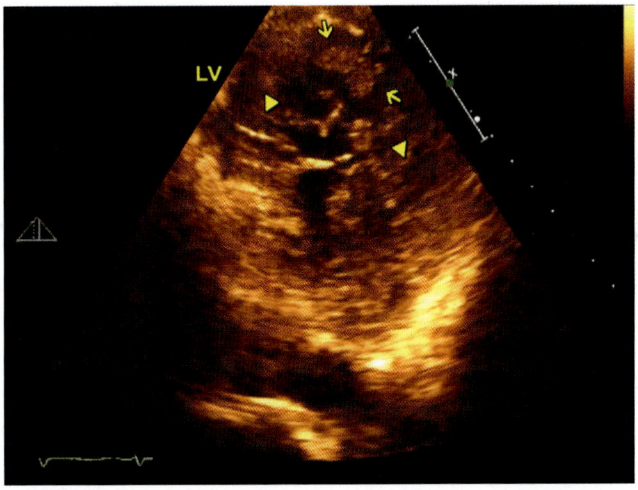

Fig. 136.2: Short-axis image of non-compaction cardiomyopathy showed thrombus (arrows) in trabecular recesses (arrowheads).

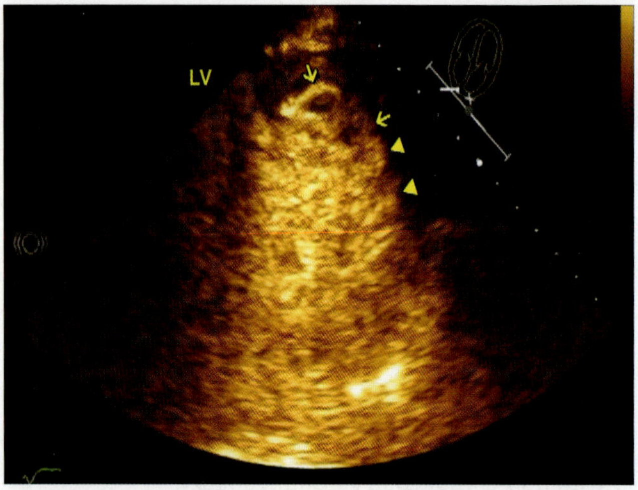

Fig. 136.3: Focused 4-chamber view of contrast echocardiogram showed unstable thrombus (arrows) in trabecular recesses (arrowheads).

c. Hypertrabeculations can develop in adulthood and are not diagnostic of cardiac non-compaction. This pattern is seen in other conditions like coronary artery disease.

d. Non-compaction cardiomyopathy can increase risk of sudden cardiac death.[2]

e. Most common genetic association of non-compaction cardiomyopathy is autosomal dominant.

MOVIE LEGENDS

441: Short-axis image of non-compaction cardiomyopathy showed hypetrabecular endocardium (arrowheads).

442: Short-axis image of non-compaction cardiomyopathy showed thrombus (arrows) in trabecular recesses (arrowheads).

443: Focused 4-chamber view of contrast echocardiogram showed unstable thrombus (arrows) in trabecular recesses (arrowheads).

REFERENCES

1. Jenni R, Oechslin E, Schneider J, et al. Echocardiographic and pathoanatomical characteristics of isolated left ventricular non-compaction: a step towards classification as a distinct cardiomyopathy. Heart. 2001;86:666.
2. Bhatia NL, Tajik AJ, Wilansky S, et al. Isolated noncompaction of the left ventricular myocardium in adults: a systematic overview. J Card Fail. 2011;17:771.

CASE 137

Bulur S, Alagic N, Elsayed M, Uygur B, Turaga NSN, Chahwala JR, Adarna LG, Nanda NC

This is a 32-year-male who presented to his family physician complaining of swollen legs. Clinical examination was negative except for 3+ pitting edema of lower extremities. 2DTTE was done (🎥 444).

1. **What does the parasternal long axis view (🎥 444) demonstrate?**
   (a) Normal LV and RV function
   (b) Echogenic LV walls with probable mild increase in wall thickness
   (c) Infiltrative disease such as amyloidosis should be considered in the differential diagnosis in addition to chronic kidney disease and hypertensive heart disease
   (d) Increased RV wall thickness could have narrowed the diagnosis to an infiltrative disease in the absence of significant pulmonary hypertension
   (e) (a), (b), (c) and (d) statements are correct
   (f) (c) is incorrect because chronic kidney disease does not result in increased LV wall echogenicity

Ans. (e)

Both chronic kidney disease with associated hypertension as well as hypertension by itself can result in increased echogenicity because of concomitant fibrosis and increased collagen deposition resulting from a reaction produced by myocyte hypertrophy. Increase in RV wall thickness would not be expected to occur in the above two conditions unless there was significant associated pulmonary hypertension (or some other independent condition producing RV hypertrophy) and therefore if present could point to infiltrative cardiomyopathy.

MOVIE 444 🎥

CASE 138

Bulur S, Alagic N, Elsayed M, Uygur B, Turaga NSN, Chahwala JR, Adarna LG, Nanda NC

Another patient with suspected amyloidosis is shown in 445 to 447. Echogenic myocardium and a small pericardial effusion (arrow in 445) are well seen. The arrow in 446 shows redundant MV chordae mimicking a small systolic anterior movement (SAM) of the MV.

MOVIES 445 TO 447

CASE 139

Bulur S, Nanda NC

This is a 42-year-old male with renal dysfunction. 2D TTE was done.

1. **What is the likely diagnosis in this patient (Figs. 139.1A and B and 448A and B)?**
   (a) LV hypertrophy due to hypertension resulting from renal dysfunction
   (b) Amyloidosis
   (c) Sarcoidosis
   (d) Hypertrophic cardiomyopathy

Ans. (b)

A likely diagnosis is amyloidosis which is laid down as sheets producing multiple interfaces (layered appearance in M-mode, Figs. 139.1A and B). These result in an echogenic myocardium. There is no real hypertrophy of LV walls in amyloidosis.

2. **Mittral inflow and tissue Doppler tracings (Figs. 139.2A to C) show:**
   (a) Decreased LV relaxation
   (b) Increased LV relaxation
   (c) Decreased left sided filling pressures
   (d) Increased left sided filling pressures

Ans. (d)

Mitral inflow pattern shows a large E wave, a very small A wave (E/A ratio around 3) and decreased MV deceleration time (120 ms, normal 160–240 ms) typical of restrictive physiology with increased left sided filling pressures. Tissue Doppler tracings show early diastolic (E') medial annular velocity of 7.80 cm/s and lateral annular velocity of 6.92 cm/s, average 7.36 cm/s. The ratio of peak MV inflow velocity (E, 160 cm/s) to average MV annular velocity (E', 7.36 cm/s) is high at 21.7 (normal ratio <14) which also indicates increased left sided filling pressures in the absence of significant MR and significant mitral annular calcification.

MOVIES 448A AND B

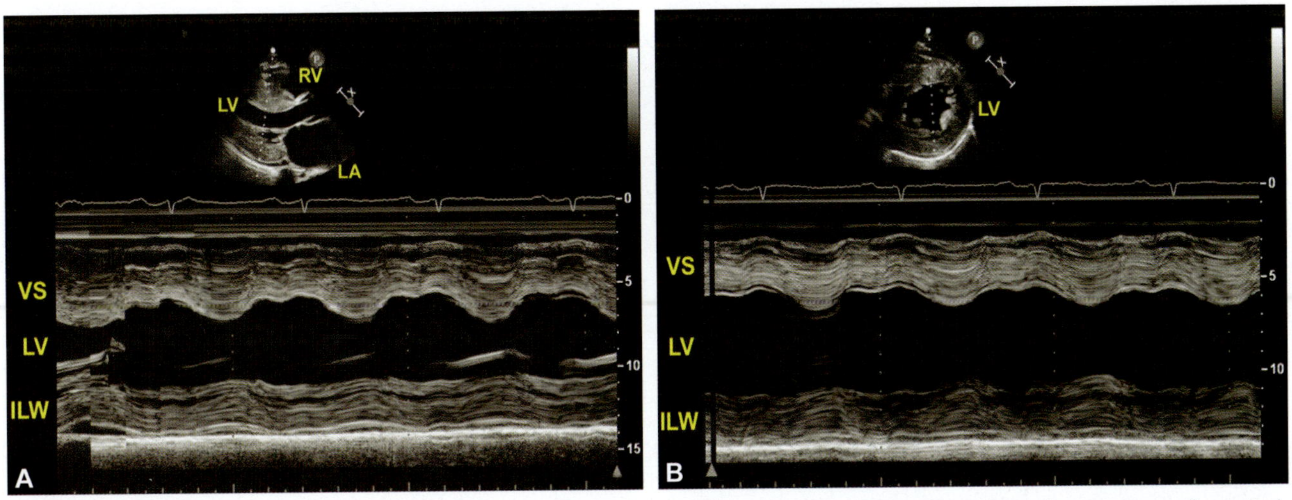

Figs. 139.1A and B: 2D directed M-mode of parasternal long (A) and short (B) axis views of LV showing a layered appearance of ventricular septum (VS) and posterior or inferolateral wall (ILW).

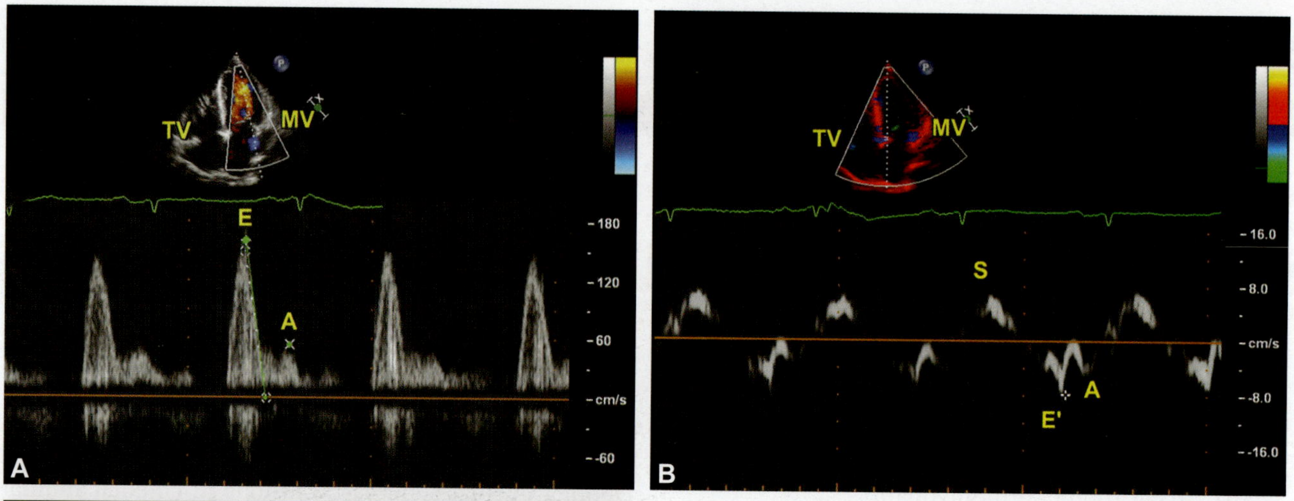

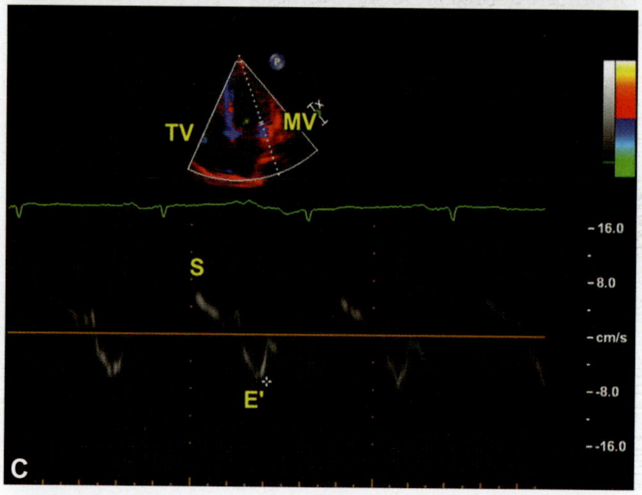

Figs. 139.2A to C: (A) Mitral inflow (B) Tissue Doppler examination of medial mitral annulus. (C) Tissue Doppler examination of lateral mitral annulus. (S: Systolic wave).

CASE 140

Taher A, Elsayed M, Adarna LG, Bulur S, Nanda NC

A 39-year-old female with heart failure.

1. **Which findings may be incorrect in the parasternal long axis view (449A and B)?**
   (a) Echogenic LV walls
   (b) Poor LV function
   (c) Thickened LV and RV walls
   (d) Hypertrophied LV and RV walls
   (e) Generalized LV hypokinesis
   (f) Segmental wall motion abnormalities
   (g) LA appears enlarged

Ans. (d and e)

In an infiltrative disease like amyloidosis which this patient may have because of echogenic LV walls, the LV walls are thickened because of amyloid deposition but are not necessarily hypertrophied. Also, the proximal inferolateral wall appears to move much better than the mid and apical segments hence the hypokinesis is not completely generalized. Segmental wall motion abnormalities may occur in cardiomyopathies of different etiologies and do not necessarily imply epicardial coronary artery disease. Thickened RV wall could be due to infiltration.

2. **What conditions you would consider in the differential diagnosis of this patient?**
   (a) Infiltrative cardiomyopathy such as amyloidosis
   (b) Chronic renal failure with coronary artery disease
   (c) End stage hypertensive heart disease with coronary artery disease
   (d) Hypertrophic cardiomyopathy
   (e) All of the above

Ans. (e)

Thick, echogenic LV walls with poor function and thickening of the RV wall would lead one to think of an infiltrative process such as amyloidosis as the most likely diagnosis. Late stage chronic renal failure, hypertensive heart disease and hypertrophic cardiomyopathy may also present with echogenic walls due to focal collagen deposition and fibrosis resulting from myocyte hypertrophy. In hypertrophic cardiomyopathy, the "higgeldy-piggeldy" appearance of the myocardium from myocardial fiber disarray may also contribute to the echogenicity. In amyloidosis there is no fibrosis but the multiple interfaces produced by layers of amyloid deposition are believed to result in echogenic walls.[1]

Thickened RV wall would narrow down the differential diagnosis to an infiltrative disease and hypertrophic cardiomyopathy since it will not develop in chronic renal failure and systemic hypertension unless pulmonary hypertension is very severe. Even in that case the RV tends to dilate considerably masking hypertrophy. 450A and B are other 2D views showing thickened RV walls.

MOVIES 449 AND 450

REFERENCE

1. Bhandari AK, Nanda NC. Myocardial texture characterization by two-dimensional echocardiography. Am J Cardiol. 1983 Mar 1;51(5):817-25.

CASE 141

Mark H Goldberger, Stephen Helmke

These are echocardiograms of four patients with a systemic disease involving the heart.

1. **What is the most likely diagnosis?**
   (a) Hypertensive heart disease
   (b) Hypertrophic cardiomyopathy
   (c) Fabry's disease
   (d) Transthyretin cardiac amyloidosis
   (e) Endomyocardial fibrosis

Ans. (d)

Patients with transthyretin (TTR) cardiac amyloidosis can present with various physical as well as echocardiographic findings. Here are four TTR cardiac amyloidosis patients with various echocardiographic findings.

The first patient is a 73-year-old active, mildly symptomatic male. Parasternal long-axis view (Fig. 141.1 and 451): Hypertrophied left ventricle (LV), moderately reduced left ventricular ejection fraction (LVEF). Apical 4-chamber view (Fig. 141.2 and 452): LV findings as in previous figure. Pacemaker is visualized in the right heart (P in 452). The interatrial septum (IAS) is thickened. Mitral inflow Doppler (Fig. 141.3A): Restrictive mitral Doppler filling pattern. LV Tissue Doppler (Fig. 141.3B), and Decreased septal E' velocity. LV longitudinal strain (Fig. 141.3C): Severely decreased global longitudinal strain with relative apical sparing pattern.

The second patient is a 76-year-old active, moderately symptomatic male. Parasternal long-axis view (Fig. 141.4 and 453): Hypertrophied LV with normal LVEF. Apical 4 chamber view (Fig. 141.5 and 454): Findings as in previous figure in addition to thickened IAS. Mitral inflow Doppler (Fig. 141.6A): Restrictive filling pattern, mitral E/A ratio greater than one. LV Tissue Doppler (Fig. 141.6B), Decreased septal E' velocity. LV longitudinal strain (Fig. 141.6C and 455), and severely decreased global longitudinal strain with some relative apical sparing pattern. Compared to the first patient, there is less apical sparing.

The third patient is a 60-year-old male, with mild 99mTc-PYP uptake, who is asymptomatic. Parasternal long-axis view (Fig. 141.7 and 456): Normal LV size and LVEF with mild left ventricular hypertrophy. Apical 4 chamber view (Fig. 141.8 and 457): Findings as in previous figure. Mitral Doppler (Fig. 141.9A): Mildly restrictive filling pattern. LV Tissue Doppler (Fig. 141.9B): Normal septal E' velocity. LV Longitudinal strain (Fig. 141.9C): Mildly decreased global longitudinal strain with relative apical sparing pattern.

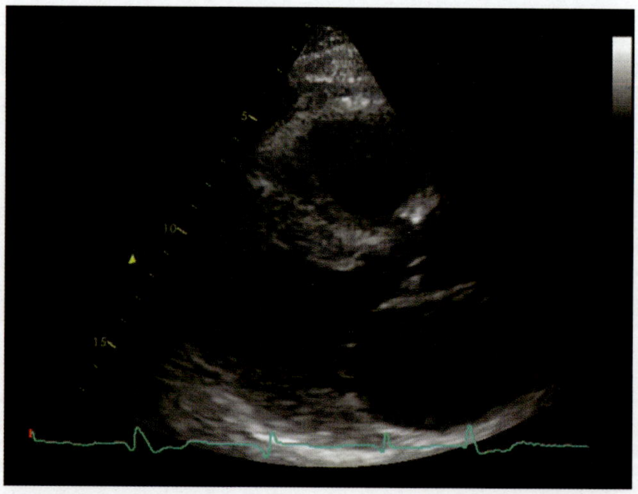

Fig. 141.1: 2D TTE. Parasternal long axis view of a 73-year-old active, mildly symptomatic male showing hypertrophied left ventricle.

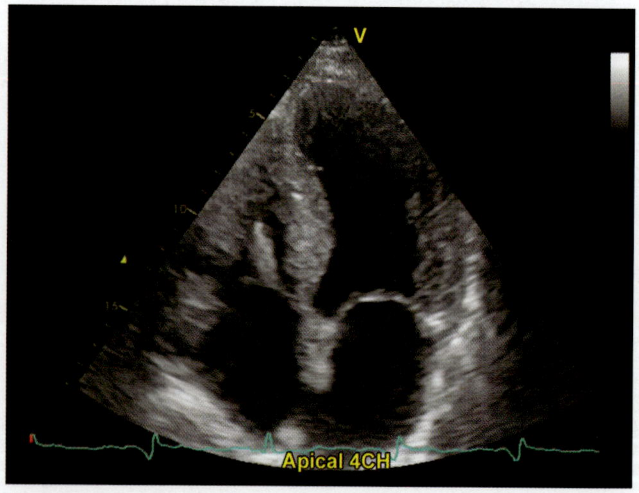

Fig. 141.2: 2D TTE. Apical 4-chamber view of a 73-year-old active, mildly symptomatic patient showing left ventricular hypertrophy and thickened interatrial septum. Pacemaker is visualized in the right side of the heart.

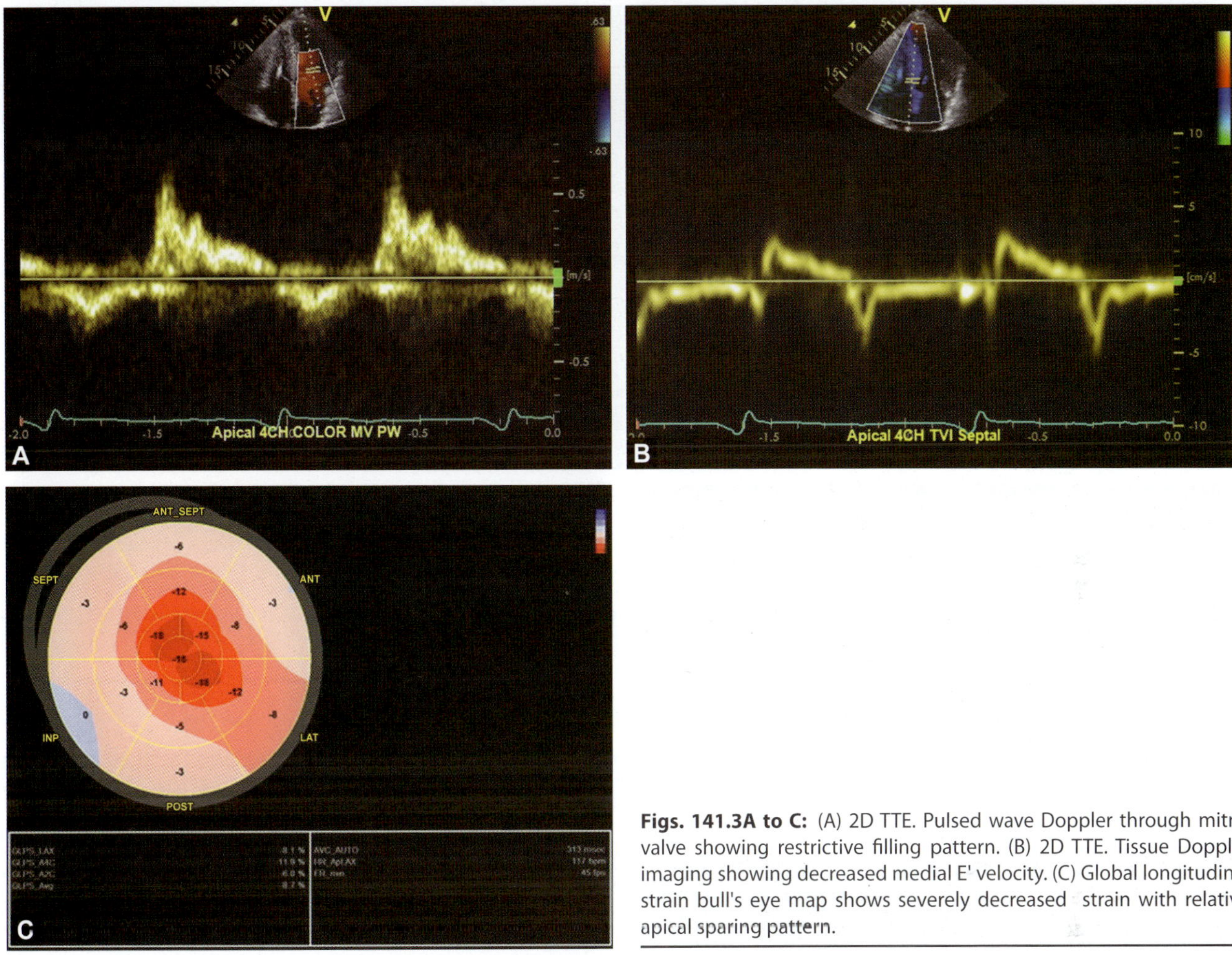

Figs. 141.3A to C: (A) 2D TTE. Pulsed wave Doppler through mitral valve showing restrictive filling pattern. (B) 2D TTE. Tissue Doppler imaging showing decreased medial E' velocity. (C) Global longitudinal strain bull's eye map shows severely decreased strain with relative apical sparing pattern.

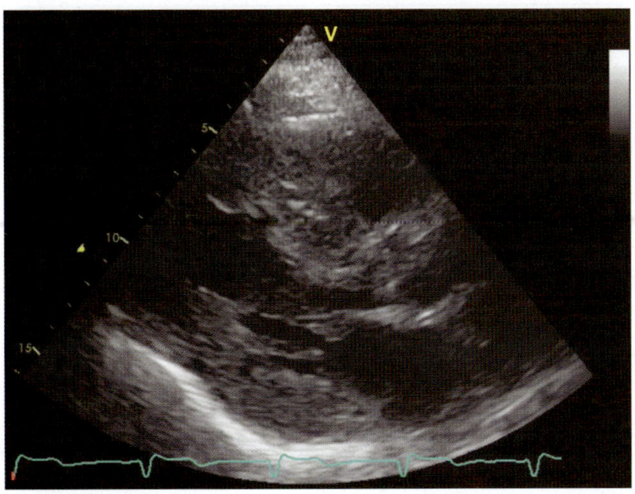

Fig. 141.4: 2D TTE. Parasternal long axis view of a 76-year-old active, moderately symptomatic male shows hypertrophied left ventricle.

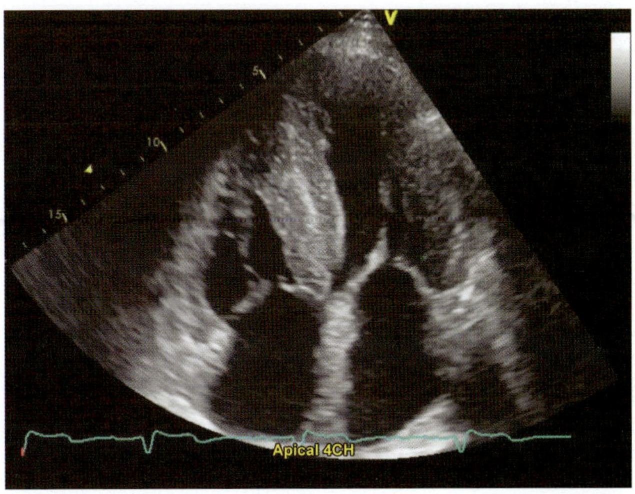

Fig. 141.5: 2D TTE apical 4-chamber view of a 76-year-old active, moderately symptomatic male showing left ventricle hypertrophy and thickened interatrial septum.

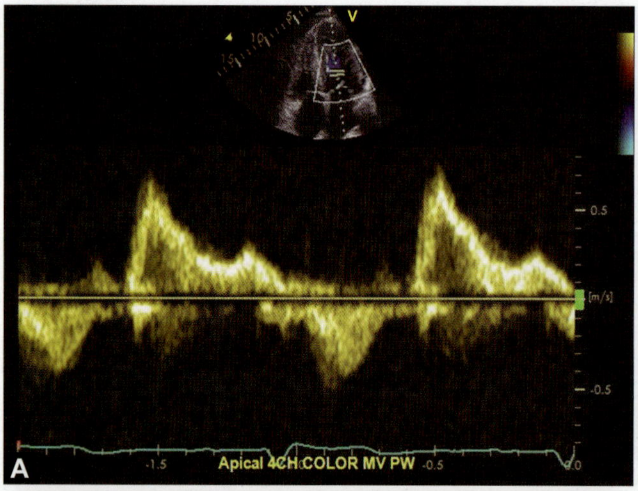

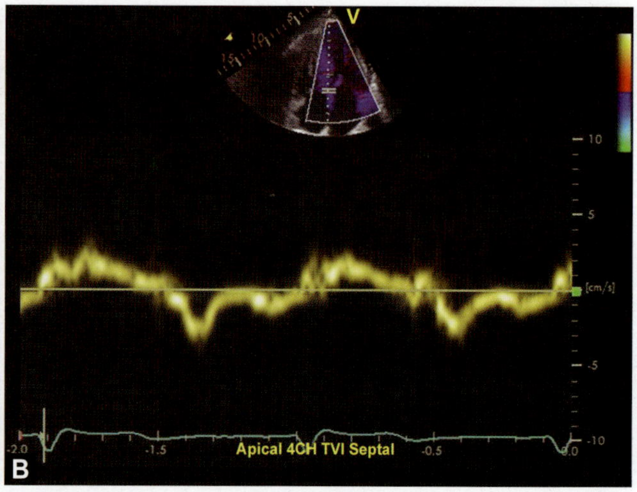

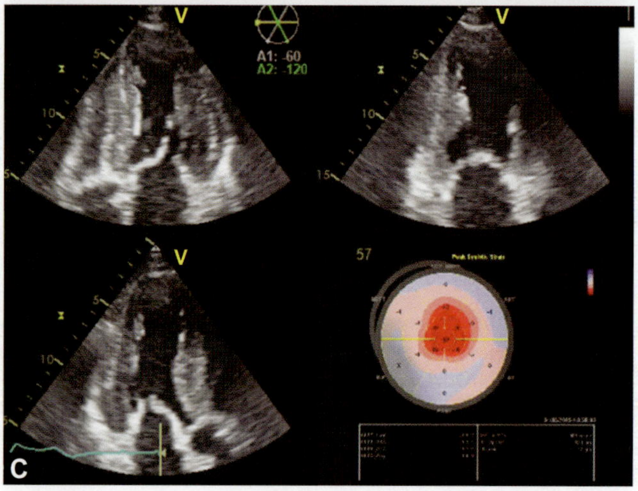

Figs. 141.6A to C: (A) 2D TTE. Pulsed wave Doppler through mitral valve showing restrictive filling pattern with mitral E/A ratio greater than two. (B) 2D TTE. Tissue Doppler imaging showing decreased mitral E' velocity. (C) 3D global longitudinal strain with bull's eye map shows severely decreased strain with some relative apical sparing pattern.

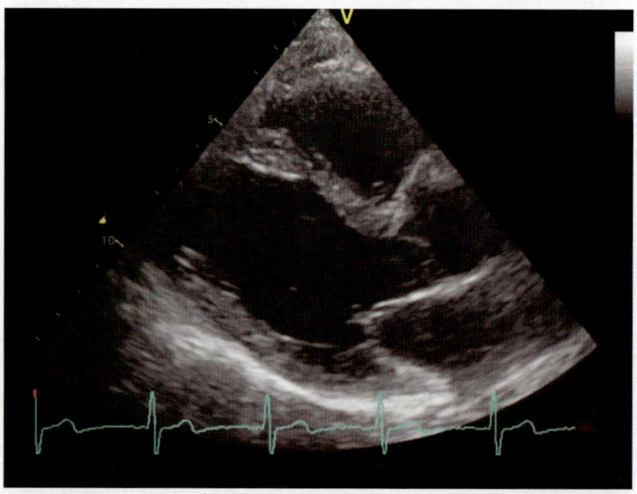

Fig. 141.7: 2D TTE. Parasternal long axis view of an asymptomatic 60-year-old male showing normal left ventricular size with mild hypertrophy.

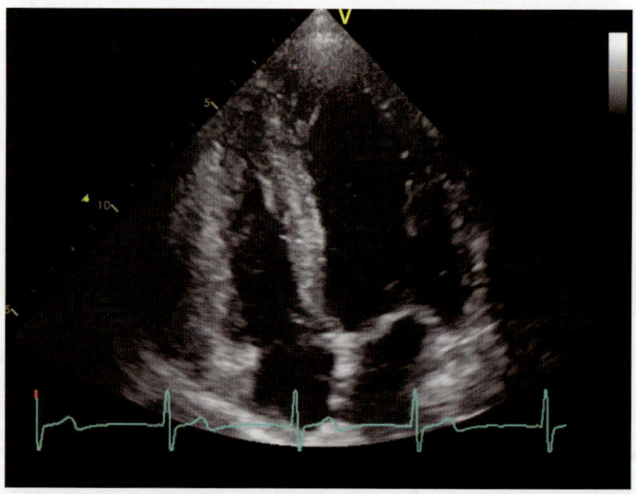

Fig. 141.8: 2D TTE. Apical 4-chamber view of an asymptomatic 60-year-old male showing mild left ventricular hypertrophy.

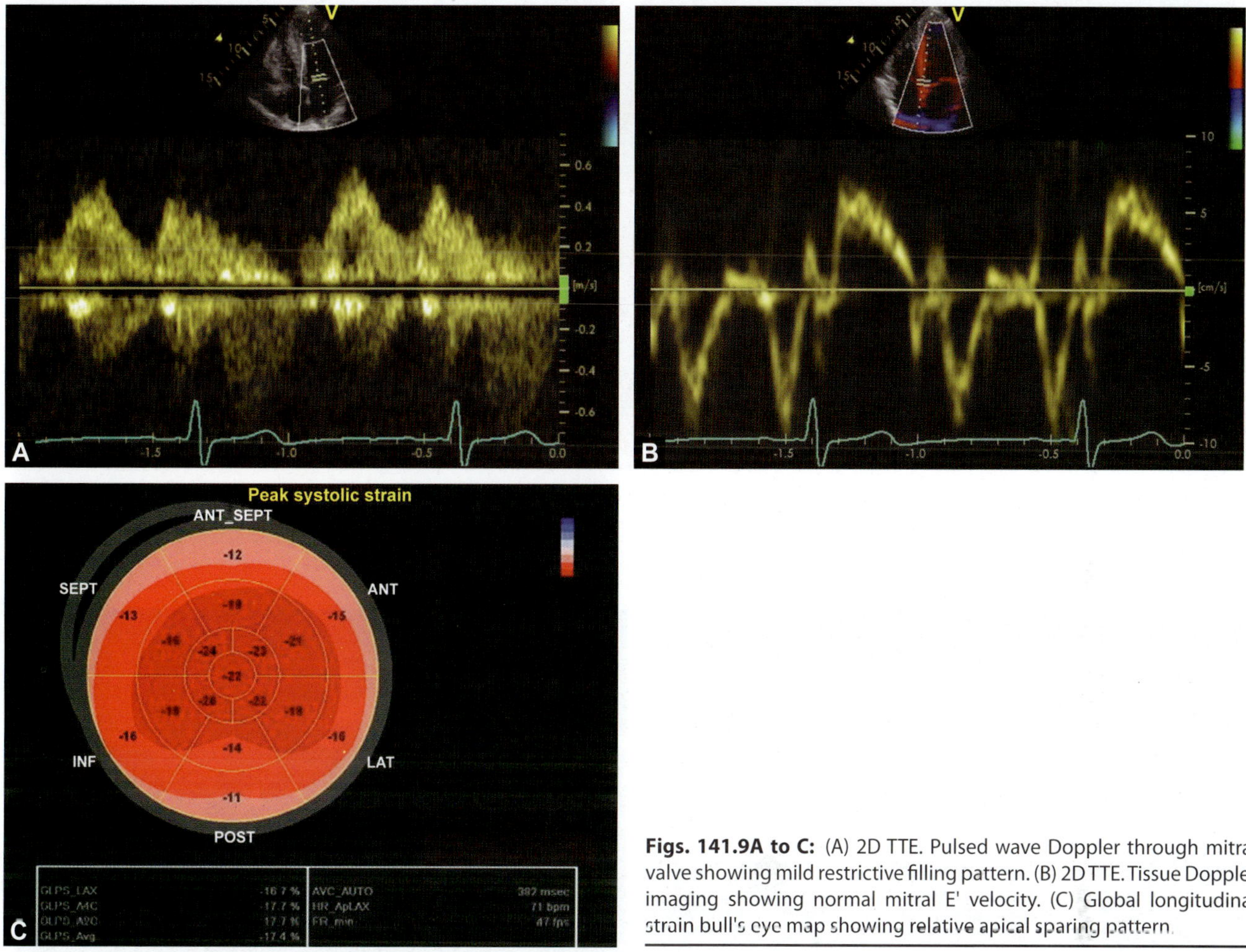

Figs. 141.9A to C: (A) 2D TTE. Pulsed wave Doppler through mitral valve showing mild restrictive filling pattern. (B) 2D TTE. Tissue Doppler imaging showing normal mitral E' velocity. (C) Global longitudinal strain bull's eye map showing relative apical sparing pattern.

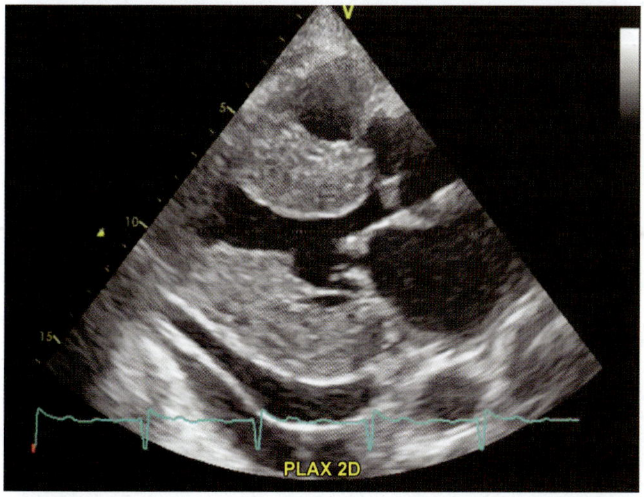

Fig. 141.10: 2D TTE. Parasternal long axis view of a 65 year-old-sendentary, severely symptomatic male showing hypertrophied left ventricle. A small pericardial and left pleural effusions are also seen.

The fourth patient is a 65-year-old sedentary, severely symptomatic male. Parasternal long-axis view (Fig. 141.10 and 458): Mildly reduced LVEF. A small pericardial effusion and a pleural effusion are visualized. Apical 4 chamber view (Fig. 141.11 and 459): LV findings and effusions as in previous figure. The left atrium is dilated. Mitral inflow Doppler (Fig. 141.12A): Restrictive filling pattern. LV Tissue Doppler (Fig. 141.12B), Decreased septal E' velocity. LV longitudinal strain (Fig. 141.12C and 460 and 461), and Severely decreased global longitudinal strain with minimal apical sparing pattern.

Classically, patients with advanced TTR cardiac amyloidosis have thickened left and right ventricular walls, but patients in the early stage of the disease may have normal or only slightly thickened ventricular walls. Choices (a), (b), and (c) are conditions typified by patients with thickened walls who exhibit diastolic

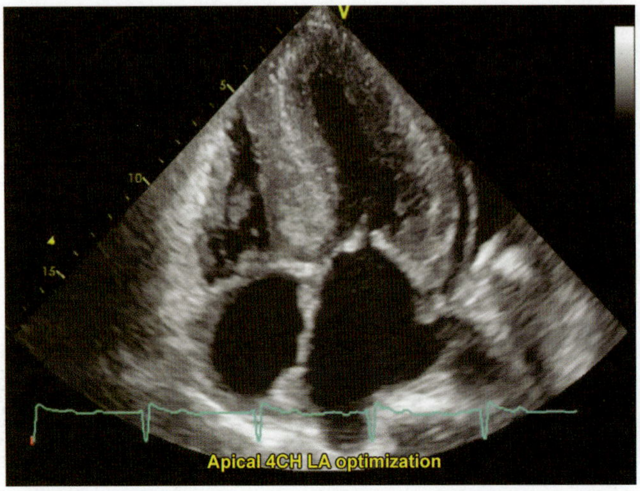

Fig. 141.11: 2D TTE. Apical 4-chamber view showing dilated left atrium. A small pericardial and left pleural effusions are also seen.

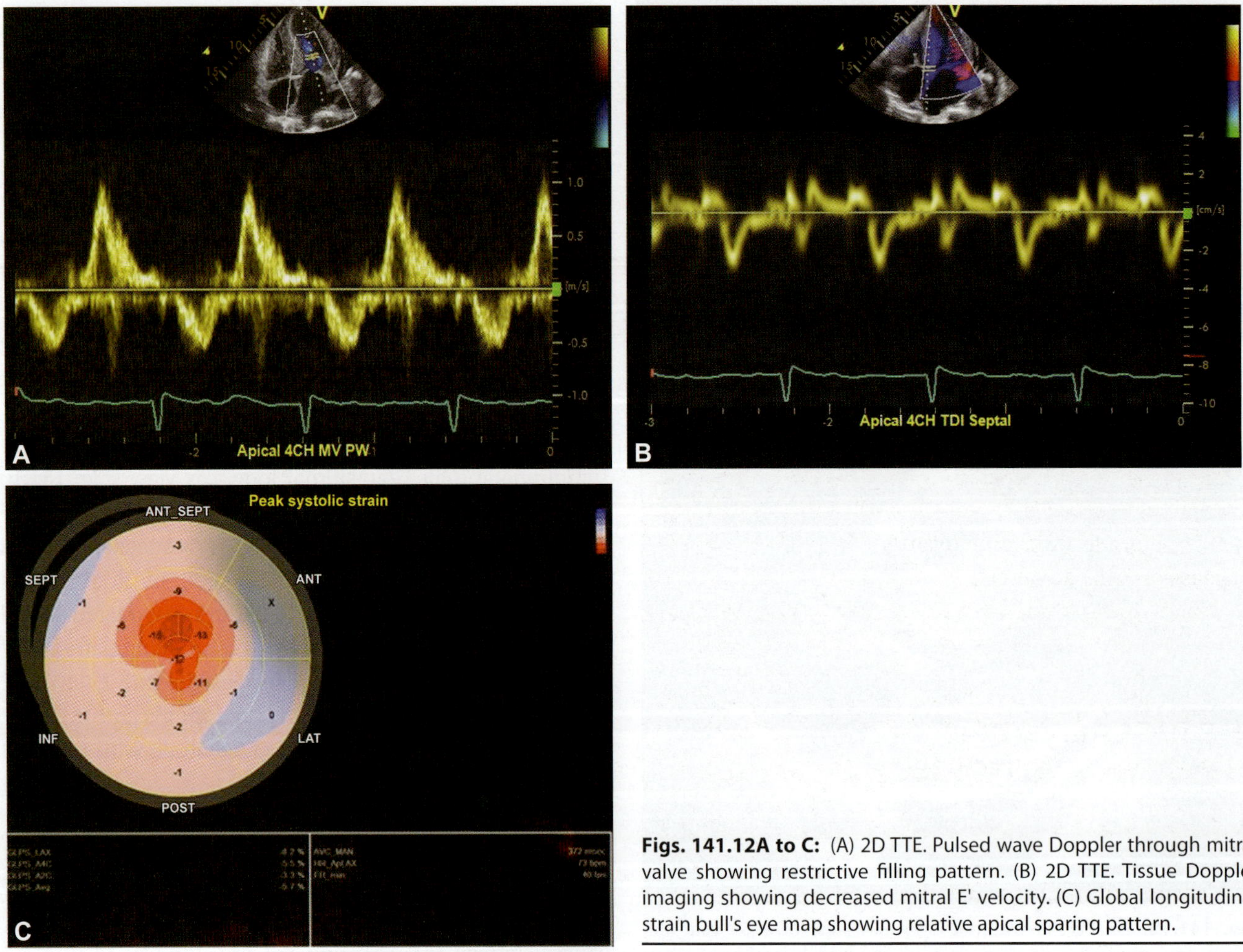

Figs. 141.12A to C: (A) 2D TTE. Pulsed wave Doppler through mitral valve showing restrictive filling pattern. (B) 2D TTE. Tissue Doppler imaging showing decreased mitral E' velocity. (C) Global longitudinal strain bull's eye map showing relative apical sparing pattern.

Table 141.1: Cardiac amyloid: Incidence/prevalence

Type	*Incidence/prevalence*
1° AL amyloid	~2,500 cases per year 50% have cardiac involvement
ATTRwt (SCA)	25% of adults > 80 years
V122I mutation	4% of African-Americans[3,4] are carriers

dysfunction but do now show echocardiographic signs of restrictive cardiomyopathy. Choice (e), endomyocardial fibrosis, does present with Doppler findings of restrictive cardiomyopathy. Other classic echocardiographic findings for endomyocardial fibrosis are apical fibrosis of the ventricles, tethering of the mitral papillary muscles and apical thrombi. Only in choice (d), TTR cardiac amyloidosis, hypertrophy, diastolic dysfunction and specific left ventricular strain patterns all are seen.

Amyloidosis is a systemic disease involving the deposition of amyloid protein in various body organs. Cardiac amyloidosis results from the deposition of amyloid proteins in the heart. TTR amyloidosis is an under diagnosed cause of heart failure, specifically heart failure with preserved ejection fraction (HFpEF). Cardiac amyloidosis results from the deposits of misfolded light chain (AL) or transthyretin (TTR) proteins. Autopsy studies have shown cardiac TTR amyloid deposits in up to 25% of individuals over the age of 80. It is also estimated that about four percent of US African-American births inherit a mutation of the TTR gene (Val122lle)[1] which may lead to cardiac TTR amyloidosis (Table 141.1).

Echocardiography continues to be an important examination for the evaluation or identification of patients with cardiac amyloidosis. Patients with early disease usually have grade I diastolic dysfunction that progresses as disease severity advances.

Classic echocardiogram findings with cardiac amyloidosis are illustrated in Figure 141.13.

ECHOCARDIOGRAPHIC FINDINGS OF CARDIAC AMYLOIDOSIS (FIG. 141.13)

- The ejection fraction is often within normal limits, although a mild to moderately reduced left ventricular ejection fraction may also noted.
- Increased left and right ventricular wall thickness. (Patients in the early stage of the disease can have normal or slightly increased wall thickness).
- Speckled or granular appearance of the myocardium. (Not sensitive or specific for the diagnosis of cardiac amyloidosis).
- Biatrial enlargement
- Interatrial septum thickening
- Thickened valves
- Pericardial and pleural effusions
- Doppler findings are consistent with restrictive cardiomyopathy

In patients with advanced disease, grade III diastolic dysfunction is present and is characterized by mitral inflow E/A ratio > 2.5, DT of E velocity < 150 msec, IVRT < 50 msec, and decreased septal and lateral E' velocities (3–4 cm/sec).

- Left ventricular longitudinal strain shows reduction in the basal and mid-wall segments, with apical sparing (Figure 141.13).

The longitudinal strain imaging pattern associated with cardiac amyloidosis is useful to differentiate from other causes of increased left ventricular wall thickness such as hypertensive heart disease and hypertrophic cardiomyopathy.[2]

Nuclear Cardiology

Radionuclide "bone" scintigraphy with technetium labeled bisphosphonates was first reported 35 years ago to bind to the myocardium in patients with cardiac amyloidosis.[5] Recent work utilizing 99mTc-PYP and 99mTc-DPD have shown a high sensitivity and specificity for the diagnosis of cardiac amyloidosis. A recent pooled group of patients from major Amyloid referral centers showed >99% sensitivity and 86% specificity for the diagnosis of cardiac TTR amyloid utilizing bone scintigraphy agents. The combination of a positive nuclear scan and a negative serum and urine immune-fixation electrophoresis and serum free light chains differentiates cardiac TTR amyloid from cardiac AL amyloidosis. The diagnostic use of technetium labeled bisphosphonates also shows promise in the early, accurate, and noninvasive diagnosis of transthyretin cardiac amyloidosis.

Cardiac Magnetic Resonance Imaging

Cardiac magnetic resonance imaging has also been investigated in the diagnosis of cardiac amyloidosis.[6] Common findings have included late, diffuse subendocardial gadolinium enhancement and abnormal T1 mapping. and abnormal blood-pool gadolinium kinetics.

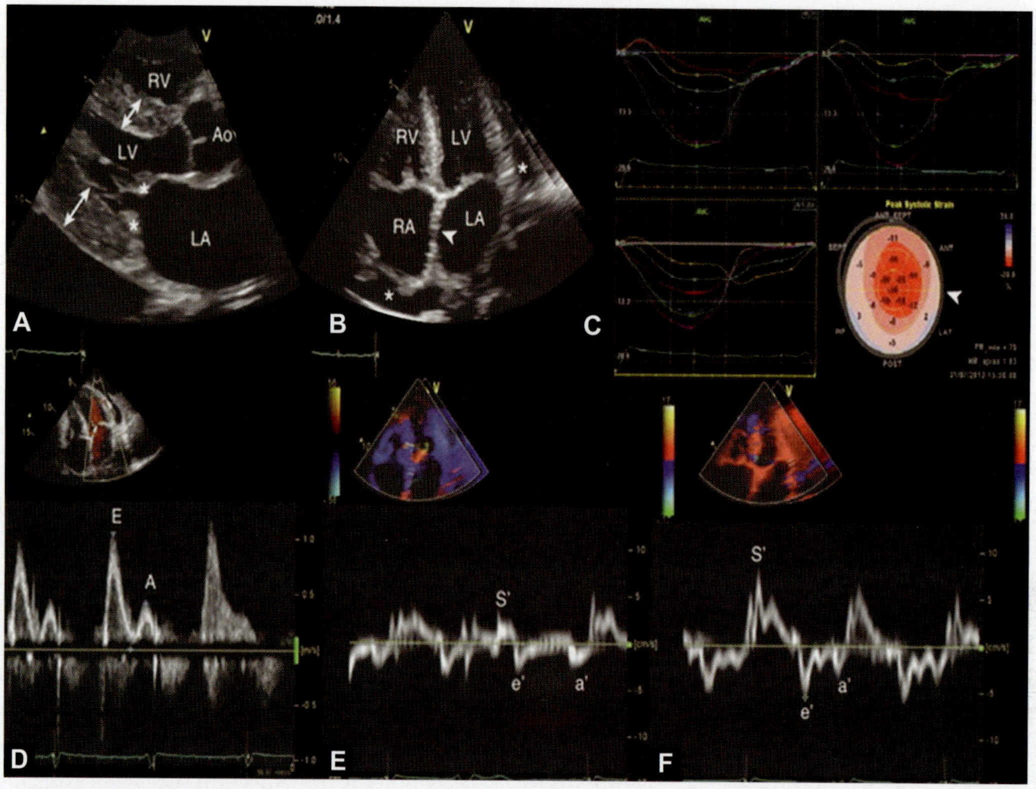

Figs. 141.13A to F: Classic echocardiographic features of cardiac amyloidosis.[2] (A) Increased left ventricular (LV) wall thickness (arrow) with granular sparkling appearance with thickening of the mitral valve (asterisk). (B) Bi-atrial enlargement, increased right ventricular (RV) wall thickness, thickening of the interatrial septum (arrowhead), and pericardial effusion (asterisk). (C) Severely decreased global longitudinal strain with relative apical sparing pattern (arrowhead) on two-dimensional speckle tracking imaging. (D) Restrictive filling pattern, mitral E/A ratio = 2.7. (E and F) Decreased medial and lateral E' velocity, consistent with restrictive cardiomyopathy and elevated LV filling pressures. (AO: Aorta; LV: Left atrium; RA: Right atrium).

MOVIES 451 TO 461

REFERENCES

1. Jacobson DR, Pastore RD, Yaghoubian R, Kane I, Gallo G, Buck FS, Buxbaum JN. Variant-sequence transthyretin (Isoleucine 122) in late-onset cardiac Amyloidosis in black Americans. N Engl J Med: 1997;336:466-73.
2. Yingchoncharoen T, Phelan D, Klein AL. Cardiac amyloidosis, echocardiographic features. In: Lang R, Goldstein S, Kronzon I, Khandheria B, Mor-Avi V, editors. ASE's Comprehensive Echocardiography, 2nd edition. Philadelphia, PA: Elsevier, 2016:343-48.
3. Kapoor P, Thenappan T, Singh E, et al. Cardiac amyloidosis: a practical approach to diagnosis and treatment. Am J Med. 2011;124:1006-15.
4. Tanskanen M, Peuralinna T, Polvikoski T, et al. Senile systemic amyloidosis affects 25% of the very aged and associates with genetic variation in alpha2-microglobulin and tau: a population-based autopsy study. Ann Med. 2008;40: 232-39.
5. Gillmore JD, Maurer MS, Falk RH, et al. Nonbiopsy diagnosis of cardiac transthyretin amyloidosis. Circulation. 2016;133(24):2404-12.
6. Wechalekar AD, Gillmore JD, Hawkins PN. Systemic Amyloidosis. Lancet. 2016;387:2641-54.

CASE 142

Amgad N Makaryus

PATIENT HH PRESENTATION

- A 66-year-old African American male with HTN and dyslipidemia presented with vague constitutional symptoms including malaise and night sweats with dyspnea on exertion and persistent dry cough.
- PMHx/PSHx/allergies: Non-contributory.
- Family Hx: pulmonary fibrosis.
- Social Hx: 2nd hand smoke, boat painting.
- No chest pain, palpitations, or orthopnea.
- Exam without heart failure or rash.
- EKG-normal sinus rhythm, 1st degree AV block.

INITIAL WORK-UP

- Initial CT chest (Fig. 142.2B) revealed bilateral perihilar and subcarinal lymphadenopathy, bilateral centrilobular micronodularity predominating along the fissures and in a peribronchovascular distribution.
- Diagnostic bronchoscopy was performed twice and was nondiagnostic.
- Etiology of the symptoms and findings remained unknown, but an exaggerated immune system response was implicated at this time.

OUTPATIENT COURSE

- Patient developed chest pain with palpitations and was admitted to the hospital.
- He was found to be in atrial fibrillation with rapid ventricular response at 160–170 bpm.
- TTE/TEE (Figs. 142.1A to C and 462) revealed no thrombus and the patient was cardioverted back into sinus rhythm.
- The LV was normal in size, wall motion and contractility. Mild LVH was present along with a dilated left atrium. Patient was discharged from the hospital.
- As the patient continued to have constitutional symptoms, he underwent repeated bronchoscopy. Repeat bronchoscopy with biopsy revealed bronchial wall tissue with non-necrotizing granulomas with multinucleated giant cells consistent with sarcoidosis. Stains were negative for microorganisms.
- Bronchial alveolar lavage with lymph flow cytometry revealed a heterogenous population of T-cells and absent B-cells, with a CD4 to CD8 ratio of 7:1, also consistent with sarcoidosis.
- Repeat CT chest revealed slightly increased micronodularity (circle in Fig. 142.2A) in the left lower lobe compared to the previous study 3 months prior.

CARDIAC MRI (FIGS. 142.3A TO C AND 463)

- Resting perfusion imaging showed no regional perfusion defect of either the right or left ventricle.
- Delayed hyperenhancement (DHE) imaging demonstrated a small patchy area of left ventricular myocardial uptake in the basal and mid-inferolateral wall denoting scar and/or infiltration in the area consistent with this patient's diagnosis of sarcoidosis (arrows in Figs. 142.4A and B).
- There was no right ventricular enlargement, aneurysm, or regional wall motion abnormality, with normal RV systolic function.
- Normal LV systolic function with an LVEF of 68%.

CARDIAC SARCOID

- Overall prevalence of sarcoidosis is 10–40 cases per 100,000 population, Sarcoidosis is 5–10 times more prevalent in Afro-American population (35.5 per 100,000) than in the white population (10.9 per 100,000).
- Cardiac sarcoidosis is reported in 25% of autopsy hearts in sarcoid patients with extracardiac involvement.
- Accounts for 13% to 25% of deaths from the disease.
- Nonspecific inflammatory changes such as infiltration of lymphocytes, interstitial edema, and damaged cardiac myocytes, resulting in interstitial fibrosis, scarring, and infiltration of noncaseating granulomas invlolving the myocardium.
- Predominantly affects the basal myocardium and the subepicardial layer and the interventricular septum is frequently affected.

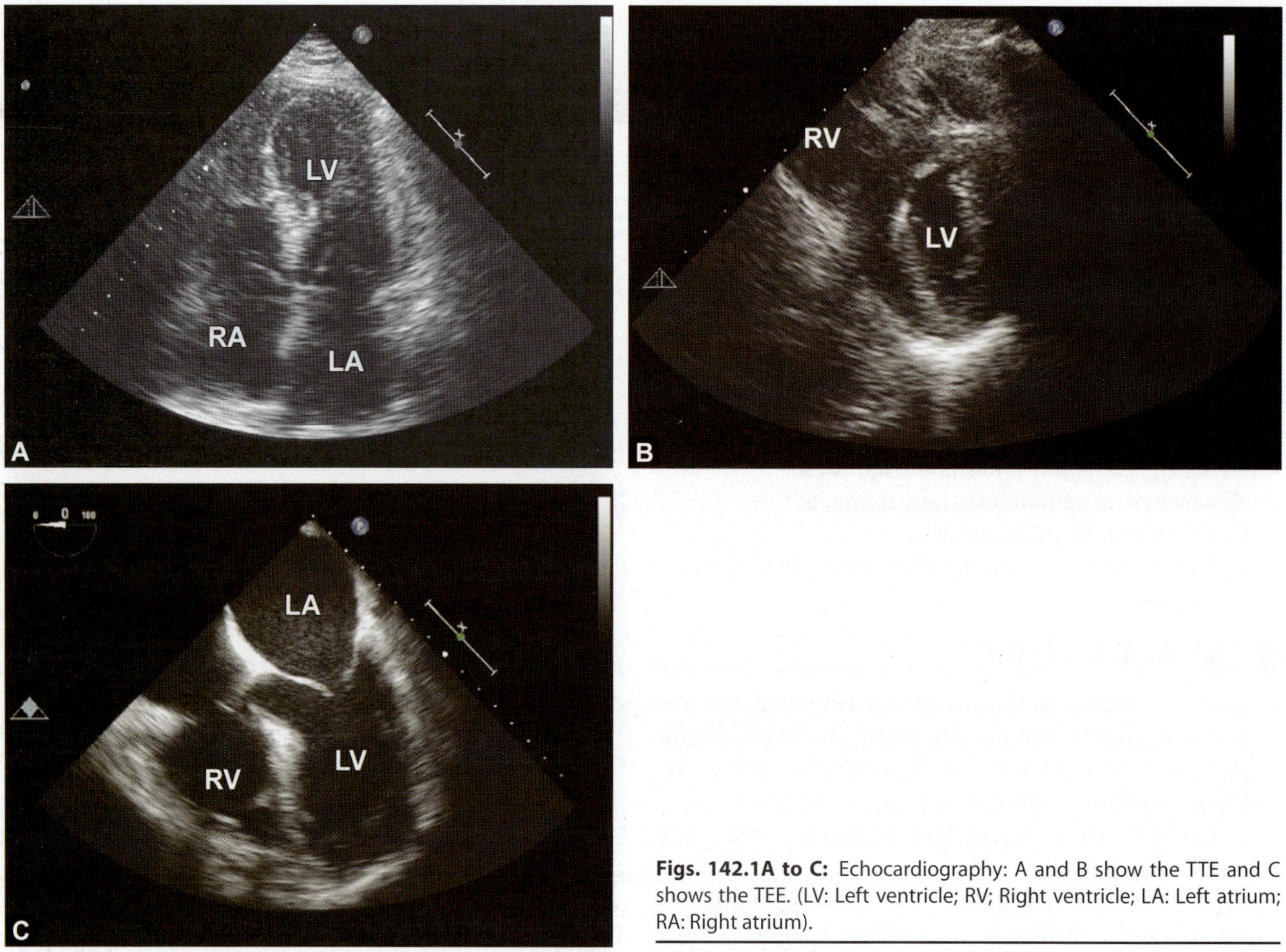

Figs. 142.1A to C: Echocardiography: A and B show the TTE and C shows the TEE. (LV: Left ventricle; RV; Right ventricle; LA: Left atrium; RA: Right atrium).

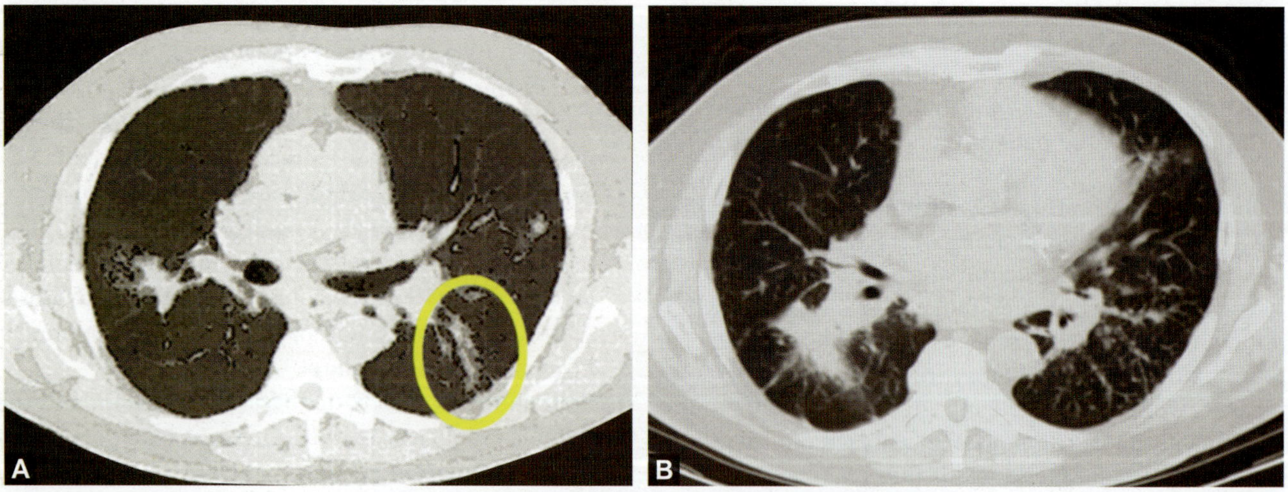

Figs. 142.2A and B: (A) Current CT chest study; (B) Prior CT chest study.

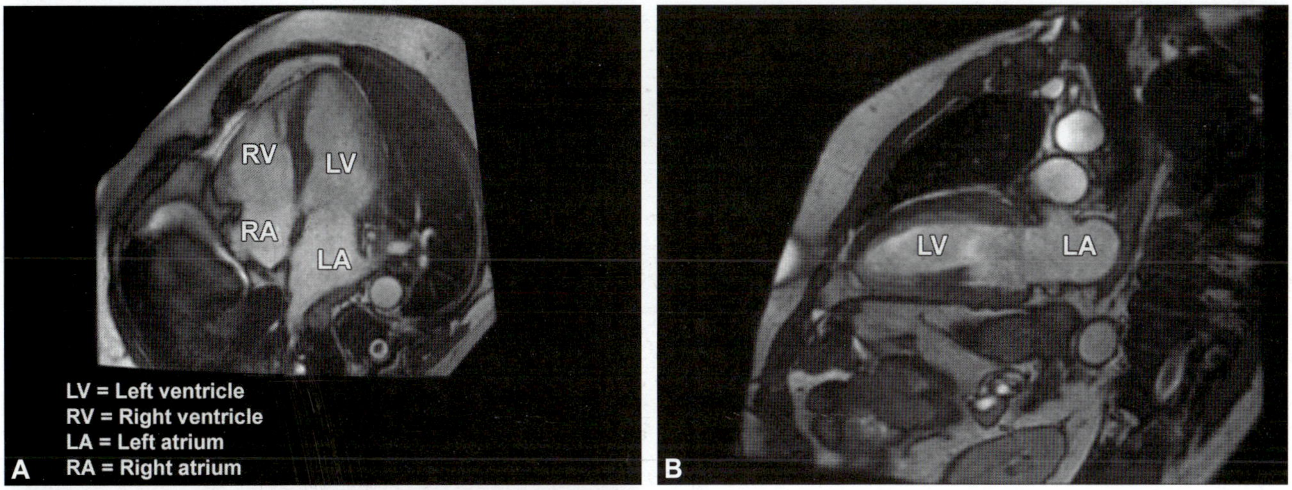

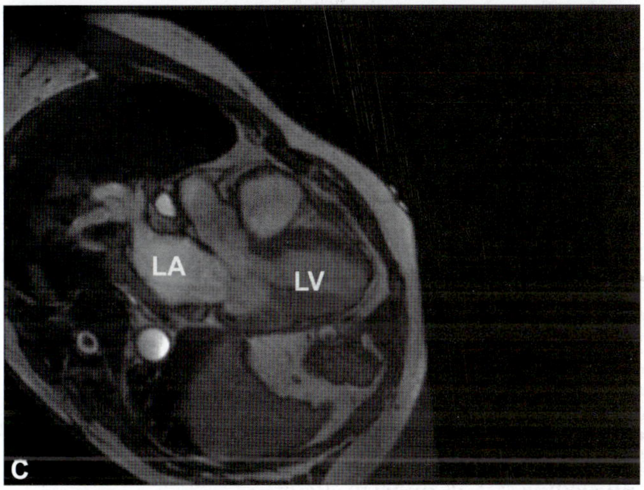

Figs. 142.3A to C: Cardiac MRI. (LV: Left vertricle; RV: Right ventricle; LA: Left atrium; RA: Right atrium).

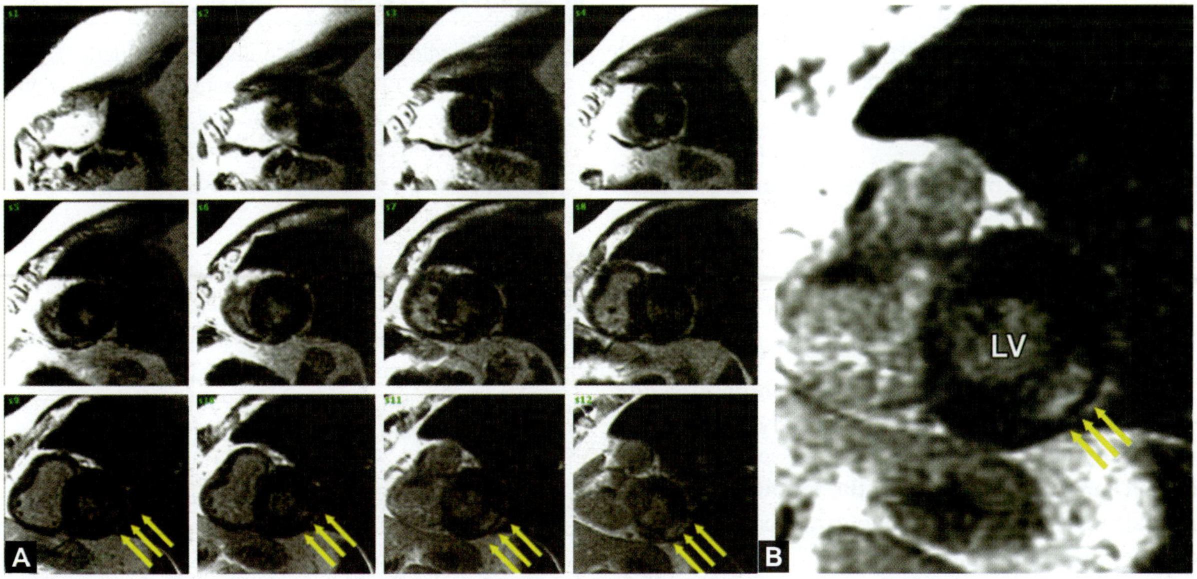

Figs. 142.4A and B: Cardiac MRI DHE images showing a small patchy area of left ventricular myocardial uptake in the basal and mid-inferolateral wall denoting scar and/or infiltration in the area consistent with this patient's diagnosis of sarcoidosis (arrows).

CARDIAC MANIFESTATIONS[1,2]

- Cor pulmonale (most common cardiac complication) caused by pulmonary fibrosis.
- Complete heart block is the most commom arrhythmia
  - Ventricular tachycardia, SVTs, bundle branch block, first degree heart block and various types of intraventricular conduction defects are also common.
- Atrial involvement alone without ventricular involvement is rare.
- Ventricular aneurysm, myocarditis, pericarditis, mitral regurgitation, aortic regurgitation, and heart failure are other manifestations.
- Decreased heart rate variability.

DIAGNOSIS AND TREATMENT[3]

- Drawbacks of achieving a diagnosis via endomyocardial biopsy of a myocardial granuloma include risks associated with an invasive technique and the possibility of obtaining a false-negative specimen (sensitivity of 20%) because of the patchy infiltration of the heart muscle.
- Echocardiography is unable to detect the intramural localization of sarcoid lesions.
- It is difficult to identify the intramural localization of sarcoid lesions using SPECT or PET because of their limited spatial resolution.
- Myocardial wall thickening and wall motion are decreased with an increase in the degree of hyperenhancement and hence myocardial involvement.
- Published sensitivity and specificity of CMR imaging are 100% and 78% respectively.
- Delayed hyperenhancement imaging CMR shows myocardial abnormalities in presumed areas of fibrosis in sarcoidosis.
- T2 weighted CMR may show areas of active inflammation.
- Typically distributed in
  - Noncoronary fashion
  - Punched out
  - Corresponds to areas of noncaseating granulomas

1. **Proposed options for treatment include steroids and possible electrophysiology study in patients with ventricular arrhythmias to assess the need for ICD or ablation. Which of the following imaging modalities has the best diagnostic capability for diagnosing cardiac sarcoid?**
   (a) Echocardiography
   (b) CCTA
   (c) CMR
   (d) SPECT myocardial perfusion imaging

Ans. (c)

Published sensitivity and specificity of CMR imaging for cardiac sarcoid are 100% and 78% respectively.

2. **Which of the following is false about the cardiac manifestations of sarcoid?**
   (a) Cor pulmonale occurs caused by pulmonary fibrosis
   (b) Atrial involvement alone without LV involvement is common
   (c) Complete heart block is the most commom arrhythmia
   (d) Decreased heart rate variability may be seen

Ans. (b)

Atrial involvement alone without LV involvement is rare.

3. **Which portion of the myocardium is predominantly affected by cardiac sarcoid?**
   (a) Epicardium
   (b) Endocardium
   (c) Parietal pericardium
   (d) Visceral pericardium

Ans. (a)

Cardiac sarcoid predominantly affects the epicardial layer of the myocardium.

MOVIE LEGENDS

462: Echocardiographic cine loops from this patient. (A) Apical 4-chamber TTE view (B) Parasternal short axis TTE view (C) Midesophageal TEE view.

463: Cardiac MRI cine loops from this patient. (A) Four chamber MRI view (B) Two chamber MRI view (C) Three chamber MRI view.

REFERENCES

1. Dubrey SW, Falk RH. Diagnosis and management of cardiac sarcoidosis. Prog Cardiovasc Dis. 2010;52(4):336-46.
2. Birnie DH, Kandolin R, Nery PB, et al. Cardiac manifestations of sarcoidosis: diagnosis and management. Eur Heart J. 2016;28.
3. Soto-Gomez N, Peters JI, Nambiar AM. Diagnosis and Management of Sarcoidosis. Am Fam Physician. 2016; 93(10):840-8.

CASE 143

Yuchi Han, Martin St John Sutton

ECHO IN CARCINOID HEART DISEASE

This is a 61-year-old gentleman who complained of mild dyspnea on exertion. He can climb one flight of stairs, runs 1–2 miles 3 days a week and lifts weights 2 days a week without any difficulty. He denies chest pain, palpitations and syncope. His other history includes atrial fibrillation requiring cardioversion and right hepatectomy.

CVS: BP 132/76, HR 54, JVP+ with a prominent V wave. Apex normal, holosystolic murmur at the left lower sternal border and an early systolic murmur and diastolic murmur heard at the left upper sternal border.

Chest: Clear, normal breath sounds.

Abdomen: Enlarged liver with palpable mass that was not tender.

EKG: NSR 56 bpm, Premature ventricular contractions (PVCs), otherwise normal

Chest CT: Unremarkable

2D TTE was done (Figs. 143.1 and 143.2; 464A to C and 465).

Patient underwent a right hepatectomy, returned to NSR, had stable liver function and finally had both pulmonary and tricuspid valve replacements with bioprostheses. He has

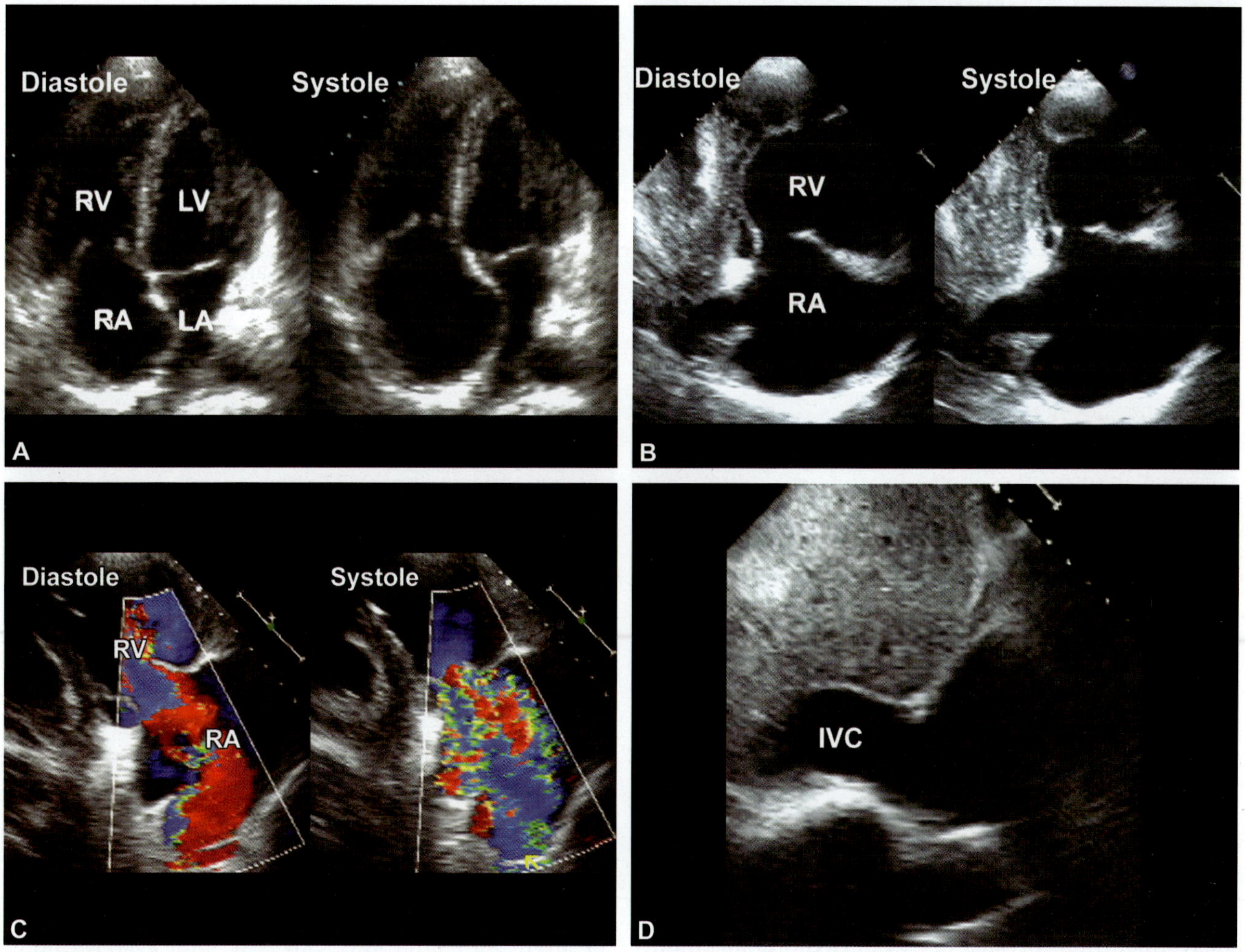

Figs. 143.1A to D: Tricuspid valve involvement. (A) Shows systolic non-coaptation of thickened TV leaflets. (B) Dilated CS and RA. (C) Severe TR. (D) Dilated IVC.

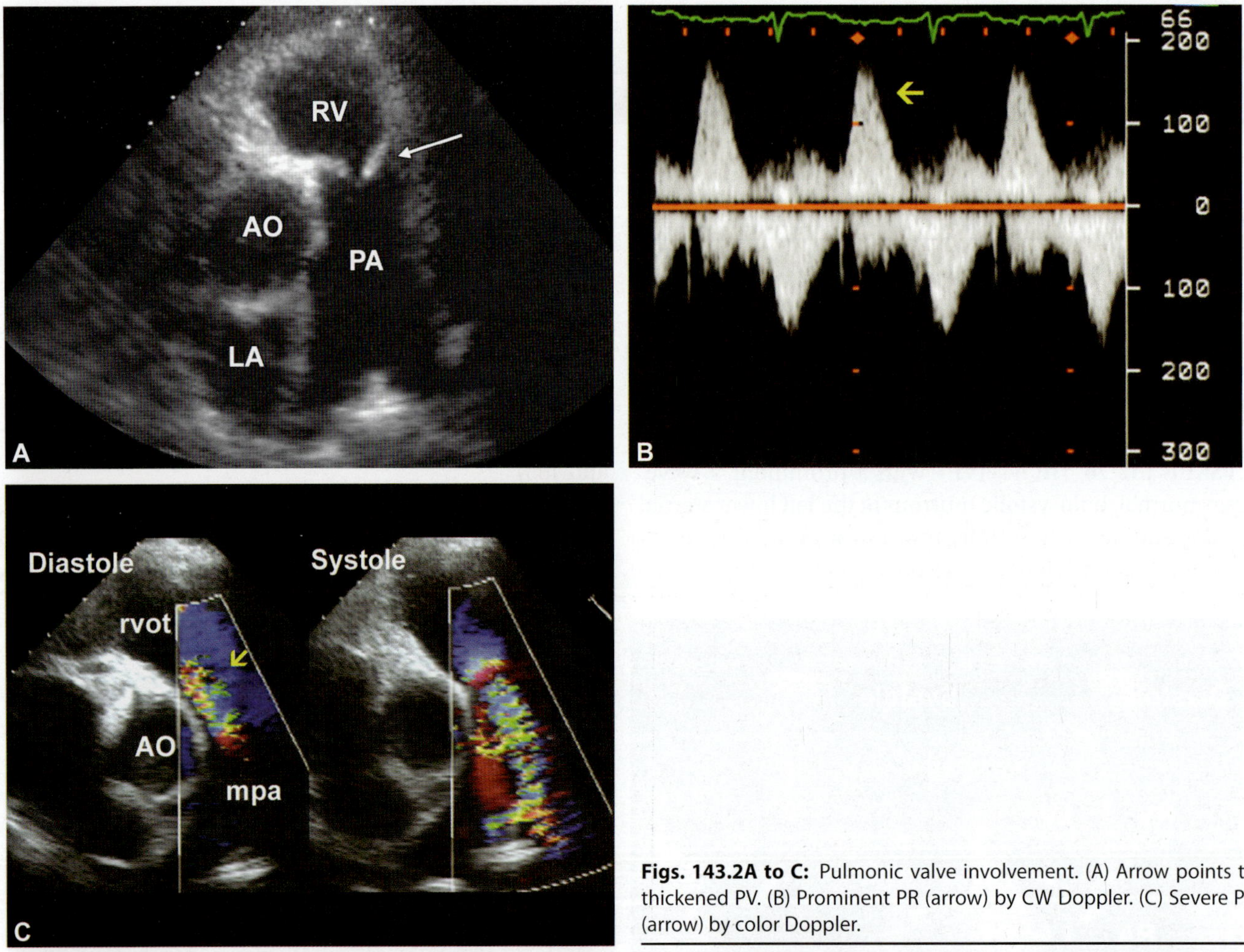

Figs. 143.2A to C: Pulmonic valve involvement. (A) Arrow points to thickened PV. (B) Prominent PR (arrow) by CW Doppler. (C) Severe PR (arrow) by color Doppler.

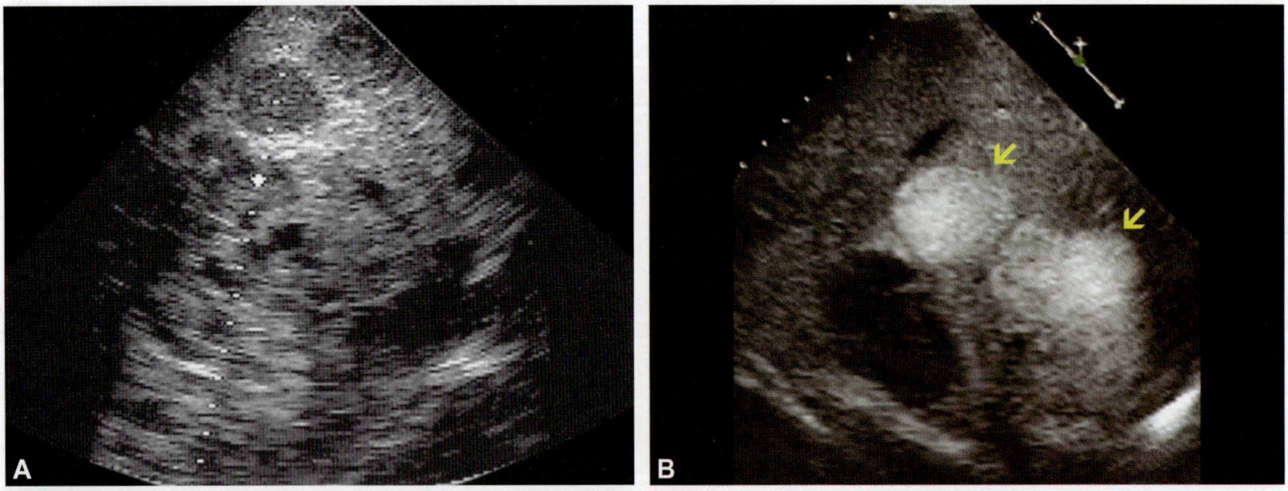

Figs. 143.3A and B: Carcinoid in the liver. Arrows point to hepatic metastasis.

metastases to the liver (Figs. 143.3A and B) but enjoys robust health running 3×/week free of any further recurrences of atrial fibrillation and with only mild exercise intolerance.

1. **The classic findings of carcinoid:**
   (a) There are fibrous plaques on all 4 valves
   (b) TR is the least common lesion
   (c) The TV and PV always need to be replaced
   (d) There is rapid downhill course
   (e) None of the above

Ans. (e)

Discussion: Carcinoid Heart Disease

Cardiac Pathology

Most common isolated lesions in order of frequency are TR, PS, PR and TS but there are varying combinations.

Echo Findings

Right-sided valve leaflets are thickened and rigid, either with varying grades of stenosis or regurgitation or both because of lack of normal leaflet coaptation (Figs. 143.1 and 143.2; 464A to C and 465).

Valve lesions do not usually occur in the left heart when there is no intracardiac shunt, because metastases only go to liver and 5-hydroxy-tryptamine is destroyed in the lungs.

The TV and PV are always both involved.

Chest pain is more common than SOB.

MOVIES 464 AND 465

CASE 144

Bhagatwala K, Elsayed M, Alagic N, Uygur B, Turaga NSN, Chahwala JR, Adarna LG, Mohamed A, Gupta N, Bulur S, Nanda NC

Apical 4 chamber and subcostal views in an adult patient.

1. **What is the most likely diagnosis (🎥 466 and 467)?**
   (a) Severe MR and TR
   (b) Restrictive cardiomyopathy
   (c) Cannot be cardiomyopathy since both LV and RV systolic function are normal

Ans. (b)

Normal-sized ventricles with markedly dilated atria are a hallmark of restrictive cardiomyopathy. Even though LV and RV systolic function are normal, diastolic dysfunction with increased filling pressures are present as reflected by enlargement of the atria.

🎥 468 is from another patient with restrictive cardiomyopathy showing similar findings. Pericardial effusion (PE) is present in this patient. The etiology of cardiomyopathy in both of these patients is currently not known.

MOVIES 466 TO 468 🎥

CASE 145

Ashley Nickerson, Vincent L Sorrell

HYPERTROPHIC CARDIOMYOPATHY

1. **Which of the following is true regarding the CMR, late gadolinium enhancement images with conventional inversion recovery [IR] sequences on left (Figs. 145.1A, 145.2A and 145.3A) and phase sensitive IR sequences on the right (Figs. 145.1B, 145.2B and 145.3B)?**
   (a) The pattern of late gadolinium enhancement (LGE) is consistent with underlying CAD.
   (b) The presence of LGE in this patient is associated with a higher mortality.
   (c) The patient meets criteria for AICD implant.
   (d) The patient meets criteria for surgical myectomy.
   (e) There is no gadolinium enhancement.

Ans. (b)

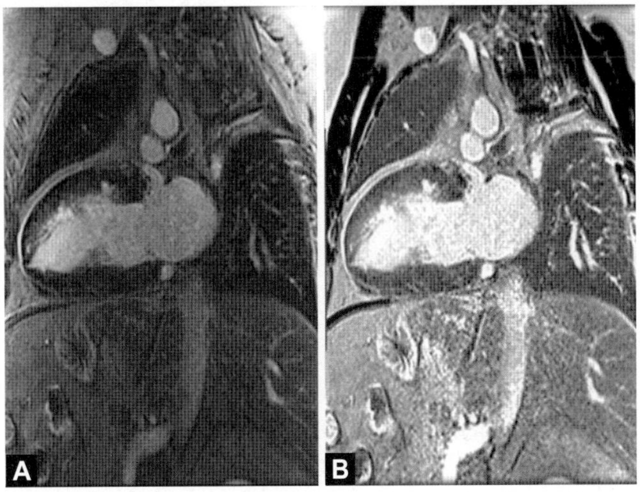

Figs. 145.1A and B: 2-chamber orientation.

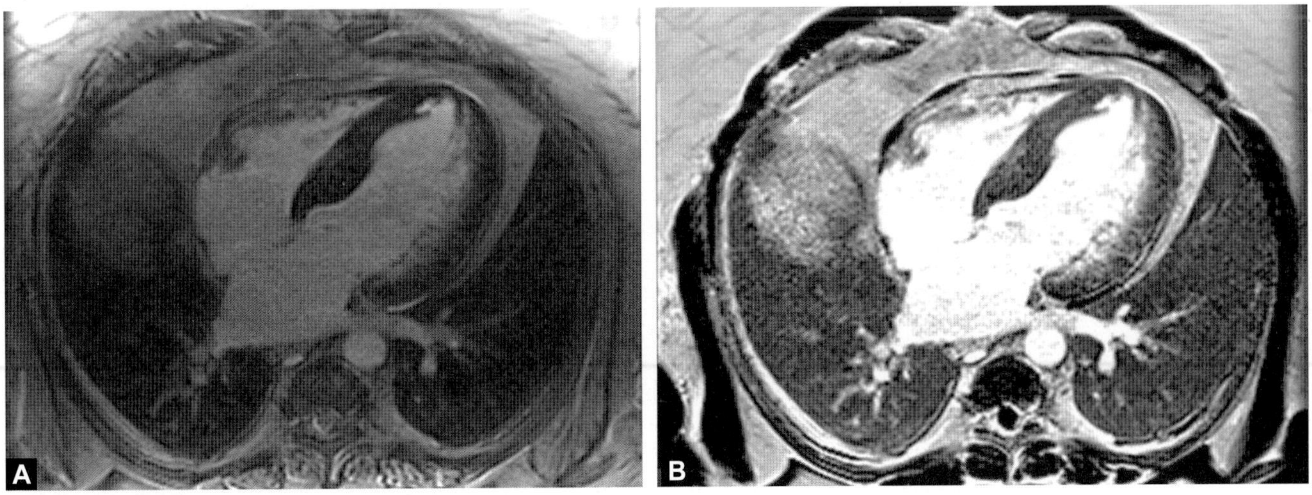

Figs. 145.2A and B: 4-chamber orientation.

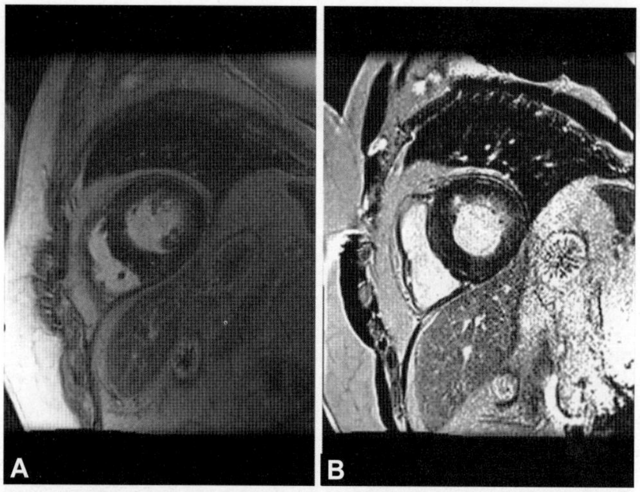

Figs. 145.3A and B: Short axis, mid-LV orientation.

This image demonstrates the classic late gadolinium enhancement (LGE) pattern seen in HCM; patchy, mid-wall enhancement with variable foci. This is typically most pronounced in hypertrophied segments and does not follow a coronary distribution. Several studies have demonstrated a significant increase in both morbidity and overall mortality in HCM patients with the presence of LGE-detected scar (but, not necessarily the extent of LGE).

DISCUSSION

(a) Incorrect since the heterogeneous, patchy enhancement throughout the hypertrophied myocardium (as demonstrated in the image) is characteristic of HCM. LGE due to CAD is more likely to have subendocardial to transmural pattern within a coronary distribution.

(c) Although literature suggests a correlation between extent of LGE enhancement and SCD, there is currently no guideline to support AICD implant in HCM based strictly on the presence or extent LGE enhancement.

(d) Indication for surgical intervention is based on clinical symptoms refractory to medical therapy (usually 2–3 drug therapy and/or documented intolerance) or resting/provoked gradients above 50 mm Hg.

(e) Incorrect since there is extensive enhancement noted in multiple myocardial regions which do not correlate well with a specific coronary anatomy.

CASE 146

Elsayed M, Gupta N, Mohamed A, Nanda NC

This is a 70-year-old female with known hypertrophic cardiomyopathy (HCM). 2D TTE was done (469 and 470).

1. What do the movies show?

(a) Maximum (MAX) resting gradient (GRD) of 27 mm Hg across the LVOT (469) increased to 67 mm Hg with the Valsalva maneuver (470).

(b) The CW Doppler velocity (VEL) waveforms with slower acceleration and rapid deceleration ("Turkish dagger shape", shown in both movies) are typical of HCM

(c) In HCM, there may be asymmetric ventricular septal hypertrophy, narrow LVOT (< 20 mm) and systolic anterior movements (SAMs) of the MV

(d) Only (a) and (c) are correct

(e) (a), (b) and (c) are correct

Ans. (e)

2. Which of the following will increase the gradient across the LVOT in patients with HCM?

(a) Increase in heart rate

(b) Increase in LV contractility

(c) Valsalva maneuver

(d) Increase in preload

(e) None of the above

(f) (a), (b) and (c)

(g) (a) and (c)

Ans. (f)

MOVIES 469 AND 470

CASE 147

Thind M, Joson M, Gaba S, Elsayed M, Bulur S, Guvenc T, Elguindy M, Nanda NC

The patient is a 42-year-old female with known history of systemic hypertension and type 2 diabetes mellitus. She was first referred to us 8 years ago complaining of exertional dyspnea (NYHA 2-3). Physical examination at that time was practically normal but EKG showed LVH and deep T-wave inversion in the left sided leads. 2D TTE showed a mildly dilated LA, mild LVH and papillary muscle hypertrophy. She was placed on beta blockers, ACE inhibitors and diuretics. Subsequently, she remained stable except for an episode of atypical chest pain one year ago. It was decided to do a coronary angiogram which did not show any stenosis. During current examination, 2D TTE demonstrated an increase in VS hypertrophy to 14 mm compared to 11 mm 8 years ago while the LV inferolateral wall thickness remained unchanged at 14 mm. Also, LV apical aneurysm (AN) was suspected. Subsequently, a contrast 2D TTE was performed and this showed LV mid-cavity obliteration at the level of papillary muscles and a large apical AN with 2 filling defects consistent with clots. A narrow channel connected the LV cavity to the AN. Figures 147.1A to D

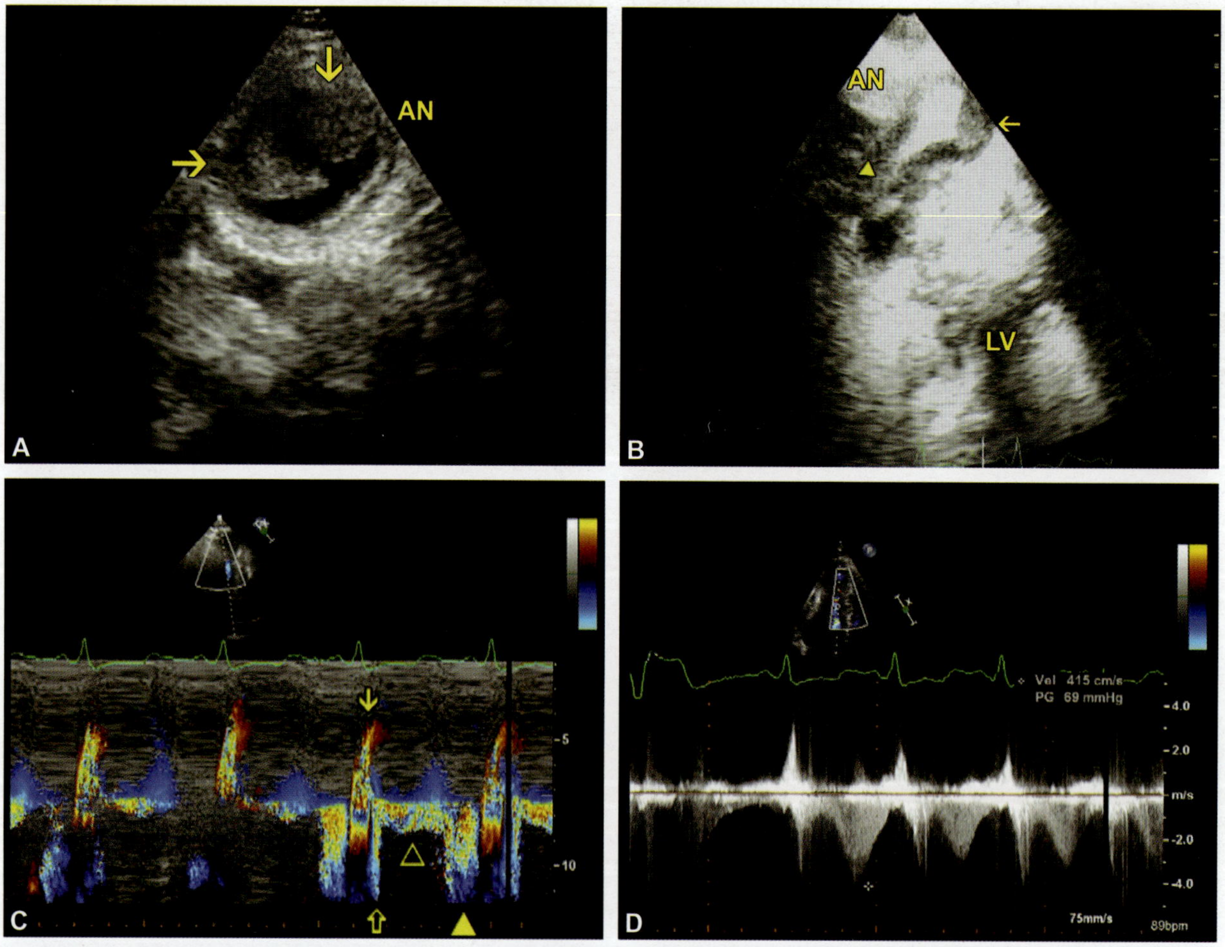

Figs. 147.1A to D: Two-dimensional transthoracic echocardiography in hypertrophic cardiomyopathy with mid-left ventricular obstruction and apical aneurysm. (A) Arrows point to what appear to be 2 thrombi in the apical aneurysm (AN). (B) Use of an echo contrast agent outlines the AN and a thrombus (arrow). Arrowhead shows the narrow channel. (C, D). Color M-mode and continuous-wave Doppler examination. Shows flow signals moving into the AN in late diastole (arrow), then into the left ventricular cavity (LV) with high velocity (hollow arrow) in early systole. Thereafter, the velocity markedly decreases in mid and late systole (hollow arrowhead). Finally, high velocity flow signals are seen moving from the AN into the LV during diastole (arrowhead) (471A to C).

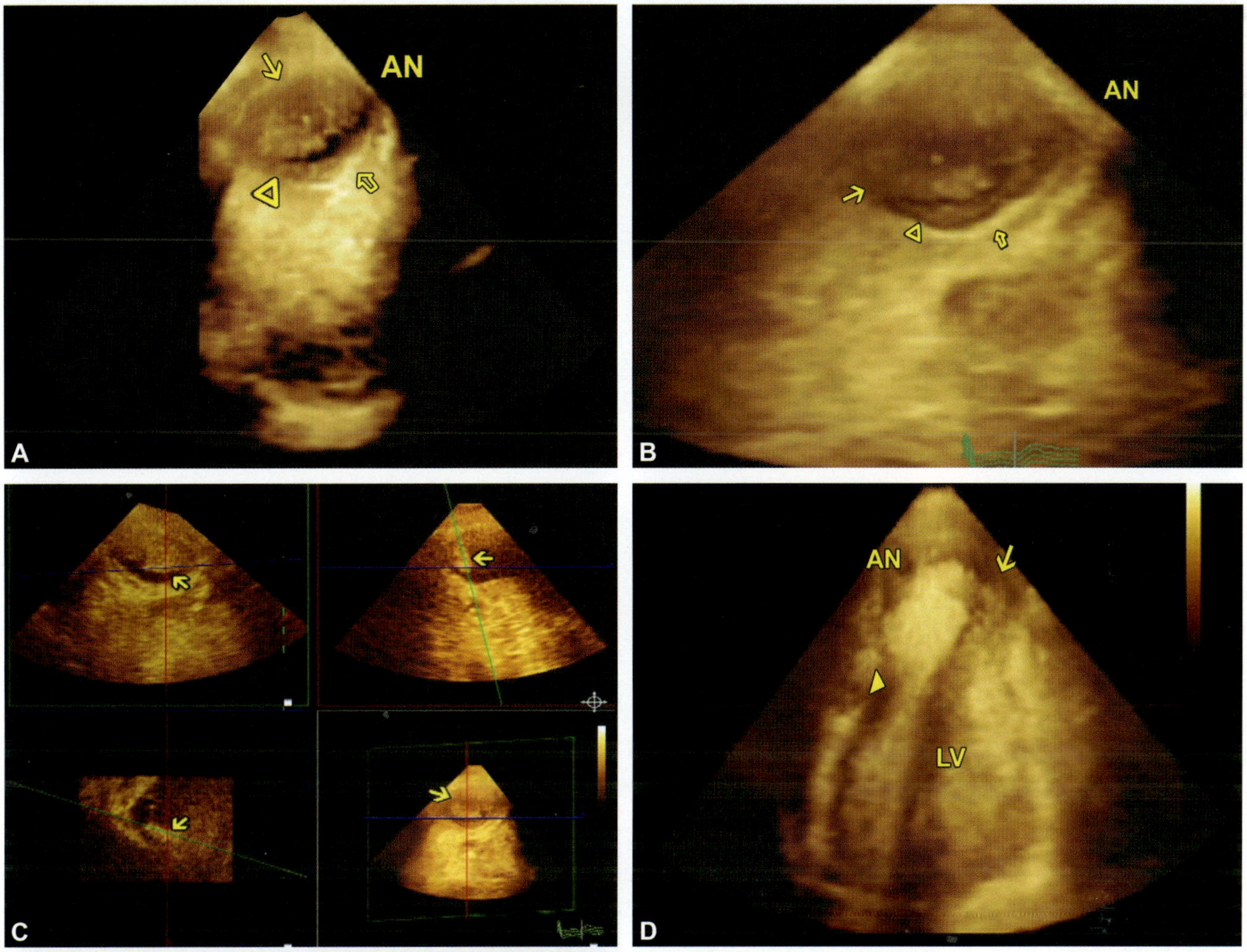

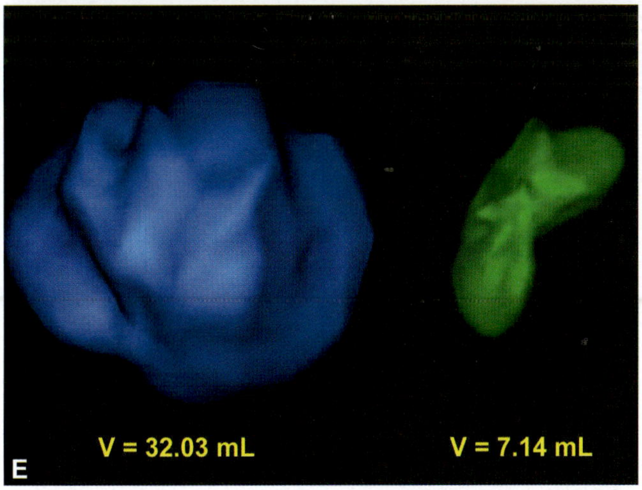

Figs. 147.2A to E: Live/real time three-dimensional transthoracic echocardiography in hypertrophic cardiomyopathy with mid-left ventricular obstruction and apical aneurysm. (A, B) Arrow points to a single large kidney-shaped thrombus in the apical AN. Hollow arrow points to a linear echogenic area posteriorly consistent with fibrosis. Hollow arrowhead shows a second thrombus lining the aneurysm posteriorly. (C) Multiplanar reconstruction (MPR) mode. A small appearing thrombus (right upper panel, red box) has been cropped (green line) to demonstrate its full extent (left upper panel, green box). (D) Contrast echocardiography shows narrowing of the mid-portion of the LV cavity (arrowhead). (E) Depicts the volume (V) of the AN (left) and thrombus (right)using an offline commercially available software (472A to D).

Case *reproduced with permission from*: Thind M, Joson M, Gaba S, Elsayed M, Bulur S, Guvenc T, Elguindy M, Nanda NC. Incremental value of live/real time three-dimensional transthoracic echocardiography over two-dimensional echocardiography in hypertrophic cardiomyopathy with mid-ventricular obstruction and apical aneurysm. Echocardiography. 2015 Mar;32(3):565-9.

471A to C). 3D TTE was also done in this patient Figures 147.2A to E and 472A to D).

The following Doppler findings were noted in this patient:

1. **How do you explain the above Doppler findings?**
   (a) In early systole, high velocity flow signals are seen moving into LV cavity from the AN
   (b) In mid and late systole the velocity of flow into LV cavity from AN markedly decreases
   (c) In diastole, high velocity flow signals move into LV cavity from the AN
   (d) In late diastole, flow signals move into AN from LV cavity

Ans.

The exact mechanism is not clear. Findings of flow signals moving into AN in late diastole and then from AN to LV cavity in systole indicate active contraction of LV apical dilatation which suggests that the dilated segment is not truly aneurysmal and the wall contains enough muscle capable of active contraction. Mitigation of flow during mid and late systole suggests that the channel connecting AN to LV cavity has become very narrow markedly limiting flow through it into LV cavity. During diastole the channel opens up and the high pressure in AN from stretching by blood trapped due to previously narrowed channel results in paradoxic high gradient flow into LV cavity.

2. **What incremental value did 3D TTE provide?**
   (a) Showed that there was only one large kidney shaped thrombus and not 2 as suspected by 2D TTE/contrast study. However, another thrombus lining the posterior wall of AN was observed only by 3D TTE
   (b) Volume of thrombus could be quantified
   (c) Echolucencies in thrombus consistent with lysis were well seen
   (d) Highly echo dense linear area consistent with fibrosis was noted in the basal wall of AN (confirmed by MRI)
   (e) All the above statements are correct.

Ans. (e)

3. **What are the different variants of hypertrophic cardiomyopathy (HCM)?**
   (a) Asymmetric LVH with narrow LVOT and SAMs of MV
   (b) Mid LV cavity obstruction
   (c) Apical HCM
   (d) Isolated papillary muscle hypertrophy
   (e) All the above statements are correct

Ans. (e)

MOVIES 471 AND 472

CASE 148

Aiman Smer, Amjad Kabach

THICK HEART WITH FAST RHYTHM

A 61-year-old man presented with symptoms of light-headedness and chest pain. Initial evaluation at the ED was remarkable for regular wide complex tachycardia with heart rate of 190 bpm (Fig. 148.1), treated successfully with electrical cardioversion. Repeat electrocardiogram showed normal rhythm with diffuse deep T wave inversion concerning for ischemia. An urgent coronary angiogram was performed to rule out acute coronary syndrome. Apart from myocardial bridging noted at the level of mid-left anterior descending artery, there was no significant stenosis or occlusion. Left ventriculogram revealed midventricular obstruction and dyskinesis of the apex resembling an "hourglass" shape (473). Transthoracic echocardiogram shows severe asymmetrical thickening of the left ventricle (Fig. 148.2), (474).

1. **Which of the following describes your diagnosis?**
   (a) Apical hypertrophic cardiomyopathy
   (b) Midventricular hypertrophic cardiomyopathy
   (c) Anderson-Fabry's disease
   (d) Athletic heart

Ans. (b)

Although the provided echocardiogram image and movie are suggestive of apical hypertrophic cardiomyopathy, these finding are not diagnostic. The use of contrast or/and other diagnostic imaging modalities in such cases is very crucial to differentiate between apical versus mid-ventricular variant of hypertrophic cardiomyopathy. In our patient, the contrast administration showed preserved left ventricular systolic function and severe left ventricular hypertrophy with midventricular obstruction and an apical aneurysm (Fig. 148.3), (475).

Moreover, cardiac magnetic resonance imaging demonstrates predominant hypertrophy at the midventricular

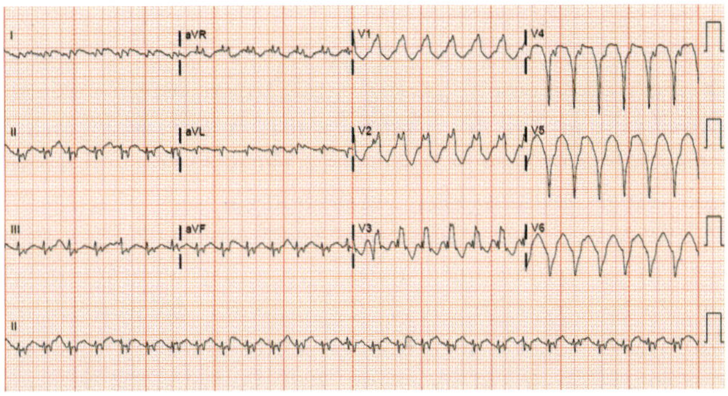

Fig. 148.1: Electrocardiogram shows regular wide QRS complex tachycardia with right bundle branch morphology.

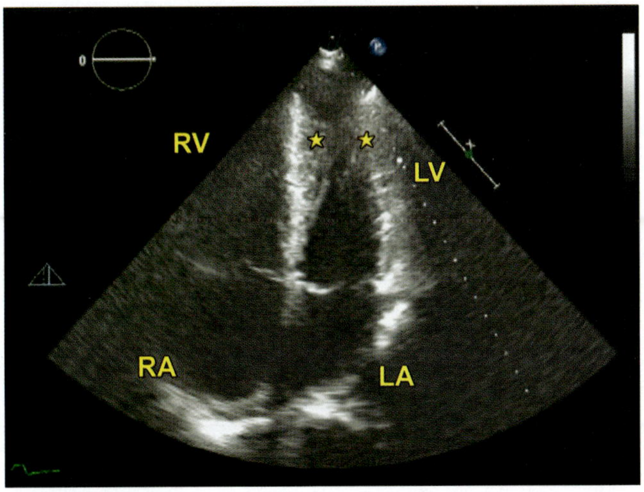

Fig. 148.2: Apical 4-chamber view shows severe left ventricular hypertrophy (*) of the mid and apical segments.

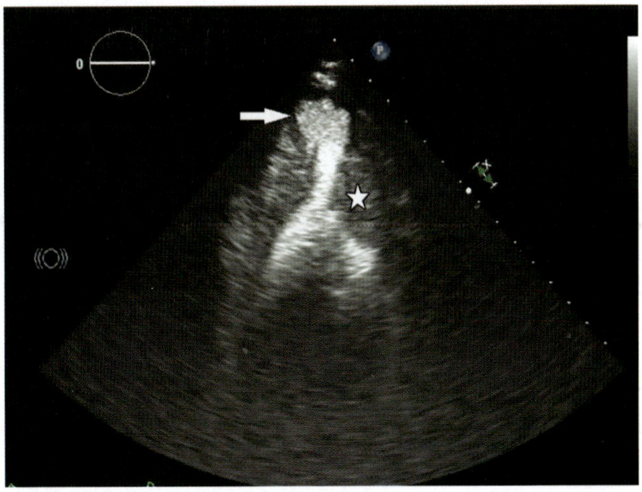

Fig. 148.3: Apical 2-chamber view with definity shows midventricular hypertrophy (*) and apical aneurysm (arrow) with no thrombus noted.

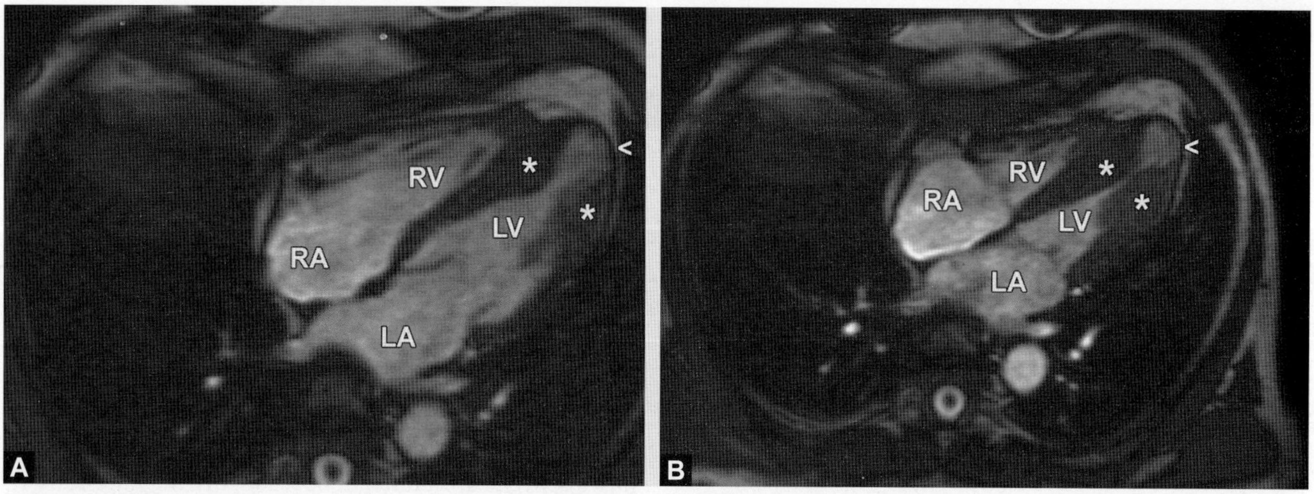

Figs. 148.4A and B: Cardiac magnetic resonance, steady state free precession (SSFP) images; Horizontal long-axis 4-chamber view (A) in diastole (B) in systole with thin-walled LV apical aneurysm (arrow head) with myocardial thickening at midventricular level (*) with near obliteration of mid-LV chamber during systole. (LV: Left ventricle; RV: Right ventricle; LA: Left atrium; RA: Right atrium).

region with maximal thickness of 31 mm, a thinned and dyskinetic apical aneurysm is also noted. Myocardial delayed enhancement is present at the midventricular and apical myocardium (Figs. 148.4A and B).

Midventricular hypertrophic cardiomyopathy is a rare variant of hypertrophic cardiomyopathy, characterized by marked hypertrophy of the midventricular myocardium associated with a high pressure gradient between the basal and apical LV cavity. This type of HCM is often complicated with apical aneurysm formation and strongly associated with ventricular arrhythmias.

MOVIE LEGENDS

473: Left ventriculogram shows severe dyskinesis of the apical wall and obstruction of the mid-left ventricle area (*).

474: Apical 4-chamber view shows normal left ventricular size and systolic function. There is severe left ventricular hypertrophy at the mid and apical segments (*).

475: Apical 2-chamber view with definity administration shows severe midventricular hypertrophy (*) and dyskinesis of the apical region with aneurysm distal to the hypertrophic segment.

CASE 149

Bulur S, Elsayed M, Nanda NC

The patient is a 39-year-old male with suspected cardiomyopathy. 2D and 3D TTE and contrast echo were done.

1. **Arrow in 🎥 476 to 478 shows:**
   (a) Apical trabeculations
   (b) Apical clot
   (c) Apical artifact
   (d) Apical trabeculations and clot
   (e) Apical trabeculations plus clot plus artifact

Ans. (a)

Apical clot would be unlikely since the LV function is essentially normal.

2. **Arrow in 🎥 479 shows:**
   (a) Apical trabeculations
   (b) Apical hypertrophic cardiomyopathy
   (c) Apical hypertrophic cardiomyopathy with possible LV non-compaction

Ans. (c)

Contrast echo clearly shows a narrow channel in the LV apex which is hypertrophied. Multiple trabeculations in LV apex were also noted in 🎥 476 to 480. Therefore, this patient has LV apical hypertrophy and in addition possible non-compaction.

MOVIES 476 TO 480

CASE 150

Anastasia Vamvakidou, Roxy Senior

A 48-year-old man with hypertension had a transthoracic echocardiogram as part of investigation for breathlessness.

1. **What do the non-contrast enhanced pictures suggest (481 to 485)?**
   (a) Concentric left ventricular hypertrophy (LVH)
   (b) Apical hypertrophic obstructive cardiomyopathy (HOCM)
   (c) HOCM
   (d) Non-compaction cardiomyopathy

Ans. (b)

There is significant increase in left ventricular (LV) wall thickness especially around the apex (Parasternal short axis [PSAX] apex level: anterior wall 1.6 cm, posterior 2.6 cm, septal 1.5 cm, lateral 1.4 cm). In the apical 4- and 2-chamber views there is obvious cavity obliteration in the apical segments. The left ventricular outflow tract (LVOT) and LV intraventricular gradients are not significantly raised (LVOT PG 10 mm Hg) (Figs. 150.1 and 150.2).

2. **What do the contrast-enhanced images suggest (486 to 489)?**
   (a) Concentric LVH
   (b) Apical HOCM
   (c) HOCM
   (d) Non-compaction cardiomyopathy

Ans. (a)

The above patient was Afro-Caribbean with resistant hypertension diagnosed 10 years ago on three different anti-hypertensives. His ECG showed small inverted T waves inferolaterally with positive Sokolow criteria for LVH. The contrast-enhanced study improved the endocardial border definition and eliminated the interference of cardiac structures, that is, chordae tendinae, papillary muscles which falsely gave the impression of asymmetric apical HOCM. The case highlights the usefulness of contrast-enhanced echocardiography as an adjunct for the diagnosis or exclusion of HOCM.[1]

MOVIES 481 TO 489

REFERENCE

1. Nagueh S, Bierig M, Butoff M, et al. American society of echocardiography clinical recommendations for multimodality cardiovascular imaging of patients with hypertrophic cardiomyopathy. J Am Soc Echocardiogr 2011;24:473-98.

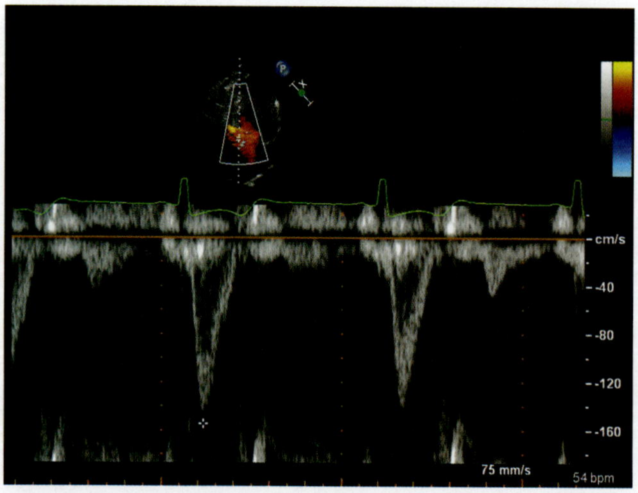

Fig. 150.1: LVOT PW Doppler assessment. The pressure gradients are not significantly raised (PG 10 mm Hg).

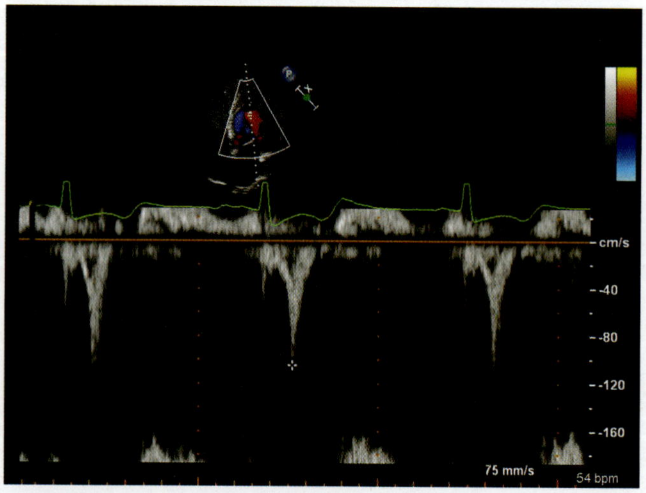

Fig. 150.2: LV intracavity PW Doppler assessment. Pressure gradients are not significantly raised (PG 4 mm Hg).

CASE 151

Elsayed M, Thind M, Joson M, Chahwala JR, Nanda NC

A 65-year-old male presented with acute heart failure. He had a prosthetic AV implanted previously. His PA systolic pressure from the TR jet was at least 60 mm Hg. Subsequently, the patient died and autopsy was not performed. 2D TTE (🎥 490 to 493) and 3D TTE (🎥 494 to 498) was done.

1. **What is the most striking finding in these movies?**
   (a) Mitral and aortic annular calcification
   (b) Prominent and calcified moderator band (MB)
   (c) Tricuspid annular calcification
   (d) Subendocardial LV calcification
   (e) False tendon in LV
   (f) Something else

Ans. (f)

The most striking feature is the presence of multiple concentric rings (arrowheads) of calcification in the LV in addition to (a)-(d) above. Arrow in 🎥 491 points to mitral annulus calcification and MR. Arrowheads in 🎥 493 demonstrate LV subendocardial calcification and calcification of basal RV free wall. Calcification also involves LA and RA walls. 3D echo cropping shows the rings plus calcification in the RV apical region which were not detected by 2D TTE. Thus this patient has calcification involving all the 4 cardiac chambers and MV, AV and TV annuli ("stone heart").

MOVIES 490 TO 498 🎥

REFERENCE

1. Rosenthal JL, Kwon DH, Soltesz EG, et al. The man with a heart of stone. J Am Coll Cardiol. 2014 Mar 4;63(8):831.

CASE 152

Bulur S, Elsayed M, Alagic N, Uygur B, Turaga NSN, Chahwala JR, Adarna LG, Nanda NC

This is an adult who underwent cardiac transplantation several years ago.

1. **What do #1 and #2 in 🎥 499 to 501 point to?**
   (a) Cor triatriatum membrane with obstruction
   (b) Cor triatriatum membrane with a wide opening
   (c) New (#1) and old (#2) LA
   (d) Need to check the relationship of LAA to the membrane before making a diagnosis of cor triatriatum sinister

Ans. (c)

#1 represents the transplanted LA and #2 a remnant of old LA.

2. **What does the arrow in 🎥 499 represent?**
   (a) Large left pleural effusion
   (b) Lung artifact
   (c) Reverberation artifact from MV
   (d) Large pericardial effusion
   (e) Ascites

Ans. (c)

It is easy to recognize this because of similar motion to the MV shown in the parasternal long axis view.

MOVIES 499 TO 501 🎥

CASE 153

Bulur S, Nanda NC

This is a 38-year-old male who underwent cardiac transplantation for dilated cardiomyopathy. He was referred for a follow-up echocardiogram.

1. **What does Figure 153.1 and 502 show?**
   (a) Poor RV function with decreased TAPSE (tricuspid annular plane systolic excursion)
   (b) Poor RV function with normal TAPSE
   (c) Mildly diminished RV function with normal TAPSE
   (d) Normal RV function with decreased TAPSE

Ans. (a)

In the apical 4-chamber view RV wall motion is considerably decreased as compared to LV wall motion. TAPSE which represents M-mode motion of the TV annulus is decreased (1.3 cm, normal >1.6 cm) which correlates with poor RV function seen on 2D echo.

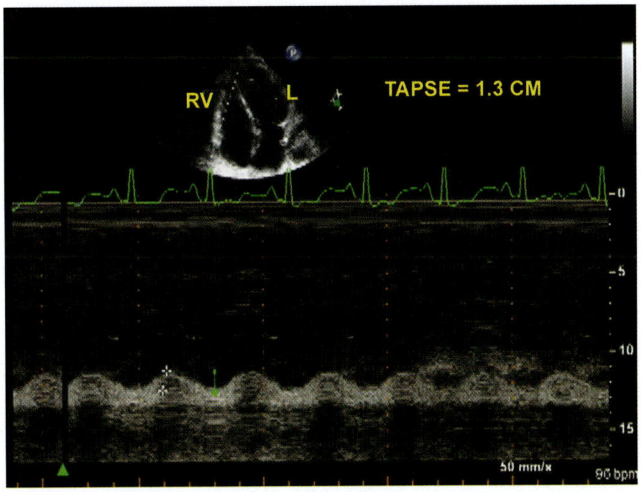

Fig. 153.1: Measurement of TAPSE by M-mode.

MOVIE 502

SECTION 8

Pericardial Disorders

CASE 154

Ajay Jindal

A 25-year-old male admitted with h/o low grade fever and palpitations for the past 10 days along with right sided chest pain. No history suggestive of specific radiation of pain. ECG shows sinus tachycardia. His chest X-ray chest revealed mild cardiomegaly. 2D TTE done (🎥 503).

1. Identify the pointed structure:
(a) Prominent eustachian valve
(b) Crista terminals
(c) Right atrial appendage
(d) Right atrial inversion
(e) Normal

Ans. (d)

The apical 4 chamber (A4C) on subcostal view shows significant pericardial effusion and right atrial inversion.

Right atrial inversion or collapse is best viewed on A4C and subcostal views.

This is an important early manifestation of increased intrapericardial pressure and is an important sign suggestive of impending cardiac tamponade commonly preceding clinical bedside signs such as hypotension and pulsus paradoxus. The duration of atrial inversion more than one third of systole increases specificity for tamponade physiology.

Eustachian valve is a flap at the distal end of IVC that directs blood into the right atrium in the fetus.

MOVIE 503 🎥

CASE 155

Taher A, Elsayed M, Bulur S, Nanda NC

A 26-year-old male patient with cardiac transplantation. Apical 5 chamber view (504) shows pericardial effusion (PE) behind both LA and LV. There is mild inversion of the LA wall.

1. **Which of the following is incorrect?**
   (a) Pleural effusion is never found behind LA
   (b) Pleural effusion may be noted behind LV
   (c) Ascites is detected in the subcostal view
   (d) Atrial inversion does not always signify cardiac tamponade

Ans. (a)

Pleural effusion, unlike pericardial effusion never occurs behind LA because of the absence of pleura in that region. However, the oblique sinus of the pericardium is located behind LA and pericardial fluid can accumulate in this area.

MOVIE 504

CASE 156

Bulur S, Elsayed M, Alagic N, Uygur B, Turaga NSN, Chahwala JR, Adarna LG, Nanda NC

Parasternal long-axis views are shown from an adult.

1. **What does arrow in 505 and 506 point to?**
   (a) Small loculated pericardial effusion (PE) behind the LA
   (b) A pulmonary vein
   (c) PE does not collect behind the LA, only left pleural effusion does
   (d) Coronary sinus
   (e) Abnormal circumflex artery

Ans. (b)

It is a small pulmonary vein which is imaged behind the LA. Color flow signals can be visualized moving from the vein into LA in 506. The patient also has mild MR. Pleural effusion is never seen behind LA. Pericardial effusion may collect behind LA (oblique sinus).

MOVIES 505 AND 506

CASE 157

Alagic N, Elsayed M, Uygur B, Turaga NSN, Chahwala JR, Adarna LG, Mohamed A, Gupta N, Bulur S, Nanda NC

A parasternal long-axis view from an adult patient is shown.

1. **What is the abnormal finding in this patient (🎥 507)?**
   (a) Mild pericardial effusion
   (b) Moderate pericardial effusion
   (c) Pericardial effusion located mainly posteriorly
   (d) There are no abnormalities and no pericardial effusion in this patient

Ans. (d)

There is no fluid behind the pericardium/lung interface denoted by an arrow in this patient. The echolucent area mimicking pericardial effusion posteriorly represents homogenous normal myocardium with no interfaces and hence it is devoid of any echo signals. Anterior echo free spaces without corresponding posterior pericardial spaces are seen even in normal individuals and result from epicardial fat pad.

MOVIE 507 🎥

CASE 158

Tevfik Fikret Ilgenli

ECHO FREE SPACE MISDIAGNOSED AS PERICARDIAL EFFUSION

A 20-year-old male admitted to our hospital with complaints of shortness of breath and angina. Blood pressure was 130/60 mm Hg and pulse was 76, regular. A systolic murmur was heard at the apical region. A difference of 45 mm Hg was noted in the blood pressure between left upper and left lower extremity.

2D TTE showed severe AR with a large LV measuring 71 mm. Aortic coarctation below the left subclavian artery was noted and confirmed by cardiac catheterization. Subsequently, AV was replaced and coarctation repaired. Two months later, he developed abdominal pain with a raised white blood cell count and abdominal ultrasound revealed choledocholithiasis. 2D TTE showed an echo free space (S) behind LV which was initially thought to be pericardial effusion but subsequently a more careful examination revealed it to be a striated dacron tube (T) graft connecting the ascending with the descending aorta and coursing behind the LV. This was used to relieve coarctation (508 to 510 and Figs. 158.1 to 158.6).

1. **Which statements are true regarding aortic coarctation?**
   (a) It is more prevalent in females
   (b) VSD, mitral stenosis, gonadal dysgenesis, bicuspid aortic valve are common associated anomalies
   (c) Possibility of coarctation should be suspected in any patient with hypertension under 50
   (d) Both (b) and (c)

Ans. (d)

2. **What are the classical findings of aortic coarctation?**
   (a) Systolic pressure in the arm is > 10 mm Hg greater than in the leg
   (b) Collaterals can be visualized and palpated over the chest
   (c) Chest X-ray may show a dilated ascending aorta and pre to post-stenotic dilation of descending aorta
   (d) Bicuspid aortic valve is the most common associated anomaly
   (e) All of the above

Ans. (e)

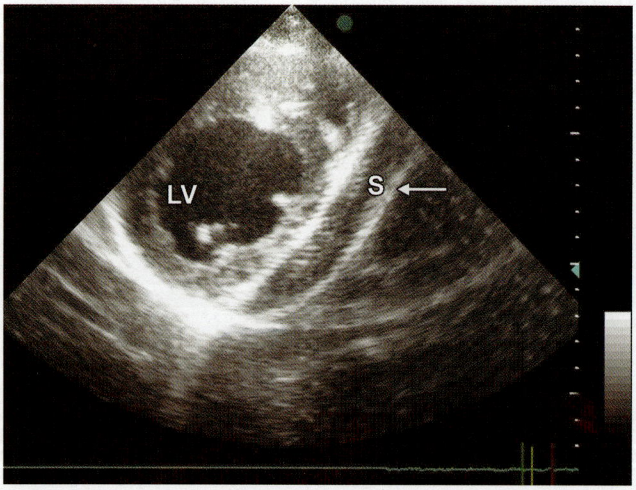

Fig. 158.1: 2D echocardiograhy. Short axis view. Arrow shows space(S), adjacent to left ventricle(LV).

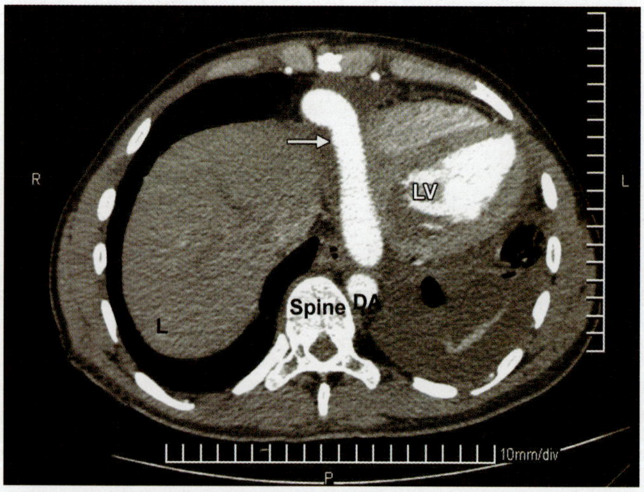

Fig. 158.2: Computerized tomography. Arrow shows dense tube like structure adjacent to heart.

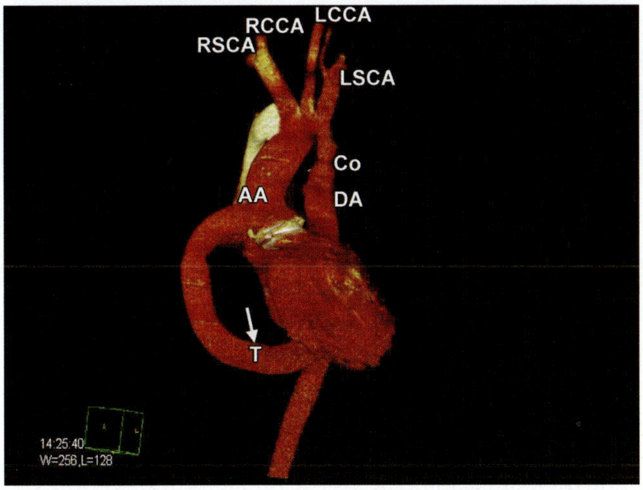

Fig. 158.3: Heart, major vessels and tube graft at MR angiography. (RSCA: Right subclavian artery; RCCA: Right common carotid artery; LCCA: Left common carotid artery; LSCA: Left subclavian artery; Co: Coarctation of Aorta; AA: Ascending aorta; DA: Descending aorta; T: Tube). Arrow shows tube graft between ascending to descending aorta.

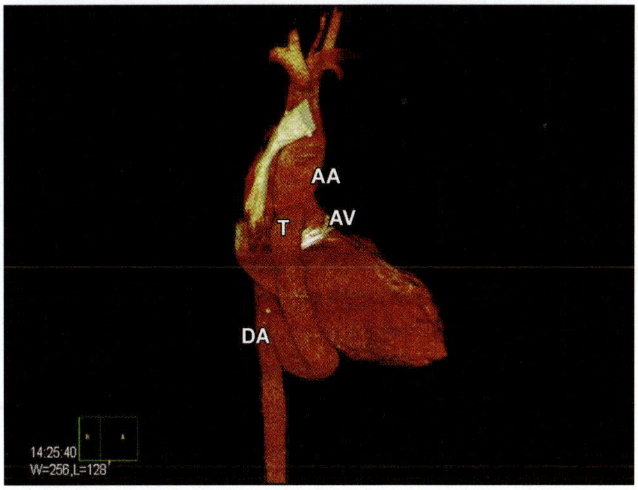

Fig. 158.4: Right lateral view of heart, major vessels and tube graft. (AA: Ascending aorta; AV: Prosthetic Aortic Valve; DA: Descending aorta; T: Tube).

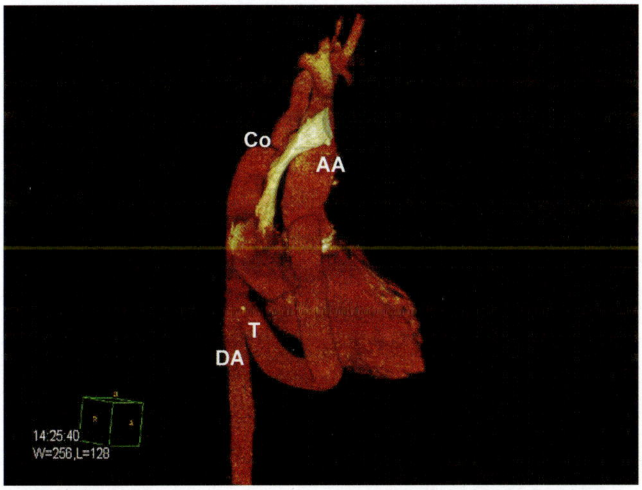

Fig. 158.5: Right anterolateral view of heart, major vessels and tube graft. (Co: Coarctation; AA: Ascending aorta; T: Tube; DA: Descending aorta).

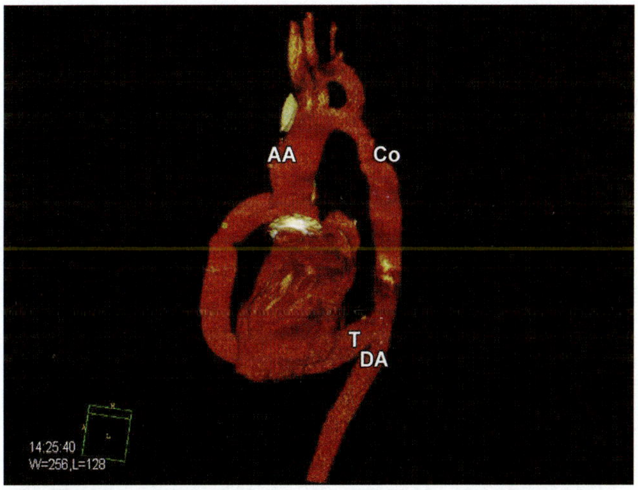

Fig. 158.6: Anterolateral view of heart, major vessels and tube graft. (Co: Coarctation; AA: Ascending aorta; T: Tube; DA: Descending aorta).

3. **Definition of significant coarctation is a pressure gradient greater than ... mm Hg across the coarctation site at angiography. What is correct pressure to fill in the gap?**
   (a) 10
   (b) 20
   (c) 30
   (d) 40
   (e) 50

Ans. (b)

4. **Intracranial aneurysms are common in patients with coarctation. Berry aneurysms of circle of Willis can be seen in approximately ... percent of patients. What is the best answer to fill in the gap?**
   (a) 10
   (b) 20
   (c) 30
   (d) 40
   (e) 50

Ans. (a)

5. Which are the foliowing are true about treatment of coarctation?

(a) Surgery can be quite challenging and residual hypertension can develop one-third of patients

(b) Complications include recurrent laryngeal nerve palsy, paraplegia, bleeding from collateral vessels and mesenteric arteritis

(c) Adult patients with coarctation of the aorta and severe AR can be treated at the same session. After AV replacement, a dacron tube graft can be used between the ascending and descending aorta

(d) All of the above

Ans. (d)

DISCUSSION

Coarctation of aorta is a discrete narrowing of distal segment of the aortic arch resulting in pathological obstruction of blood flow to systemic circulation.[1] The characteristic lesion is a deformity of the media of the aorta usually resulting in a curtain-like infolding of the left posterolateral aspect of aortic wall. This causes lumen obstruction which can be eccentric. It was described over 200 years ago by Prussian anatomist Johann Friedrich Meckel.[2] Only 20% of cases are diagnosed for the first time in adolescents or adults. 95% of cases are below the left subclavian artery and above ductus arteriosus (preductal). 5% of cases are localized either proximal to the left subclavian artery or rarely in the abdominal aorta.

The most important consequence of coarctation of aorta is systemic proximal hypertension with abnormal differences between upper and lower extremity pulses and systolic blood pressures.[3] It is two to five times more common in males.

The diagnosis of coarctation is frequently overlooked:

1. Possibility of coarctation of the aorta should be suspected in any patient under the age of 50 who has systemic hypertension.
2. Simultaneous palpation of the radial and femoral pulses should be performed as a part of any routine cardiovascular examination.

The initial clue to coarctation of the aorta in the adolescent or young adult is the discovery of systemic hypertension or an abnormality on a routine chest X-ray, particularly notching of the ribs. EKG can be normal. Echocardiogram is particularly useful in diagnosis and determining the associated abnormalities. Discrete coarctation may be demonstrated by 2D TTE. In addition to echo and Doppler studies, MRI may be helpful to diagnose the disease. Catheterization and angiography are also useful but they are invasive modalities. Coarctation can be relieved using transcatheter interventions or surgery.

Simple coarctation which is the most common form represents absence of associated lesions such as AS, bicuspid AV, AR, VSD and MS.

Surgical correction of coarctation in adults includes patch grafting or resection of the coarcted segment with end-to-end anastomosis. Occasionally, a tubular prosthesis is required to bridge the gap between the two ends of the aorta when the coarcted segment is long. Rarely, a tube graft connecting the ascending and descending segments of the aorta may be used as was done in our patient.[4]

Exposure of the descending aorta through a median sternotomy and posterior pericardium was first described by Vijayanagar et al.[5] They described an adult patient with coarctation of the aorta and severe AR. This technique allows AV replacement and coarctation repair in the same session.

MOVIES 508 TO 510

REFERENCES

1. The Heart. 9th Edition.1998. Chapter 70. Congenital Heart Disease. Pages: 1951-55.
2. Mayo Clinic Practice of Cardiology. 3rd Edition.1997. Chapter 45. Coarctation of Aorta. Pages: 1572-80.
3. Heart Disease. 7th Edition. 2005. Chapter 56. Congenital Heart Disease. Pages:1532-5.
4. Goksel OS, Inan K, Ucak A, et al. Posterior Pericardial Ascending to Descending Aortic Bypass through Median Sternotomy. J Card Surg. 2008;23:515-8.
5. Vijayanagar R, Natarajan P, Eckstein P, et al. Aortic valvular insufficiency and postductal aortic coarctation in the adult: combined surgical management through median sternotomy: a new surgical approach. J Thorac Cardiovasc Surg. 1980;79:266-68.

CASE 159

Bulur S, Elsayed M, Nanda NC

A 14-year-old female who underwent cardiac transplantation. 2D TTE done.

The parasternal long-axis view shows thickening of the posterior pericardium (arrow in 🎥 511). She does not have any clinical or other echocardiographic evidence of constriction.

1. **Which of the following is correct?**
   (a) Pericardial calcification is present in all patients with constriction
   (b) Mild pericardial thickening can be confused with normally highly refractile interface between the epicardium and lung
   (c) Pericardial thickening is never localized
   (d) It is impossible for constrictive pericarditis to develop after cardiac surgery

Ans. (b)

Normally the interface between the LV epicardium and lung is highly refractile and echogenic because of the high acoustic impedance produced by lung tissue which prevents penetration of the ultrasound beam. Therefore, less severe thickening of the pericardium can be missed by echocardiography. Constriction can present as multiple localized areas of patchy thickening. Pericardial thickening without calcification is not infrequent in constrictive pericarditis cases. Constrictive pericarditis can develop after cardiac surgery.

MOVIE 511

CASE 160

Bulur S, Nanda NC

This is a 58-year-old female with nonspecific chest pains. 2D TTE was done (512 and 513).

1. **What do the arrows show?**
   (a) Thickened anterior and posterior pericardium with no obvious constriction
   (b) Thickened anterior and posterior pericardium but constriction cannot be ruled out
   (c) There is no real thickening of the pericardium and the echogenic pericardium results from high acoustic impedance between the heart and lung tissue

Ans. (a)

The pericardium may appear thickened posteriorly because of the normally high acoustic impedance between cardiac tissue and lung. However, in this patient the anterior pericardium is also echogenic and somewhat thickened. The IVC in this patient was not well-imaged but it appeared normal in size which would go against the diagnosis of the constriction. The small echo free space anteriorly represents normal epicardial fat pad. There is no echo free space posteriorly and hence, this patient does not have pericardial effusion.

MOVIES 512 AND 513

CASE 161

Juliet Ryan, Nicholas Furiasse, Michael Cuttica, Hyde Russell, Vera H Rigolin

CONSTRICTIVE PERICARDIAL DISEASE

Clinical History

A previously healthy 25-year-old male initially presented with fevers, myalgia, dyspnea, and chest pain. A small pericardial effusion and bilateral pleural effusions were noted on additional workup. A thoracentesis was performed demonstrating a transudative effusion leading to a diagnosis of presumptive viral pericarditis and pleuritis. Laboratory testing confirmed antibodies to Coxsackie virus. Colchicine was initiated for treatment of pericardial-related chest pain with improvement in his symptoms. The patient returned one month later with recurrent chest pain and shortness of breath in setting of viral-type symptoms. A recurrent pericardial effusion and large pleural effusions were noted. A repeat thoracentesis was performed again showing transudative fluid. All microbiologic, rheumatologic, and neoplastic systemic studies were negative. Ultimately, the patient presented once again with myalgias, fatigue, and dyspnea. A recurrent large right pleural effusion was noted with negative diagnostic testing. The patient's breathlessness persisted despite therapeutic thoracentesis. Additional diagnostic workup with echocardiography and cardiac magnetic resonance imaging was then performed.

Transthoracic/Transesophageal Echocardiogram and Cardiac MRI Findings

A two-dimensional, transthoracic Doppler echocardiogram demonstrated normal left and right ventricular size and systolic function. LV ejection fraction was 62%. There was biatrial enlargement and an aneurysmal interatrial septum. A subtle interventricular septal bounce (arrowhead), small pericardial effusion (arrow) and aneurysmal interatrial septum (open arrow) were also noted (514). The parasternal short-axis view also shows the septal bounce (arrowhead) as well as septal flattening (515). Color and spectral Doppler demonstrated mild tricuspid regurgitation and left to right flow across an interatrial septal defect. Pulmonary artery systolic pressure was estimated at 39 mm Hg (mildly elevated) with a severely elevated right atrial pressure of 15 mm Hg. Tissue Doppler septal and lateral E' velocities were at the upper limit of normal (16 cm/s). Mild respirophasic variation was noted at the mitral inflow position on pulse-wave interrogation (Fig. 161.1). A subsequent two- and three-dimensional transesophageal echocardiogram confirmed the presence of a bidirectional secundum-type atrial septal defect measuring 8 mm in diameter.

A cardiac MRI confirmed preserved left ventricular ejection fraction and biatrial enlargement. The calculated Qp: Qs shunt ratio was 1:1.2 in the setting of the atrial septal defect. There was no evidence of myocarditis, however, there was diffuse thickening and enhancement of the pericardium. (arrow, Fig. 161.2). Additionally, interventricular septal discordance with respiration was again noted suggesting possible constrictive physiology.

Given these findings and the patient's recurrent symptoms, the patient underwent pericardiectomy and atrial septal defect closure. The findings at the time of surgery indicated dense mediastinal inflammation with adherent parietal and visceral pericardium (arrow, Fig. 161.3). Following surgery, the patient had complete resolution of his symptoms.

Role of Imaging

This case demonstrates the importance of supportive diagnostic testing when constrictive pericarditis is sus-

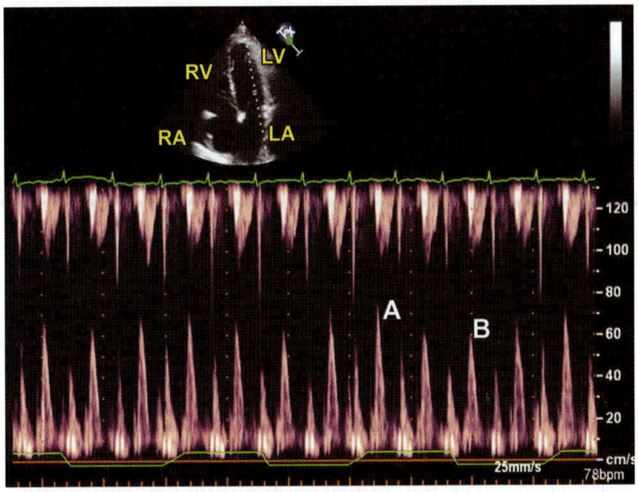

Fig. 161.1: Mild respirophasic variation of mitral inflow E wave velocity is shown. (A: Expiration; B: Inspiration).

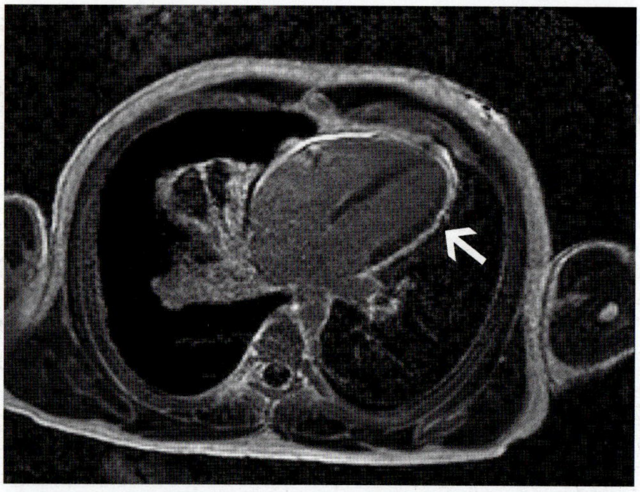

Fig. 161.2: Cardiac MRI PSIR (phase sensitive inversion recovery) post gadolinium contrast imaging demonstrating a small pericardial effusion, pericardial thickening with evidence of enhancement (arrow).

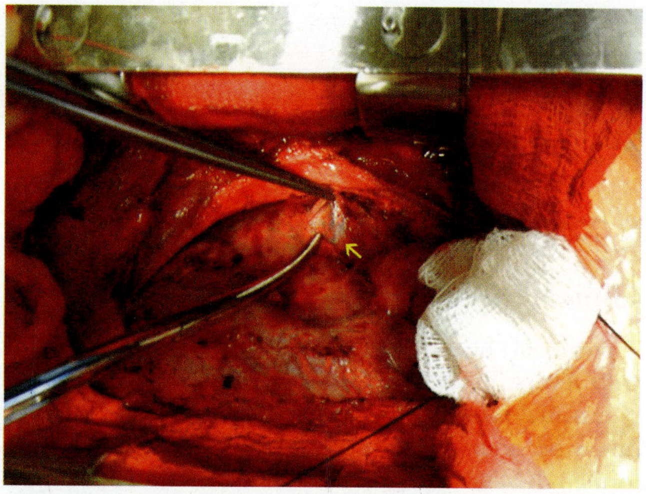

Fig. 161.3: Parietal and visceral pericardium at the time of surgery. The two layers are thickened and inflamed with adhesion to one another.

pected. Echocardiography has proven to be a useful tool in the evaluation of dyspnea, particularly in the setting of pericardial disease. There are a host of "classic" echocardiographic findings that may be seen including a preservation of left ventricular ejection fraction, possible biatrial enlargement, abnormal interventricular septal motion ("bounce'), increased early diastolic filling (higher E wave, shorter deceleration time), exaggerated variation of E-wave velocities with respiration at the mitral and tricuspid inflow interrogation, minimal respiratory variation of the inferior vena cava due to elevated right atrial pressures, and an increase in septal e' velocity on tissue Doppler examination.[1] Despite the "clues" provided with echocardiography to the diagnosis, recently cardiac MRI has proved to be a useful complementary imaging modality. The benefit of cardiac MRI allows for future classification of the pericardium with a determination of thickness, presence of calcifications, identification of pericardial effusion, and qualitative assessment of pericardial enhancement. Additional free-breathing sequences allow for assessment of interventricular septal motion. Finally, cardiac MRI allows for characterization of the myocardium in the assessment of myopericardial processes.[2]

SUMMARY

Constrictive pericarditis most commonly is the sequela of pericardial inflammation/injury that results from infectious (viral/bacterial/fungal), radiation exposure, prior cardiac surgery, malignancies, or rheumatologic diseases. A high index of suspicion for constrictive pericardial disease should be maintained in the presence of the correct clinical setting. This case is a prime example of a "real world" experience of pericardial disease in which the clinical symptoms drove the initial suspicion of the disease with support from echocardiography and cardiac MRI. Commonly, diagnostic testing will demonstrate some but not all features of constriction. This condition is important to diagnose since it can be life threatening with progression to heart failure and end-organ dysfunction if left untreated. A high index of suspicion is commonly needed in the diagnosis of this disease, which is curative with surgical pericardiectomy in most cases.

1. **Which of the following are NOT echocardiographic findings associated with constrictive physiology?**
   (a) Decreased septal and lateral E' velocities on tissue Doppler measurement
   (b) Interventricular discordant movement (septal bounce)
   (c) Exaggerated variation in mitral and tricuspid valve inflow E-wave velocities
   (d) Preserved left ventricular ejection fraction

Ans. (a)

In the setting of constrictive pericardial disease, the left ventricle is dependent on early diastolic filling with accentuated longitudinal motion of the ventricle leading an increase in septal E' velocity relative to lateral E' velocity, not a decrease in tissue velocities which is classically seen with restrictive myocardial disease.

2. **Which therapy is NOT recommended in the initial treatment of acute pericarditis?**

(a) High dose aspirin
(b) Indomethacin
(c) Colchicine
(d) Prednisone

Ans. (d)

Anti-inflammatories are first-line therapy in the treatment of acute pericarditis. Colchicine, high dose aspirin, and nonsteroidal anti-inflammatory drugs including indomethacin are all reasonable first line therapy. Steroids, while decreasing inflammation and symptoms are associated with recurrent pericarditis with discontinuation of therapy. Therefore, they are not recommended in the initial treatment of acute pericarditis.[3]

3. Ventricular septal shift with which other echocardiographic finding has been associated with a high sensitivity and specificity in the diagnosis of constrictive pericarditis in a surgically confirmed cohort of patients?

(a) Left atrial enlargement
(b) Elevated pulmonary artery systolic pressure
(c) Elevated right atrial pressure
(d) Hepatic vein expiratory diastolic reversal ratio ≥0.79

Ans. (d)

In a retrospective analysis of 130 patients with surgically confirmed constrictive pericarditis at the Mayo Clinic, the presence of a ventricular septal shift and either a hepatic vein expiratory diastolic reversal ratio ≥0.79 or septal E' tissue velocity ≥ 9 cm/s was associated with a sensitivity of 87% and specificity of 91% in the diagnosis of constrictive pericarditis.[1]

MOVIE LEGENDS

514: Two-dimensional echocardiography with an apical 4-chamber view demonstrating an interatrial septal aneurysm with increased mobility, biatrial enlargement, normal biventricular size and function. Also note the interventricular septal bounce (arrowhead).

515: Parasternal short-axis view demonstrating septal flattening and the septal bounce (arrowhead).

REFERENCES

1. Oh J, et al. Echocardiographic Diagnosis of Constrictive Pericarditis: Mayo Clinic. Circ Cardiovasc Imaging. 2012; 7:526-34.
2. Francone M, Bogaert J. Cardiac Magnetic Resonance in Pericardial Disease. J of Card Mag Resonance Imaging. 2009;11:14.
3. Adler Y, et al. A Randomized Trial for Colchicine for Acute Pericarditis. N Eng J Med. 2013;369:1522-8.

CASE 162

Edgar Argulian, Farooq Chaudhry

A 51-year-old male comes to the emergency room with progressive exertional dyspnea over the last several weeks. His past medical history is insignificant. He is a lifetime non-smoker and he has no personal or family history of cancer. He is diagnosed with a large pericardial effusion (arrows, Fig. 162.1) which was successfully drained. After the drainage, he describes improvement of his symptoms but he is still dyspneic on exertion. Repeat echocardiogram is performed. Please review the findings of 2D echocardiogram (Fig. 162.2 and 516A and B), M-mode (Fig. 162.3), tissue Doppler at the medial and lateral mitral annulus (Fig. 162.4), and Doppler findings for mitral inflow and hepatic vein flow (Fig. 162.5).

1. **Which of the following best describes septal motion observed in this patient?**
   (a) Beat-to-beat 'shudder' only
   (b) Respiratory septal shift only
   (c) Both beat-to-beat 'shudder' and respiratory septal shift
   (d) Normal septal motion

Ans. (c)

2. **Based on Mayo Clinic findings, which of the following has the strongest association with constrictive pericarditis compared to restrictive cardiomyopathy and severe tricuspid regurgitation?**
   A. Annulus reversus
   B. Inferior vena cava dilation and absence of respiratory collapse
   C. Respiratory variation in mitral E velocity
   D. Systolic hepatic venous flow reversal
   E. Ventricular septal shift

Ans. (e)

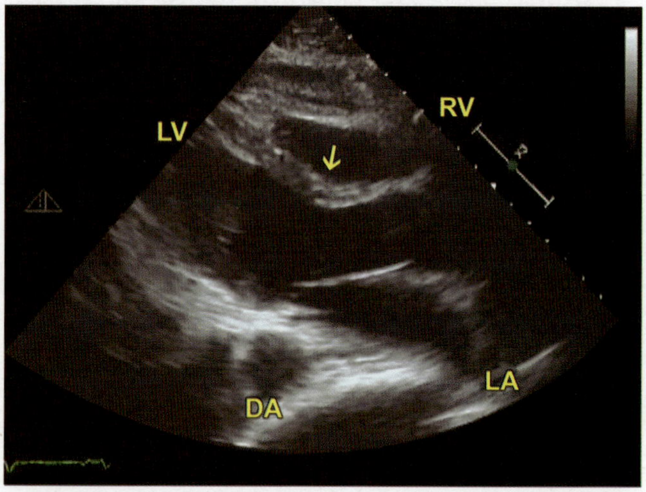

Fig. 162.2: 2D echocardiogram after pericardial effusion drainage. Arrow points to ventricular septum.

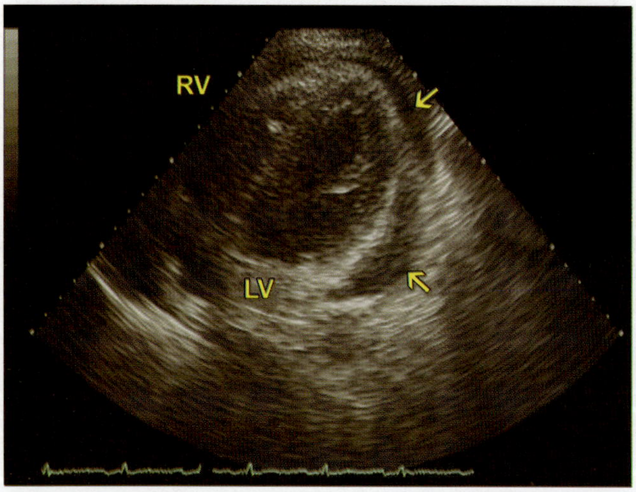

Fig. 162.1: 2D echocardiogram before pericardial effusion drainage.

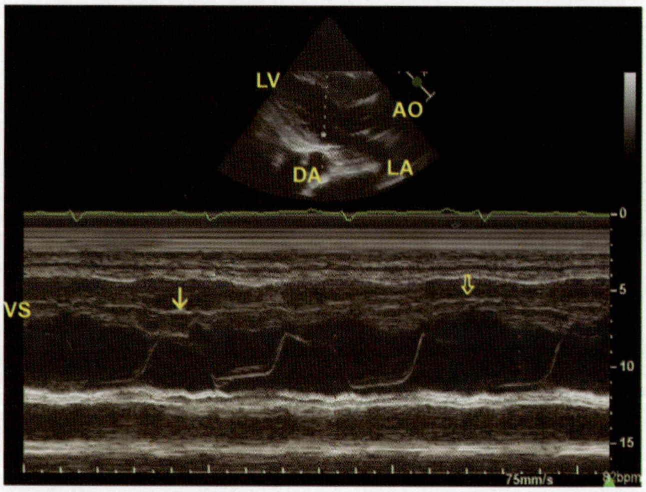

Fig. 162.3: M-mode findings.

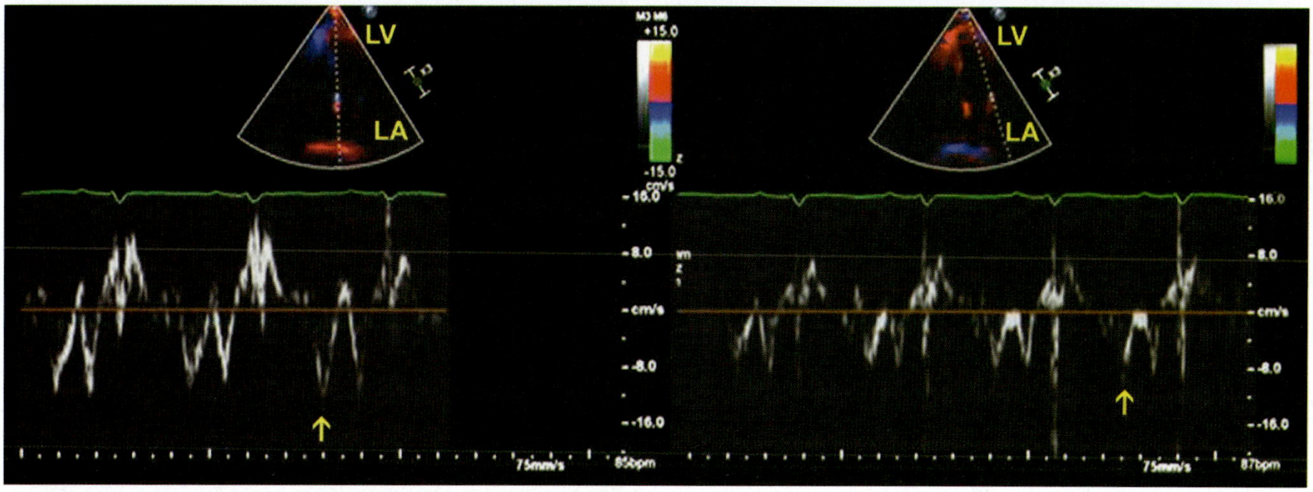

Fig. 162.4: Tissue Doppler findings. Septal E' velocity is higher than lateral E' velocity.

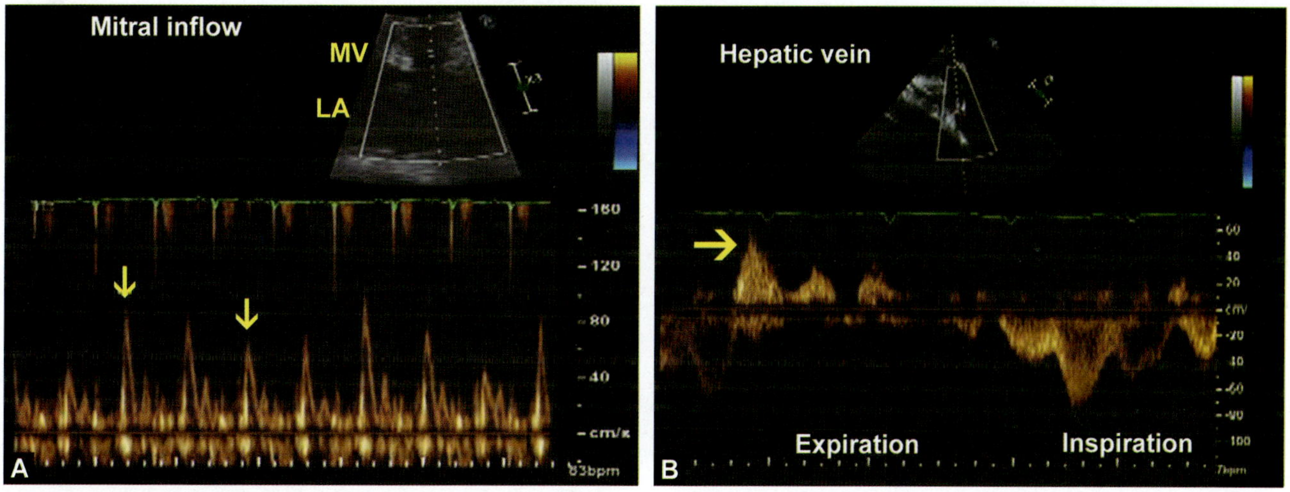

Figs. 162.5A and B: Spectral Doppler findings.

This patient's clinical presentation and echocardiographic findings are consistent with effusive-constrictive pericarditis.[1] He presented initially with a large pericardial effusion (Fig. 162.1) which was drained but he had persistent symptoms. Subsequent echocardiographic findings are suggestive of constrictive pericarditis. Evaluation of wall motion (arrow in 516A and B) shows two distinct abnormalities of interventricular septal motion: beat-to-beat 'shudder' and cyclical movement of the septum with respiration. The latter can also be appreciated on M-mode tracing (Fig. 162.3) showing septal motion toward the left ventricle with inspiration (left arrow) and toward the right ventricle with expiration (right arrow). Also, tissue Doppler data (Fig. 162.4) shows preserved medial mitral E' velocity exceeding that of the lateral mitral annulus (annulus reversus). Marked variation in the mitral E velocity was seen (arrows, Figs. 162.5A and B). In addition, expiratory reversal (arrow) of the hepatic venous flow was demonstrated (Figs. 162.5A and B). Based on Mayo Clinic data, three echocardiographic variables have been independently associated with constrictive pericarditis: ventricular septal shift, medial mitral E' and hepatic vein expiratory flow reversal ratio; ventricular septal shift has been shown to have the strongest association.[2]

MOVIES 516A AND B

REFERENCES

1. Sagrista-Sauleda J, Angel J, Sanchez A, et al. Effusive-constrictive pericarditis. N Engl J Med. 2004;350:469-75.
2. Welch TD, Ling LH, Espinosa RE, et al. Echocardiographic diagnosis of constrictive pericarditis: Mayo Clinic criteria. Circ Cardiovasc Imaging. 2014;7:526-34.

CASE 163

Naveen Garg, Kanwal K Kapur

RIGHT DIAGNOSIS

An African male age about 42 years admitted with complaints of breathlessness, pedal edema, abdominal distention and weakness. On examination HR 90/min, BP 90/70 mm Hg, edema and ascites. Laboratory tests showed deranged LFT and reversed albumin globulin ratio of 3:4.5. His viral markers were negative. His diagnosis was cryptogenic cirrhosis and liver transplant surgery was planned.

2D TTE reveals—(Figs. 163.1 to 163.4 and 517 to 519)

1. What do these (Figs. 163.1 to 163.3) findings indicate?

Ans. Echo findings are:

- Small ventricles, large atria
- Fair LV systolic function
- Low cardiac output
- Calcified pericardium
- Jerky interventricular septum (septal bounce)

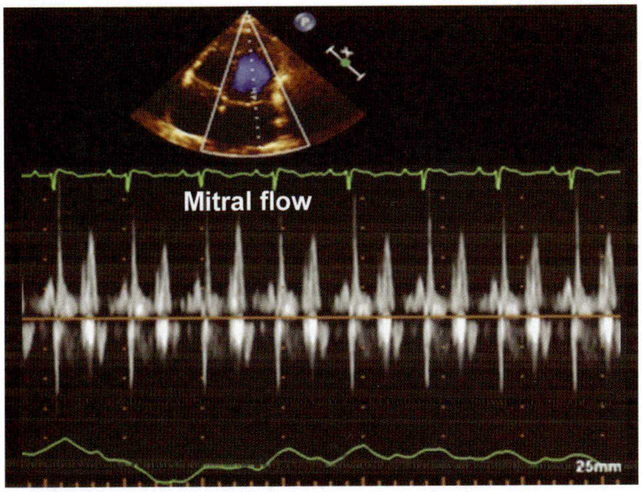

Fig. 163.1: Mitral flow Doppler.

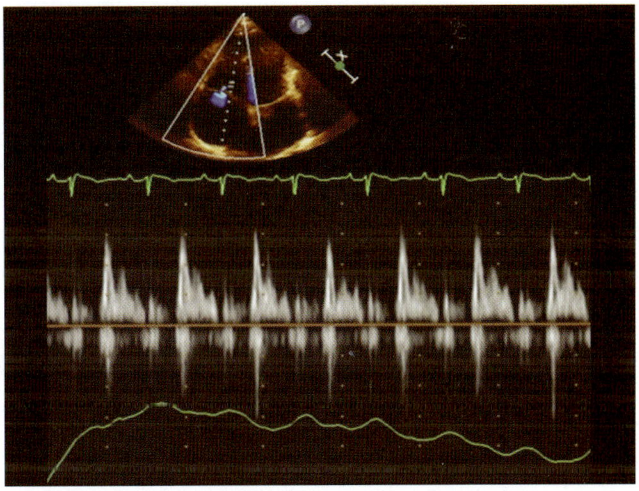

Fig. 163.2: Tricuspid flow Doppler.

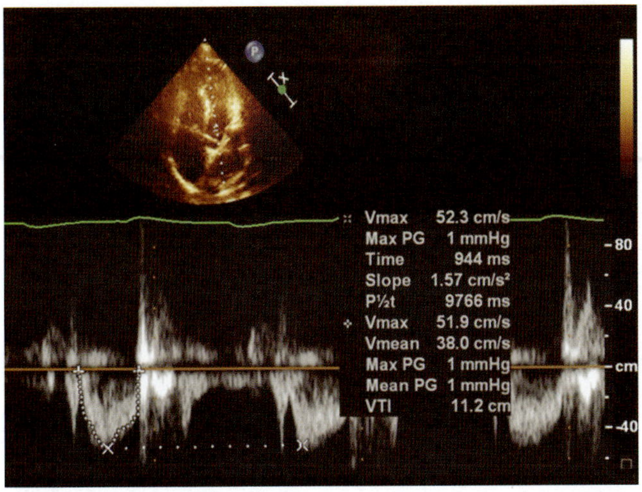

Fig. 163.3: LVOT flow Doppler.

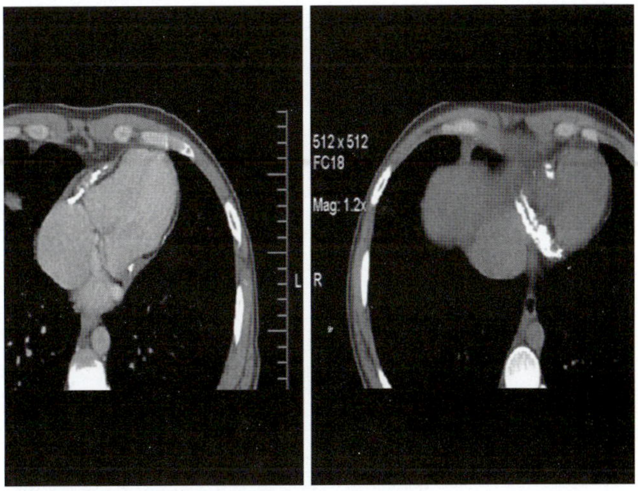

Fig. 163.4: CT scan shows calcified pericardium.

- Dilated IVC
- Respiratory variations across valves (25% change)

DIAGNOSIS

Constrictive Pericarditis

This was the reason for his symptoms. Patient did not need any transplant!! ECHO helped in making the right diagnosis. Patient underwent pericardiectomy and the signs of pericardial constriction gradually resolved over a period of 4–5 weeks.

MOVIE LEGENDS

517. 4C view
518. SAX view
519. IVC

CASE 164

Ahmad S Omran

CONSTRICTIVE PERICARDITIS

This 32-year-old man presented to our center with a 2-month history of fatigue, shortness of breath and peripheral edema. Past medical history was unremarkable. He had transthoracic echocardiography (TTE) which showed all the classical signs of constrictive pericarditis including septal bounce (520), supernormal tissue Doppler imaging (TDI) of septal mitral annulus, respiratory variation of mitral and tricuspid inflow Doppler, and inferior vena cava (IVC) plethora (521). Cardiac CT confirmed thickening of the pericardium. Echocardiographic assessment of cardiac mechanics using speckle tracking technique was performed which showed decreased global circumferential strain values. Net left ventricular (LV) twist was also decreased (Figs. 164.1A and B).[1,2]

Patient underwent pericardiectomy. Both parietal and visceral pericardium were severely thickened. Total pericardial stripping was performed (Figs. 164.3A and B). He was discharged home in good general condition a week later. Follow-up visit after 2 years showed the patient was doing fine and was able to go back to his original work. Peripheral edema and all previous symptoms had disappeared and conventional TTE returned to normal (522 and 523). In cardiac mechanics assessment, all values including net LV twist and global circumferential strain had returned back to normal (Figs. 164.2A and B, 524 to 529).

1. **In echocardiographic assessment of cardiac mechanics for differentiation between constrictive pericarditis and restrictive cardiomyopathies, all of the followings are correct *except*:**
   (a) In cardiac amyloidosis at an early stage, net left ventricular (LV) twist is normal
   (b) In dilated cardiomyopathy LV twist remains normal
   (c) In constrictive pericarditis net LV twist is severely reduced
   (d) In constrictive pericarditis LV global circumferential strain is reduced while global longitudinal strain is preserved

Ans. (b)

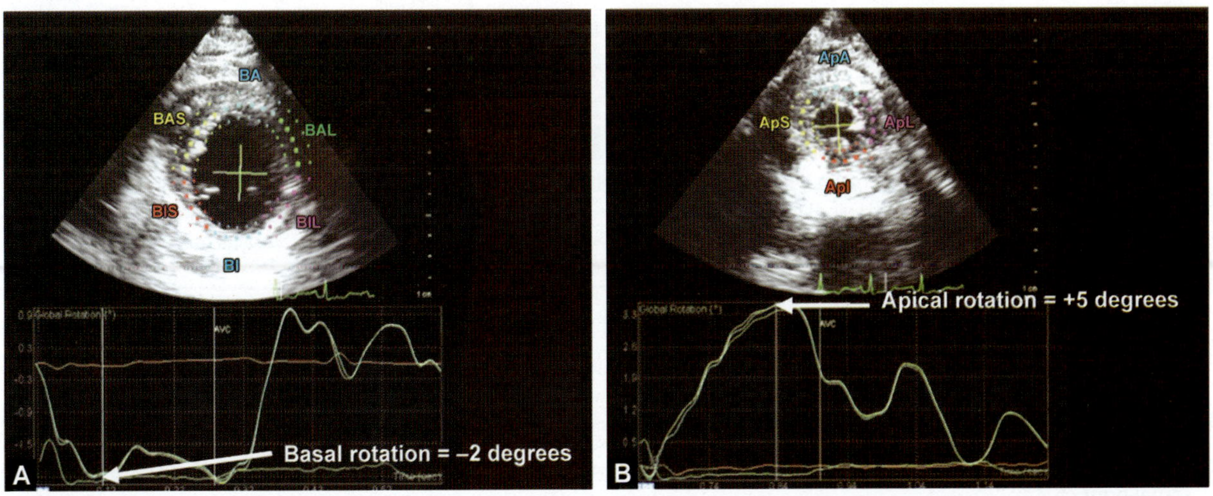

Figs. 164.1A and B: Assessment of left ventricular (LV) rotation using speckle tracking echocardiography (STE). (A) Basal LV rotation is about – 2 degrees (clockwise rotation). (B) LV apical rotation is about +5 degrees (counter-clockwise rotation). Net LV twist which is calculated as absolute apex-to-base differences in LV rotation would be 7 degrees in this patient. Normal value for net LV twist is about 20 degrees. Decrease in LV twist and torsion is an important finding that differentiates constrictive pericarditis from restrictive cardiomyopathy.

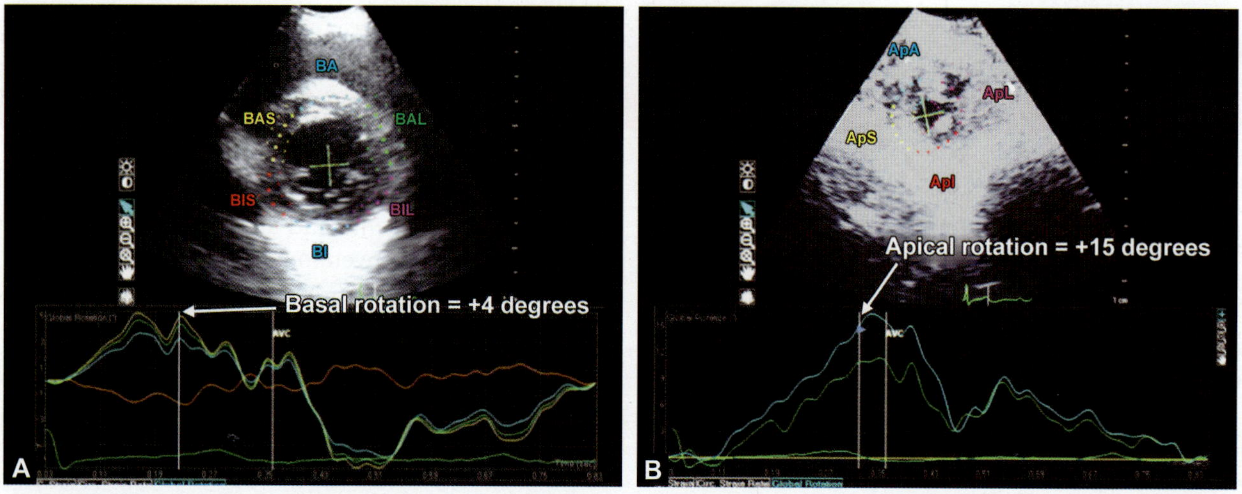

Figs. 164.2A and B: Assessment of left ventricular (LV) twist 2 years after pericardiectomy. (A) Basal LV rotation is about +4 degrees (counterclockwise rotation). This rotation is in abnormal direction. Normal value for basal LV rotation is –7 degrees. (B) LV apical rotation is about +15 degrees which is above the normal values. Net LV twist is calculated as 11 degrees (normal value is about 20 degrees). Comparison between preoperative and postoperative assessment of LV rotation by STE shows that 2 years after pericardiectomy, LV apical rotation returned to normal in this patient but the basal rotation was still abnormal.

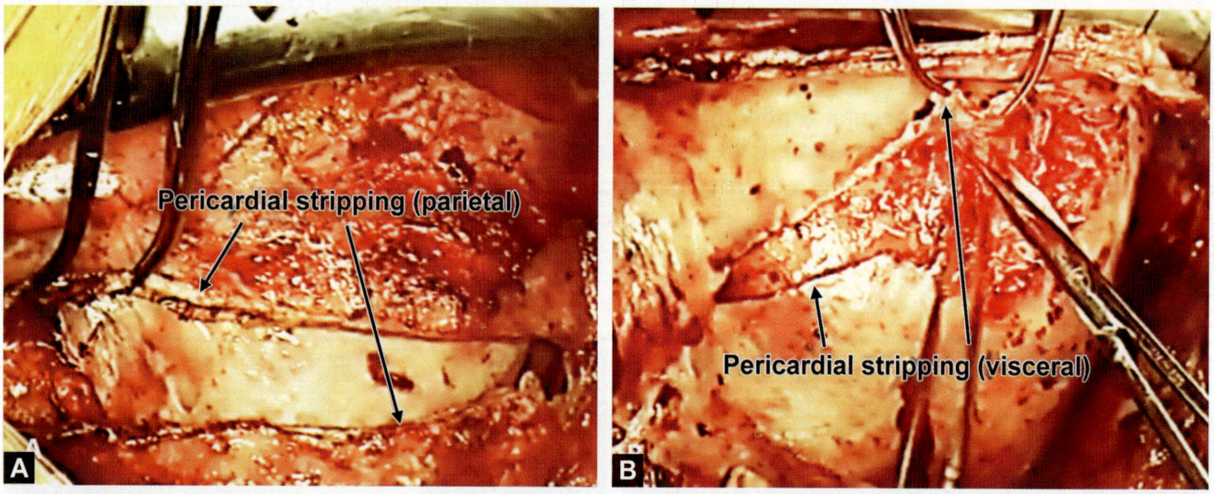

Figs. 164.3A and B: Surgical exploration. (A) Very thick parietal pericardium was stripped carefully. (B) Thickened visceral pericardium was also removed. Pericardiectomy (pericardial stripping) is a surgical option for constrictive pericarditis and is usually subtotal (from phrenic nerve to phrenic nerve). Surgery is a lengthy operation and usually is performed without cardiopulmonary bypass. Surgical mortality in an experienced center is about 2–3%.

MOVIE LEGENDS

520: Preoperative TTE in short-axis view showing ventricular septal bounce.

521: Preoperative TTE showing dilated noncollapsing IVC (IVC plethora).

522: Follow-up TTE after 2 years showing normal motion of the ventricular septum (no septal bounce).

523: Follow-up TTE after 2 years showing small size IVC with good respiratory collapse.

524: Preoperative assessment of left ventricular global circumferential strain (GCS) at the basal LV = –18.5% which is lower than normal.

525: Postoperative basal LV strain, GCS = –21% which is in the normal range.

526: Preoperative assessment of left ventricular global circumferential strain (GCS) at the apical level = –15.1% which is severely reduced.

527: Postoperative GCS at apical LV = –55% which is super normal.

528: Preoperative assessment of left ventricular global longitudinal strain (GLS) is –16.4% which is slightly below normal.

529: Postoperative GLS = –18% which is in the normal range.

REFERENCES

1. Sengupta PP, Tajik J, Chandrasekaran K, et al. Twist mechanics of the left ventricle: Principles and applications. JACC Cardiovascular Imaging. 2008;3:366-76.
2. Russel IK, Gotte MJW, Bronzwaer JG, et al. Left ventricular torsion: An expanding role in analysis of myocardial dysfunction. JACC Cardiovascular Imaging. 2009;2(5):648-55.

CASE 165

Mohamed A, Gupta N, Elsayed M, Nanda NC

This is a 44-year-old male with cirrhosis of liver. 2D TTE was done to evaluate LV and RV function which was found to be normal.

1. **Why was examination performed from the left and right back in this patient (530 and 531)?**
   (a) To check for left and right pleural effusion
   (b) To check for ascites
   (c) To check for pericardial effusion
   (d) To check for lung carcinoma

Ans. (a)

This is the most reliable technique to assess for both left and right pleural effusions (arrows in 530 and 531). Examination is performed by placing the transducer in the lower back with the patient sitting up so that the pleural fluid gravitates towards the bottom. When large, left pleural effusion may also be detected in the parasternal long axis view as a posterior echo free space (arrow in 532) extending beyond the descending aorta (DA).

MOVIES 530 TO 532

CASE 166

Mohamed A, Gupta N, Elsayed M, Nanda NC

Another adult patient with left pleural effusion (PLE) is shown in 🎥 533 to 535. In 🎥 533, the large echo free space behind the LV in the parasternal long-axis view clearly extends beyond the descending AO typical of left PLE. This is confirmed by examining the patient from the left back while sitting up and finding a large echo free space beneath the back wall. No echo free space is noted subcostally (🎥 535). Arrows in 🎥 534 point to fibrin strands in PLE.

MOVIES 533 TO 535 🎥

CASE 167

Bulur S, Nanda NC

The patient is a 62-year-old male with chronic renal failure. Subcostal 2D echo examination was done.

1. **What does the arrow show (🎥 536 and 537)?**
   (a) Fibrinous material in right pleural effusion
   (b) Fibrinous material in ascites
   (c) Typical echo artifact seen during subcostal examination
   (d) Falciform ligament

Ans. (d)

Presence of a vertically oriented band of tissue called falciform ligament in a fluid space between liver and the heart is considered diagnostic of ascites. This ligament runs between liver and the anterior abdominal wall. This patient also has associated pericardial effusion (PE).

2. **What is the best way to diagnose pleural effusion?**
   (a) Fluid space behind the heart extending beyond the level of the descending aorta (parasternal long axis view)
   (b) Subcostal examination
   (c) Examination of the back

Ans. (c)

Since pleural effusion is gravity dependent, it is best to ask the patient to sit up so the fluid gravitates to the bottom and then place the transducer in the posterior intercostal spaces on both left and right sides. Normally no fluid is noted but when pleural effusion is present a clear space would be detected between the back wall and lung. A large left sided pleural effusion would also be detected behind the descending aorta in the parasternal long-axis view but a small one and pleural effusion on the right side would be missed.

MOVIES 536 AND 537

CASE 168

Elsayed M, Nanda NC

This is a 62-year-old male with cirrhosis of liver. 2D TTE was done. Subcostal examination and bubble study in the apical four chamber view are shown.

1. The arrow in the subcostal four chamber view (Fig. 168.1 and 🎥 538) points to:

(a) Pericardial effusion
(b) Ascites
(c) Pleural effusion
(d) Pericardial cyst

Ans. (b)

Ascites is identified by the presence of the falciform ligament (arrowhead). Ascites appears to be small.

2. Which of the following statements is correct (🎥 539)?

(a) Bubble study is negative
(b) Bubble study is positive for intracardiac shunt
(c) Bubble study is positive for intrapulmonary shunting
(e) Bubble study is positive for both intracardiac and intrapulmonary shunting
(e) Bubble study is positive for neither intracardiac nor intrapulmonary shunting

Ans. (c)

Bubbles (arrow in 🎥 539) are seen in the LA/LV at least 3 beats following first appearance in the right heart. This is suggestive of intra-pulmonary shunting unlike a PFO/ASD where the bubbles will appear in the left heart within 3 beats. Intrapulmonary shunting in patients with cirrhosis of liver is generally due to dilatation of pulmonary arterioles and not due to a large pulmonary arteriovenous fistula.

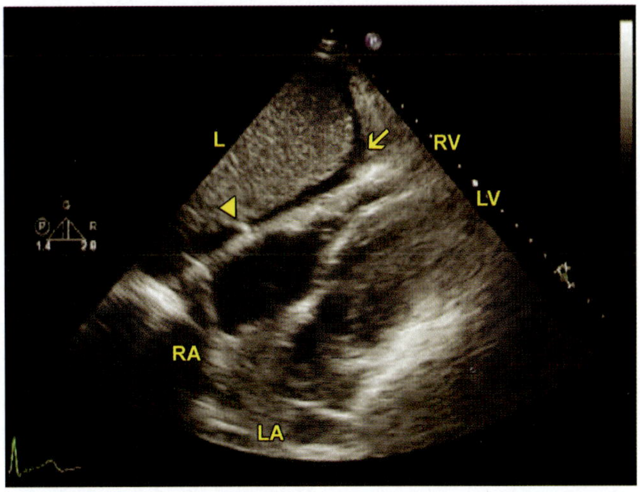

Fig. 168.1: Subcostal examination. Arrow points to ascites and the arrowhead to falciform ligament.

MOVIES 538 AND 539 🎥

CASE 169

Mohamed A, Gupta N, Elsayed M, Nanda NC

This is a 47-year-old male with cirrhosis of liver. 2D TTE was done.

1. **What is the echo free space due to (arrowhead in 540 to 542)?**
   (a) Malignant fluid
   (b) Ascites
   (c) Bilateral pleural effusion
   (d) Massive pericardial effusion

Ans. (b)

Visualization of coils of intestine (arrows) during abdominal examination provides a clue that the fluid (arrow head) collection is ascites.

MOVIES 540 TO 542

CASE 170

Adarna LG, Elsayed M, Alagic N, Uygur B, Turaga NSN, Chahwala JR, Mohamed A, Gupta N, Bulur S, Nanda NC

This is an adult patient presenting with shortness of breath. 2D TTE was done (Fig. 170.1 and 543 to 546, L = Liver).

1. **What findings are noted in this patient (Fig. 170.1 and 543 to 546)? All statements below are correct *except*:**
   (a) Presence of pericardial effusion (PE) behind LV, LA (arrow in 543), RA (arrow in 544) and RV (horizontal arrow in 544, vertical arrow in 546)
   (b) Presence of ascites (transverse arrow in 546) with falciform ligament (hollow arrow in 546)
   (c) Dilated coronary sinus (CS in 544)
   (d) Normal LV function (543, 545 and 546)
   (e) Both left and right pleural effusion

Ans. (e)

The arrow in Figure 170.1 (M-mode) shows flattening of RV wall with atrial systole but there is no collapse or downward motion during the remainder of diastole which would have been suggestive of cardiac tamponade.

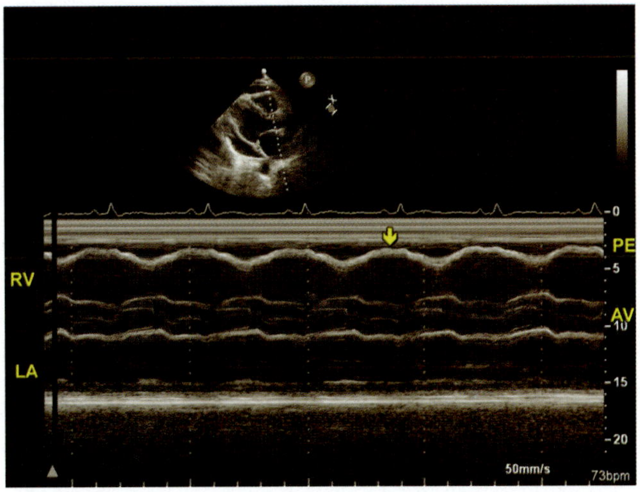

Fig. 170.1: M-mode echocardiogram showing flattening of RV wall with atrial systole (arrow) but there is no downward motion.

2. **Which of the following parameters is not an echocardiographic finding for tamponade?**
   (a) RV early diastolic collapse
   (b) RV mid systolic collapse
   (c) Decreased in mitral inflow E velocities by at least 25% during respiration
   (d) Dilated IVC with minimal or no collapse during respiration
   (e) Prominent septal bounce (ventricular interdependence)

Ans. (b)

MOVIES 543 TO 546

CASE 171

Bulur S, Adarna LG, Alagic N, Elsayed M, Uygur B, Turaga NSN, Chahwala JR, Taher A, Mohamed A, Arisha MJ, Elkaryoni A, Nanda NC

The patient is a 73-year-old female complaining of shortness of breath. She is known to have hepatitis C virus infection.

1. **What is the echo free space due to (arrow in 🎥 547 to 549)?**
   (a) Ascites
   (b) Loculated pericardial effusion
   (c) Pleural effusion
   (d) Echo lucent tumor or hematoma
   (e) Something else

Ans. (e)

This echo free space is produced by breast implants. The arrowhead in 🎥 550 is an artifact from the breast implant.

MOVIES 547 TO 550

SECTION 9

Tumors and Masses

CASE 172

Mohamed Ayan, Jitendra Pandya, Aiman Smer

An 82-year-old gentleman presented to ER with severe right-sided chest pain associated with significant shortness of breath of 4 hours duration. Physical exam showed tachycardia, tachypnea, and blood pressure of 129/78. Oxygen saturation was 94% on 3 L of oxygen. Chest and cardiovascular exam were normal. EKG showed sinus tachycardia with non-specific ST-T changes. Initial lab result showed D-dimer of 10.4 mg/L, troponin I of < 0.04 ng/mL. A transthoracic echocardiogram (TTE) at the bedside showed a free-floating 4.75 × 2.65 cm large size RA mass (arrow), severe RV dilatation and reduced RV systolic function (Fig. 172.1 and 551). CT angiogram showed extensive bilateral pulmonary emboli (PE) in interlobar arteries.

1. **What is the most likely diagnosis?**
   (a) Right atrial myxoma
   (b) Right atrial thrombus
   (c) Intracardiac lipoma
   (d) Secondary metastatic cardiac tumor

Ans. (b) Right atrial thrombus

The patient was started on IV heparin. Thrombolytic therapy was not a good option because he was hemodynamically stable. A repeat TTE on the second day showed complete disappearance of the thrombus (Fig. 172.2 and 552). Patient remained hemodynamically stable and his oxygen requirement remained unchanged. Extensive PE secondary to RA thrombus carry grave prognosis. The choice of treatment depends mainly on the patient's hemodynamics. In hemodynamically unstable patient thrombolytic therapy is the best initial treatment. Surgery and interventional techniques may be considered. However, in hemodynamically stable patient IV heparin could be tried first with close monitoring of the patient hemodynamics and good results have been reported.

MOVIE LEGENDS

551: TTE. Subcostal view showing a free-floating 4.75 × 2.65 cm size large RA thrombus (arrow).

552: TTE. Apical four chamber view showed complete disappearance of the thrombus.

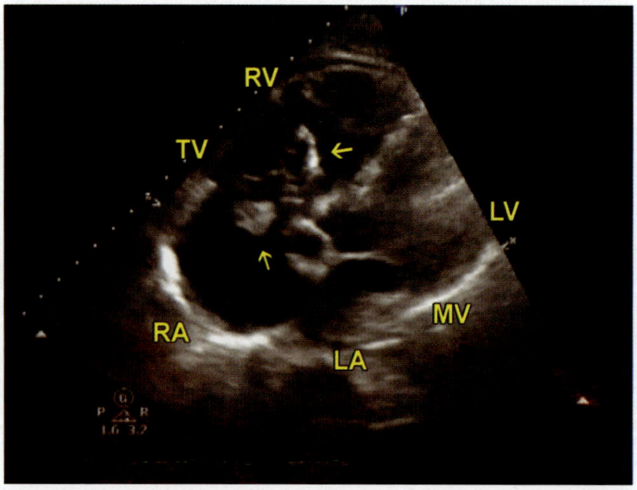

Fig. 172.1: TTE. Subcostal view showing a free-floating 4.75 x 2.65 cm size large RA thrombus (arrow).

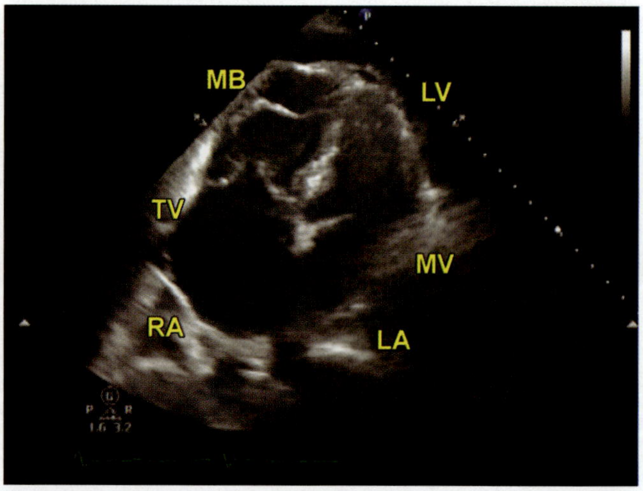

Fig. 172.2: TTE. Apical four chamber view showed complete disappearance of the thrombus.

CASE 173

Roomi AU, Elsayed M, Bulur S, Nanda NC

A 34-year-old obese male referred from a remote area with complaints of SOB NYHA (class II /III). He had 2 episodes of TIA.

He is known to have dilated cardiomyopathy with LVEF 25%, s/p implantable cardioverter-defibrillator lead inserted in a local hospital four months prior to presentation. 2D TTE and 2D TEE were done to rule out cardiac source of embolization (Figs. 173.1 to 173.6 and 553 to 558).

1. **What do you think caused the TIA in this patient?**
   (a) Carotid atherosclerosis

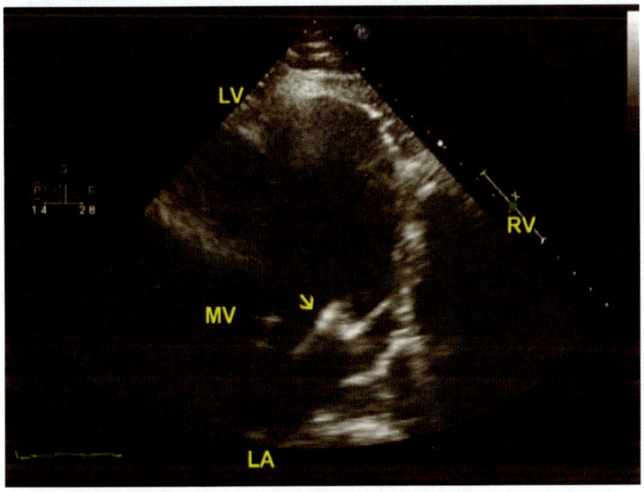

Fig. 173.1: Transthoracic apical view. Arrow points to implantable cardioverter defibrillator lead going through the MV.

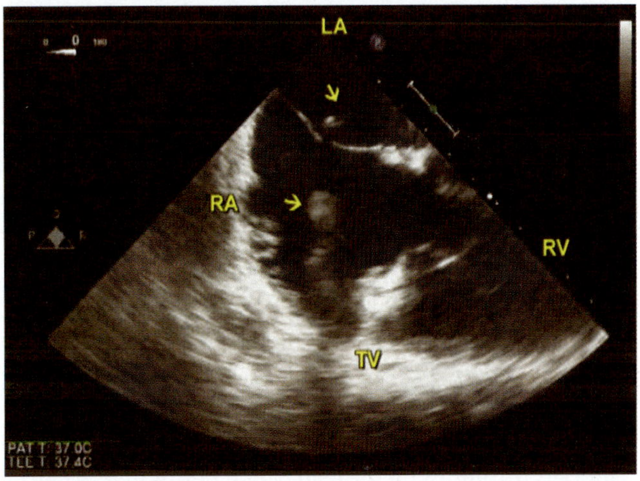

Fig. 173.2: Transesophageal echocardiography. Upper arrow points to the lead in LA while the lower arrow shows the RA lead.

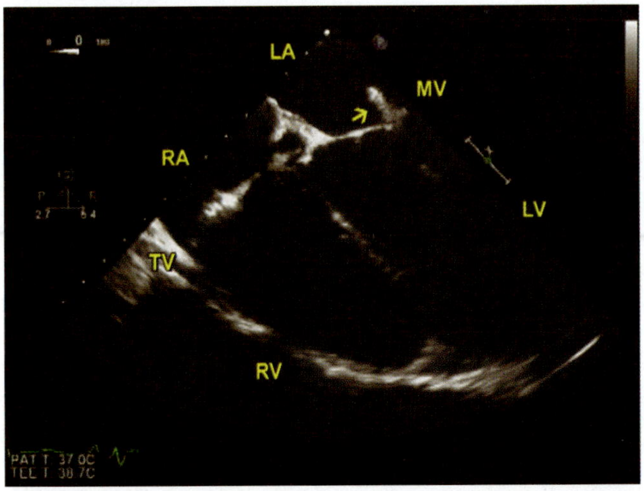

Fig. 173.3: Transesophageal echocardiography. Arrow points to the lead going through the MV.

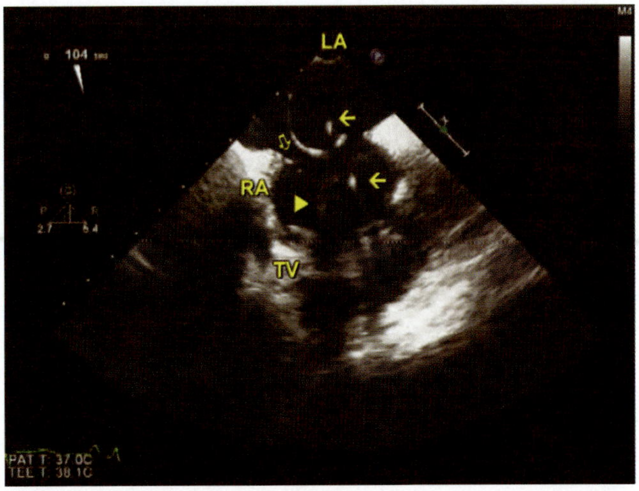

Fig. 173.4: Transesophageal echocardiography. Upper arrow points to the lead in LA while the lower arrow shows the lead in RA. Arrowhead points to thrombus attached to the lead. Hollow arrow points to Eustachian valve.

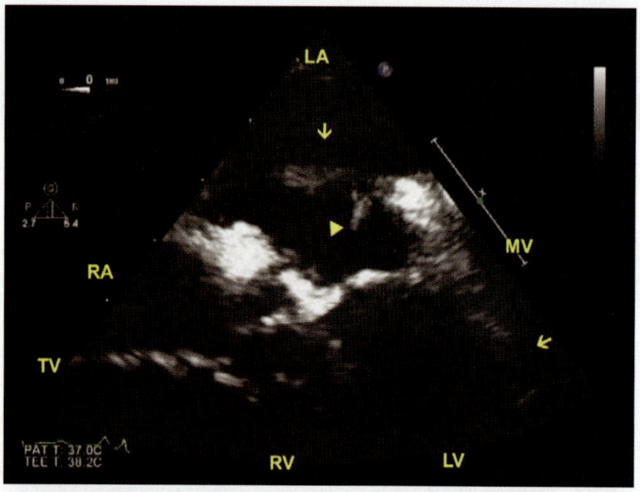

Fig. 173.5: Transesophageal echocardiography. Arrow points to the lead. Arrowhead demonstrates the thrombus attached to the lead.

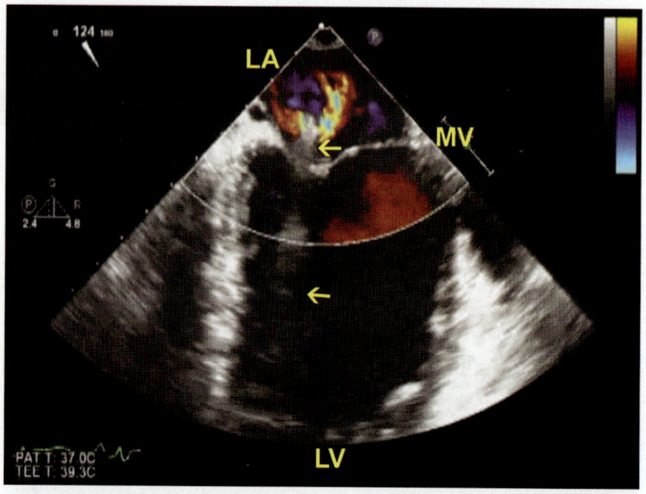

Fig. 173.6: Transesophageal echocardiography. Upper and lower arrows point to the lead in LA and LV, respectively.

(b) Cardioverter-defibrillator lead embolization

(c) Cardioverter-defibrillator lead thrombus embolization

(d) Lower extremity deep vein thrombosis

Ans. (c)

This is the most likely etiology given clear visualization of a mobile thrombus on the lead which perforated the atrial septum and entered the left heart.

Postoperative findings:

1. Mitral valve repair
2. LV lead extraction and reposition
3. ASD closure

MOVIE LEGENDS

553: Transthoracic apical view. Arrow points to implantable cardioverter defibrillator lead going through the MV.

554: Transesophageal echocardiography. Upper arrow points to the lead in LA while the lower arrow shows the RA lead.

555: Transesophageal echocardiography. Arrow points to the lead going through the MV.

556: Transesophageal echocardiography. Upper arrow points to the lead in LA while the lower arrow shows the lead in RA. Arrowhead points to thrombus attached to the lead. Hollow arrow points to Eustachian valve.

557: Transesophageal echocardiography. Arrow points to the lead. Arrowhead demonstrates the thrombus attached to the lead.

558: Transesophageal echocardiography. Upper and lower arrows point to the lead in LA and LV, respectively.

CASE 174

Elsayed M, Kalra R, Mustafa IA, Uygur B, McGiffin DC, Chahwala JR, Nanda NC

A 50-year-old female was referred to our hospital from an outside facility for neurosurgical evaluation of epidural abscesses. Her past medical history was notable for pulmonary embolism and end stage renal disease with dialysis through a tunneled (Groshong) catheter.

The patient had initially been noted to have methicillin-resistant *Staphylococcus aureus* bacteremia at an outside hospital, complicated by an epidural abscess. At the referring hospital, 2DTTE revealed a linear, mobile right atrial mass suggestive of thrombus with mild tricuspid regurgitation. No valvular vegetations were seen. Next, 2DTEE revealed a large, pedunculated, and mobile echodensity attached to the catheter tip and extending into the superior vena cava (SVC). Vegetations were not noted on 2DTEE.

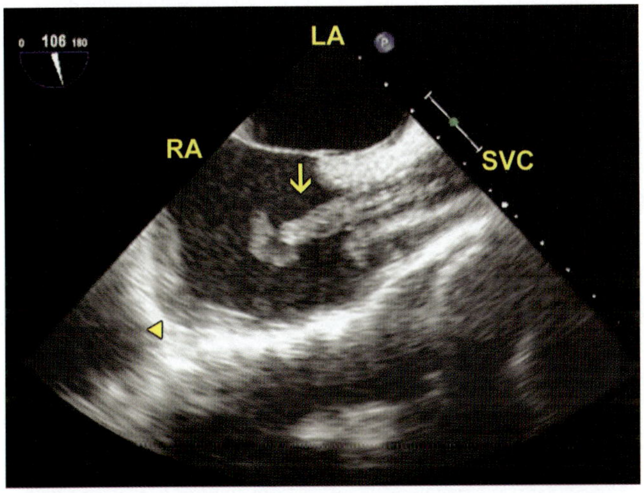

Fig. 174.1: Post catheter removal. Arrow points to a thrombus in the SVC extending into the RA. The RA component of the thrombus is mobile. Arrowhead points to another thrombus lining the RA wall.

After transfer to our hospital, the patient underwent successful thoracic laminectomy and excision of thoracic epidural phlegmon. Tunneled catheter removal was then planned due to persistence of the right atrial mass. In the operating room, the Groshong catheter was first removed with 2DTEE guidance. Right atriotomy revealed thrombus and total thrombectomy was performed. The fibrin sheath was then removed through meticulous dissection from the posterior wall of the SVC. Following a prolonged stay in the intensive care unit for management of hypertension and encephalopathy, the patient was discharged to her home.

2D (Fig. 174.1 and 559) and 3D (Figs. 174.2A and B and 560 and 561) TEE were done in the operating room.

1. **What incremental value did 3D TEE provide over 2D TEE?**
   (a) Much better visualization of the thrombus.
   (b) Volume of the thrombus and therefore assessment of thrombus burden

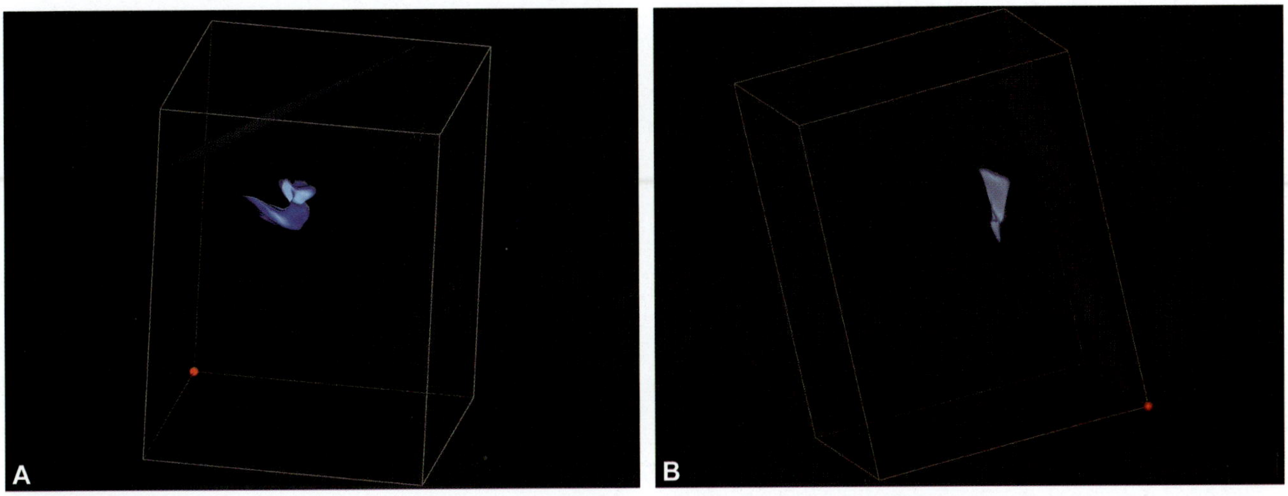

Figs. 174.2A and B: Volume measurement of the thrombus in RA (A) and SVC (B) using 3D TEE. Cropping of the 3D data set in Movie 560 shows prominent echolucencies within the SVC thrombus (arrow) viewed in short axis due to liquefaction and lysis. In Movie 561, the mobile component of the RA thrombus (arrow) is viewed in cross-section.

(c) Short axis view of the thrombus
(d) (b) and (c)
(e) All of the above

Ans. (d)

Cropping of thrombus using multiple planes and angulations provides its inside view which permits visualization of echolucencies resulting from thrombus liquefaction (lysis). The natural lytic elements in blood tend to dissolve the thrombus from inside and this dissolution is further facilitated by anticoagulants like warfarin. On the other hand, with thrombolytic therapy the thrombus tend to dissolve from outside. Volume measurement of thrombus by 3D is a much better parameter of size than dimensions estimated by 2D. The volume of the thrombus by 3D was 2.04 mL in RA (Fig. 174.2A) and 1.25 mL in SVC (Fig. 174.2B). The total volume of thrombus was 3.29 mL.

MOVIES 559 TO 561

CASE 175

Mohamed A, Gupta N, Elsayed M, Nanda NC

The patient is a 31-year-old female with end stage renal disease and a hemodialysis catheter in the SVC. 2D (562-566) and 3D (567-569) TTE were done. 562-564 and 567 are obtained from apical and left parasternal windows while 565, 566, 568 and 569 are taken using the right parasternal approach.

1. **What does the arrow most likely point to (562-566)?**
   (a) RA thrombus
   (b) RA tumor suggestive of myoxma
   (c) RA/TV vegetations
   (d) RA tumor of uncertain etiology since it is not a myxoma which would have been attached to the inter-atrial septum (IAS)

Ans. (a)

The association of the RA mass with a permacath makes thrombus a likely diagnosis. Main, left and right (origin) pulmonary arteries were also examined using a high left parasternal window and found to be clear without any thrombus (564).

2. **What incremental value one would expect 3D TTE (567-569) to have over 2D (562-566) TTE in this patient? All, but one of the following statements are accurate.**
   (a) More comprehensive assessment of RA mass and its size and volume.
   (b) Potential for looking inside the RA mass and evaluating its morphology.
   (c) Cropping of 3D datasets of RA thrombus would give a good idea of the number and extent of echolucencies which denote clot lysis/liquefaction.
   (d) May show the relationship of the RA thrombus to the permacath.
   (e) 3D provides better quality images than 2D TTE.
   (f) Assessment of attachment of RA mass to RA wall/IAS.

Ans. (e)

3D provides inferior quality images compared to 2D and therefore it is important to obtain best quality 2D images for 3D acquisition. Arrow in both 2D and 3D movies point to the RA thrombus, arrowhead to permacath in the SVC and asterisk to the crista terminalis. This case also demonstrates the usefulness of the right parasternal approach in assessing RA pathologies.

MOVIES 562 TO 569

CASE 176

Soung Ick Cho, Zarina Alam, Alma Tozaj, Mohsin Alam

Filling Defect or Lack of Flow?

A 60-year-old African American male with past medical history significant for HTN, COPD, CKD, alcohol and opioid abuse, and combined systolic/diastolic nonischemic cardiomyopathy, presented with worsening dyspnea on exertion and fatigue over the 2 days prior to admission, with increased lower extremity swelling and paroxysmal nocturnal dyspnea as well as weight gain, after running out on his blood pressure medications. He had previously been hospitalized for hypertensive emergency 4 months ago with asymmetric pulmonary edema, with improvement of symptoms with diuresis and BP control.

In the ED, he was noted to be hypertensive with BP 170/120, with prominent jugular veins and trace bibasilar crackles, with CXR revealing cardiomegaly with small bilateral pleural effusions, and was restarted on his home BP medications including Hydralazine, Isosorbide mononitrate, Metoprolol succinate and Nifedipine. He was determined to be volume overloaded and treated with IV diuresis, with Furosemide drip and restarted on Methadone and given possible withdrawal symptoms received Lorazepam IV and admitted to the general floors for further management.

His initial Cr was 3.22 mg/dL (from baseline of 1.9–2.1 on previous admission) with anion gap of 21, and BUN of 46 mg/dL, with LFTs consistent with congestive hepatopathy, and BNP of 2933 pg/mL.

His transthoracic echocardiogram from 4 months ago revealed LVEF 34%, moderate hypokinesis of the entire left ventricle wall, Grade 2 diastolic dysfunction, low normal RVSF, PASP estimated at 62 mm Hg, large Chiari network, (arrow in Figs. 176.1 and 176.2) and moderate to severe MR, eccentric, up to left pulmonary veins. A SPECT MPI performed for new onset HF evaluation showed no evidence of ischemia or infarction, but severely dilated left ventricle, moderate LV dysfunction, LVEF 38%, consistent with nonischemic dilated cardiomyopathy (Figs. 176.1 to 176.3 and 570–572).

After admission to the general floors, in the evening the patient was found non-responsive, with a very weak pulse, bradycardic in the 30s, agonal breathing, and unobtainable pulse oximetry or BP readings. He was given Atropine (0.5 mg IV) by the code team with HR improvement to the 50s, he was intubated for airway protection and given naloxone over concern of opiate overdose. He was transferred to the MICU and was started on high dose norepinephrine for hypotension. 12 hours later, the patient went onto asystole

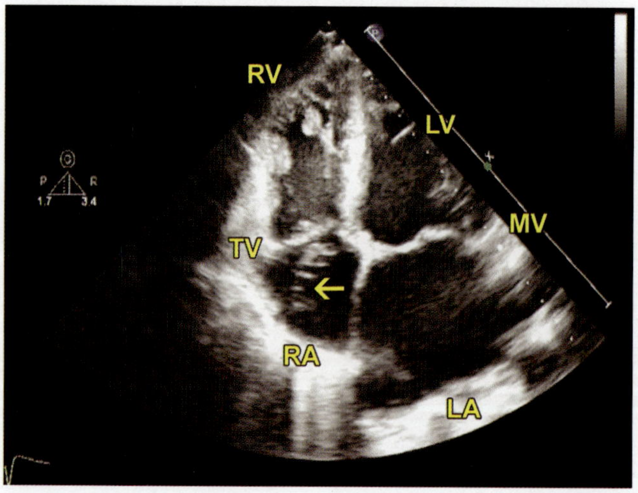

Fig. 176.1: Apical 4 chamber.

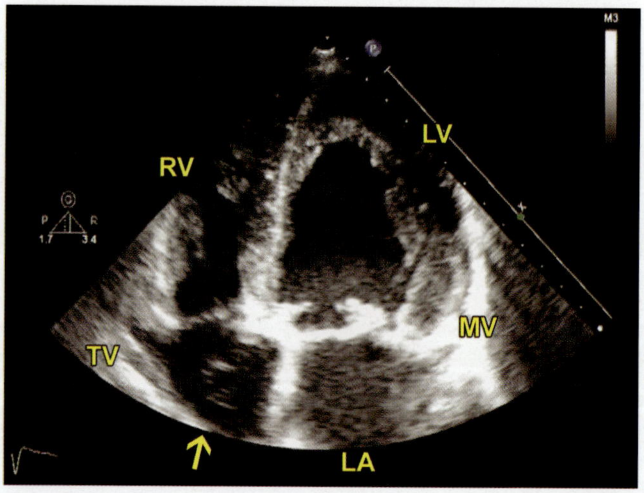

Fig. 176.2: Apical 4 chamber zoomed.

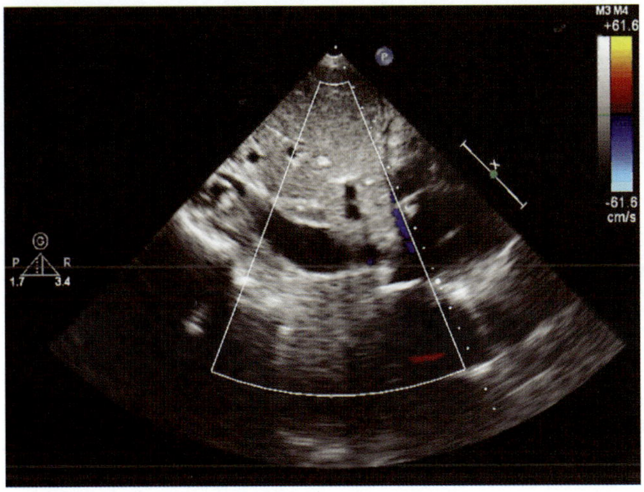

Fig. 176.3: Subcostal view, IVC.

and underwent CPR with ACLS protocol with ROSC achieved after several minutes, and requiring multiple high dose pressors including norepinephrine, dopamine and vasopressin. Also was started on broad spectrum antibiotics for possible septic shock. ECG post arrest did not reveal any significant ST segment changes.

An emergent echocardiographic evaluation was requested which was performed at the bedside and revealed the following images (573A and B).

1. **How would you explain the clinical presentation and the new echocardiographic findings?**
   (a) RCA territory infarct leading to acute RV failure
   (b) Worsening biventricular failure from progression of the NICM
   (c) Massive pulmonary embolism from DVT leading to acute RV failure
   (d) Stress cardiomyopathy due to administration of exogenous catecholaminergic agents/post cardiac arrest findings
   (e) Embolism of the Chiari's network leading to acute RV failure.

Ans. (c)

Transient LV systolic dysfunction in the absence of obstructive CAD can occur in patients with acute medical illness, especially those treated in intensive care units. The transient wall motion abnormalities associated with acute medical illness can present as global LV hypokinesis, apical and/or midventricular hypokinesis, or isolated apical and anterior hypokinesis.

Sepsis is a well-recognized cause for transient, global LV systolic dysfunction. It is estimated that up to 50% of patients with severe sepsis develop an associated reversible cardiomyopathy affecting both the left and right ventricles, with recovery of ventricular function within 7 to 10 days if the patient survives the acute phase of the illness.

Transient LV dysfunction can result from endogenous overproduction of catecholamines by neuroendocrine tumors (pheochromocytoma, neuroblastoma) and with the administration of exogenous catecholamines and catecholamine analogues. The LV wall motion abnormality in patients with pheochromocytoma crisis is generally global in nature, although apical sparing and Takotsubo-like wall motion abnormalities have been reported.

Transient cardiomyopathy resulting from administration of exogenous catecholamines has been reported after administration of beta-agonists and methylxanthines in those presenting with exacerbations of underlying obstructive airway disease, including asthma, and in those given intravenous and subcutaneous epinephrine in life-threatening situations.[1]

The Chiari network is a mobile, net-like structure occasionally seen in the right atrium near the opening of the inferior vena cava and coronary sinus. This is usually of no clinical significance and is often diagnosed incidentally.[2]

Sometimes it poses diagnostic difficulties during echocardiography where it could be misdiagnosed as right atrial thrombi, tumors and vegetations.[3,4]

The Chiari network protruding into the right ventricle may produce significant tricuspid regurgitation.[5]

By maintaining an embryonic right atrial flow pattern into adult life and directing the blood from the inferior vena cava preferentially toward the interatrial septum, Chiari's network may favor persistence of a patent foramen ovale and formation of an atrial septal aneurysm and facilitate paradoxic embolism.[6,7]

It may be associated with thrombi formation, and part of the strands may embolize. Infective endocarditis has been reported in association with the Chiari network.[8-12]

Interestingly, the Chiari network has been described to play a protective role in special situations, such as an inferior vena cava filter in patients with thrombophilia, and holding thrombus in the network preventing embolization.[13-15]

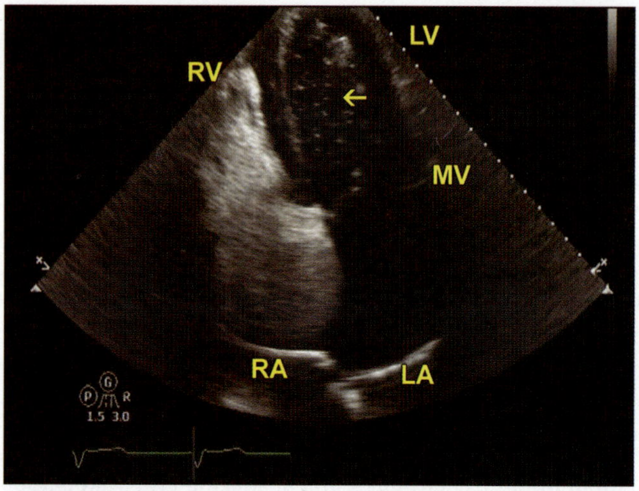

Fig. 176.4: Apical 4 chamber with ultrasound contrast. Arrow points to bubbles appearing in the LV.

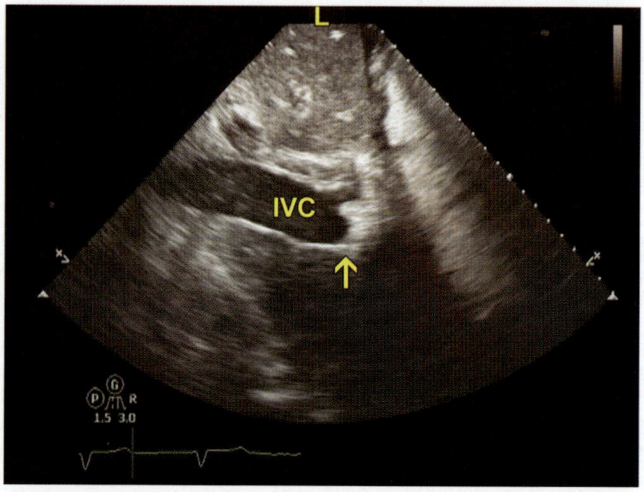

Fig. 176.5: Subcostal/IVC view with ultrasound contrast with delayed filling of the IVC. Arrow shows appearance of bubbles in the IVC.

Decision was made to administer perflutren ultrasound contrast agent in order to better define the wall motion abnormalities (Fig. 176.4 and 574).

2. **How would you explain the echocardiographic findings?**
   (a) Microspheres crossing R to L demonstrating the presence of PFO associated with the Chiari network
   (b) Delayed appearance of bubbles demonstrating R to L shunt due to intrapulmonary shunting/arteriovenous malformations (AVMs)
   (c) Normal pattern of L ventricular filling with ultrasound contrast agent
   (d) Low flow state/significant hemodynamic obstruction on the RV Outflow, delaying passage of microspheres from R to L circulation.

Ans. (d)

The presence of the severely enlarged right ventricle and severely reduced global RV systolic function, with the interatrial septum bowing from the Right to Left, which are new finding not seen in previous study, correlates with the diagnosis of acute RV failure with pressure/volume overload, which could be due to an acute obstruction of the RVOT, such as a large pulmonary embolism.

Use of second-generation perflutren-based echocardiographic contrast agents (perflutren) is currently contraindicated in patients with known right-to-left, bidirectional, or transient right to-left intracardiac shunts (intracardiac shunts) according to the US Food and Drug Administration. This contraindication is primarily a result of concerns related to neurological complications and/or systemic embolism from animal data describing entrapment of perflutren lipid microspheres (>5 mm in diameter) within small arterioles and capillaries in skeletal muscles after intra-arterial injection. To date, no definitive evidence demonstrates patient safety concerns from perflutren use in humans with intracardiac shunts.[16,17]

The microspheres are stable and small enough to pass through the pulmonary capillaries, and fill the endovascular space uniformly including the LA and LV which usually occurs within the first couple of cardiac cycles after being injected on the venous system. The isolated filling of the right sided chambers with only few microbubbles appearing in the left sided chambers is consistent with a low flow state/significant hemodynamic obstruction on the RV outflow, delaying passage of microspheres from R to L circulation.

The next set of Figure 176.5 and 575 and 576, demonstrated the presence of mass or thrombus occluding the inferior vena cava (revealing as contrast defect) and delayed filling of the IVC with minimal forward movement, with the contrast seen back flowing onto the hepatic veins, consistent with the diagnosis of acute RV failure with pressure/volume overload, due to a large pulmonary embolism with large emboli in transit in the IVC.

The use of perflutren-based echocardiographic contrast agent was fundamental in this case to differentiate a large thrombus in the IVC from stasis/low flow state in the IVC, and demonstrates other potential utilities of the echocardiographic contrast agents, besides assisting in the apex-endocardial border enhancement, cavity filling and myocardial perfusion imaging.

MOVIES 570 TO 576

REFERENCES

1. Bybee KA, Prasad A. Stress-related cardiomyopathy syndromes. Circulation. 2008;118:397-409.
2. Islam et al. Chiari Network: A case report and a brief overview. J Saudi Heart Assoc 2013;25:225-9.
3. Werner JA, Cheitlin MD, Gross BW, et al. Echocardiographic appearance of the Chiari network: differentiation from right heart pathology. Circulation. 1981;5:1104–9.
4. Payne DM, Baskett RJF, Hirsch GM. Infectious endocarditis of a Chiari network. Ann Thorac Surg 2003;76:1303–5.
5. Jen-Ping Chang JP. Tricuspid regurgitation as a result of Chiari network attachment. J Thorac Cardiovasc Surg. 2012; 143:235.
6. Schneider B, Hofmann T, Justen MH, et al. Chiari's network: normal anatomic variant or risk factor for arterial embolic events. J Am Coll Cardiol. 1995;26:203–10.
7. Lagunaa G, Arcea N, Blancoa M. Giant Chiari Network, Foramen Ovale, and Paradoxical Embolism. Rev Esp Cardiol. 2015;68:273.
8. Payne DM, Baskett RJF, Hirsch GM. Infectious endocarditis of a Chiari network. Ann Thorac Surg. 2003;76:1303–5.
9. Yater WM. The paradox of Chiari's network. Am Heart J 1936;1936(11):542–53.
10. Powell EDU, Mullaney JM. The Chiari network and the valve of the inferior vena cava. Br Heart J. 1960;22:579–84.
11. Mousavi N, Bhagirath K, Ariyarajah V, Fang T, Ahmadie R, Lytwyn M, et al. Chiari network endocarditis: not just an innocent bystander. Echocardiography. 2008;25(6):642-5.
12. Lejko-Zupanc T, Kozelj M, Pikelj F. Right sided endocarditis: clinical and echocardiographic characteristics. J Clin Basic Cardiol. 1999;2:81–4.
13. Obaji SG, Cooper R, Somauroo J. Chiari network: a protective filter against pulmonary embolism in a case of polycythaemia. BMJ Case Rep 2012. http://dx.doi.org/ 10.1136/ bcr.05.2011.4289.
14. Motovska Z, Widimsky P, Bilkova D, Penicka M, Linkova H, Kautznerova D, et al. An embolus in the right atrium caught in the Chiari network and resistant to thrombolysis. J Thromb Thrombolysis. 2010;30(1):114–8.
15. Goedde TA, Conetta D, Rumisek JD. Chiari network entrapment of thromboemboli: congenital inferior vena cava filter. Ann Thorac Surg. 1990;49(2):317–8.
16. Parker JM, Weller MW, Feinstein LM, et al. Safety of ultrasound contrast agents in patients with known or suspected cardiac shunts. Am J Cardiol. 2013;112:1039–45.
17. Porter TR, et al. Guidelines for the Cardiac Sonographer in the Performance of Contrast Echocardiography: A Focused Update from the American Society of Echocardiography. J Am Soc Echocardiogr. 2014;27:797-810.

CASE 177

Ramdas G Pai

HISTORY

- A 27-year-old female, multiparous, 37 week gestation
- She had no other medical history
- She was confined to bedrest for several weeks because of antepartum hemorrhage and uterine contractions
- Developed shortness of breath on exertion, no other symptoms
- On physical examination: Obese, 1-2+ edema of the legs, no murmurs, ECG unremarkable
- Echocardiogram was obtained

1. **What does the arrow point to in Figure 177.1?**
   (a) Left atrial myxoma
   (b) Paradoxical embolism
   (c) Artifact from ascending aorta
   (d) Fossa ovalis aneurysm

Ans. (d) Fossa ovalis aneurysm

2. **What will you do next? (See Figure 177.2 and 577 and 578)**
   (a) Perform immediate TEE to evaluate left atrial mass
   (b) Start IV heparin and perform chest CT with contrast
   (c) Diurese with IV lasix
   (d) Send the patient to surgery

Ans. (b) Start IV heparin and perform chest CT with contrast

3. **What does the chest CT show? (Figs. 177.3A and B)**
   (a) Pulmonary emboli
   (b) Aortic dissection
   (c) Nothing abnormal

Ans. (a) Pulmonary emboli (pointed by the arrows in the CT images) (Fig. 177.4)

DISCUSSION

Note the dilated and hypokinetic RV in 577 and 578. In a pregnant patient (who is hypercoagulable) confined to bed and short of breath, it should raise the possibility of pulmonary embolism. The "mass" in the left atrium is the aneurysmal atrial septum bulging to the left (because of elevated right atrial pressure) and cut tangentially. The patient is not hemodynamically compromized to warrant thrombolytics. There is no absolute contraindication for thrombolytics in pregnancy and can be used if necessary.

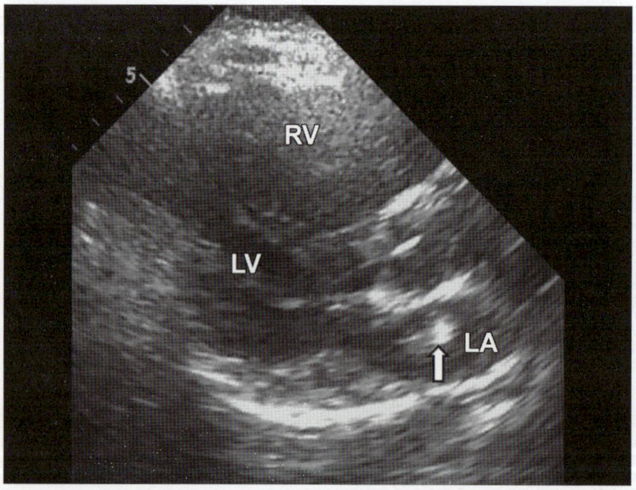

Fig. 177.1: Transthoracic parasternal long axis view. Arrow points to fossa ovalis aneurysm.

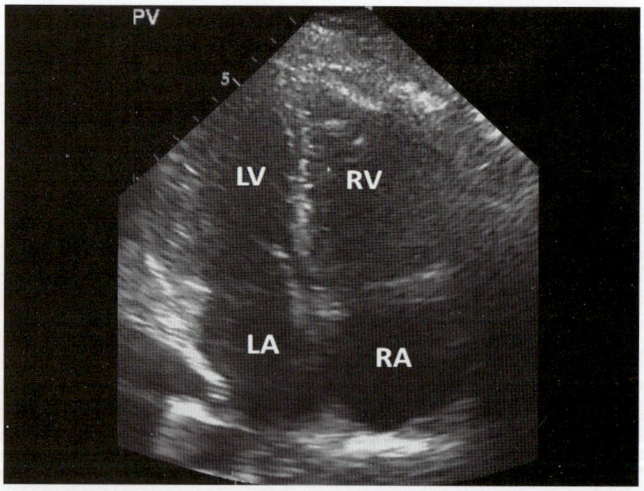

Fig. 177.2: Transthoracic apical 4 chamber view showing similar findings as above.

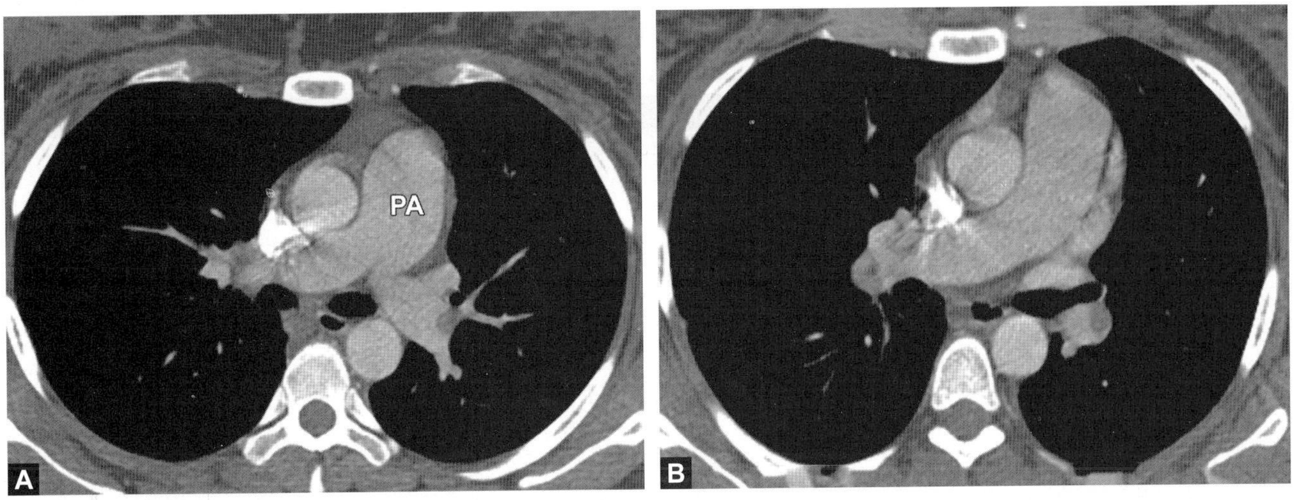

Figs. 177.3A and B: CT pulmonary angiography.

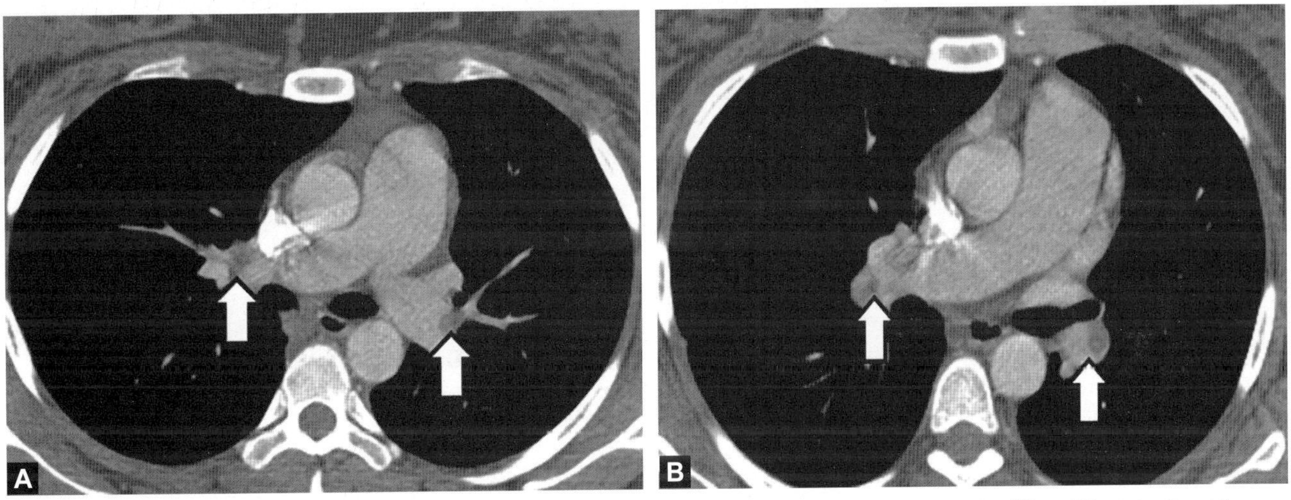

Figs. 177.4A and B: Same CT pulmonary angiography as in Figures 177.3 A and B with arrows pointing to filling defects in the pulmonary arteries suggestive of multiple pulmonary emboli.

MOVIE LEGENDS

577: Transthoracic parasternal long axis view. Arrow points to fossa ovalis aneurysm.

578: Transthoracic apical 4 chamber view showing similar findings as above.

CASE 178

Elsayed M, Hsiung MC, Meggo-Quiroz LD, Elguindy M, Uygur B, Tandon R, Guvenc T, Keser N, Vural MG, Bulur S, Chahwala JR, Abtahi F, Nanda NC

This is a 54-year-old male presented with left-sided hemiplegia. Magnetic resonance imaging findings were suggestive of ischemic stroke. Both 2DTEE and 3DTEE demonstrated a large mass measuring more than 2 cm in a left sided atrial septal pouch (LASP). The mass contained multiple echolucencies similar to those visualized in thrombi and suggestive of clot lysis and liquefaction. The patient was placed on warfarin and repeat 2DTEE and 3DTEE performed a month later showed complete resolution of the mass without any clinical or laboratory evidence of embolization. These findings suggest the mass was most likely a thrombus (Figs. 178.1–178.6 and 579–581).

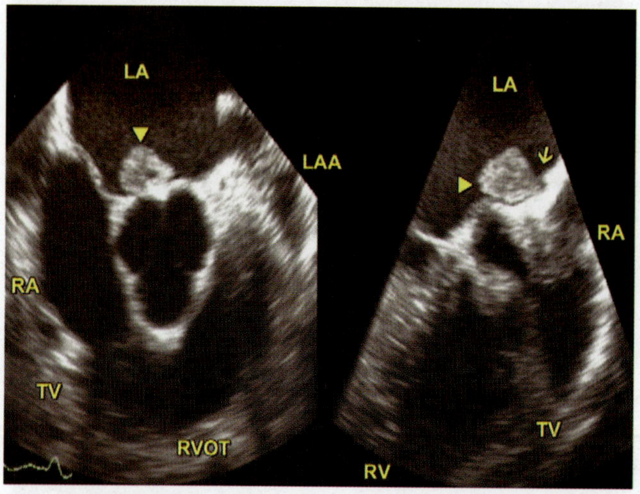

Fig. 178.1: 2DTEE. Arrow points to the atrial septal pouch and the arrowhead to the thrombus.

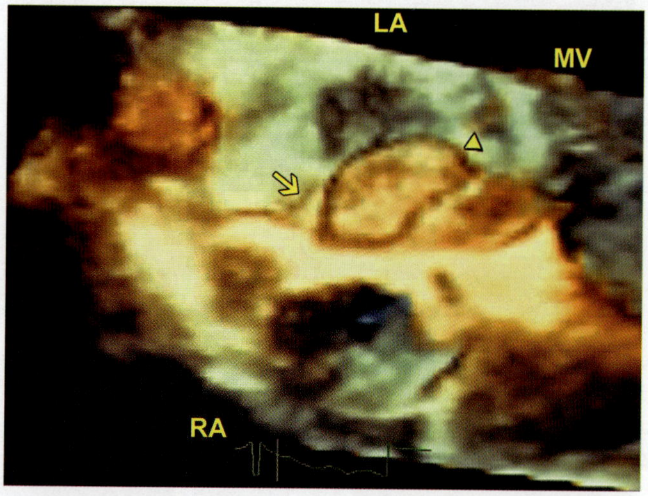

Fig. 178.2: 3DTEE. Arrow points to the atrial septal pouch and the arrowhead to the thrombus. Note the presence of echolucencies in the thrombus consistent with lysis.

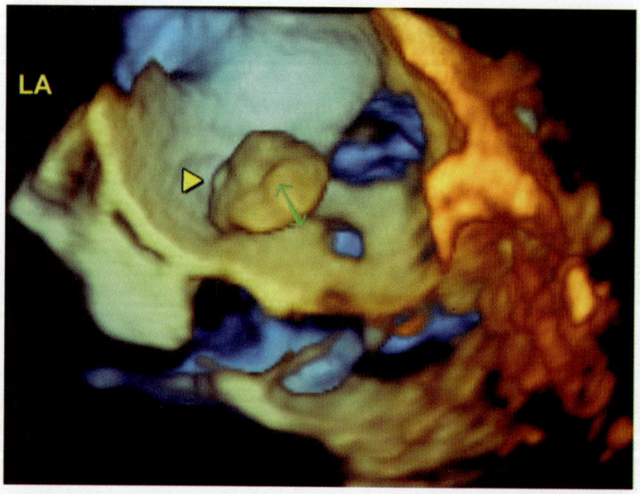

Fig. 178.3: 3DTEE. Arrowhead points to the mass in the atrial septal pouch.

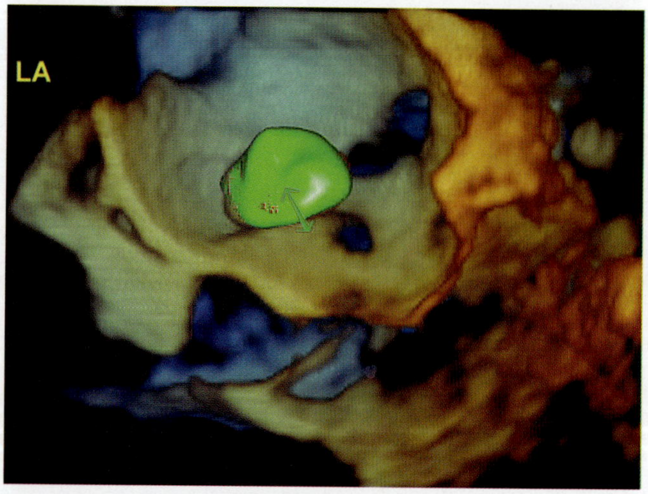

Fig. 178.4: 3DTEE. The green colored mass represents a thrombus.

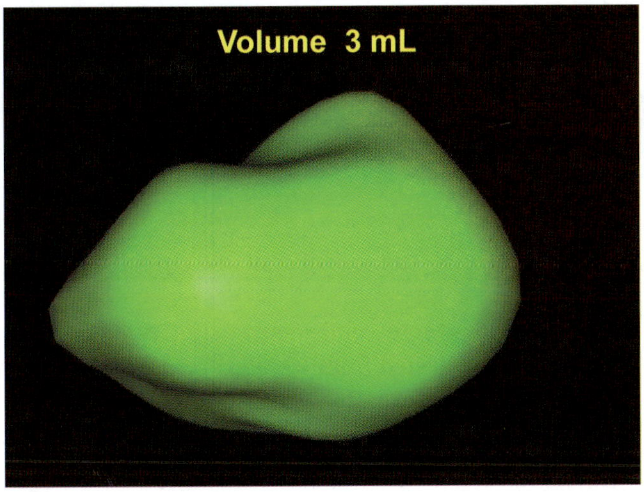

Fig. 178.5: 3DTEE. The volume of the thrombus measured 3.0 mL.

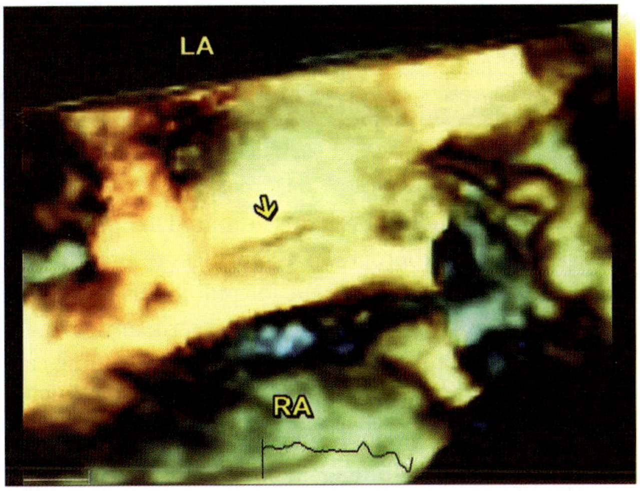

Fig. 178.6: 3DTEE. Arrow points to complete resolution of the thrombus following anticoagulation therapy.

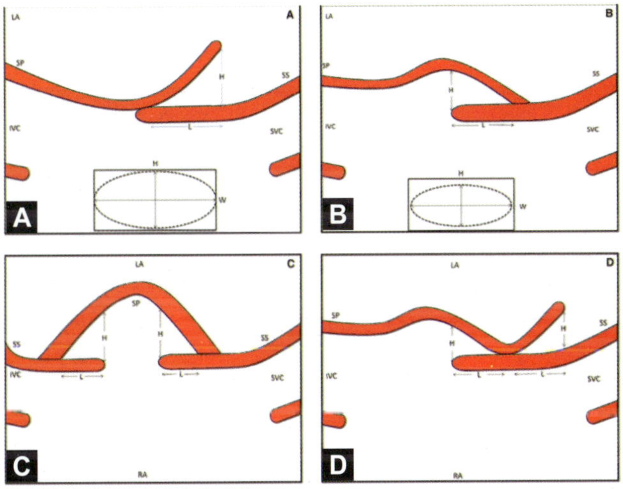

Figs. 178.7A to D: Schematic drawing of atrial septal pouches as demonstrated by transesophageal echocardiography. (A) Left atrial septal pouch. (B) Right atrial septal pouch. (C) Two right atrial septal pouches in the same patient. (D) Right and left atrial septal pouches in the same patient. The length (L) and height (H) of the pouches were measured by both two and three-dimensional transesophageal echocardiography. In addition, three-dimensional echocardiography facilitated measurements of width (W), area and volume of the pouch. (IVC: Inferior vena cava; LA: Left atrium; RA: Right atrium; SP: Septum premium; SS: Septum secundum; SVC: Superior vena cava). *Courtesy*: This case is reproduced with permission from: Elsayed M, Hsiung MC, Meggo-Quiroz LD, Elguindy M, Uygur B, Tandon R, Guvenc T, Keser N, Vural MG, Bulur S, Chahwala JR, Abtahi F, Nanda NC. Incremental Value of Live/Real Time Three-Dimensional over Two-Dimensional Transesophageal Echocardiography in the Assessment of Atrial Septal Pouch. Echocardiography. 2015 Dec;32(12):1858-67.

DISCUSSION

An atrial septal pouch (ASP) is defined as an incomplete fusion of the septum primum and the septum secundum, which can be visualized in the standard or modified bicaval view by 2D TEE. The fusion at the caudal limit of the zone of overlap results in a left atrial septal pouch (LASP). Reversely, the fusion at the cranial limit of the zone of overlap results in a right atrial septal pouch (RASP). An additional fusion of the overlap zone at some other point would theoretically create a second atrial septal pouch (Fig. 178.7). Prospective and retrospective studies have not yet conclusively established an association between LASP and strokes but the ASP is a potential location for stasis and therefore it needs to be routinely visualized to rule out the presence of a thrombus especially in patients with embolic stroke.

MOVIE LEGENDS

579: 2DTEE. Arrow points to the atrial septal pouch and the arrowhead to the thrombus.

580: 3DTEE. Arrow points to a margin of the pouch which contains the thrombus (arrowhead) which measured larger than two-dimensional imaging. The volume of the mass measured 3 mL.

581: 3DTEE. It shows complete disappearance of the thrombus in the pouch (arrow) one month after anticoagulant therapy with warfarin.

CASE 179

Thind M, Ahmed MI, Gok G, Joson M, Elsayed M, Tuck BC, Townsley MM, Klas B, McGiffin DC, Nanda NC

A 68-year-old female patient was admitted to our hospital with chest pain and progressive shortness of breath. Past medical history was significant for pulmonary thromboembolism for which she received short-term anticoagulation therapy. 2D and 3D TEE were done. The findings are illustrated in Figures 179.1A to C and 582A-C (2D TEE) and Figures 179.2A to J and 583A-I (3D TEE).

1. **How would you manage a patient with a thrombus in-transit:**
   (a) Anticoagulant therapy
   (b) Antiplatelet therapy
   (c) Emergency surgery
   (d) Thrombolytic therapy

Ans. (c)

This is because the chances of systemic embolization are very high.

Echo findings were confirmed at surgery and a long thrombus was resected from RA, PFO and LA (Fig. 179.3 and 584). Large thrombi were also removed from LPA and RPA. The PFO was closed. She did well and was discharged without any neurological or other deficits. She was begun on long-term anticoagulation with warfarin but was subsequently diagnosed with metastatic gastric carcinoma. Later, she suffered embolic stroke with multiple cerebral infarcts and was discharged to a rehab facility.

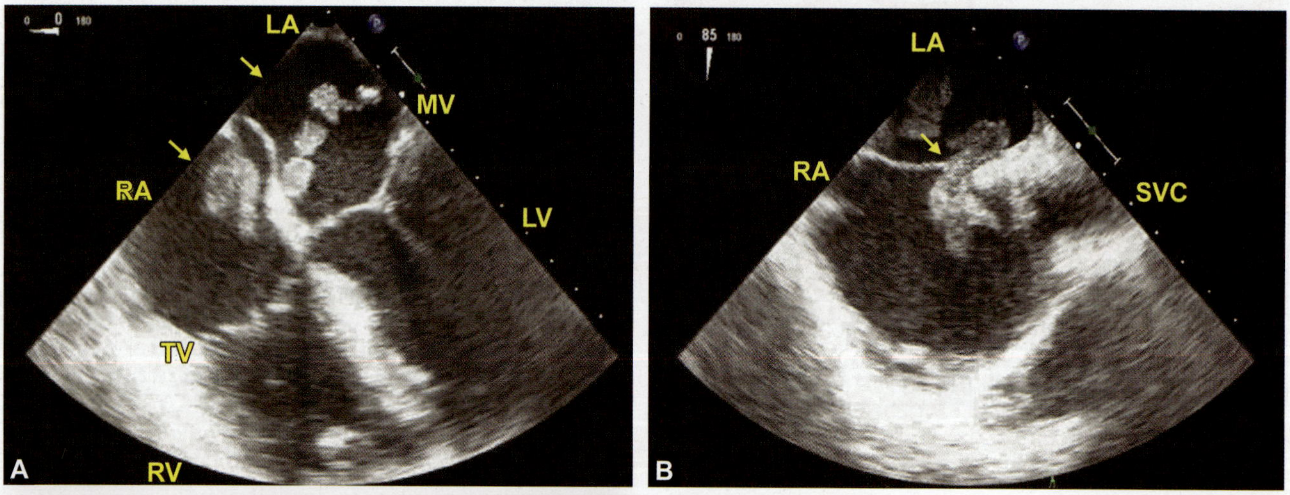

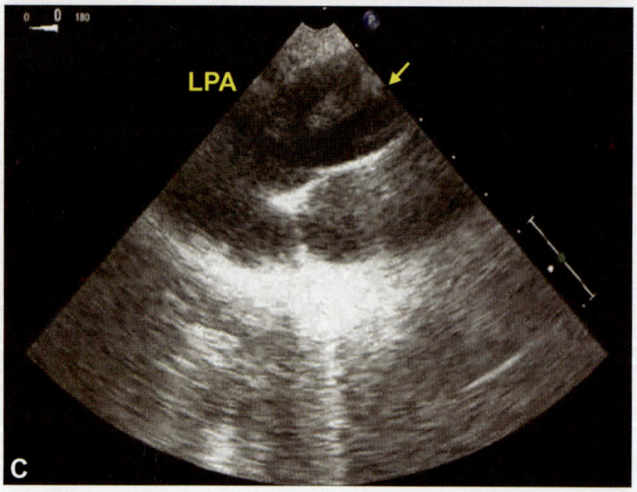

Figs. 179.1A to C: Two-dimensional transesophageal echocardiography of a thrombus in transit through a patent foramen ovale. (A) Arrows show a mass in the right atrium (RA) and multiple masses in the left atrium (LA). The tricuspid valve (TV), right ventricle (RV), mitral valve (MV) and left ventricle (LV) are also seen. (B) Arrow shows point where mass is stretching open patent foramen ovale when transiting from the RA to the LA. The superior vena cava (SVC) is also seen. (C) Arrow shows the mass within the left pulmonary artery (LPA).

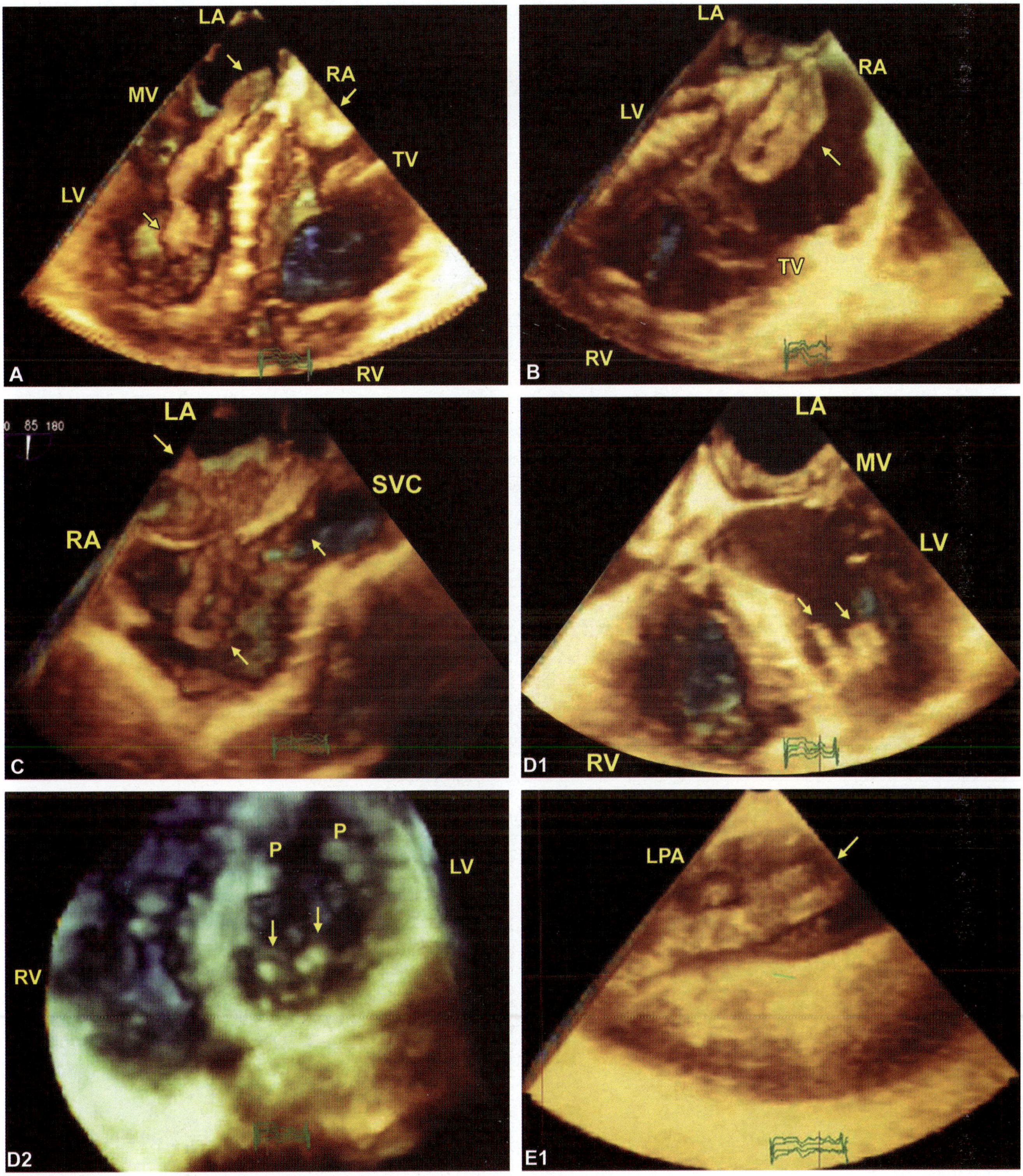

Figs. 179.2A to E1

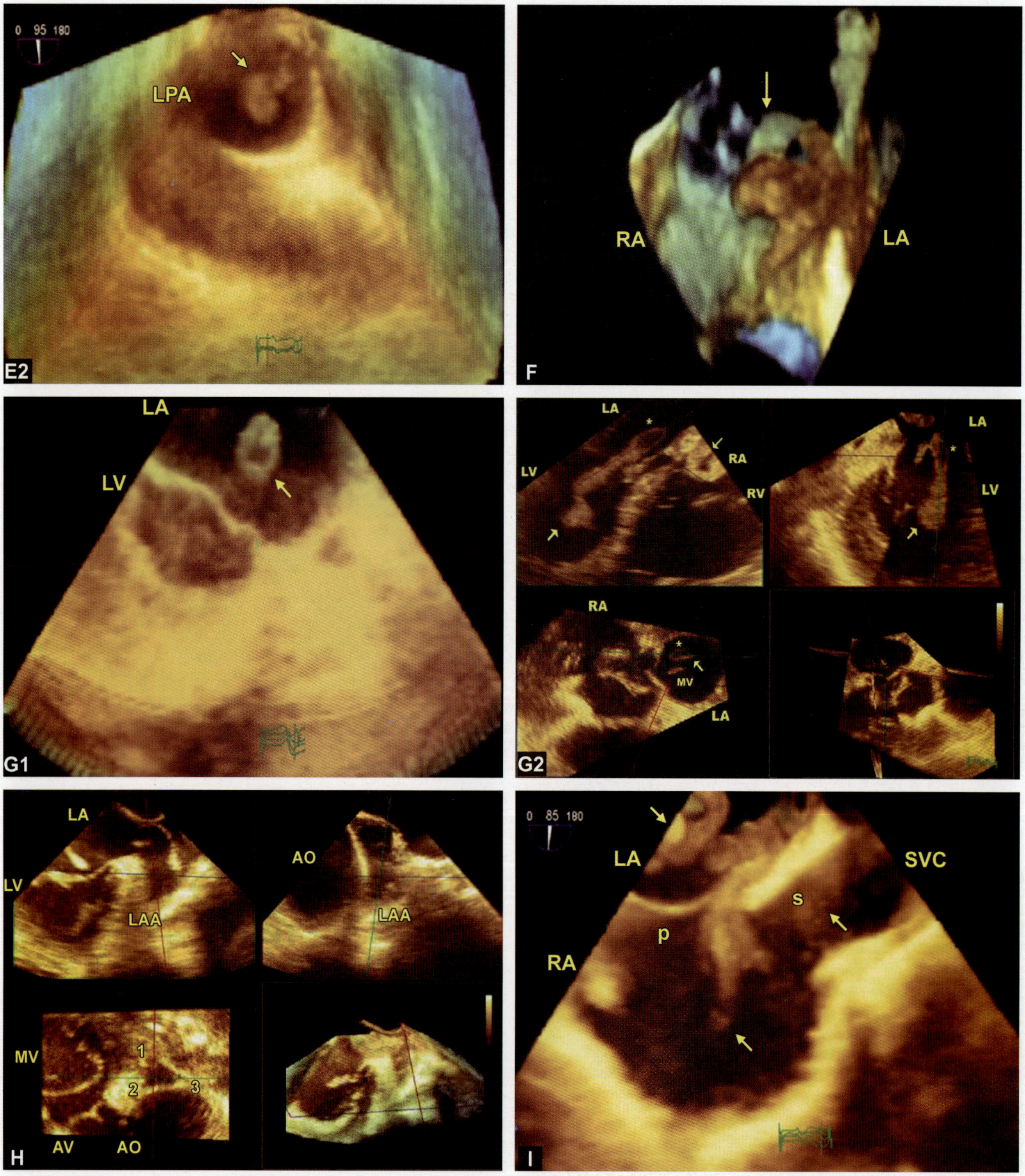

Figs. 179.2E2 to I

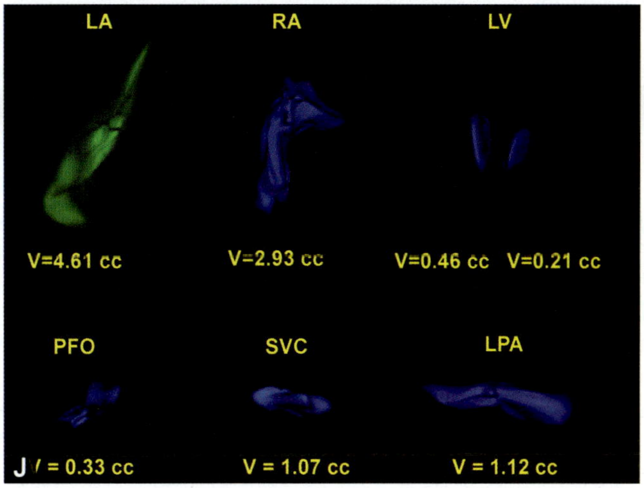

Figs. 179.2A to J: Three-dimensional transesophageal echocardiography of a thrombus in transit through a patent foramen ovale. (A) Arrows show a looped mass in the right atrium (RA) and a serpentine mass extending from the left atrium (LA), through the mitral valve (MV), into the left ventricle (LV) during diastole. The tricuspid valve (TV) and right ventricle (RV) are also seen. (B) Arrow points to a looped mass in the RA. (C) Arrows show mass in the superior vena cava (SVC), RA, transiting through the patent foramen ovale and in the LA. (D1) Two masses seen lodged in the apex of the LV. (D2) This short-axis view of the LV apex clearly shows two distinct masses (arrows) separate from the papillary muscles (P). (E1) Arrow points to the mass in the left pulmonary artery (LPA). (E2) Arrow points to the mass in the short-axis view of the LPA. (F) Arrow shows mass in the RA suspended across the interatrial septum. (G1) This cross-section of the mass (arrow) in the LA shows an echolucent area within the mass consistent with thrombus lysis. (G2) Multiplanar reconstruction (MPR) mode. The green box (upper left panel) shows a four chamber view with arrows pointing to the mass. The red box (upper right panel) shows a two chamber view at the level of the red line in the green box. The blue box (lower left panel) is a short-axis view of the atria at the level of the blue line in the green box. The asterisk in each panel marks the echolucent area within the mass consistent with thrombus lysis. (H) Multiplanar reconstruction (MPR) mode. The green box (upper left panel) shows the LA, LV and left atrial appendage (LAA). The red box (upper right panel) shows the LAA at the level of the red line in the green box (upper left panel). The aorta (AO) is also seen. The blue box (lower left panel) shows a short-axis view of the LAA at the level of the blue line in the green box. Three lobes (1, 2, 3) of the LAA can be seen free of mass. (I) Arrows point to the mass traversing the patent foramen ovale (PFO). The mass can be seen separating septum primum (P) from septum secundum (S). (J) Depicts the volumes (V) of the mass in the LA, RA, LV, PFO, SVC and LPA. Movies 582A to C, 583A1, 583A2, 583B to 583.1. *Source*: This case is reproduced with permission from Thind M, Ahmed MI, Gok G, Joson M, Elsayed M, Tuck BC, Townsley MM, Klas B, McGiffin DC, Nanda NC. Incremental Value of Three-Dimensional Transesophageal Echocardiography over the Two-Dimensional Technique in the Assessment of a Thrombus in Transit through a Patent Foramen Ovale. Echocardiography. 2015;32(5):848-54.

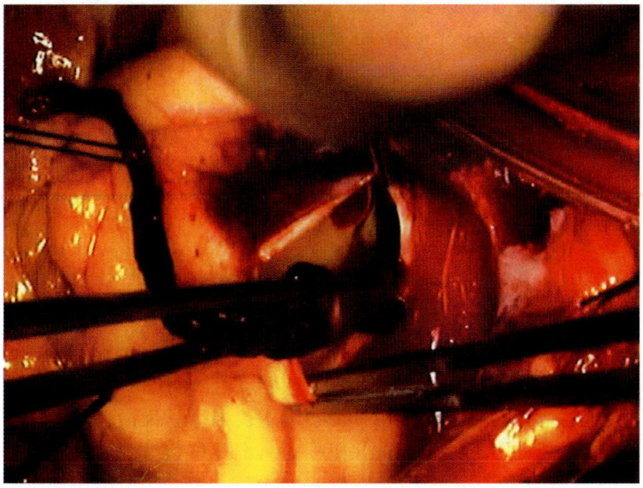

Fig. 179.3: Shows removal of the thrombus during surgery.

MOVIES 582 TO 584

CASE 180

Omer Iqbal, Paul O'Malley

THROMBUS IN TRANSIT

A 23-year-old female was admitted with a history of transient ischemic attacks. The patient's medical history indicates that two years ago she had an incident of deep vein thrombosis which after further testing was believed to be as a result of a deficiency in protein C and S. Since then she has been taking warfarin. TEE revealed a thrombus crossing a patent foramen ovale (PFO) (Fig. 180.1 and 585)

Based on the above scenario answer the following:

1. **The percutaneous PFO closure devices which were investigated in randomized trials include:**
   (a) Amplatzer (AMP)
   (b) STARFlex (STF)
   (c) HELLEX (HLX)
   (d) All of the above
   (e) None of the above

Ans. (d)

The three percutaneous PFO closure devices investigated in randomized trials were Amplatzer PFO Occluder (AMP, St Jude Medical, Plymouth, MN, USA; STARFlex Septal Occluder (STF), NMT Medical, Boston, MS, USA; and HELEX PFO Occluder (HLX, W.L. Gore and Associates, Flagstaff, AZ, USA.[1]

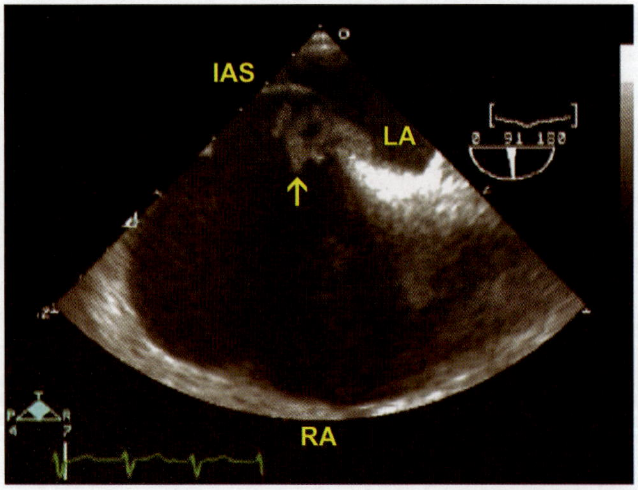

Fig. 180.1: Transesophageal echocardiography: Arrow points to a large mass of thrombi, some with mobile components, wedged in the PFO.

2. **Recently published randomized trials established superiority of percutaneous PFO closure over medical therapy in patients with cryptogenic stroke or embolism.**
   (a) True
   (b) False

Ans. (b)

Recently published randomized trials failed to establish superiority of percutaneous PFO closure over medical therapy in patients with cryptogenic stroke or embolism.[2-4] Possible reasons include unrealistically large treatment effects assumed for sample size considerations and lower event rates than anticipated (1); variation of effectiveness and safety between different devices, with potential differences in the effectiveness of the device to close the PFO (1); the risk of thrombus formation due to the thrombogenecity of the surface material[5,6]; and the risk of onset of atrial fibrillation associated with device implantation.[7]

3. **The potential complications of using percutaneous PFO closure devices is:**
   (a) Excessive bleeding
   (b) Thrombus formation on device
   (c) Both
   (d) None of the above

Ans. (c)

The potential complication of using the percutaneous PFO closure devices is the risk of thrombus formation due to the thrombogenicity of the surface material (also see explanation given for Q2).

4. **The ideal PFO closure device should be able to:**
   (a) Minimize bleeding
   (b) Minimize risk of atrial fibrillation (AF)
   (c) Provide higher rates of effective closure
   (d) Minimize thrombus formation
   (e) B, C, D only

Ans. (e)

The ideal PFO closure device should minimize the risk of thrombogenicity, minimize the risk of atrial fibrillation and increase the rates of effective closure. There is no reported incidence of bleeding with the use of PFO closure devices. However, the doses of anticoagulants given for thrombogenicity due to PFO closure devices should be carefully calibrated to avoid the risk of bleeding complications.

5. According to GLORIA-AF Registry (n = 3415), patients with non-valvular AF who were at a high risk of stroke were found to be undertreated with oral anticoagulants. Of the patients studied the percentage of patients who had AF and the percentage of patients who did not receive oral anticoagulants included:

(a) 65.9% had paroxysmal AF- 21.9% did not receive warfarin or newer oral anticoagulant drugs (NOAD).

(b) 29.5% had persistent AF- 12.4% did not receive warfarin or NOAD

(c) 4.6% had permanent AF- 11.2% did not receive warfarin or NOAD

(d) All of the above

Ans. (d)

Oral anticoagulants are reported to be underused for stroke prevention in non-valvular atrial fibrillation. As per GLORIA-AF Registry, new data suggest that patients with non-valvular AF at high risk of stroke with a CHA2DS2-VASc Score of 2 are undertreated with oral anticoagulants and that the initial therapy is not prescribed in accordance with the guidelines recommendation. Of the 3415 patients studied in this registry, 65.9% had paroxysmal AF- 21.9% did not receive warfarin or NOAD; 29.5% had persistent AF- 12.4% did not receive warfarin or NOAD; and 4.6% had permanent AF- 11.2% did not receive warfarin or NOAD.[8]

6. New oral anticoagulants have a favorable risk-benefit profile with significant reductions in stroke, intracranial hemorrhage and mortality and with similar major bleeding as for warfarin but increased gastrointestinal bleeding:

(a) True

(b) False

Ans. (a)

As per the results of a meta-analysis of randomized trials, a comparison of the efficacy and safety of new oral anticoagulants with warfarin in patients with atrial fibrillation, new oral anticoagulants had a favorable risk-benefit profile with significant reductions in stroke, intracranial hemorrhage and mortality and with similar major bleeding as for warfarin but increased gastrointestinal bleeding.[9]

7. Which of the following is not an ideal candidate for new oral anticoagulants?

(a) Over the age of 75

(b) Mechanical valve

(c) Pregnant

(d) All of the above

(e) The above indications still allow for new oral anticoagulant therapy

Ans. (d)

The ideal candidates for new oral anticoagulant therapy are the patients with unstable INR on warfarin which is not due to poor compliance; have good renal and hepatic function; have no mechanical valve; not pregnant (drugs cross placenta); under the age of 75 years; have no history of lower gastrointestinal bleeding; and not at high risk for acute coronary syndrome.

MOVIE LEGEND

585: Transesophageal echocardiography. Arrow points to thrombus in transit through a patent foramen ovale.

REFERENCES

1. Stortecky S, da Costa BR, Mattle HP, et al. European Heart Journal 2015;36:120-8.
2. Furlan AJ, Reisman M, Massaro J, et al. Closure or medical therapy for cryptogenic stroke with patent foramen ovale. N Engl J Med. 2012;366:991-9.
3. Meier B, Kalesan B, Mattle HP, et al. Percutaneous closure of patent foramen ovale in cryptogenic embolism. N Engl J Med. 2013;368:1083-91.
4. Carroll JD, Saver JL, Thaler DE, et al. Closure of patent foramen ovale versus medical therapy after cryptogenic stroke. N Engl J Med. 2013;368:1092-1100.
5. Anzai H, Child J, Natterson B, et al. Incidence of thrombus formation on the cardioSEAL and the Amplatzer interatrial closure devices. Am J Cardiol. 2004;93:426-31.
6. Krumsdorf U, Ostermayer S, Billinger K, et al. Incidence and clinical course of thrombus formation on atrial septal defect and patent foramen ovale closure devices in 1,000 consecutive patients. J Am Coll Cardiol. 2004;43:302-9.
7. Johnson JN, Marquardt ML, Ackerman MJ, et al. Electrocardiographic changes and arrhythmias following percutaneous atrial septal defect and patent foramen ovale closure. Catheter Cardiovasc Interv. 2011;78:254-61.
8. Halperin JL, et al. Abstracts 1246-122 and 1246-124 presented at ACC Scientific Session; March 14-16, 2015, San Diego, CA, USA.
9. Ruff CT, Giugliano RP, Braunwald E, et al. Comparison of the efficacy and safety of new oral anticoagulants with warfarin in patients with atrial fibrillation: a meta-analysis of randomized trials. Lancet. 2014;383:955-62.

CASE 181

Sibel Catirli Enar

LEFT RETINAL VEIN OCCLUSION IN SINUS RHYTHM

A 67-year-old man was referred to the cardiology department from the ophthalmology department. One week prior he developed severe sight impairment. He was diagnosed as having left retinal vein occlusion and sent to our department for further evaluation.

History: Newly diagnosed hypertension and smoker for 20 years. Family history was positive for coronary artery disease.

Lab findings: Total cholesterol: 215 mg/dl, LDL cholesterol: 140 mg/dL, Homocystein: 29.2 µmol/L, CRP 5 mg/L Protein C and Protein S: Normal, Uric acid: 7.3 mg/dL. ECG: Sinus rhythm, LVH, negative T waves in V4-6.

Carotid ultrasound: No stenosis was diagnosed, atheromatous plaques were present. Rhythm Holter: no paroxysmal atrial fibrillation (PAF) was detected. 2DTTE (586) and TEE (587) were performed.

1. **What is the diagnosis and what treatment should be advised?**
   (a) Pectineate muscle, no anticoagulation is needed
   (b) Clot or smudge, anticoagulation with coumadine
   (c) Clot or smudge, anticoagulation with NOAC
   (d) Clot or smudge, acetlysalicic acid, antiagregation therapy
   (e) Artifact, no anticoagulation is needed

Ans. (b)

Coumadin 5 mg was started. Ophthalmology: laser photocoagulation therapy given. Six weeks later TEE was repeated.

Coumadin was stopped and coraspin 300 mg was begun. Coronary angiography was planned.

DISCUSSION

Left heart related thrombi may be seen in patients with sinus rhythm. Enlargement of left atrial appendage, left atrium and left ventricle play a role in thrombus formation.[1] In this case, a dilated left atrium was present.

LAA function impairment is also responsible for thrombus formation in sinus rhythm. Other than the decrease in LAA flow velocity, recent studies suggest the role of speckle tracking echocardiography to predict impaired LAA function. Impaired LA deformation parameters were found to be associated with the presence of LAA thrombus in stroke patients without overt structural abnormalities and with sinus rhythm.[2,3]

3DTEE provides additional information for evaluation of LAA morphology and measurement of size.[4,5] It may also be useful for thrombus detection, and to differentiate thrombus from trabeculae and pectineate muscles.[6]

Contrast echocardiography is also another method which may be used to visualize thrombi.[7]

Antithrombotic therapy: In heart failure patients with reduced LVEF who are in sinus rhythm there is no evidence for overall benefit of vitamin K antagonists on mortality. Risk factors associated with increased risk of thromboembolic events should be identified and decision regarding use of anticoagulation individualized. New oral anticoagulants may be an attractive therapeutic option, but this needs to be confirmed in clinical trials.[8]

MOVIES 586 AND 587

REFERENCES

1. Prevalence of left chamber cardiac thrombi in patients with dilated left ventricle at sinus rhythm: the role of transesophageal echocardiography. Bakalli A, Georgievska-Ismail L, Koçinaj D, Musliu N, Krasniqi A, Pllana E. J Clin Ultrasound. 2013;41(1):38-45.
2. Left atrial strain as evaluated by two-dimensional speckle tracking predicts left atrial appendage dysfunction in patients with acute ischemic stroke. Sasaki S, Watanabe T, Tamura H, Nishiyama S, Wanezaki M, Sato C, Yamaura G, Ishino M, Arimoto T, Takahashi H, Shishido T, Miyamoto T, Kubota I. BBA Clin. 2014;2:40-7.
3. Left atrial strain: a new predictor of thrombotic risk and successful electrical cardioversion. Costa C, González-Alujas T, Valente F, Aranda C, Rodríguez-Palomares J, Gutierrez L, Maldonado G, Galian L, Teixidó G, Evangelista A. Echo Res Pract. 2016;3(2):45-52.

4. Real-time three-dimensional transesophageal echocardiography of the left atrial appendage initial experience in the clinical setting. Shah SJ, Bardo DM, Sugeng L et al. J Am Echocardiologr. 2008;21(129):1362-8.
5. Analysis of the left atrial appendage by three-dimensional transesophageal echocardiography. Nakajima H, Seo Y, ishizu T. Am J Cardiol. 2010;106(6):885-92.
6. Real-time three-dimensional transesophageal echocardiography is more specific than the two-dimensional transesophageal echocardiography in the assessment of the left atrial appendage thrombus. Mareh D, Vindis D, Kocinova E, et al. Biomed Pap Med Fac Univ Palacky Olomuc Czech Reub. 2013;157(1):22-6.
7. CUTE-CV: a prospective study of enhanced left atrial appendage visualization with microbubble contrast agent use during transesophageal echocardiography-guided cardioversion. Bernier M, Abdelmoneim SS, Stuart Moir W, et al. Echocardiography. 2013;30(9):1091-7.
8. Thromboembolism and antithrombotic therapy for heart failure in sinus rhythm: an executive summary of a joint consensus document from the ESC Heart Failure Association and the ESC Working Group on Thrombosis. Lip GY, Piotrponikowski P, Andreotti F, Anker SD, Filippatos G, Homma S, Morais J, Pullicino P, Rasmussen LH, Marín F, Lane DA; Heart Failure Association (EHFA) of the European Society of Cardiology (ESC) and the ESC Working Group on Thrombosis. Thromb Haemost. 2012;108(6):1009-22.

CASE 182

Pasquale Palmiero, Annapaola Zito, Fiorella Devito, Roberta Romito, Maurizio Campaniello, Ottavio Di Cillo, Maria Maiello, Marco Matteo Ciccone

AN UNCOMMON CASE OF LEFT ATRIAL APPENDAGE THROMBUS DURING DABIGATRAN THERAPY

Abstract

We describe a rare case of a left atrial appendage thrombus in a 65-year-old man, with non-valvular atrial fibrillation (AF) which was noted while the patient was on therapy with dabigatran 150 mg twice a day. Shifting to warfarin therapy resulted, after twenty days, in the disappearance of the thrombus, as assessed by transesophageal echocardiography.

This case of dabigatran resistance underlines the importance of paying attention to the possible phenomenon of pharmacologic resistance and to administer appropriate anticoagulant therapy to a patient with non-valvular AF, for the prevention of thrombus and stroke.

Warfarin is an effective anticoagulant used to reduce the risk of stroke and prevent or dissolve a left atrial thrombus in patients with AF.[1] Recent studies have shown dabigatran to be a valid alternative to warfarin and have demonstrated its effectiveness for the prevention of stroke in patients with AF.[2]

CASE REPORT

A 65-year-old man, with a history of hypertension and dyslipidemia, was admitted to our Hospital after the onset of arrhythmic palpitations. The electrocardiogram showed AF with a ventricular rate of 120 beats per minute. Five years before, the patient presented with an episode of non-valvular AF which was reversed with electrical cardioversion. After one year, the atrial arrhythmia relapsed, but it was reversed by pharmacological cardioversion. After the last episode of AF, six months earlier, the patient was placed on dabigatran 150 mg twice a day, for the prevention of stroke. The patient was still on dabigatran when a new relapse of AF necessitated admission to the Chest Pain Unit. At the time of admission, the blood pressure was 145/85 mm Hg, pulmonary examination was normal, and cardiac examination showed irregular heart sounds. Laboratory tests showed mild renal impairment (Glomerular Filtration Rate: 50 mL/min), D-dimer: 0.05 mg/L, troponins: 0 ng /ml, activated partial thromboplastin time (APTT): 34.3 seconds and prothrombin time/international normalized ratio: 1.03. Lipid and glycemic assessment were in the normal range. Echocardiography examination showed atrial septal aneurysm, dilated left atrium, good systolic function (left ventricular ejection fraction -LVEF: 60%) and moderate tricuspid regurgitation. Infusion of amiodarone was initiated, with the aim of restoring normal sinus rhythm and therapy with dabigatran was continued.

After 6 days, because of the persistence of the arrhythmia, transesophageal echocardiography (TEE) was performed and demonstrated an atrial septal aneurysm, patent foramen ovale, dilated left atrial appendage and the presence of a mobile oval mass (1.2 × 0.8 cm) consistent with a thrombus in the main lobe of the left atrial appendage (Fig. 182.1; 588).

Laboratory tests showed an increase in D-dimer (0.61 mg/L), APTT of 38 seconds and prothrombin time/international normalized ratio of 1.06. Screening test markers for thrombophilia (Factor V Leiden, Factor II, Fibrinopeptide) were negative.

To reach a target prothrombin time/international normalized ratio of between 2.0 and 3.0, therapy with dabigatran was discontinued and replaced first with enoxaparin and warfarin, then only warfarin.

After ten days of hospitalization, the patient was discharged with a diagnosis of permanent AF, thrombus in the left atrial appendage, arterial hypertension and dyslipidemia.

TEE performed at discharge revealed a small reduction in the thrombus size.

The discharge medications included warfarin, bisoprolol 2.5 mg/day, irbesartan 150 mg/day, lansoprazole 30 mg/day and diuretics.

After twenty days the patient was re-evaluated by TEE which demonstrated a complete resolution of the thrombus. D-dimer was in the standard normal range.

DISCUSSION

Sargento-Freitas et al. has described a case of pharmacologic resistance to dabigatran in a patient with cardioembolic stroke.[3] Tabata et al.[4] described a case of a 74-year-old man with thrombus in the left atrial appendage that increased in size after dabigatran therapy (110 mg twice

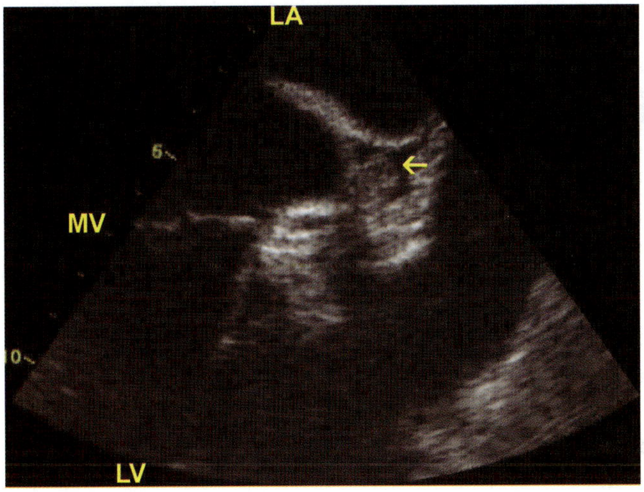

Fig. 182.1: Transesophageal echocardiography. Arrow points to left atrial appendage thrombus measured 0.8 × 1.2 cm.

daily). Sunbul et al[5], in a recent clinical case reported an episode of cardiac thrombus and pulmonary embolism in patient with AF while on dabigatran therapy.

The present report highlights the importance of paying attention to the possible phenomenon of pharmacologic resistance and administer an appropriate anticoagulant therapy for the prevention of thrombus and stroke when managing a patient with non-valvular AF.

1. **According to current guidelines when it is recommended to perform a TEE in a patient affected by AF?**
   (a) In all patients affected
   (b) Only in patients waiting to be submitted to cardioversion
   (c) Only in patients affected by paroxysmal AF

Ans. (b)

2. **A mass observed in a dilated left atrial appendage leads one to suspect :**
   (a) Atrial thrombus
   (b) Atrial tumor
   (c) None of them

Ans. (a)

MOVIE LEGEND

588: Transesophageal echocardiography. Arrow points to left atrial appendage thrombus measured 0.8 × 1.2 cm.

REFERENCES

1. Hart RG, Pearce LA, Aguilar MI. Meta-analysis: Antithrombotic therapy to prevent stroke in patients who have non-valvular atrial fibrillation. Ann Intern Med. 2007; 146:857-67.
2. Schulman S, Kearon C, Kakkar AK, Mismetti P, Schellong S, Eriksson H, et al. Dabigatran versus warfarin in the treatment of acute venous thromboembolism. N Engl J Med. 2009;361:2342-52.
3. Sargento-Freitas J, Silva F, Pego J, Duque C, Cordeiro G, Cunha L. Cardioembolic stroke in a patient taking Dabigatran Etexilate: The first case report of clinical and pharmacologic resistance. J Neurol Sci. 2014;346 (1-2):348-9.
4. Emi Tabata, Masahiro Yasaka, Yoshiyuki Wakugawa, Motohiro Komori, Kohta Mori, Yuichiro Tsurusaki, et al. Increase in the Size of an Intracardiac Thrombus during Dabigatran Therapy (110 mg b.i.d.) in an Acute Cardioembolic Stroke Patient. Cerebrovasc Dis Extra. 2013;3(1):78-80.
5. Sunbul M, Cincin A, Mammadov C, Mutlu B. Is Dabigatran as effective as warfarin on cardiac thrombus in a patient with atrial fibrillation? A challenging question. Am J Ther. 2014 Nov 21. [Epub ahead of print]

CASE 183

Giove GC, Singla I, Mishra J, Nanda NC

The patient is a 61-year-old female with paroxysmal atrial fibrillation, who was scheduled for ablation. 2D TEE was done to rule out LA/LAA thrombus.

1. **What are the echo findings (Figs. 183.1A and B and 589)?**
   (a) Mass (thrombus) in LAA
   (b) Mass (thrombus) just outside LAA
   (c) No mass or thrombus. Clear the patient for ablation
   (d) Tumor in transverse sinus of pericardium

Ans. (c)

A 1.5 cm echo density consistent with a mass lesion in or adjacent to LAA is demonstrated. An MRI was done which suggested a tumor in the LAA region. The patient was placed on warfarin and repeat TEE was scheduled after 6 weeks. At that time also, the same echo density was demonstrated with no change in size. To further define this, the probe was slightly withdrawn and rotated so that the echo density was practically centered in the middle of the viewing monitor screen. The transducer was then rotated from 0° to 180° and it became clear there was no mass in or around the appendage. The mass-like effect was produced by the ultrasonic beam transversing the top surface of a lobe of the LAA, which was visualized en face (Figs. 183.2A and B, 590). The presence of a small amount of fluid in the transverse sinus of the pericardium facilitated this effect of a circumscribed mass. Thus, an erroneous diagnosis of a thrombus or tumor was avoided and the patient underwent successful ablation. Our case highlights the importance of careful examination of the LA and LAA during 2D TEE. If the 2D TEE is inconclusive, 3D TTE or 3D TEE may be indicated. This case is reproduced with permission from: Giove GC, Singla I, Mishra J, Nanda NC. Transesophageal echocardiographic finding of left atrial appendage lobe mimicking a mass lesion. Echocardiography. 2011;28(6):684-5.

MOVIES 589 AND 590

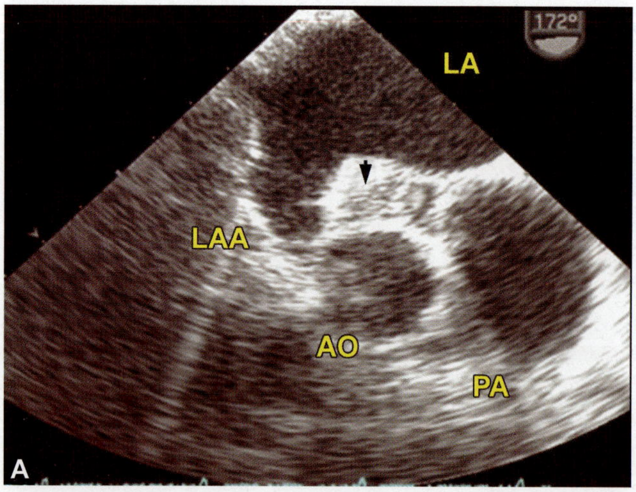

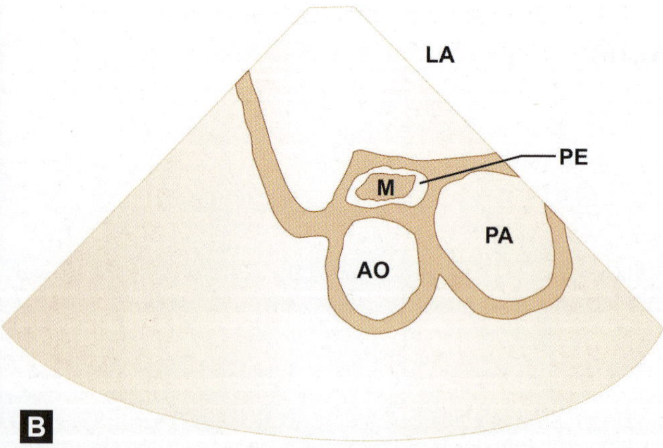

Figs. 183.1A and B : Transesophageal echocardiographic finding of left atrial appendage lobe mimicking a mass lesion. (A) The arrowhead in this figure and Movie 589 points to what appears to be a mass in or adjacent to left atrial appendage (LAA). (B) Schematic. (AO: Aorta; LA: Left atrium; M: Mass; PA: Pulmonary artery; PE: Fluid in the transverse sinus of pericardium).

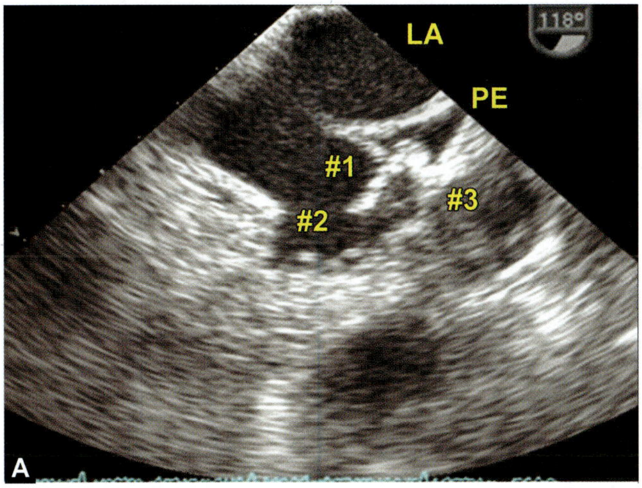

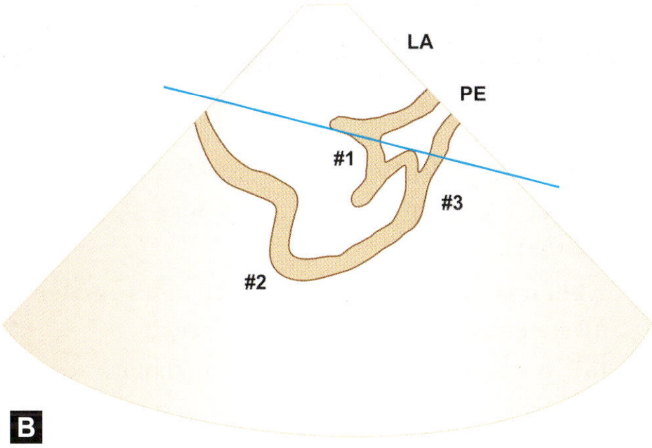

Figs. 183.2A and B: Transesophageal echocardiographic finding of left atrial appendage lobe mimicking a mass lesion. (A) Keeping the mass-like lesion in the middle of the monitor screen and rotating the transducer from 0° to 180° shows that the mass-like effect is produced by a lobe (#3) of the left atrial appendage. (B) Schematic. Numbers 1 and 2 denote the other two lobes of the left atrial appendage. Other abbreviations as in Figure 183.1.

CASE 184

Taher A, Elsayed M, Nanda NC

This is an adult patient with dilated cardiomyopathy. 2D TTE showed a large thrombus in the LV apex. 3D TTE was done (591).

1. **What was the need to do a 3D TTE in this patient? All statements below are correct *except*:**
   (a) It will show the thrombus (arrow) more beautifully
   (b) The size of the thrombus can be more reliably assessed and its volume quantified
   (c) 3D cropping is valuable in finding lytic/liquefied areas in the thrombus which herald thrombus dissolution
   (d) Any additional thrombi in the LV can be detected more reliably

Ans. (a)

The arrow in 591 shows the large thrombus in LV apex which shows some areas of lysis on cropping (sectioning).

MOVIE 591

CASE 185

Ahmad S Omran

RIGHT ATRIAL MYXOMA

This 46-year-old woman presented to our ER with rapid atrial fibrillation in 2001. Initial transthoracic echocardiography showed a large highly mobile mass in the right atrium (Figs. 185.1A and B, 592 and 593). Mass was prolapsing into the right ventricle during diastole. Severe tricuspid regurgitation (TR) was noted with a right ventricular systolic pressure of 60–70 mm Hg. Pulmonary CT was negative for pulmonary embolism. Transesophageal echocardiography (TEE) was done which showed a large highly mobile cauliflower-shaped mass in the right atrium (RA) attached to the junction of the superior vena cava (SVC) with the RA by a long pedicle (Figs. 185.2A and B, 594 and 595). Although the mass was highly suspicious of a RA myxoma but due to the presence of atrial fibrillation, RA clot could not be ruled out. Cardiac MRI was not available in our center at that time for tissue characterization. A careful history taken from the patient elicited that two years previously she was told to have a mass in the heart at another hospital but had refused surgery. This past history was not supportive of the diagnosis of RA clot.

Patient was taken to the operating room the following week. Surgical exploration was performed via a right atriotomy. A very large myxoma attached to the junction of the SVC with the RA by a long pedicle was resected. Mass showed gelatinous appearance with multiple fronds (Figs. 185.3A and B). Mass weighed about 90 grams. Microscopic examination confirmed the diagnosis of right atrial myxoma. Patient was discharged home in good condition. Follow up echocardiography 14 years after surgery showed no sign of recurrence of myxoma but moderate TR and high pulmonary artery systolic pressure were still present.

1. **In cardiac tumors of the right heart which of the following statements is correct?**
   (a) Cardiac lymphomas are the most common malignant primary tumors of the right heart.
   (b) About 18% of cardiac myxomas are located in the right atrium.
   (c) Rhabdomyomas of the right heart are more common in adults than in children.
   (d) Mesotheliomas always arise in the pleura and can metastasize into the right atrium.

Ans. (b)

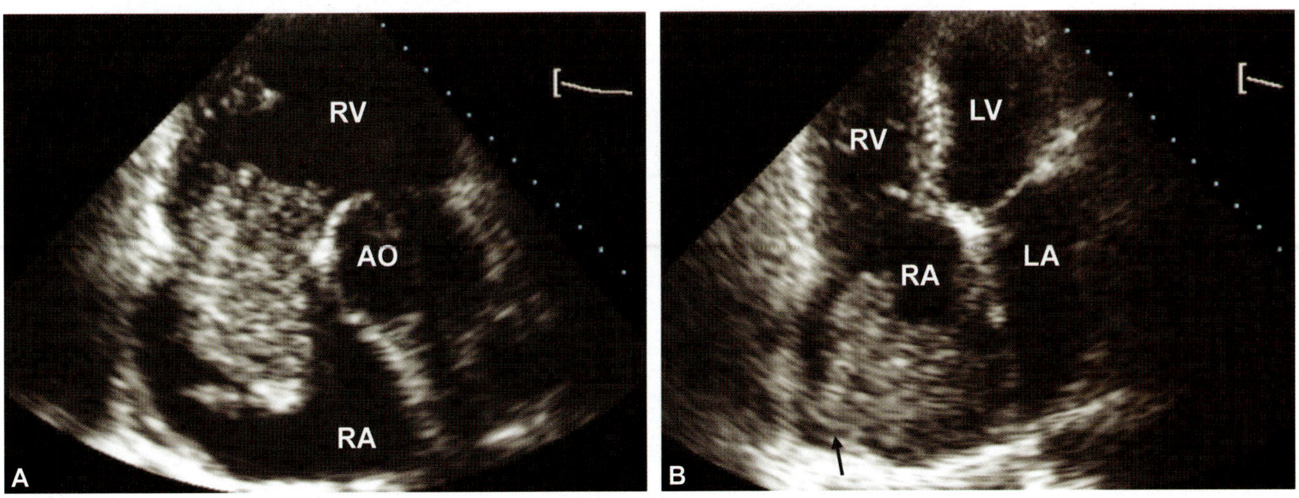

Figs. 185.1A and B: Transthoracic echocardiography (TTE). (A) TTE in short-axis view shows a large mass in the RA prolapsing into the RV through the tricuspid valve; (B) TTE 4-chamber view shows attachment of the mass to the SVC junction (black arrow). (RV: Right ventricle; LV: Left ventricle; LA: Left atrium; RA: Right atrium; SVC: Superior vena cava).

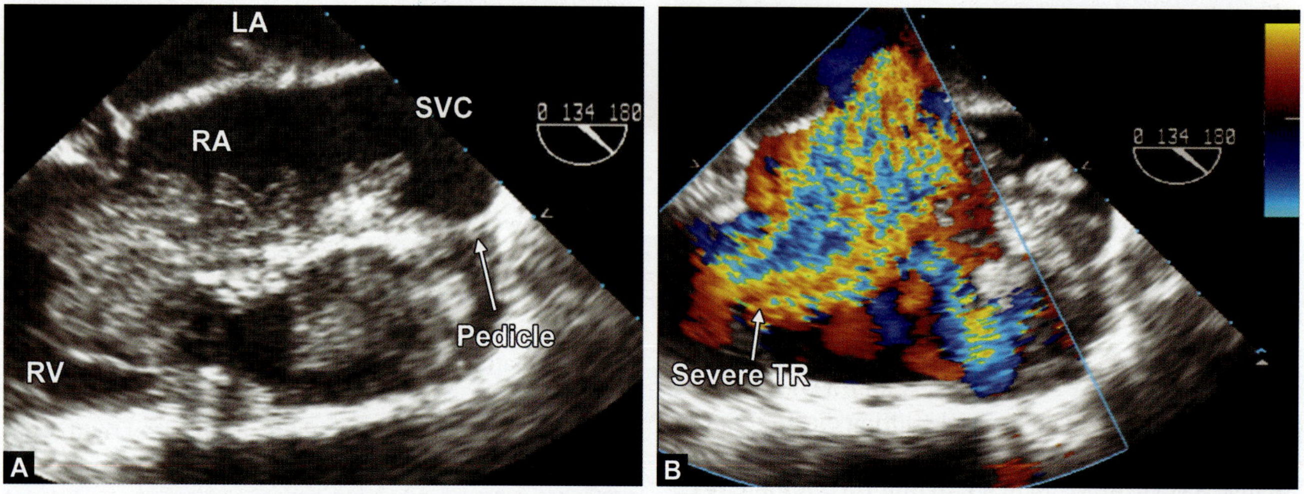

Figs. 185.2A and B: Transesophageal echocardiography (TEE). (A) TEE long-axis view showing right atrium, junction of SVC and the mass with the pedicle. Mass is prolapsing into the RV through the tricuspid valve. (B) Severe tricuspid regurgitation is seen, likely due to long-term damage to the valve. (RV: Right ventricle; LA: Left atrium; RA: Right atrium; SVC: Superior vena cava).

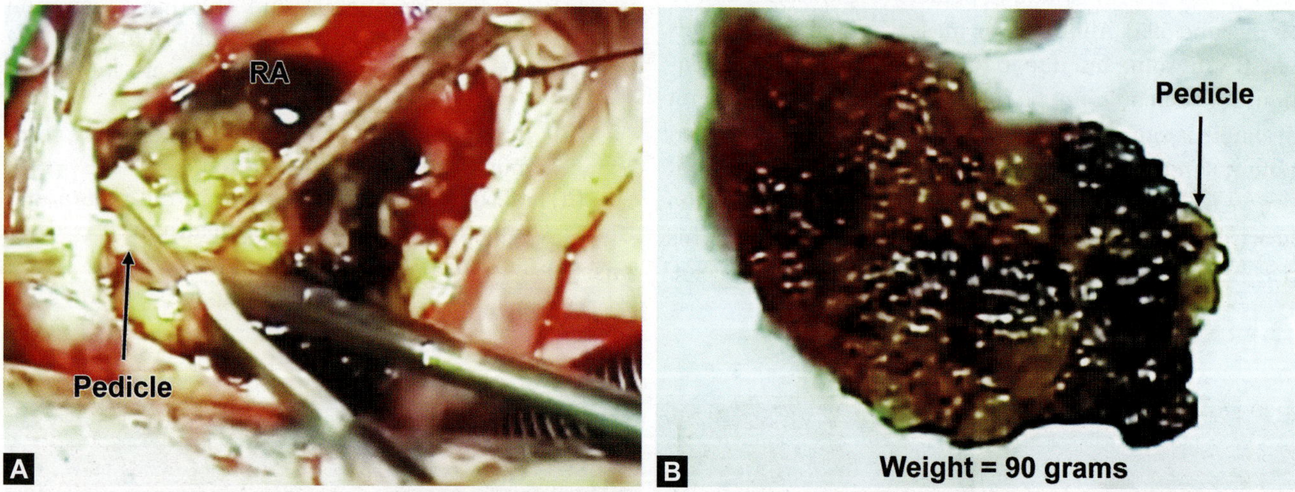

Figs. 185.3A and B: Surgical inspection of the right atrium. (A) Myxoma was resected from the junction of right atrium and superior vena cava. (B) Large jelly-like villous mass weighing about 90 grams. (RA: Right atrium).

MOVIE LEGENDS

592: Transthoracic RV inflow view showing the large RA myxoma attached to the SVC junction.

593: Transesophageal echocardiography (TEE) showing the large RA myxoma prolapsing through the tricuspid valve in diastole.

594: TEE bicaval view showing the RA myxoma attached to the junction of SVC and RA by a long pedicle.

595: TEE 4 chamber view showing severe tricuspid regurgitation.

CASE 186

Desiree M Younes, Smadar Kort

HEMOPTYSIS DURING PREGNANCY

Ms S is a 25-year-old female with no past medical history who presents in her 27th week of pregnancy with coughing. Symptoms started 10 days prior to presentation. She was prescribed a one week course of azithromycin and prednisone. Following the completion of treatment, she noted hemoptysis with nearly one cup of bright red blood and dyspnea with exertion. She did not have fevers, chills, sick contacts, recent travel, orthopnea, or lower extremity edema.

Other than two C-sections for uncomplicated pregnancies, Ms S had no prior surgeries or medical illnesses. Her only medication was a multivitamin. She did not smoke tobacco but did engage in occasional marijuana use prior to her pregnancy. She had no family history of cardiac disease or cancer.

In the emergency room she was afebrile with a heart rate of 91 beats per minute and blood pressure of 118/57 mm Hg. Her oxygen saturation was 98% on room air. She was resting comfortably. Her cardiac exam demonstrated a normal S1/S2 and was negative for jugular venous distention, gallops, rubs, or murmurs. She had bilateral rales on pulmonary exam. Abdomen was soft and non-tender, and she had trace non-pitting bilateral pedal edema. Her electrocardiogram was remarkable for left atrial enlargement. Her chest X-ray was remarkable for pulmonary vascular congestion and enlargement of the left heart border. Echocardiogram was done (Figs. 186.1 to 186.8 and 596-599).

1. **What is the best next step in determining the diagnosis?**
   (a) Immediate cardiac computed tomography with shielding over the abdomen.
   (b) Cardiac computed tomography after delivery
   (c) No further testing is required; transthoracic echocardiography has established the diagnosis
   (d) Percutaneous transeptal biopsy of the mass

Ans. (c)

Atrial myxomas are benign neoplasms of multipotent mesenchymal cells and make up 50 to 70% of all primary cardiac tumors. They are found more commonly in females between the ages of 30 and 60.

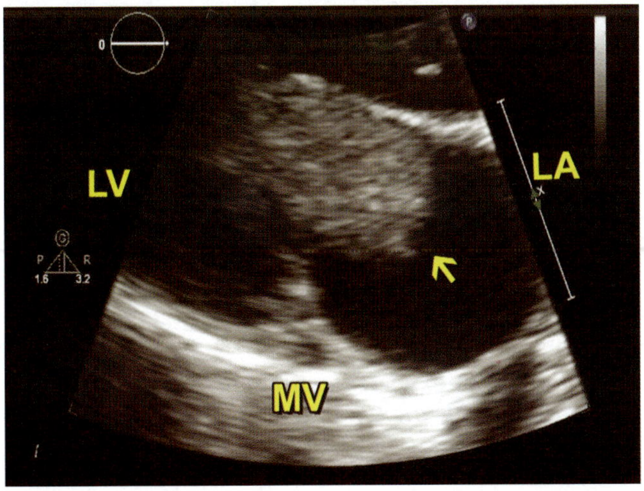

Fig. 186.1: Transthoracic echocardiography. Parasternal long axis view of the mitral valve. (LA: Left atrium; LV: Left ventricle). Arrow points to a large mass within the left atrium and protruding into the left ventricle.

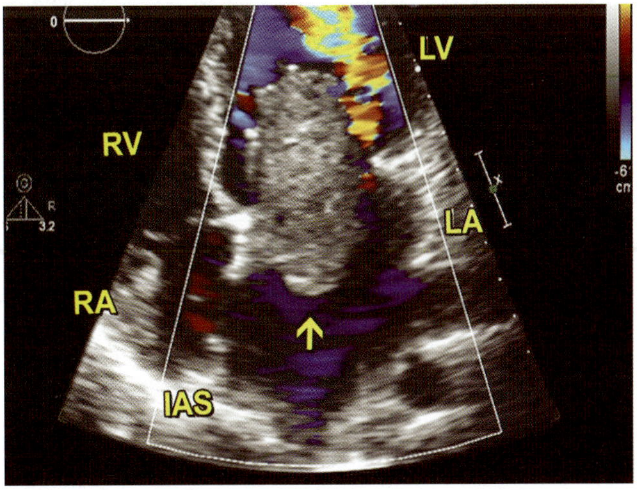

Fig. 186.2: Transthoracic echocardiography. Apical four chamber view. (LA: Left atrium; LV: Left ventricle; IAS: Interatrial septum; RA: right atrium; RV: Right ventricle). Arrow points to a large mass within the left atrium and protruding into the left ventricle.

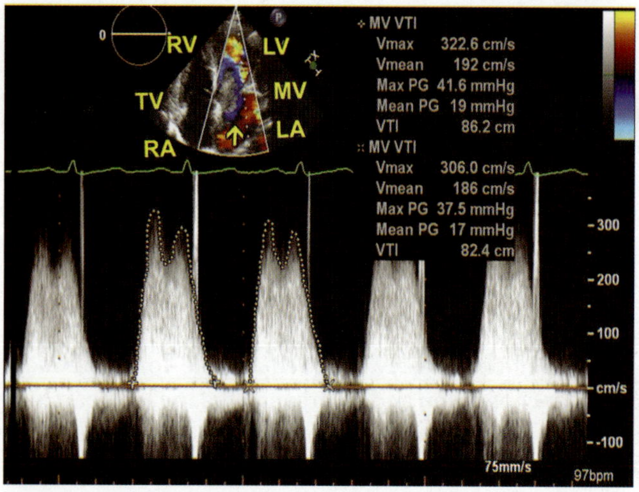

Fig. 186.3: Continuous wave Doppler through mitral valve inflow.

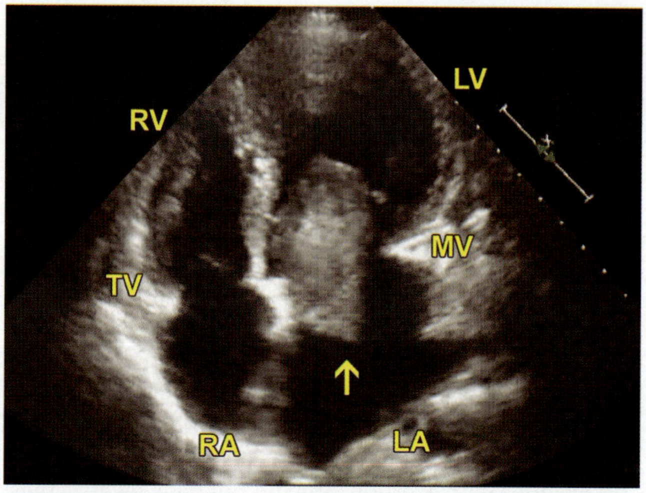

Fig. 186.4: Transthoracic echocardiography. Apical four chamber view. (LA: Left atrium; LV: Left ventricle; RA: Right atrium; RV: Right ventricle). Arrow points to a large mass within the left atrium and protruding into the left ventricle.

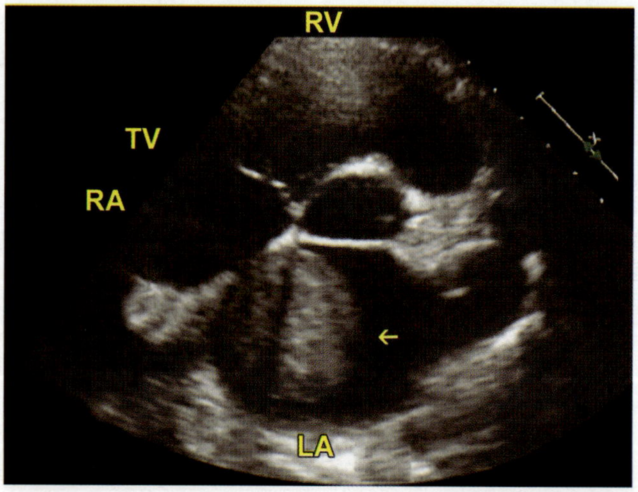

Fig. 186.5: Transthoracic echocardiography. Parasternal short axis around the level of the aortic valve. (RA: Right atrium; LA: Left atrium; RV: Right ventricle; TV: Tricuspid valve). Arrow points to a mass attached to the left atrial surface of the interatrial septum.

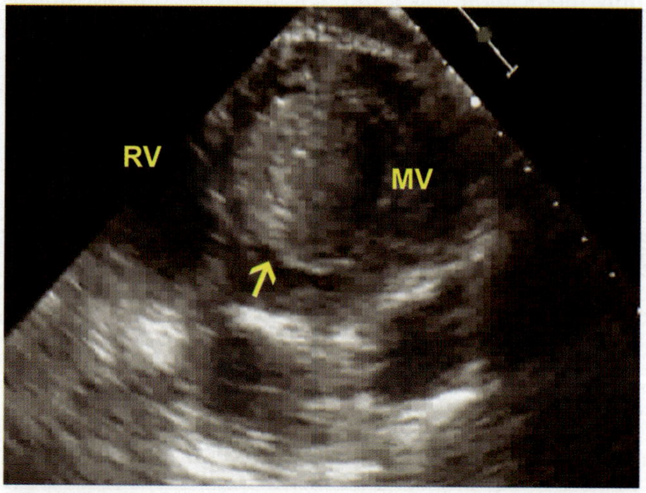

Fig. 186.6: Transthoracic echocardiography. Parasternal short axis at the level of the mitral valve. (RV: Right ventricle; MV: Mitral valve). Arrow points to the myxoma protruding through MV.

The diagnosis of myxomas can almost always be made by echocardiography alone. Over 75% are located in the left atrium, and the majority are attached to the interatrial septum around the border of the fossa ovalis. Myxomas normally have a heterogenous consistently, unlike thrombi which are typically homogenous, and may have a smooth or friable surface. If the diagnosis is unclear on echocardiography, such as in cases of myxomas originating in the left atrial appendage (5%), other forms of cardiac imaging such as magnetic resonance imaging should be considered.[1-5]

2. **What is the expected course during pregnancy in patients with the hemodynamic properties shown in Figure 186.3?**
   (a) No hemodynamically significant abnormality is seen in this patient.
   (b) The majority of patients respond well to low doses of oral loop diuretics and undergo routine follow-up until delivery

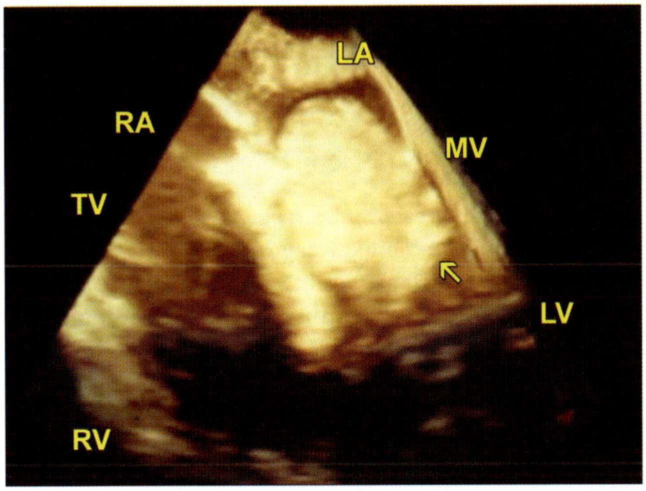

Fig. 186.7: Transesophageal three-dimensional echocardiography rendering of the four chamber mid-esophageal view. (LA: Left atrium; LV: Left ventricle; RA: Right atrium; RV: Right ventricle). Arrow points to the large myxoma.

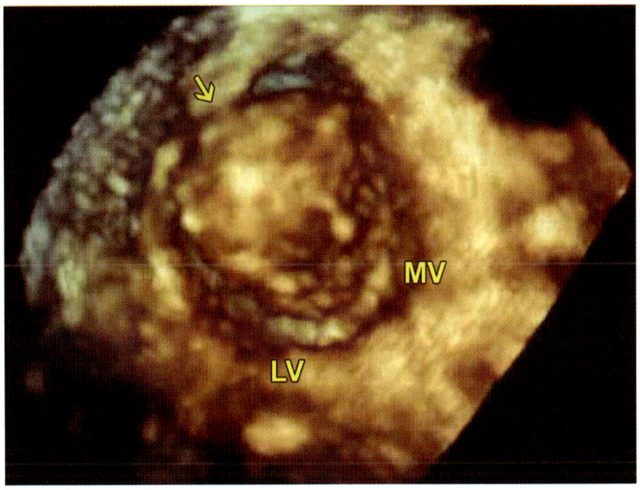

Fig. 186.8: Transesophageal three-dimensional echocardiography rendering of the mitral valve viewed from the left atrium ("surgeon's view"). Arrow points to the myxoma as it is protruding through the mitral valve.

(c) Decrease in peripheral vascular resistance as the pregnancy progresses results in an improvement in cardiac output and symptoms in the majority of patients without the need for continual use of loop diuretics.

(d) The majority of patients develop New York Heart Association class III or IV heart failure symptoms by their third trimester of pregnancy and require hospitalization for cardiac symptoms.

Ans. (d)

Patients with left atrial myxomas most often present with heart failure symptoms due to tumor obstruction of the mitral valve. Doppler ultrasound in our case reveals a mean gradient of 19 mm Hg across the mitral valve, consistent with severe functional mitral stenosis.

Left atrial myxomas diagnosed during pregnancy are rare, with only a small number of cases reported in the literature.[6] However, the outcome of pregnant women with severe mitral stenosis (MS) secondary to rheumatic heart disease is well described.[7,8] Increase in plasma volume and heart rate with pregnancy leads to the development of heart failure or atrial arrhythmias in over 2/3 of women with severe MS. Many require repeated or continual hospitalizations for cardiac symptoms. Mitral valvoplasty may need to be considered in those with symptoms despite medical therapy.

Case (*contd...*)

Ms S was admitted to the hospital and started on intravenous loop diuretics and unfractionated heparin. Her heart failure symptoms decreased to New York Heart Association class I/II. Cardiothoracic surgery consult was obtained.

3. What are the indications for surgical resection in newly diagnosed atrial myxomas?

(a) Increase in tumor diameter by more than 0.5 cm per year on follow-up echocardiography

(b) Recurrent embolization despite systemic anticoagulation

(c) Heart failure symptoms that do not respond to diuretic therapy

(d) All atrial myxomas should be resected promptly in patients who are not high risk for cardiac surgery

(e) A, B and C

Ans. (d)

Patients with atrial myxomas commonly present with heart failure secondary to intracardiac obstruction, systemic tumor embolization or constitutional symptoms such as fevers or weight loss. Although myxomas are benign, cardiac symptoms and high risk of embolization (30-40%) necessitate surgical resection promptly after diagnosis in patients who are surgical candidates.[1-5]

Case (*contd...*)

The patient was taken to the operating room on hospital day 5. Transesophageal echocardiogram was obtained (Figs. 186.7 and 186.8 599 and 600). She was found to have a smooth, glistening, 2.5 × 1.5 cm tumor attached to the left atrial surface of the interatrial septum on a stalk.

This was resected via a left atriotomy. Normothermia was maintained and she remained on cardiac bypass for 18 minutes.

4. What syndrome or condition should be suspected if preoperative transesophageal echocardiogram revealed a second cardiac myxoma in the right atrium?

(a) Barlow's syndrome
(b) Carney complex
(c) Tuberous sclerosis
(d) Non-cardiac malignancy with metastases to the heart.

Ans. (b)

Carney complex is an autosomal dominant genetic disorder consisting of multiple cardiac, endocrine, mucosal and cutaneous tumors. Cardiac myxomas, when present, may be multiple or in atypical locations. Other manifestations of the syndrome include a number of cutaneous pigmented lesions such as lentigines, blue nevi, and café-au-lait spots. Neoplasms of the breast, thyroid, adrenal gland, pituitary gland, or gonads are also seen. Genetic mutations on chromosomes 2 and 17 have been implicated with this syndrome.[9]

Barlow's syndrome refers to myxomatous changes of the mitral leaflets with diffuse severe prolapse of multiple scallops. Tuberous sclerosis is a genetic disorder associated with multi-system neoplasms; the cardiac neoplasm typically seen in this disorder is cardiac rhabdomyoma, not myxoma. Although most intracardiac masses are metastatic rather than primary cardiac tumors, the echocardiographic findings in this case are consistent with the diagnosis of myxoma.

5. What is the risk of tumor recurrence in patients with sporadic myxomas?

(a) 1-3%
(b) 22%
(c) 35%
(d) 50%

Ans. (a)

Resection is considered curative and recurrence is rare in those with isolated atrial myxomas. Potential risk factors for recurrence include incomplete resection, intraoperative displacement of tumor material, embolization, and malignant conversion.[5] Patients with Carney syndrome often have recurrent myxomas, and this diagnosis should be considered in patients presenting with recurrency.

Case (*contd...*)

The remainder of Ms. S.'s hospital course was uneventful. She was discharged on hospital day 5. She described symptom resolution on follow-up and her pregnancy was otherwise uncomplicated. She underwent a C-section on her expected due date.

MOVIE LEGENDS

596: Transthoracic echocardiography. Apical four chamber view. (LA: left atrium; LV: left ventricle; RA: right atrium; RV: right ventricle).

597: Transthoracic echocardiography. Parasternal short axis around the level of the aortic valve. (RA: right atrium; LA: left atrium).

598: Transthoracic echocardiography. Parasternal short axis at the level of the mitral valve. Shows the myxoma protruding through MV.

599: Transesophageal three-dimensional echocardiography rendering of the four chamber mid-esophageal view. (LA: left atrium; LV: left ventricle; RA: right atrium; RV: right ventricle).

600: Transesophageal three-dimensional echocardiography rendering of the mitral valve viewed from the left atrium ("surgeon's view").

REFERENCES

1. Shapiro LM. Cardiac tumours: diagnosis and management. Heart. 2001;85:218-22.
2. Reynen K. Cardiac myxoma. N Eng J Med. 1995;333:1610-17.
3. Butany J, Nair V, Naseemudin A, et al. Cardiac tumours: diagnosis and management. Lancet Oncol. 2005;6:219-28.
4. Oliveira R, Banco L, Galrinho A, et al. Cardiac myxoma: a 13-year experience in echocardiographic diagnosis. Rev Port Cardiol. 2010;29:1087-1100.
5. Pinede, Duhaut P, Loire R. Clinical presentation of left atrial cardiac myxoma. A series of 112 consecutive cases. Medicine. 2001;80:159-72.
6. John AS, Connolly HM, Schaff HV, Klarih K. Management of cardiac myxoma during pregnancy: A case series and review of the literature. Inter J Cardiol. 2012;155:177-80.
7. Silversides CK, Colman JM, Sermer M, Sui SC. Cardiac risk in pregnant women with rheumatic mitral stenosis. The Amer J Cardiol. 2003;91:1382-85.
8. Lesniak-Sobelga A, Tracz W, Kostkiewicz M, Podolec P, Pasowicz M. Clinical and echocardiographic assessment of pregnant women with valvular heart diseases-maternal and fetal outcome. Inter J Cardiol. 2004;94:15-23.
9. Stratakis CA, Kirschner LS, Carney JA. Clinical and molecular features of the Carney complex: diagnostic criteria and recommendations for patient evaluation. J Clin Endocrinol Metab. 2001;86:4041-6.

CASE 187

Ahmad S Omran

LEFT ATRIAL MYXOMA

This 54-year-old woman was referred to our center for surgical intervention. Patient has a history of palpitations and shortness of breath for 2 months. Transthoracic echocardiography showed large left atrial (LA) myxoma occupying entire LA (Figs. 187.1A and B). ECG showed normal sinus rhythm. CT angiography showed normal coronary arteries. Patient was transferred to cardiac operating room one day after for surgical resection. Preoperative transesophageal echocardiography (TEE) confirmed attachment of the myxoma to the interatrial septum with a broad-based short pedicle (Figs. 187.2A and B, 601 to 604). Mitral valve was normal. Surgical exploration of the myxoma was performed via a right atriotomy. Resection of the entire tumor was done including part of interatrial septum (IAS) which was attached to the pedicle to prevent chance of recurrence of the myxoma (Figs. 187.3A and B). IAS then was patched by a bovine pericardium. Microscopic examination of the mass confirmed the diagnosis of LA myxoma. Patient was discharged home with good condition.

1. **In cardiac tumors, which of the following statements is correct?**
   (a) Primary cardiac tumors are more common than metastatic involvement of the heart
   (b) Myxomas are the most common benign tumors in adults and children
   (c) Approximately 80% of myxomas originate in the left atrium
   (d) Renal cell carcinoma is the most common metastatic tumor to the left atrium

Ans. (c)

MOVIE LEGENDS

601: Intraoperative TEE (4 chamber view) demonstrates large atrial myxoma with no obstruction to the mitral inflow.
602: 3D TEE full volume acquisition shows large myxoma occupying the entire left atrium.
603: 3D TEE full volume acquisition demonstrates basal attachment of the myxoma to the fossa ovalis with a broad-based short pedicle.
604: 3D TEE demonstration of the left atrial myxoma with MPR (multiplanar reconstruction) mode.

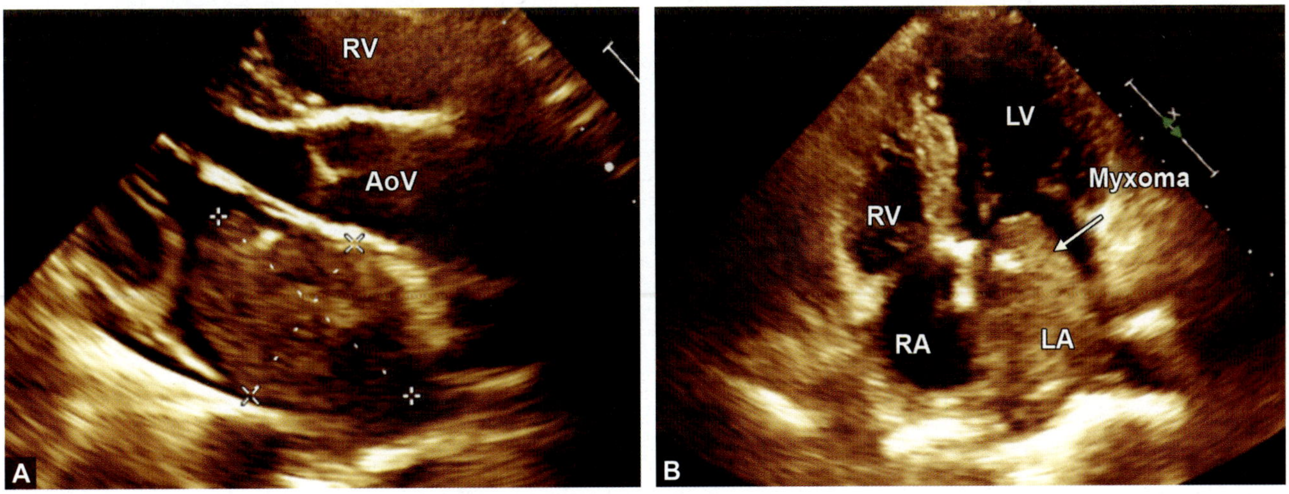

Figs. 187.1A and B: Transthoracic echocardiography demonstrating left atrial mass (myxoma). (A) Parasternal long axis view demonstrates large mass which is occupying entire left atrium. Mass is measured at 5 × 7 cm in diameter. Mass shows a few rarefactions and some bright areas as well due to liquefactions and calcifications. (B) Apical 4-chamber view demonstrates atrial septal attachment of the LA myxoma and prolapsing of the mass into mitral inflow. (RV: Right ventricle; AoV: Aortic valve; LV: Left ventricle; RA: Right atrium; LA: Left atrium).

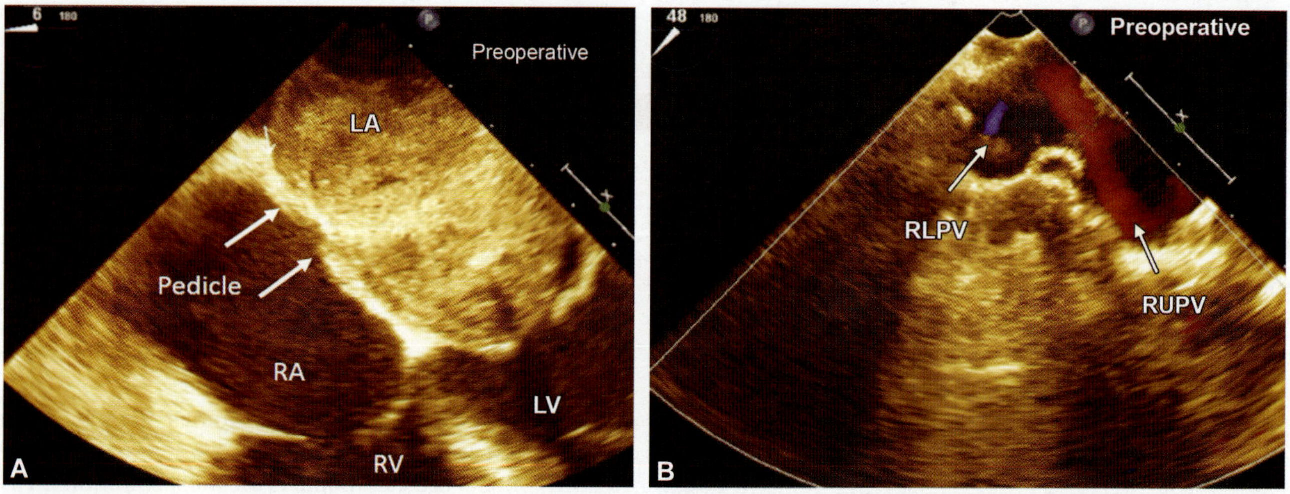

Figs. 187.2A and B: Intraoperative transesophageal echocardiography demonstrates location of the LA myxoma. (A) Four-chamber view shows myxoma is attached to upper limbus of fossa ovalis with a broad-based short pedicle. (B) Right upper and lower pulmonary veins are visualized with laminar flow into LA. This interrogation is necessary to rule out possible metastatic tumors to the LA originating from pulmonary veins. (RUPV: Right upper pulmonary vein; RLPV: Right lower pulmonary vein; RV: Right ventricle; LV: Left ventricle; RA: Right atrium; LA: Left ventricle).

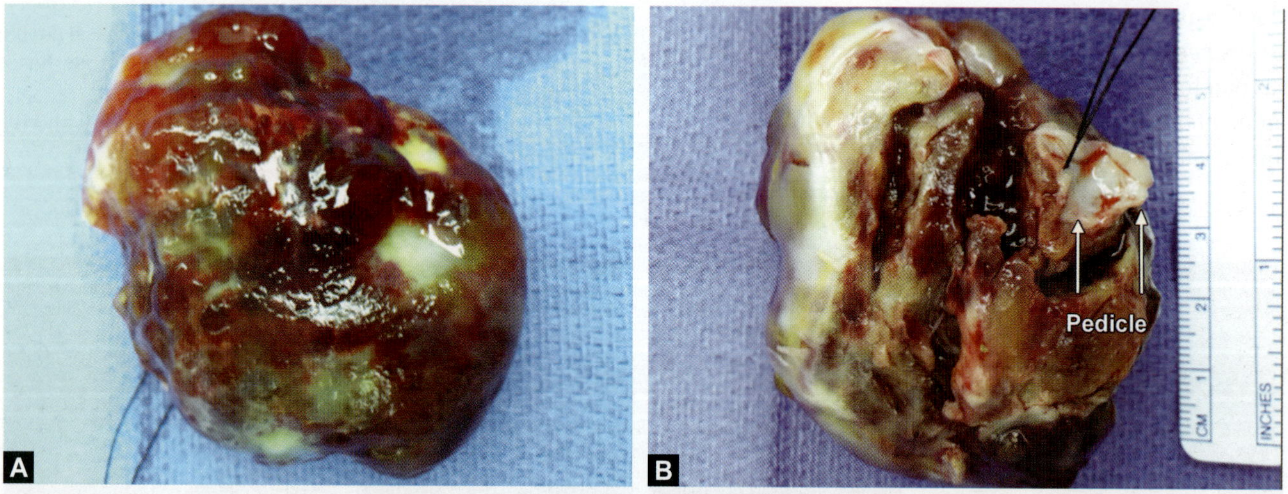

Figs. 187.3A and B: The excised mass is shown from LA side (A) and attachment side (B). Mass is measured approximately at 5 × 7 × 4 cm. (A) Typical myxoma appearance with relatively smooth, and gelatinous surface. (B) Mass was resected via the right atrium through the fossa ovalis. The entire base of the myxoma was excised with portion of atrial septum (arrows).

CASE 188

Roomi AU, Elsayed M, Bulur S, Nanda NC

LA MYXOMA

This middle aged male presented with near syncope. Past history, family history and physical examination were unremarkable. 2D TTE was done and showed a large mass in the LA protruding into the LV during diastole. A diagnosis of LA myxoma was made (Figs. 188.1, 188.2, 605 and 606).

1. **The following echo features could help distinguish a myxoma from other cardiac tumors in the same location *except*?**
   (a) Mobile and attachment to the mid portion of atrial septum
   (b) Presence of localized areas of hyperechogenicity in the mass suggestive of calcification (myxomas generally grow slowly and therefore calcification is not uncommon)
   (c) Common presence of localized areas of echolucencies due to hemorrhage, occasionally necrosis
   (d) Myxomas may be familial, may occur simultaneously or at different times in a second cardiac chamber and rarely may get infected
   (e) Constitutional symptoms such as fever may be present
   (f) Numerous localized echolucencies extending all the way to the periphery of the tumor.

Ans. (f)

This is a typical feature of a hemangioma which is a completely vascular tumor and therefore the tumor practically consists of numerous echolucencies which are seen even at the periphery.

MOVIE LEGENDS

605: TTE. Parasternal long axis view. A large mobile mass (arrow) is seen in the LA. Arrowhead points to mild MR.

606: TTE. Apical 4 chamber view. The mass (arrow) is attached to the atrial septum.

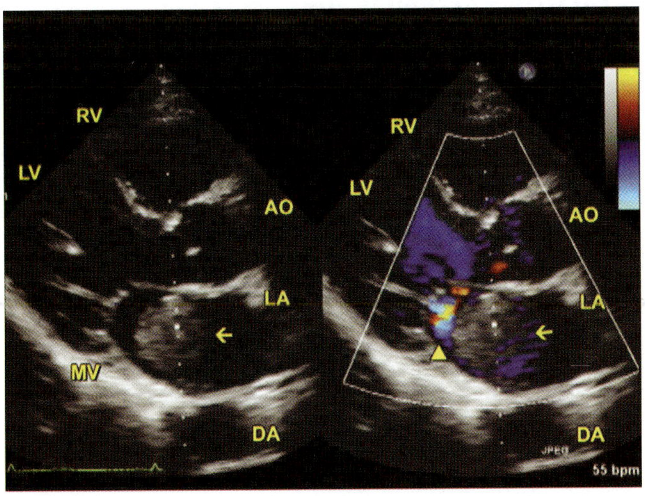

Fig. 188.1: TTE. Parasternal long axis view. A large mass (arrow) is seen in the LA.

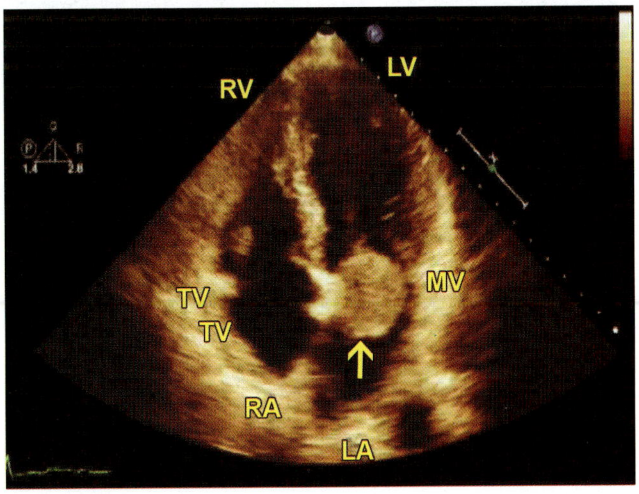

Fig. 188.2: TTE. Apical 4 chamber view. The mass (arrow) is attached to the atrial septum.

CASE 189

Muhammad Soubhi Azzouz, Aiman Smer

INCIDENTAL FINDING OF LEFT ATRIAL MASS

A 61-year-old man with a history of hypothyroidism and no prior cardiac history presented with chest pain and exercise intolerance. His EKG was unremarkable and his cardiac enzymes remained negative. Transthoracic echocardiogram (TTE) showed large left atrial mass (Fig. 189.1 and 607). The patient has no constitutional symptoms and he did not have any current or prior history of cerebrovascular events.

1. **Which of the following best describes your diagnosis?**
   (a) Left atrial thrombus
   (b) Cardiac angiosarcoma
   (c) Left atrial myxoma
   (d) Primary cardiac lymphoma

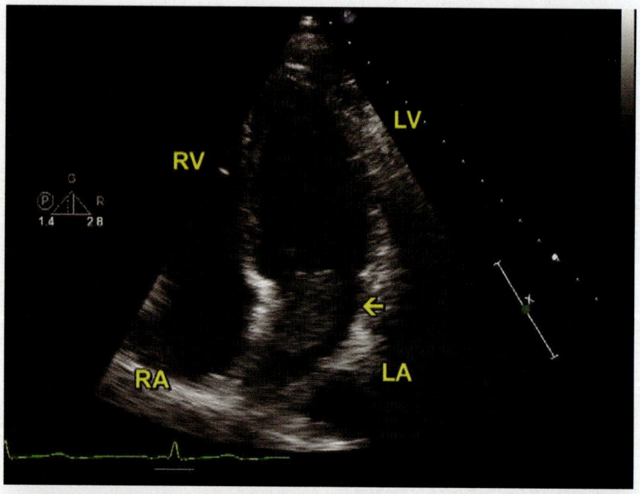

Fig. 189.1: Transthoracic echocardiogram apical four chamber view of the left atrial mass (arrow).

Ans. (c) Left atrial myxoma.

The patient underwent transesophageal echocardiogram (TEE) for further evaluation of the left atrial mass (608). We also obtained three dimensional images (609) revealing large mobile left atrial mass measuring 3 × 2.5 cm attached to the interatrial septum.

Cardio-thoracic surgery was consulted and patient underwent surgical resection of the left atrial mass. Intraoperatively, he was found to have a large 3 × 4 cm left atrial mass with a pedicle attached to the fossa ovalis, he underwent complete surgical excision of the mass with a full septal thickness excision of the pedicle stalk without any complication. Gross pathology examination showed a red-brown papillary cystic nodular gelatinous mass measuring 4.1 × 3.1 × 2.2 cm. The microscopic exam of this mass showed spindle cell proliferation in a myxoid stroma favoring atrial myxoma. Patient did remarkably well after the surgery and is now able to run 2 miles a day without any cardiopulmonary complaints.

MOVIE LEGENDS

607: Transthoracic echocardiogram apical four chamber view revealed large mobile left atrial mass (arrow) measuring 3.5 × 3 cm.

608: Transesophageal echocardiogram midesophageal view with X-plain mode showing large mobile left atrial mass (arrow) attached to the interatrial septum.

609: Three dimensional transesophageal echocardiogram in biatrial en face view demonstrating large mobile left atrial mass (arrow) attached to the interatrial septum.

CASE 190

Ahmad S Omran

UNUSUAL ANATOMIC LOCATION OF A LEFT ATRIAL MYXOMA

This 46-year-old woman presented to our center with a 2-month history of palpitations. She had an echocardiogram done 2 years ago which was reported as normal. Transthoracic echocardiography at this admission showed a large highly mobile mass in the left atrium (LA) suspicious for a LA myxoma (Figs. 190.1A and B). Mitral valve appeared normal. Preoperative TEE showed attachment of the mass to the ridge between left atrial appendage (LAA) and left upper pulmonary vein (coumadin/warfarin ridge) with a calcified pedicle. This is an unusual location for a LA myxoma attachment (🎥 610 to 613). Although there were no predisposing factors to have a LA clot in this patient but cardiac MRI was requested for tissue characterization which was consistent with the diagnosis of LA myxoma (Figs. 190.2A and B). Patient underwent cardiac surgery and the mass was resected via a left atriotomy. Mass was attached to the base of the LAA by a long pedicle exactly as was described by preoperative 3D TEE (Fig. 190.3A). Mass was measured at 3 × 3 × 4 cm, weighing about 40 gm (Fig. 190.3B). Microscopic examination of the mass confirmed the diagnosis of LA myxoma. Patient was discharged home in good condition.

Cardiac myxoma is defined by WHO as a neoplasm composed of stellate to plump, cytologically bland mesenchymal cells in a myxoid stroma (Figs. 190.4A and B).[1] Etiology of cardiac myxomas is not clear. Although genetic factors clearly play a role in myxoma syndromes (Carney complex), they do not appear to offer a consistent explanation in sporadic cases.[2] Classic triad of symptoms relates to the obstructive, embolic and constitutional effects of the tumor. However, myxomas are often asymptomatic.

1. In left atrial myxoma, which of the following statements is correct?

(a) Only 15% of times LA myxomas are not attached to the interatrial septum. They may be attached to posterior wall of the LA, anterior wall of LA or LAA

(b) In individuals with Carney complex, myxomas are more common in LA

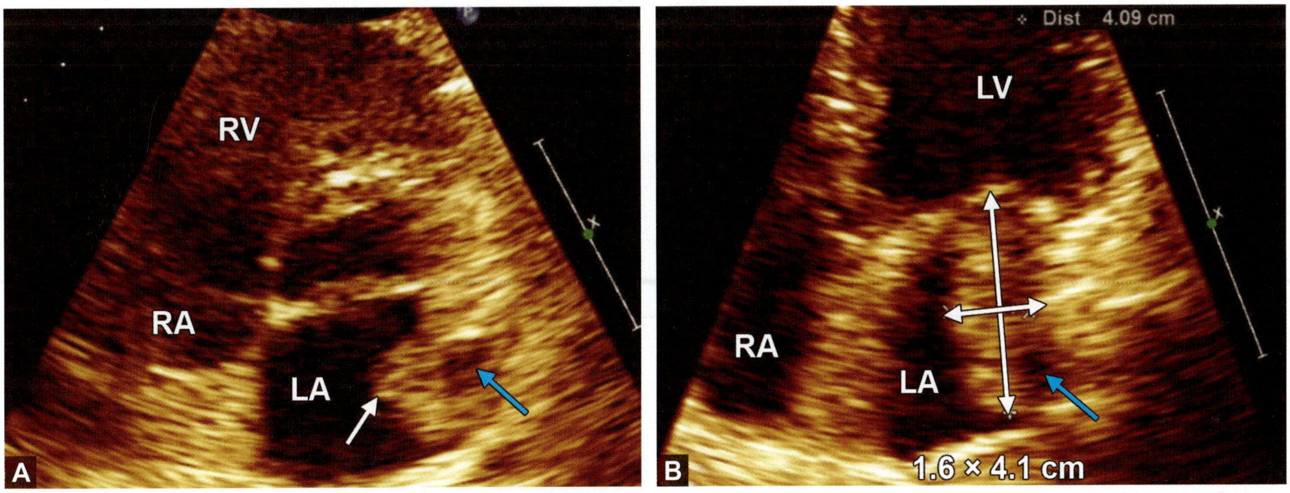

Figs. 190.1A and B: Transthoracic echocardiography (TTE) demonstrating a left atrial mass (myxoma). (A) Parasternal short axis view (off axis) showing a large LA myxoma (white arrow) probably attached to the left atrial appendage. The consistence of the mass is fairly uniform although there may be a few rarefactions due to liquefaction (necrosis) and hemorrhage (blue arrows). (B) TTE in apical 4-chamber view. (RV: Right ventricle; LV: Left ventricle; RA: Right atrium; LA: Left atrium).

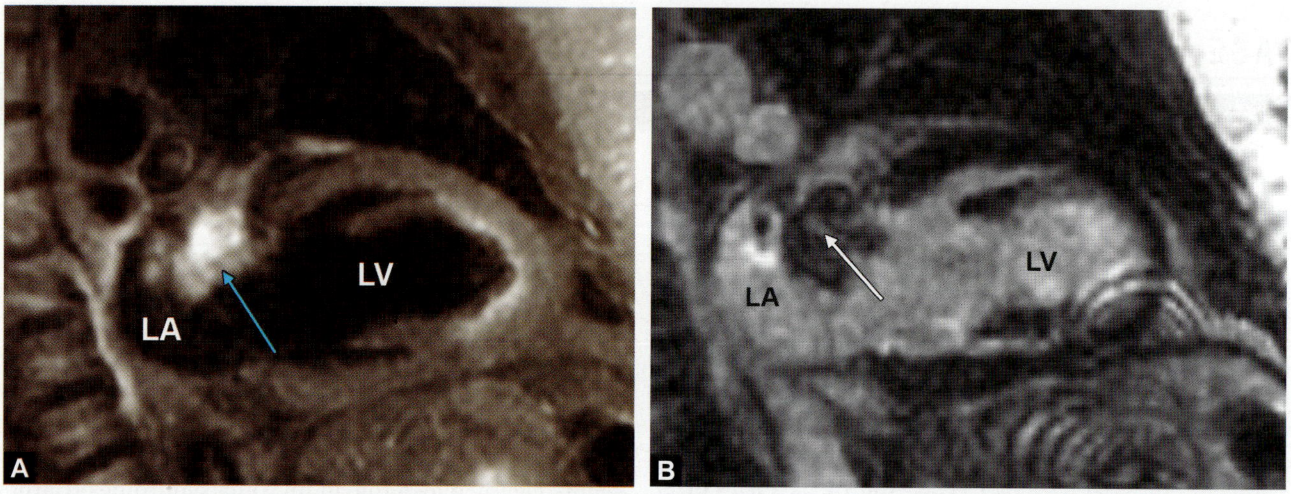

Figs. 190.2A and B: CMR tissue characterization. (A) T2 weighted image of the left atrium (LA) and left ventricle (LV) shows the mass at the base of the LA appendage with increased (bright) signal intensity (blue arrow) indicating increased water content which is against the diagnosis of thrombus. (B) T1 weighted delayed enhancement image showing the mass with areas of increased signal intensity (bright) indicating fibrosis (white arrow). The dark area may represent necrosis/hemorrhage within the mass typically seen in myxomas.
Courtesy: Dr. Ahmed Alsaileek, KACC.

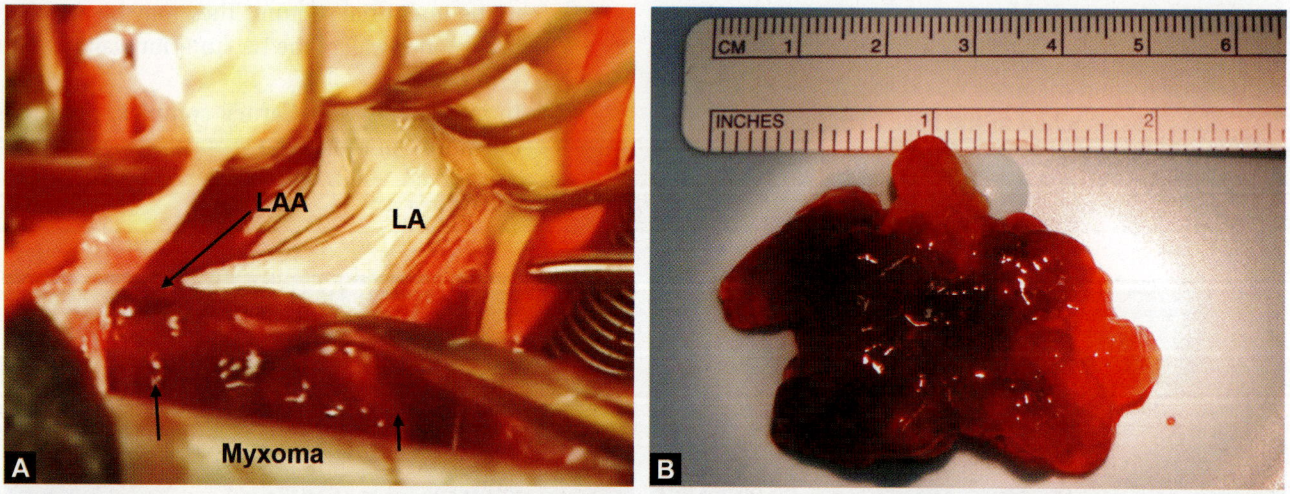

Figs. 190.3A and B: Surgical resection of the myxoma from left atriotomy. (A) Easily fragmented mass with jelly like appearance attached to the base of the left atrial appendage (coumadin ridge) was excised with the pedicle. (B) Myxoma measured 3 × 3 × 4 cm, weighing about 40 grams. Mass shows gelatinous, villous, and friable appearance.

(c) Surgical resection of LA myxoma is recommended only if patient is symptomatic
(d) Chance of recurrence of myxoma after surgical resection is about 20%

Ans. (a)

MOVIE LEGENDS

610: Preoperative TEE in 4-chamber view demonstrates a large highly mobile cauliflower shaped myxoma (arrow) attached to the ridge between left atrial appendage and left upper pulmonary vein (LUPV) with a calcified pedicle.

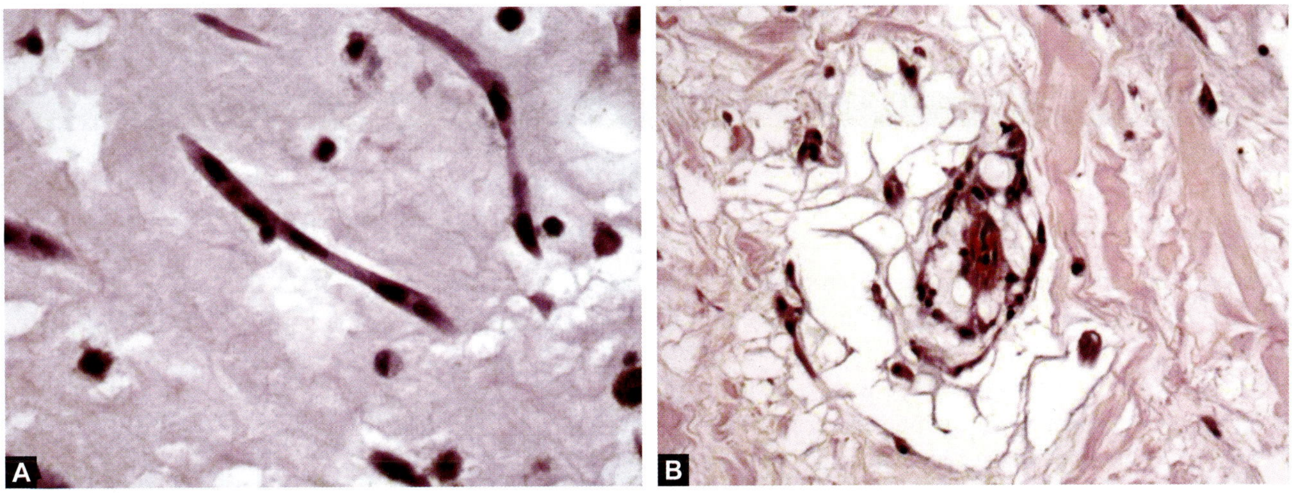

Figs. 190.4A and B: Microscopic appearance of the myxoma. (A) Stellate myxoma cells. (B) Myxoma cells forming rings.

611: 3D TEE full volume acquisition in surgical views shows a large myxoma prolapsing towards the mitral valve (MV).

612: 3D TEE full volume acquisition in surgical view with 2 orthogonal corresponding 2D TEE display.

613: Immediate postoperative TEE showing total resection of the myxoma. Note: bright calcified muscle ridge (Coumadin Ridge, CR) between left upper pulmonary vein and the LAA.

REFERENCES

1. Burke A, Tavora F. The 2015 WHO classification of tumors of the heart. Journal of Thoracic Oncology. 2016;11(4): 441-52.
2. Havrankova E, Stenova E, Olejaroval I, et al. Carney complex with biatrial myxoma. Ann Thorac Cardiovasc Surg. 2014; suppl: 890-92.

CASE 191

Naveen Garg, Kanwal K Kapur

EVALUATION OF LV MASS

A 31-year-old male reported with sudden onset of pain and numbness of left leg. There was no h/o chest pain or breathlessness. His BP was 120/70 mm Hg, and pulse 80/min sinus rhythm. Left femoral pulse was weak, left popliteal pulse was absent and distal pulses were also absent on left side. Right sided lower limb pulses were normal. Upper limb pulses were normal bilaterally. Examination of chest, CVS and abdomen were normal. ECG finding as in Figure 191.1.

His transthoracic echocardiography (🎥 614A to C) reveals:

What could be the possibilities:

1. Anterior- Septal Myocardial infarction with Clot—Left leg embolization?
2. Non-thrombotic LV Mass - Embolization?

What could be the management:

1. Thrombolysis?
2. Peripheral embolectomy?
3. CAG and excision LV mass?

COURSE IN HOSPITAL

Thrombolysis was started but later discontinued because of no relief. Peripheral femoral + popliteal embolectomy was performed. Embolus/clot was a whitish tissue (Figs. 191.2, 191.3A and B).

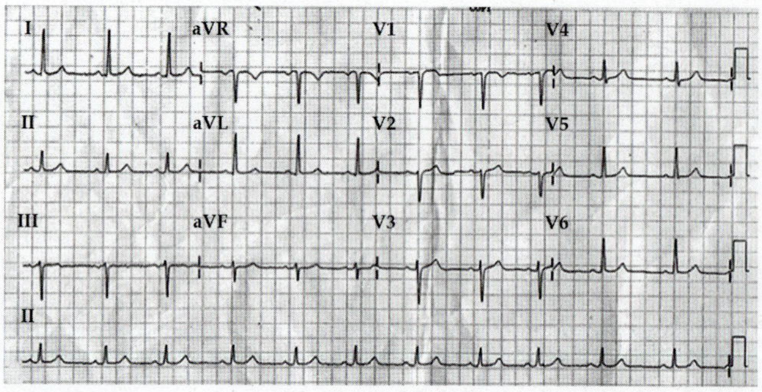

Fig. 191.1: ECG.

TEE was then performed

🎥 615A and B

What could it be:

1. LV Clot?
2. LV Myxoma?
3. LV Fibroma?

Findings Favoring LV Myxoma (Figs. 191.4A and B):

- Well defined, hypermobile, pedunculated mass.
- Relatively preserved IVS wall motion.
- Mobile pseudopodia like extensions.
- Expansion and contractions.
- Heterogeneous Echo texture

Patient was taken to surgery. His coronary angiography showed a discrete radiolucent obstruction in mid LAD suggestive of a myxomatous embolism.

Intraoperative Findings were:

🎥 616A to D

🎥 617

Postoperative findings were:

🎥 618A to C

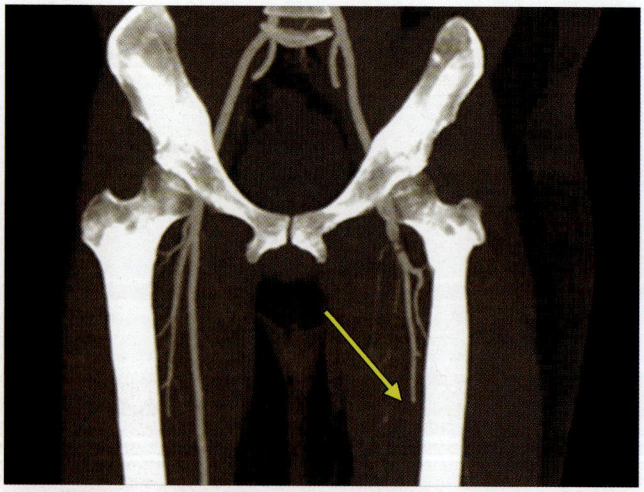

Fig. 191.2: Lower limb angiography (left lower limb angiogram shows blunt cut-off due to embolus or clot).

DISCUSSION

- LV tumors are rare. Of them myxoma is the most common primary intracardiac tumor.
- Myxoma of LV – 2.5 to 4% of all myxomas. Myxomas are most common in LA>RA>LV=RV. As compared to LA myxomas, LV myxomas are more likely to embolization and this happens to be the presenting feature in our case.
- LV myxoma – most patients are <30 years. Female > male (3:1).
- More commonly attached to IVS. Constitutional symptoms are usually absent.
- Myxoma with villous surface is more likely to embolise. Cerebral embolization is most common followed by peripheral embolization.Coronary embolization-extremely rare.
- In our case—Coronary embolization which were revealed on the angiogram as a radiolucent discrete mid LAD block. However this appeared to be only

Histopathology reports confirmed the diagnosis...

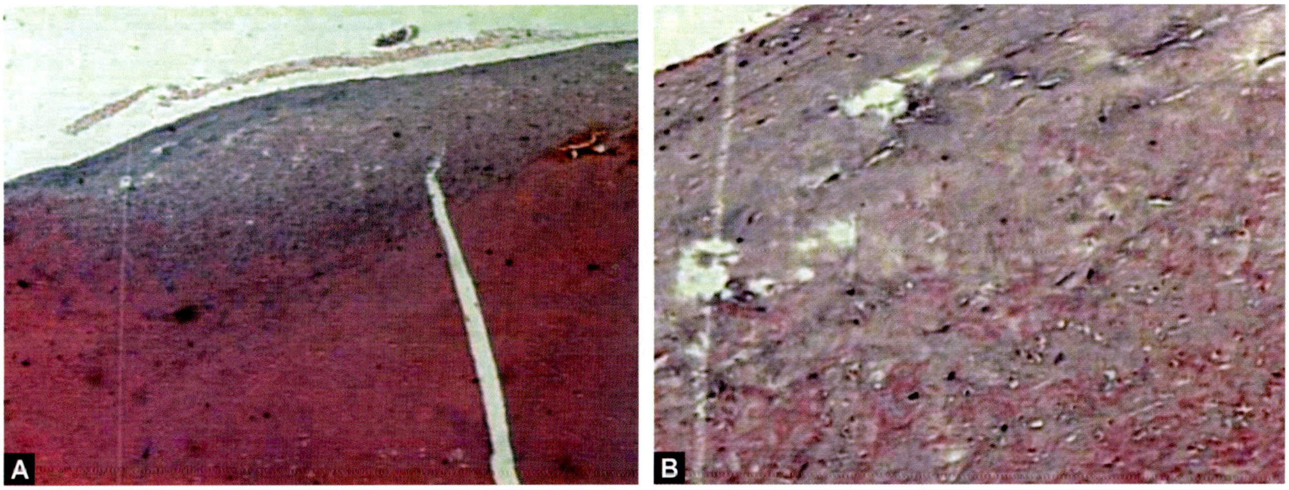

Figs. 191.3A and B: Histopathology of tissue material taken out from embolectomy showed both fibrin (part of clot) as well as a myxoid stroma (bluish gray) with vacuolated cells.

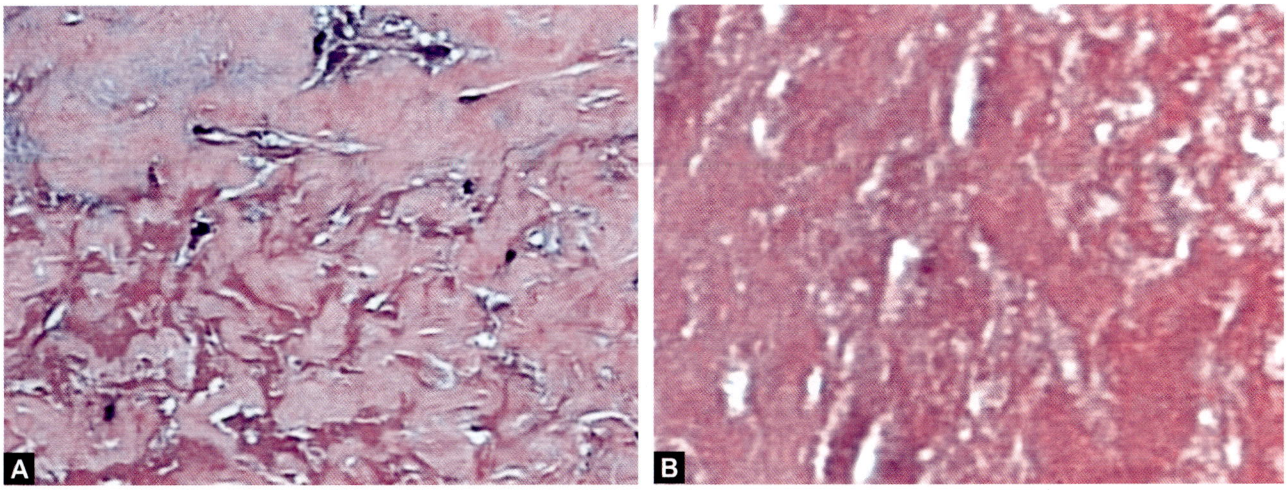

Figs. 191.4A and B: Histopathology of mass removed from LV revealed myxoid stroma with fibrin.

an incidental finding with no corresponding clinical events. Moreover, coronary flow could be observed immediately beyond this block. Therefore no revascularization procedure was performed at the time of excision (619A to D).

MOVIES 614 TO 619

614A: TTE 4C-view showing mass in LV
614B: TTE SAX view showing mass in LV
614C: TTE PLAX view showing mass in LV
615A: TEE 5C view showing mass in LV
615B: TEE zoomed view showing mass in LV attached to IVS
616A: TEE ME-Mitral commissural view; LV mass attached to IVS
616B: Mass attached to IVS
616C: TG-SAX view
616D: TG 2C view
617: Surgical removal of mass
618A: TEE 4C view showing complete resection of LV mass.
618B: Uninterrupted flow across the valve and LV cavity.
618C: TEE-TG view showing complete resection.
619A,B,C: Coronary angiography showing mid LAD radiolucent shadow with distal flow
619D: Flow across RCA appears normal.

CASE 192

Ahmad S Omran

MITRAL VALVE FIBROELASTOMA (A "SEA ANEMONE" WITHIN THE HEART)

This 54-year-old man with a history of stroke was referred to the echo lab for stroke protocol investigation. There was no history of fever or other clinical manifestations of endocarditis. Blood culture was negative. Transthoracic echocardiography (TTE) showed a large highly mobile mass which measured 1.5 cm in length attached to the atrial side of the posterior mitral leaflet (Fig. 192.1A). Transesophageal echocardiography (TEE) confirmed the TTE finding and showed the mass was attached to the atrial side of the posterior mitral valve leaflet (PMVL) with a long stalk (Fig. 192.1B). No mitral regurgitation or other echocardiographic signs of endocarditis were detected. Cardiac MRI was performed which confirmed the echo findings. Patient was discussed in our heart team meeting and the consensus was that it was a mitral fibroelastoma. Surgical intervention was recommended 3-4 weeks following the stroke. In the operating room 3D TEE was done which showed the mass was still present with the same dimensions (Figs. 192.2A and B). No signs of mitral leaflet destruction or mitral regurgitation were present (620-623). At surgery, via a left atrial approach the mass was easily excised from the PMVL (Figs. 192.3A and B). Posterior mitral leaflet was intact and appeared normal. After resection, the mass was immersed in normal saline and showed a "sea anemone-like appearance", characteristic of papillary fibroelastoma (Figs. 192.4A and B). Microscopic examination of the mass confirmed the diagnosis of fibroelastoma. Patient was discharged home in good condition.

Papillary fibroelastomas are the second most common primary cardiac tumors in adults, their appearance is often compared to sea anemones. Mean age at detection is 60 years. Size, location and number varies from 2–70 mm in size, over 80% of them are found on valves (aortic 36%, mitral 29%, tricuspid 11%, pulmonic 7%, multiple 9%). Symptoms are usually due to embolization (stroke, TIA, angina, myocardial infarction, sudden death, heart failure, syncope, pulmonary embolism). Thirty percent of patients with fibroelastoma are asymptomatic and diagnosed incidentally by echo, cardiac surgery or autopsy. Recurrence of cardiac papillary fibroelastoma following surgical resection has not been reported.[1,2]

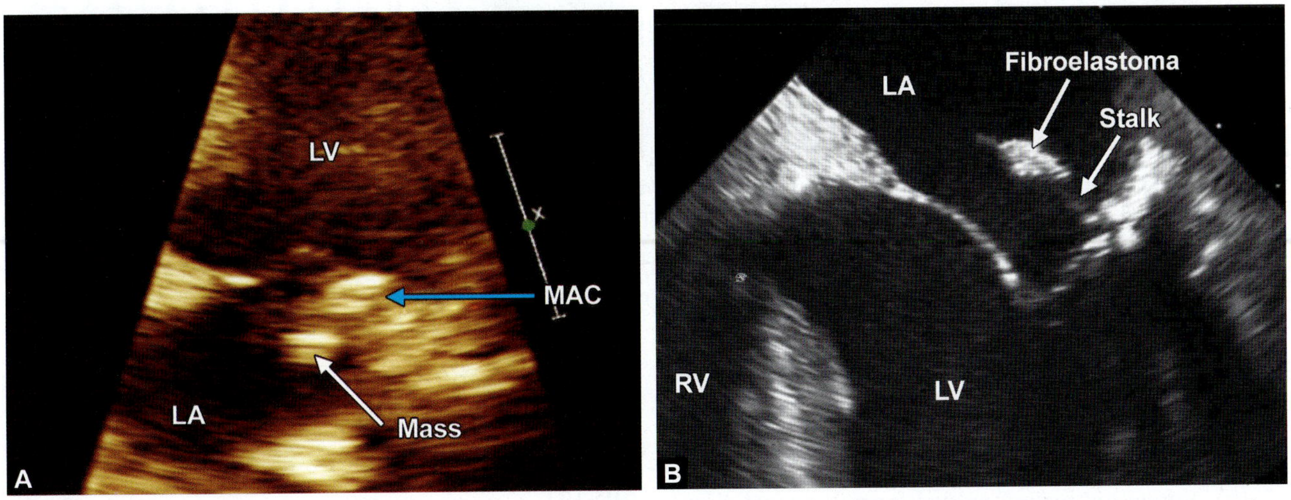

Figs. 192.1A and B: Transthoracic and transesophageal echocardiography (TTE and TEE). (A) TTE apical 4-chamber view demonstrates a large echo dense mass in LA attached to the posterior mitral leaflet. (B) TEE showing the same mass with a long stalk. (RV: Right ventricle; LV: Left ventricle; LA: Left atrium; MAC: mitral annular calcification).

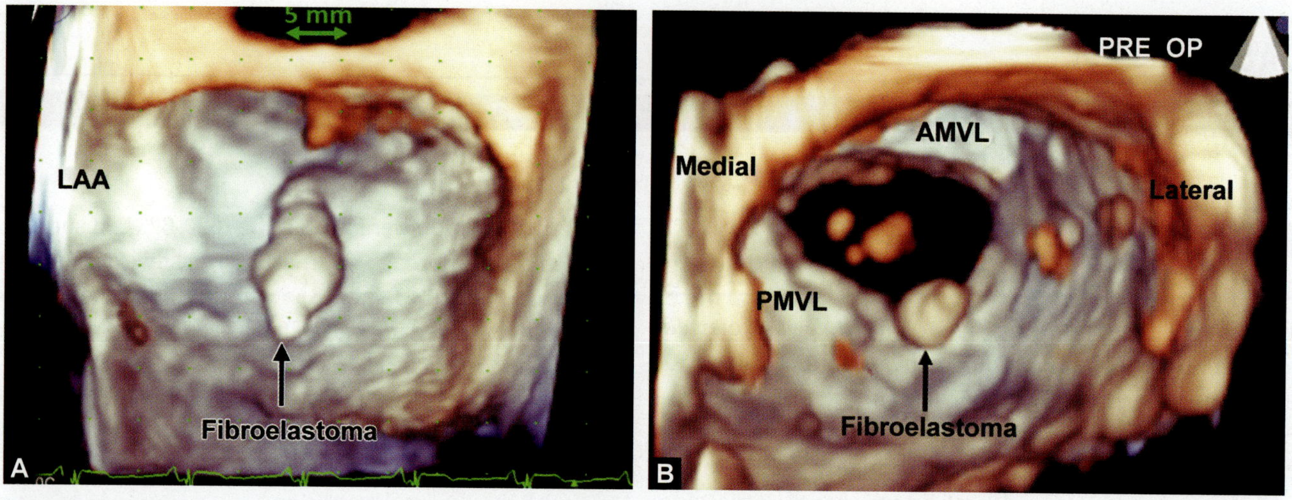

Figs. 192.2A and B: Intraoperative 3D TEE. (A) 3D zoom mode acquisition of the mitral valve in surgical view shows the mitral valve in closed position (systole) with a large mass attached to the tip of posterior leaflet. Length of the mass measured by 3D grid is approximately 1.5 cm. (B) 3D TEE view of the mitral valve from LV perspective demonstrates the mass prolapsing into the left ventricle. (LAA: left atrial appendage; AMVL: Anterior mitral valve leaflet; PMVL: Posterior mitral valve leaflet).

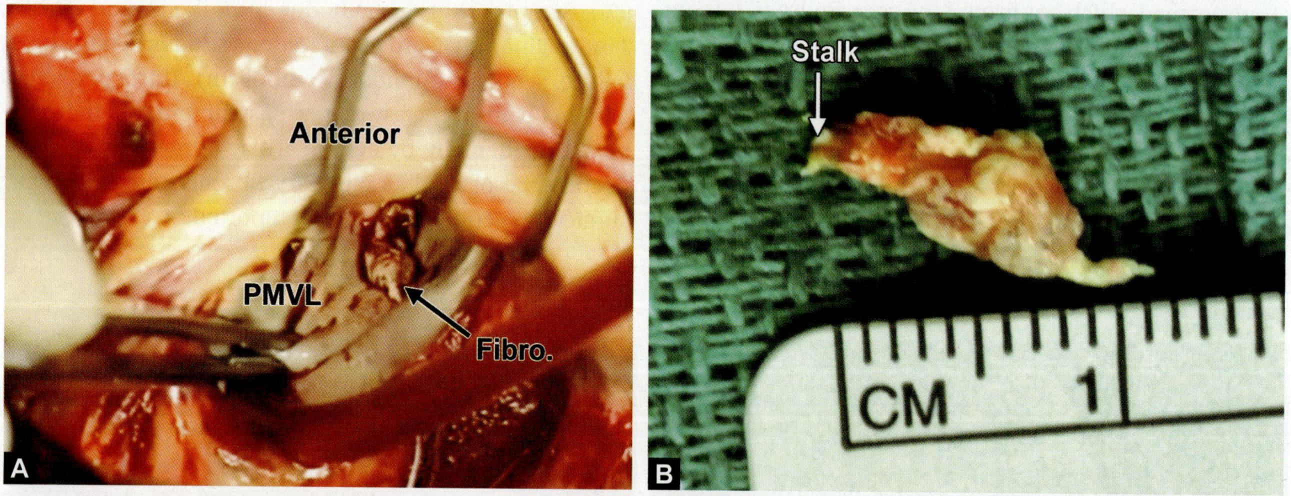

Figs. 192.3A and B: Surgical inspection of the left atrium and mitral valve. (A) Mass is attached to the tip of the posterior mitral leaflet. Mass was easily resectable without damaging the leaflet. (B) Well-delineated, pedunculated mass which measured about 1.5 cm in length. (PMVL: Posterior mitral valve leaflet; Fibro: Fibroelastoma).

1. **Regarding surgical intervention for cardiac fibroelastoma which of the following is correct?**
   (a) Surgery is recommended for patients who had embolic events.
   (b) Surgery is recommended for patients who had complications directly related to tumor mobility (e.g. coronary ostial occlusion).
   (c) Surgery is recommended for patients with a highly mobile mass or larger than 1 cm.
   (d) All of the above.

Ans. (d)

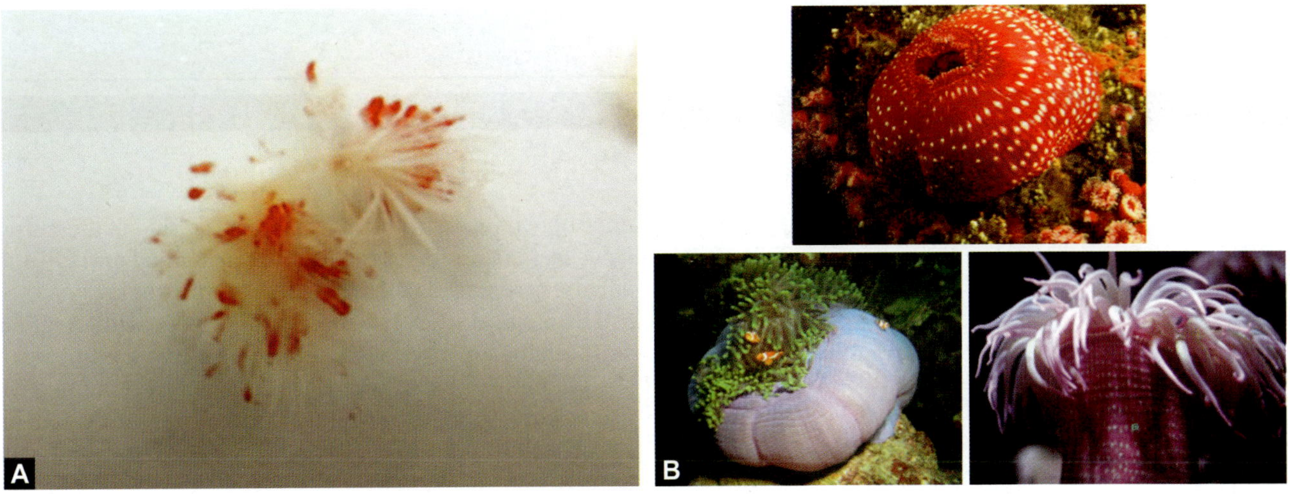

Figs. 192.4A and B: (A) Multiple small fronds are noted after immersion of the mass in normal saline giving the appearance of a sea anemone. (B) Actual sea anemone (for comparison).

MOVIE LEGENDS

620: TEE 4 chamber view showing a highly mobile pedunculated mass attached to the atrial side of the posterior mitral leaflet prolapsing into the left ventricle.

621: 3D TEE zoom mode acquisition of the mitral valve showing the fibroelastoma.

622: 3D TEE full volume acquisition (higher frame rate) in surgical view of the left atrium showing the highly mobile fibroelastoma.

623: 3D TEE full volume acquisition of the surgical view of the mitral valve shows no mitral regurgitation which is against the differential diagnosis of infective endocarditis.

REFERENCES

1. Evans AJ, Butany J, Omran AS, David TE. Incidental detection of an aortic papillary fibroelastoma by echocardiography in an asymptomatic patient presenting with hypertension. Can J Cardiol19997; 13(10):905-8.
2. Gowda RM, Khan IA, Nair CK, et al. Cardiac papillary fibroelastoma: a comprehensive analysis of 725 cases. Am Heart J. 2003; 146(3): 404.

CASE 193

Alberto Barón Castañeda

WHAT IS AROUND THE MITRAL VALVE?

A 47-year-old woman presented to the hospital because of a sudden loss of strength and muscular tone of her right arm, while working at her office. The paresis began to recover spontaneously, leaving no sequelae after 6 hours. She had no previous history of muscular disorders. In the past, she had sporadic episodes of migraine controlled with symptomatic treatment. She had normal blood pressure, 120/80 mm Hg, and the heart rate was 80/min. The only abnormal finding on physical examination was a soft grade II/VI systolic murmur, suggestive of mitral regurgitation. The blood tests were normal, with normal white and red blood cell count, and normal biochemistry. There was no evidence of brain infarct on magnetic resonance imaging (MRI).

To study the cause of the transient ischemic attack, a transesophageal echocardiogram (TEE) was performed. The cardiac chambers were normal in size, with normal systolic and diastolic function. The most relevant finding was the presence of an intracardiac mass, attached to the posterior mitral leaflet, in the P2 scallop. The size was about 10 mm diameter, and was moderately mobile. A smaller mass with similar characteristics was identified at the tip of the anterior leaflet (Figs. 193.1, 193.2, 624 and 625). Color Doppler confirmed grade III/IV central mitral regurgitation (Fig. 193.3, 626, arrow shows mitral regurgitation). In pursuit of a more precise definition of the mass and its relationship with cardiac structures, three-dimensional echocardiographic images were obtained using live 3D and zoom 3D techniques. The surface of the mass was irregular, with the presence of small mobile filaments, and the attachment pedicle was short (Figs. 193.4, 193.5, 627 and 628).

1. **What is the diagnosis?**
   (a) Thrombus
   (b) Vegetation
   (c) Papillary fibroelastoma
   (d) Myxoma
   (e) Lipoma

Ans. (c) Papillary fibroelastoma.

With the clinical history of severe transient ischemic attack, no brain infarction on MRI, and one of the masses with at least 1 cm diameter, surgery was performed soon. Macroscopical inspection of the valve confirmed the presence of two masses attached to the atrial side of the mitral valve leaflets similar to the findings described on TEE. The valve was replaced with a mechanical prosthesis.

Histological study revealed small tumors, with irregular surface due to finger-like projections that resembled a sea anemone. The structure was formed by a connective tissue core, with no evident blood vessels, covered by hypertrophic endothelial cells (Fig. 193.6), consistent with papillary fibroelastoma.

DISCUSSION

Papillary fibroelastoma is a benign endocardial tumor, the cause is not clear; some authors have proposed the hypothesis of inflammatory reaction consequence. The size is usually small with a mean diameter of about 8 mm. The surface is irregular with multiple frond-like projections resembling a sea anemone. The attachment is usually by a small pedicle, more frequently to the heart valves. The lesion is exclusively on the endocardial surface; is more common on the valve leaflets but may occur in any part of the heart.

The tumor is generally asymptomatic but non-specific symptoms such as fever may occur. The most serious symptoms are related to mechanical effects that may cause systemic embolization of tumor fragments or thrombus attached to the fibroelastoma, myocardial infarction,

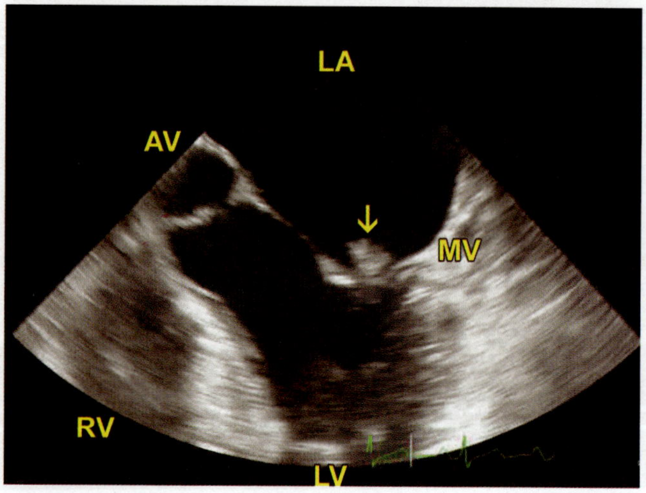

Fig. 193.1: Transesophageal echocardiogram at mid esophagus level. Notice the mass attached to the mitral valve (arrow).

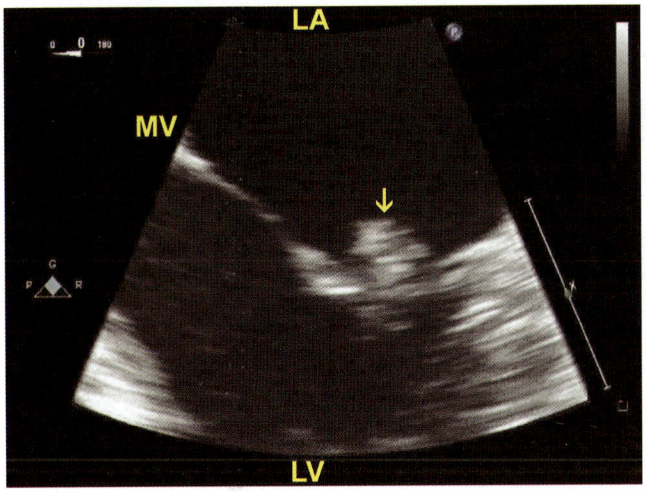

Fig. 193.2: Transesophageal echocardiogram at mid esophagus, zoom at the mitral valve. Notice the mass attached to the mitral valve (arrow).

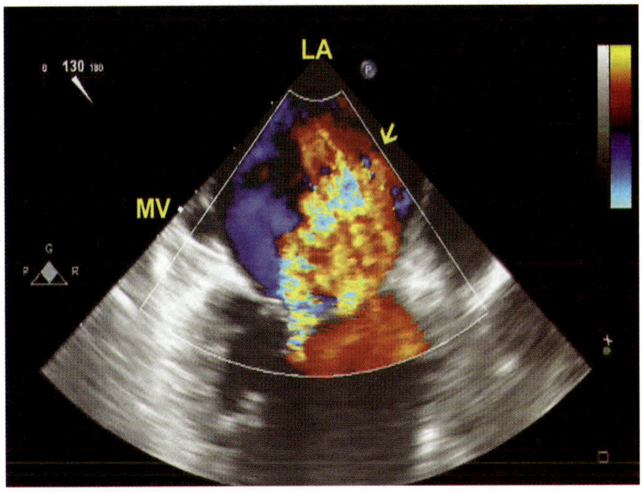

Fig. 193.3: Transesophageal echocardiogram at mid esophagus level. Color Doppler imaging shows mitral regurgitation (MR) (arrow).

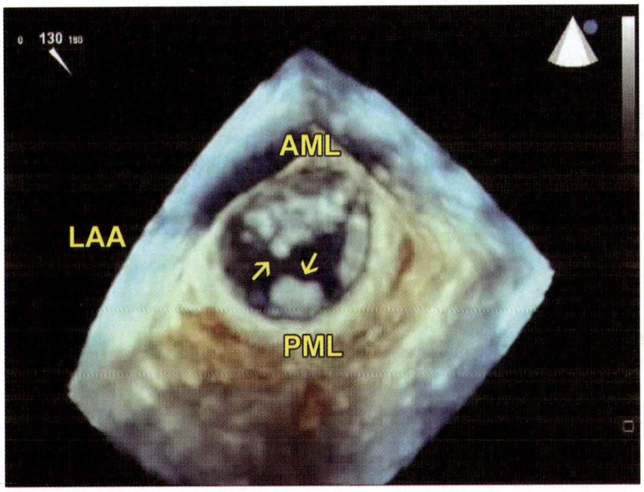

Fig. 193.4: Transesophageal 3D imaging of the mitral valve. Notice the masses attached to the mitral valve, at P2 and A2 scallops (arrows).

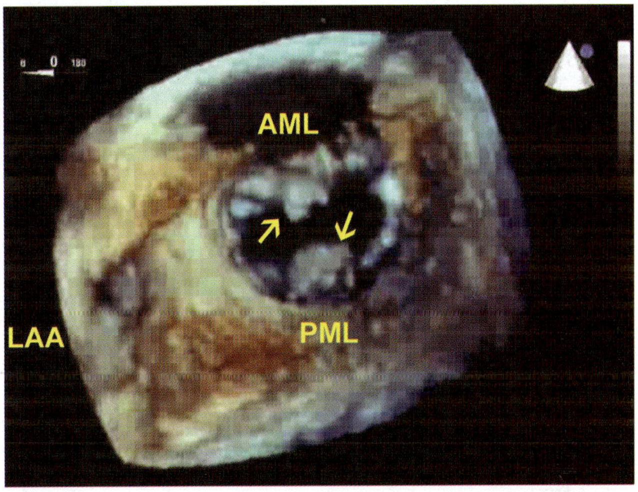

Fig. 193.5: Transesophageal zoom 3D imaging of the mitral valve. Notice the masses attached to the mitral valve, at P2 and A2 scallops (arrows).

syncope or sudden death as a consequence of coronary ostium occlusion by a mobile tumor.[1]

Because of lack of symptoms in many cases, the diagnosis is made by an incidental finding on echocardiographic studies. Its true prevalence is unknown, but it is the second most common cardiac tumor, after cardiac myxomas. In large series, papillary fibroelastoma constitutes 5 to 10% of all tumors of the heart.[2-4] Papillary fibroelastomas are the second most common primary neoplasm, after myxomas, and they are the most common valve tumor. They have been described in all age groups but it is more common in adults and the mean age of presentation is around 60 years.

The largest series have confirmed their location on left sided valves, about 70 to 80% of all fibroelastomas. They are more common on the aortic valve, about 40%.[5,6] Some are located on the right heart valves, and non-valvular locations have been described. The tumors are usually single but multiple fibroelastomas have been noted.[7]

The microscopic characteristics include a connective tissue core, composed of components derived from the endocardium. Usually there are no visible blood vessels.

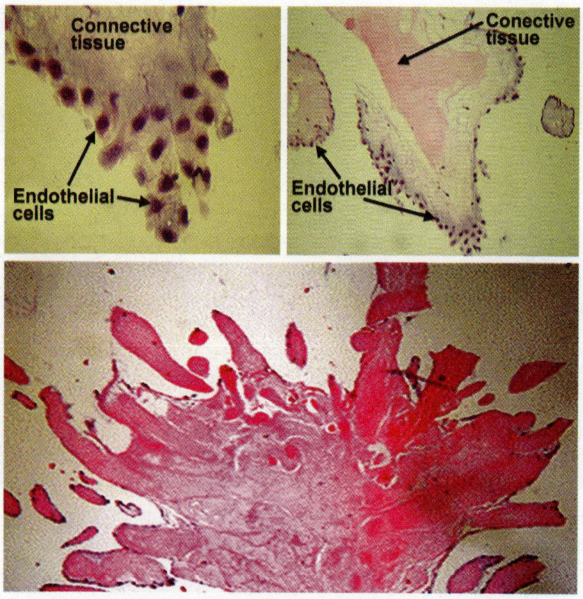

Fig. 193.6: Low magnification histological study of the cardiac mass attached to the posterior mitral leaflet. Observe the multiple finger-like projections that correspond with papillae.

The distribution is in form of papillae made of a muchopolysaccharide matrix surrounded by elastic fibers, loose connective tissue, and covered with hyperplastic endocardial cells.

Echocardiography is the ideal screening test for cardiac tumors with good overall accuracy, about 88%, even with transthoracic echo. The false negatives are due to masking by an associated lesion, very small tumors, association with degenerative valve disease, and in some cases due to poor quality examination.[7] According to the echocardiographic characteristics, the papillary fibroelastoma is described as a small homogeneous echo-dense mass, with irregular surface, attached to valves or endocardium by a short pedicle. The irregular surface may give a "vibration" appearance that differentiates it from a thrombus.

The differential diagnosis must include endocarditis, thrombus, fibroma, myxoma, Lambl's excrescences and valvular fenestrations.

In conclusion, papillary fibroelastoma is the second most common tumor of the heart, it has a small size and is usually related to cardiac valves. Diagnosis should be made not only by imaging as clinical presentation is important. Surgical excision is recommended when symptoms are present or with a size about 10 mm. Echocardiography is the ideal non-invasive screening test because it defines its location, size, movement, and relationships. Three-dimensional echocardiography gives more details about the mass.

MOVIE LEGENDS

624: Transesophageal echocardiogram at mid esophagus level. Notice the mass (arrow) attached to the mitral valve.

625: Transesophageal echocardiogram at mid esophagus, zoom at the mitral valve. Notice the mass (arrow) attached to the mitral valve.

626: Transesophageal echocardiogram at mid esophagus level. Color Doppler imaging shows mitral regurgitation (MR arrow).

627: Transesophageal 3D imaging of the mitral valve. Notice the masses attached to the mitral valve, at P2 (lower arrow) and A2 (upper arrow) scallops.

628: Transesophageal zoom 3D imaging of the mitral valve. Notice the masses attached to the mitral valve, at P2 (lower arrow) and A2 (upper arrow) scallops.

REFERENCES

1. Erdoes G, Stalder M, Basciani R, Gugger M, Carrel T, Eberle B. An Uncommon Cause of Coronary Artery Ostial Obstruction: Papillary Fibroelastoma. Echocardiography 2010;27:337-40.
2. Burke A, Jeudi J, Virmani R. Cardiac tumours: Cardiac tumours: an update. Heart 2008;94(1):117-23.
3. Edwards FH, Hale D, Cohen A, Thompson L, Pezzella AT, Virmani R. Primary cardiac tumors. An Thorac Surg 1991; 52(5):1127-31.
4. Tazelar HD, Locke TJ, McGregor CG. Pathology of surgical excised primary cardiac tumors. Mayo ClinProc 1992; 67: 957-65.
5. Gowda RM, Khan IA, Nair CK, Mehta NJ, Vasavada BC, Sacchi TJ. Cardiac papillary fibroelastoma: A comprehensive analysis of 725 cases, Am Heart J 2003;146:404–10.
6. Sun JP, Asher CR, Yang XS, Cheng GG, Scalia GM, et al. Clinical and Echocardiographic Characteristics of Papillary Fibroelastomas: A Retrospective and Prospective Study in 162 Patients. Circulation. 2001;103:2687-93.
7. Klarich KW, Enriquez-Sarano M, Gura GM,Edwards WD, Tajik AJ, Seward JB. Papillary fibroelastoma: echocardiographic characteristics for diagnosis and pathologic correlation. J Am Coll Cardiol. 1997; 30:784–90.

CASE 194

Jiang Leng, Mara Slawsky

PAPILLARY FIBROELASTOMAS

A 61-year-old female transferred from a local hospital for evaluation of chest pain. She is an ex-smoker, with past medical history of dyslipidemia and family history of premature coronary artery disease (CAD), father died of heart attack in the 60s and two brothers were diagnosed CAD in the 50s. She has been having recurrent intermittent chest pain over the past 9 months. The chest pain was substernal, angina in nature, but no clear association with exertion. Nine months ago, she underwent cardiac catheterization for chest pain associated with positive troponin, but did not find any coronary artery lesion. A week ago, she underwent a successful treadmill stress test in her cardiologist's office; however she developed cardiac arrest during recovery. She received CPR and was immediately transferred to our hospital for emergent cardiac catheterization. Again, there was no evidence of CAD, and LVEF was normal. She was discharged with medications for suspected vasospasm. But she continued having recurrent episodes of chest pain despite the medical treatment. Five days later, having been in severe prolonged chest pain, she presented in the local hospital, where she was diagnosed non-ST elevation myocardial infarction, with troponin peaked to 1.3 and CK 422. A bedside Echo was performed (Fig. 194.1, 629).

1. **What would you do next?**
   (a) More aggressive medical treatment
   (b) Repeat cardiac catheterization
   (c) Repeat a TTE echo
   (d) Oder a CTA
   (e) Perform a TEE

Ans. (e)

After the TEE (Figs. 194.2, 194.3 and 630 and 631), the patient underwent emergent cardiac surgery. While placing a retrograde catheter in the RA, the patient developed profound hypotension (SBP 40 mm Hg), marked ST depression, and marked global LV hypokinesis. Cardiopulmonary bypass was immediately commenced. A large papillary fibroelastomas was seen partially occluding the ostial left main coronary artery (Figs. 194.4 and 194.5).

Take Home Message

- Papillary fibroelastomas, although rare and generally benign, can result in life-threatening complications,

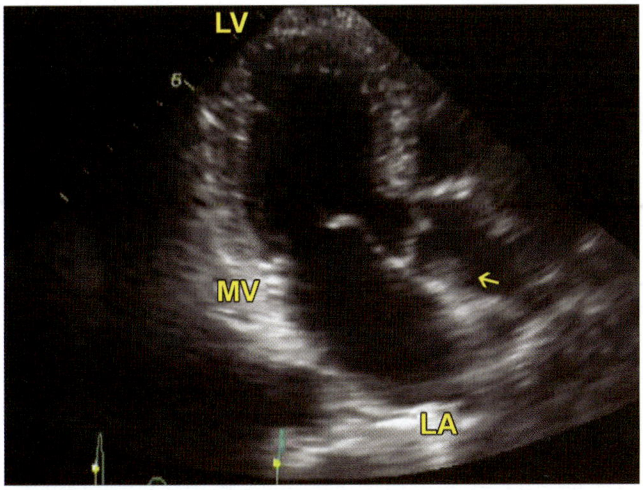

Fig. 194.1: Transthoracic apical view. Arrow points to a mass in the ascending aorta.

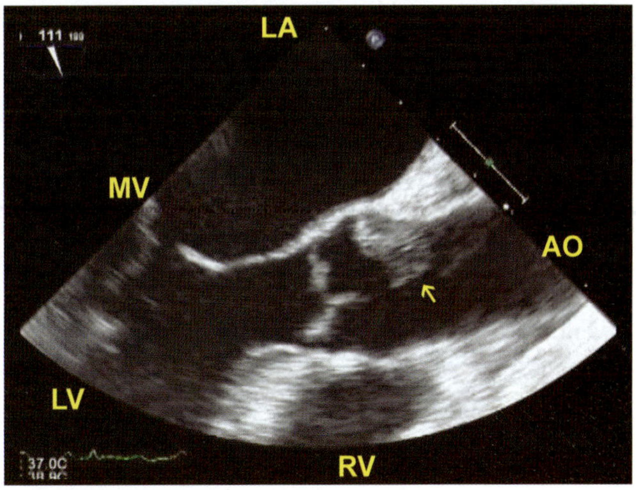

Fig. 194.2: Transesophageal echocardiography showing a mass in the ascending aorta (arrow).

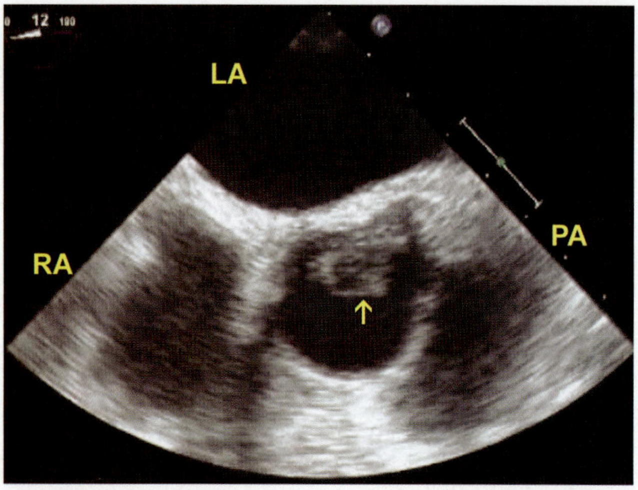

Fig. 194.3: Transesophageal short axis of the ascending aorta showing a mass (arrow) partially occluding the left coronary artery.

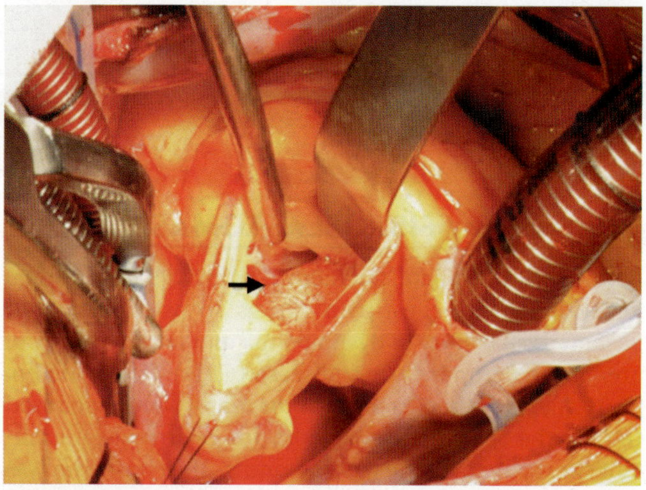

Fig. 194.4: Intraoperative view. Arrow points to the mass in the ascending aorta.

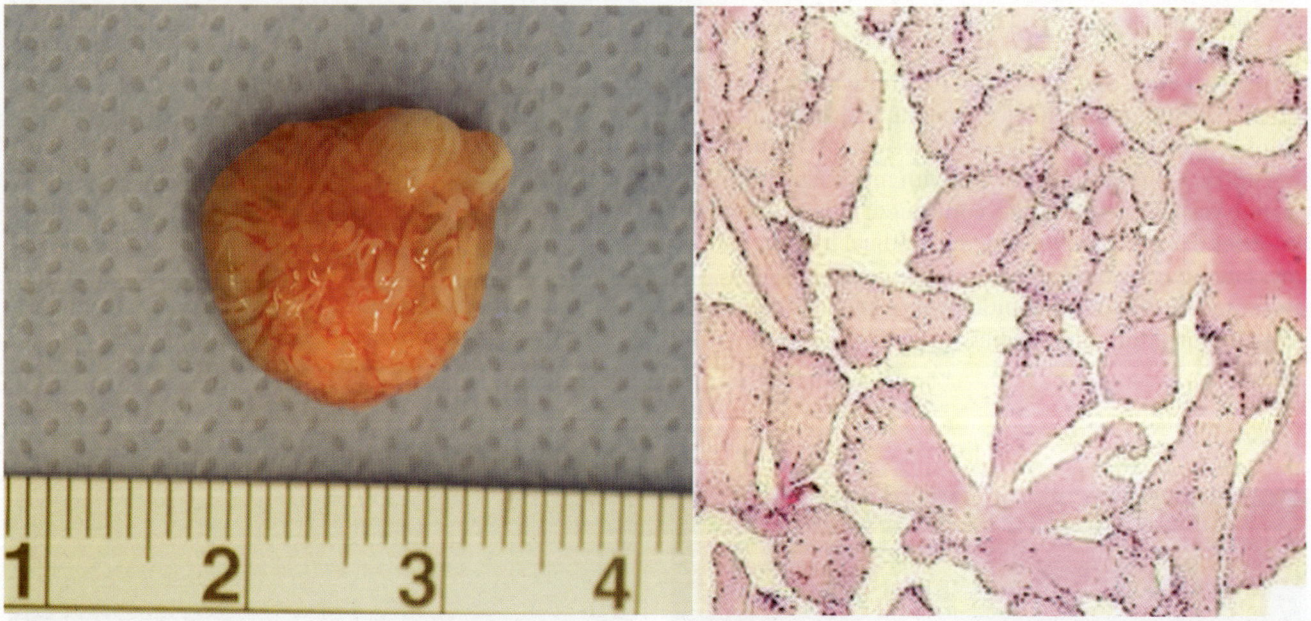

Fig. 194.5: Gross picture (left) and microscopic picture (right) of the resected mass.

such as acute coronary syndrome, stroke, embolism, ventricular fibrillation and sudden death.

- Patients with cardiovascular events (dynamic angina) that are not explained by the commonly seen cardiovascular diseases should undergo TTE/TEE, if necessary, to exclude other possible sources.

MOVIE LEGENDS

629: Transthoracic apical view. Arrow points to a mass in the ascending aorta.

630: Transesophageal echocardiography showing similar findings as above.

631: Transesophageal short axis of the ascending aorta showing a mass (arrow) partially occluding the left coronary artery.

CASE 195

Rajiv Patel, Jayant Patel, Julius M Gardin

HISTORY

This 54-year-old woman presented with chest pain and syncope while working in the OR.

ER findings: BP 177/98 mm Hg, pulse 83 bpm (regular), T 99°F, O_2 sat 100%

Mucus membranes were dry

Cardiovascular exam was normal

EKG: Normal Cardiac enzymes: Positive

Echocardiographic Findings (Figs. 195.1 to 195.3A and B and 632 to 634A and B)

Transthoracic and transesophageal long and short axis views demonstrate a round mass attached to the left coronary leaflet of the aortic valve.

CT Angiogram (Figs. 195.4A and B)

- No aortic dissection
- Small hypoattenuating structure arising from the left coronary cusp, measuring 4 mm × 4 mm

Operative Report

- Reddish-appearing mass, 8 mm in diameter, no stalk, on the free edge of the left coronary cusp, extending to the commissure with the non-coronary cusp
- Mass was excised and aortic leaflet defect was repaired.

Surgical Pathology Report

Aortic valve fibroelastoma measuring 3 mm × 3 mm × 2 mm.

Cardiac Papillary Fibroelastoma

Cleveland Clinic Series (Sun JP, et al. Circulation. 2001; 103:2687-93)

- Age/gender: 60 years (mean), 46% male
- Of 158 fibroelastomas, 48 were not seen by echo (< 2 mm)
- Among 110 fibroelastomas seen on echo
  - Average size: 9 ± 5mm
  - Mobility: 44% mobile
  - 48 had stalks

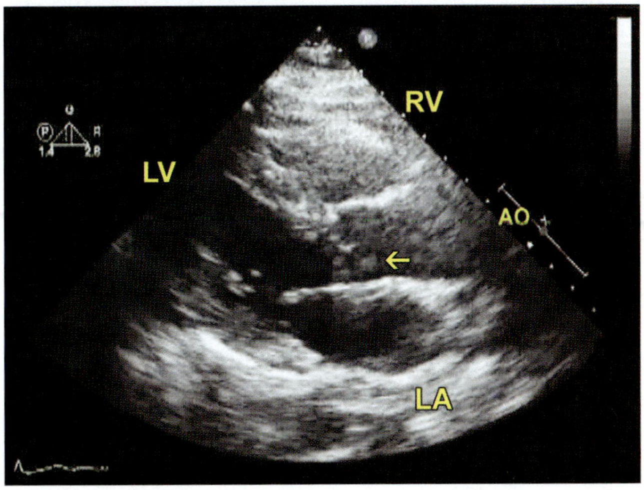

Fig. 195.1: Transthoracic parasternal long axis view. Arrow points to a mass attached to aortic valve leaflet.

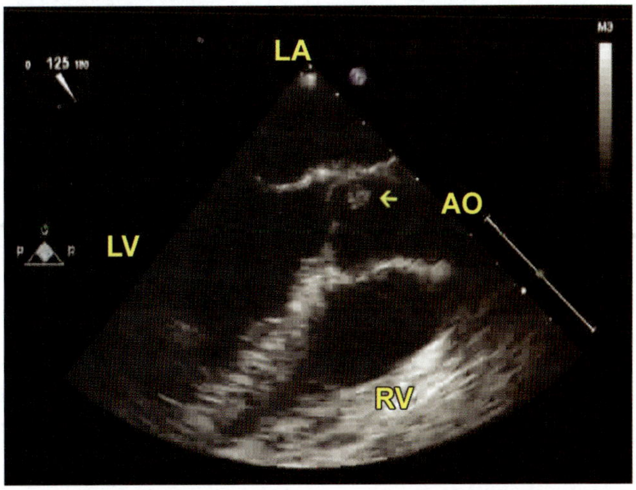

Fig. 195.2: Transesophageal long axis view showing a mass (arrow) attached to aortic valve leaflet.

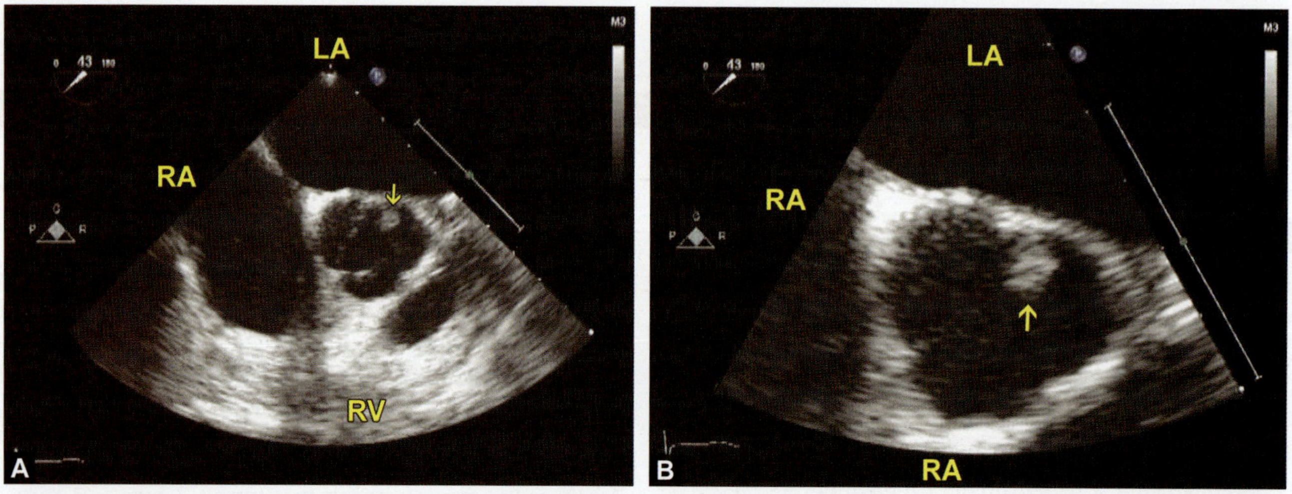

Figs. 195.3A and B: Transesophageal short axis view. (A) Arrow points to a mass attached to left coronary leaflet of the aortic valve. (B) Zoomed view of the aortic valve with similar findings.

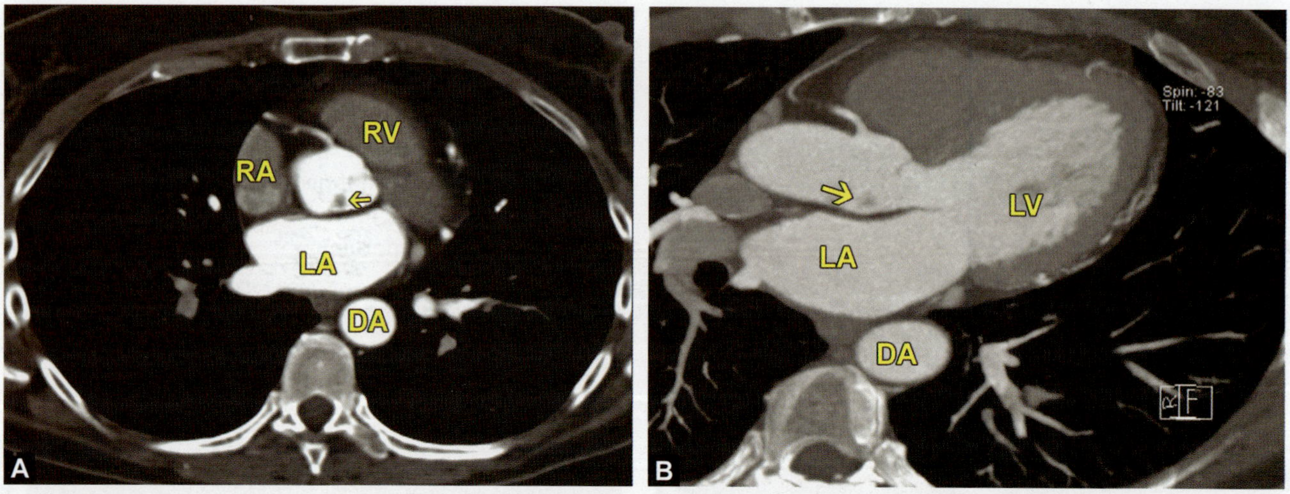

Figs. 195.4A and B: Computed tomography (CT) scan with contrast. Arrow points to a mass attached to aortic valve leaflet.

- Location (by echo)
  - 49 were on aortic valve
    - 24 on right, 6 on left and 19 on non-coronary cusps
    - 40 on aortic side and 9 on LV side of valve
  - 40 were on mitral valve
    - 23 on anterior and 17 on posterior leaflet
    - 32 on LA surface and 8 on LV surface
- During follow-up (552 ± 706 days) of 45 patients with echo diagnosis of fibroelastoma
  - One stroke
  - Two TIAs

MOVIE LEGENDS

632: Transthoracic parasternal long axis view. Arrow points to a mass attached to aortic valve leaflet.

633: Transesophageal long axis view showing a mass (arrow) attached to aortic valve leaflet.

634A and B: Transesophageal short axis view. (A) Arrow points to a mass attached to left coronary leaflet of the aortic valve. (B) Zoomed view of the aortic valve with similar findings.

CASE 196

Elsayed M, Hsiung MC, Kalra R, Mustafa IA, Uygur B, Chahwala JR, Nanda NC

THYMOMA

The patient is a 35-year-old male. Chest X-ray showed a mediastinal mass and he underwent median sternotomy with mediastinal tumor resection which was found to be a malignant thymoma on pathology. He was placed on chemotherapy. 2D (635) and 3D (636) TEE were done during surgery.

1. **Which of the following statements is incorrect (635 and 636)?**
   (a) The arrowhead shows echogenic areas consistent with calcifications, solid arrow shows echolucencies surrounded by echogenic rings (doughnut appearance) and the hollow arrow shows localized echolucencies consistent with tumor necrosis. A diagnosis of malignancy can be suggested on the basis of one or two of these findings.
   (b) A diagnosis of malignant nature of the tumor can never be suggested on the basis of the above findings.
   (c) Calcification seen in this mass may point to a relatively slow growth of the tumor.
   (d) Echolucencies may not always mean necrosis. They may be due to hemorrhages and in case of a clot result from clot lysis or liquefaction.

Ans. (b)

There is a case report in the literature (1) which demonstrated a doughnut appearance suggestive of malignancy with correlation with histology. The doughnut appearance is caused by small echolucencies suggestive of tumor necrosis surrounded by rings of fibrous/collagen tissue. Areas of calcification may be present in any tumor if the growth is slow. Echolucencies in a tumor are consistent with hemorrhage as in a myxoma or necrosis due to malignancy. Echolucencies involving the whole tumor including extension to the periphery point to vascular channels in a hemangioma. In this patient the LV function is normal hence clot formation would not be expected (Figs. 196.1A to D).

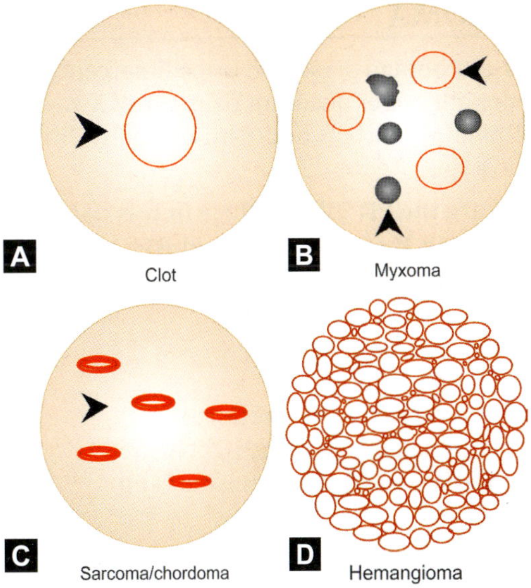

Figs. 196.1A to D: Schematics drawing of (A) clot, (B) myxoma, (C) sarcoma/chordoma, and (D) hemangioma. The horizontal arrowhead in (A) points to central lysis in a clot, in (B) it points to an area of hemorrhage/necrosis in a myxoma, and in (C) to an area of necrosis surrounded by thick, band-like tissue containing collagen, giving a doughnut-like appearance seen with chordoma and sarcoma. The vertical arrowhead in (B) points to dense calcification in the myxoma. (D) demonstrates a hemangioma that is completely vascular and the echolucencies involve the whole tumor, including periphery.
Source: Reproduced with permission from Nanda NC. Editor: Comprehensive Textbook of Echocardiography (2014). Page: 1505, Fig. 70.48E. Jaypee Brothers Medical Publishers (Limited). New Delhi, London, Philadelphia and Panama.

MOVIES 635 AND 636

REFERENCE

1. Suwanjutah T, Singh H, Plaisance BR, et al: Live/real time three-dimensional transthoracic echocardiographic findings in primary left atrial leiomyosarcoma. Echocardiography 2008;25:337-39.

CASE 197

Thind M, Hsiung MC, Gok G, Elsayed M, Joson M, Nanda NC

LYMPHOMA

A 63-year-old woman presented to the Emergency Department with right upper quadrant pain. Chest X-ray showed bilateral pleural effusion and cardiomegaly. 2D and 3D TEE were done.

1. **What are the 2D TEE findings in this patient (Figs. 197.1A and B and 637A and B)? All except one statement are correct:**
   (a) Pericardial effusion (PE)
   (b) Left pleural effusion
   (c) Mass infiltrating IAS
   (d) Mass encasing the aortic root
   (e) Pacemaker lead in the right heart
   (f) Mass probably involving the Q tip

Ans. (b)

The figure and movie show the above findings. This patient was found to have diffuse, large B-cell lymphoma on open epicardial biopsy. Chemotherapy with various agents was instituted but the patient died before the course could be completed.

2. **What incremental value was provided by 3D echo (Figs. 197.2A-K and 638A-J)?**
   (a) More comprehensive assessment of tumor burden by showing involvement of additional structures
   (b) Quantification of tumor volume
   (c) Differentiation of tumor involvement of IAS from lipomatous hypertrophy. In both cases the fossa ovalis is usually spared
   (d) All of the above are correct
   (e) Only A and B are correct

Ans. (d)

All the 3D figures and movies bring the above points home convincingly. They also provide valuable educational insight into the technique of careful and systematic cropping of the 3D data sets resulting in a comprehensive examination. Figures 197.3A and B are CT scan images of the lymphoma.

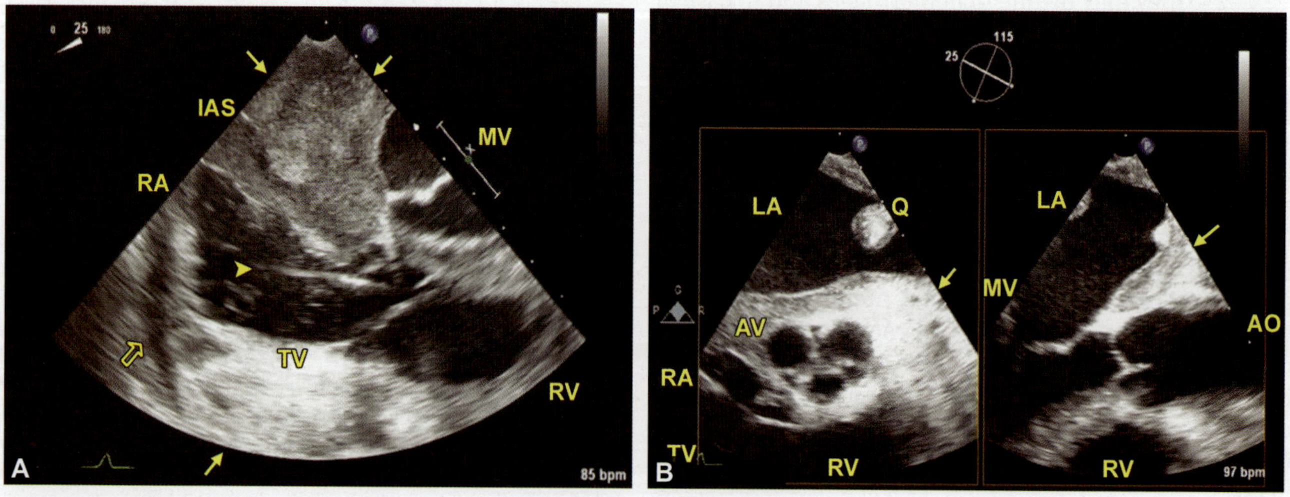

Figs. 197.1A and B: Two-dimensional transesophageal echocardiography in cardiac lymphoma. (A) Arrows point to a mass infiltrating the interatrial septum (IAS) and right atrioventricular groove consistent with a tumor. Hollow arrow shows pericardial effusion. Arrowhead points to pacemaker lead in the right atrium (RA). Mitral valve (MV), tricuspid valve (TV), and right ventricle (RV) are shown. (B) Arrows point to a mass encasing the aortic valve (AV) annulus and between left atrium (LA) and aorta (AO). The "Q" tip (Q) appears thickened. MV, TV, RA, and RV are shown.

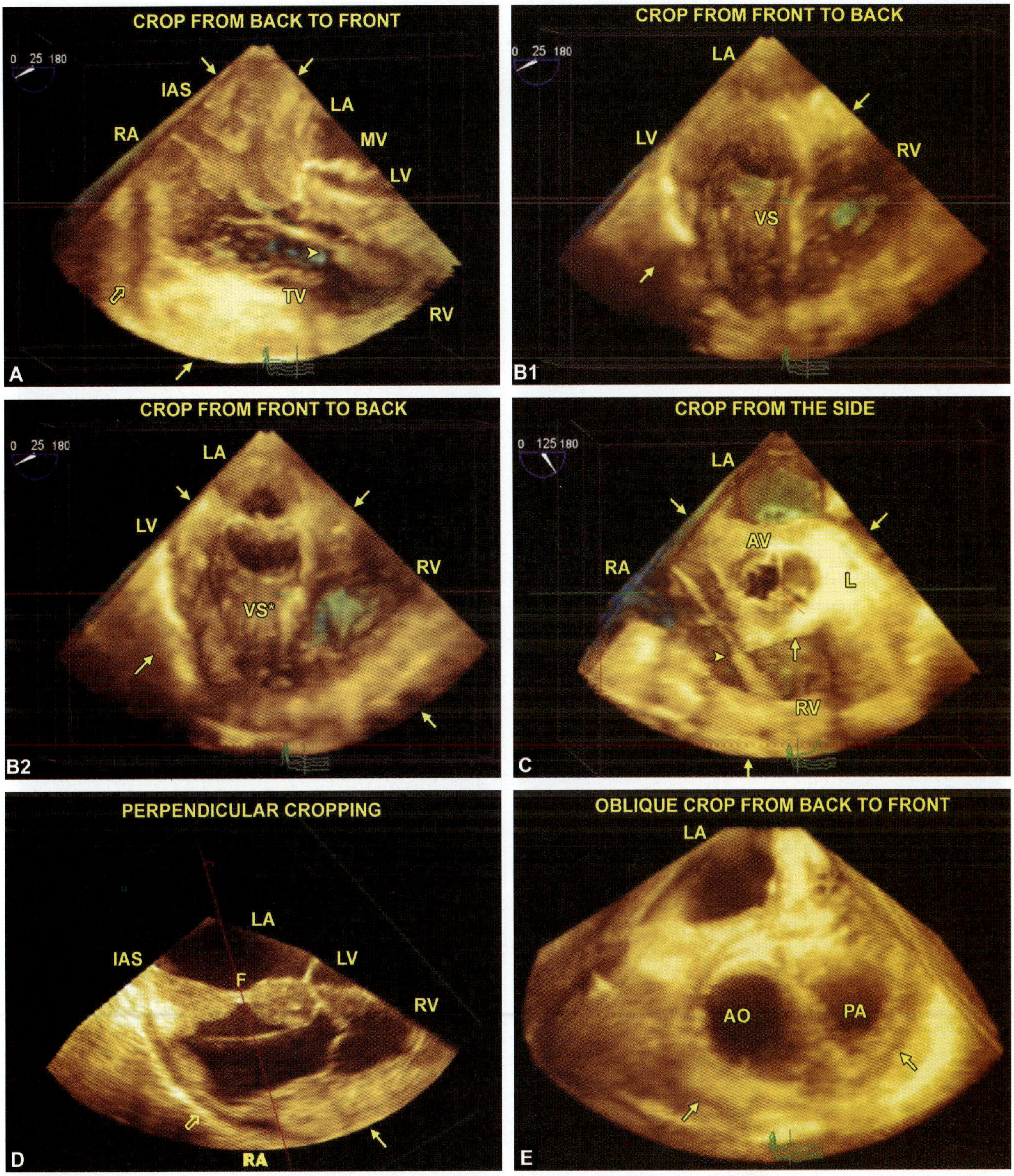

Figs. 197.2A to E: Three-dimensional transesophageal echocardiography in cardiac lymphoma. (A) Extensive inhomogeneity and lobularity can be seen between RA and LA (arrows). The pacemaker lead (arrowhead) and pericardial effusion (hollow arrow) can be seen. Infiltrated tissue (arrow) can also be seen in the free wall of the RA and RV. (B1) Infiltrated tissue can be seen in the walls of the LV and LA (arrows). There is slight thickening of this anterior portion of the ventricular septum (VS). (B2) There is greater involvement of this posterior portion of the ventricular septum (VS*). (C) Infiltrated tissue (arrows) can be seen surrounding the aortic annulus and encasing the left main coronary artery (L). The pacemaker lead (arrowhead) can be seen in the RV chamber, and infiltrated tissue (arrow) can be seen in the wall. (D) The thickened interatrial septum is infiltrated by the mass (arrow) with relative sparing of the fossa ovalis (F). (E) The mass (arrows) has encased the AO and PA causing marked thickening of their walls.

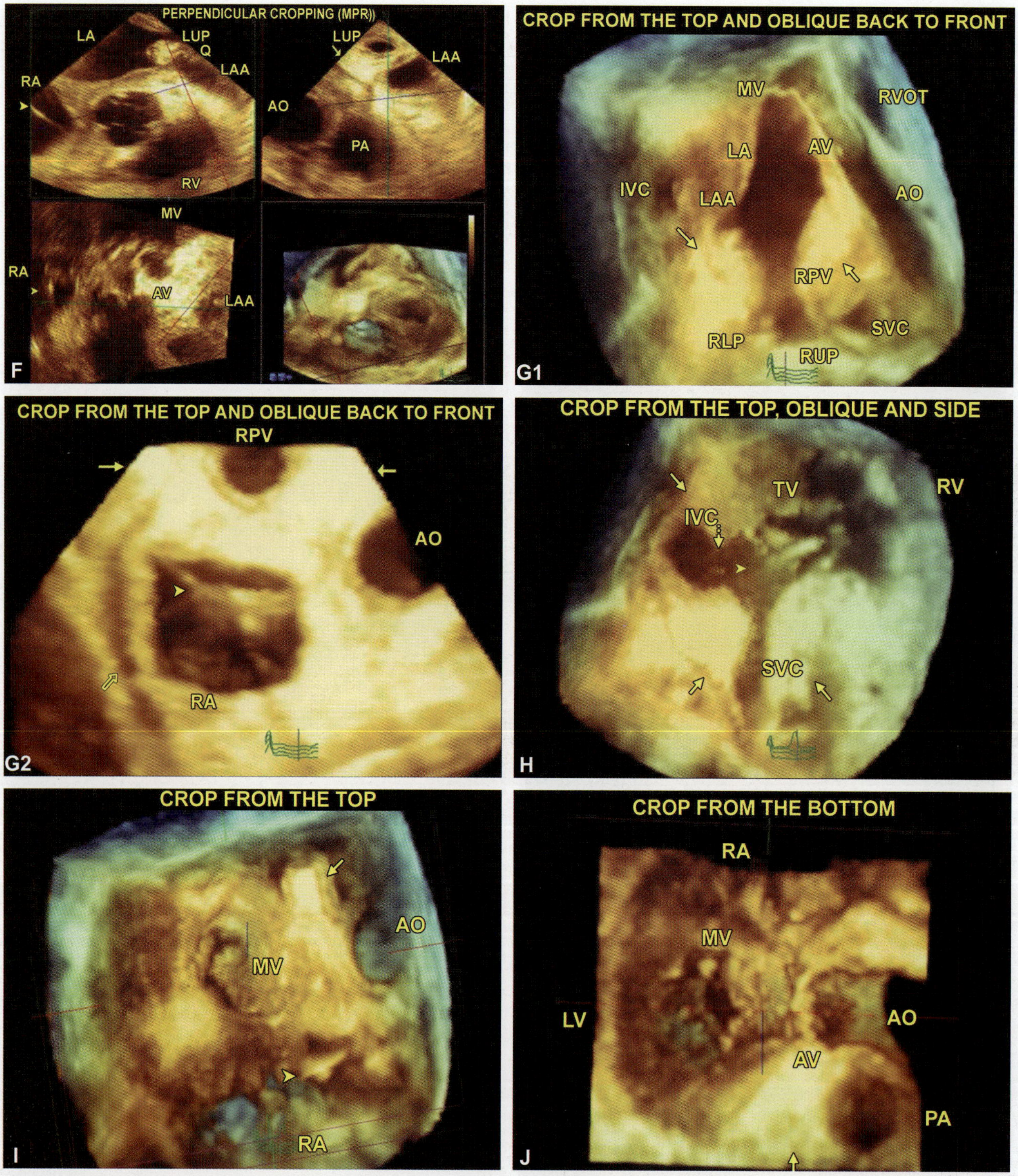

Figs. 197.2F to J: (F) Multiplanar reconstruction (MPR) mode. In the green box (left upper panel), a long-axis view of the left upper pulmonary vein (LUP), Q, and LAA can be seen. The blue line within the green box indicates the level at which the dataset was cropped to view the LAA in short axis (blue box, left lower panel). Four lobes of LAA can be seen with adjacent infiltrated tissue. The red line within the green box indicates the level at which the dataset was cropped to view the LUP in short axis (red box, right upper panel). Infiltrated tissue can be seen adjacent to but not invading the LUP lumen. (G1) Infiltrated tissue (arrows) is seen on each side of the right upper (RUP) and right lower (RLP) pulmonary veins, which join to form a confluent right pulmonary vein (RPV). LA, MV, AV, AO, LAA, superior vena cava (SVC), inferior vena cava (IVC), and RV outflow tract (RVOT) are also seen. (G2) Infiltrated tissue can be seen surrounding the RPV in this short-axis view. (H) Infiltrated tissue (arrows) can be seen surrounding the SVC and IVC. The dotted arrow points to the Eustachian valve. The TV and RV are also seen. (I) Infiltrated tissue (arrow) can be seen encasing the MV annulus. (J) Infiltrated tissue (arrow) can be seen encasing the aortic valve.

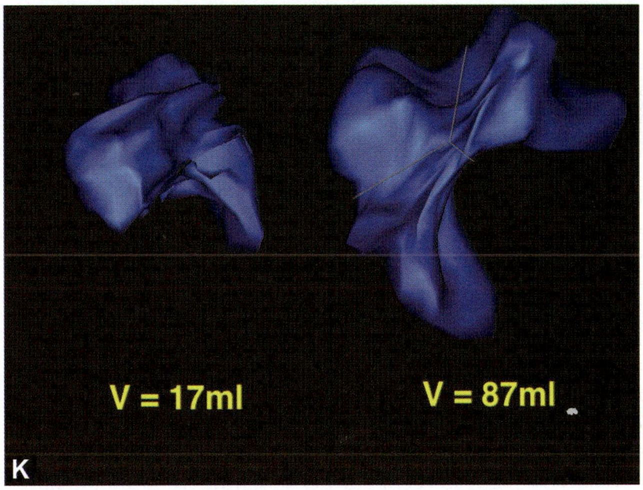

Fig. 197.2K: The total mass burden of 104 mL was calculated by combining the volume of infiltrated tissue between the AO, LA, and PA (17 mL) with the volume of infiltrated tissue extending from the right atrioventricular groove, around the SVC, and encasing the other great vessels (87 mL).

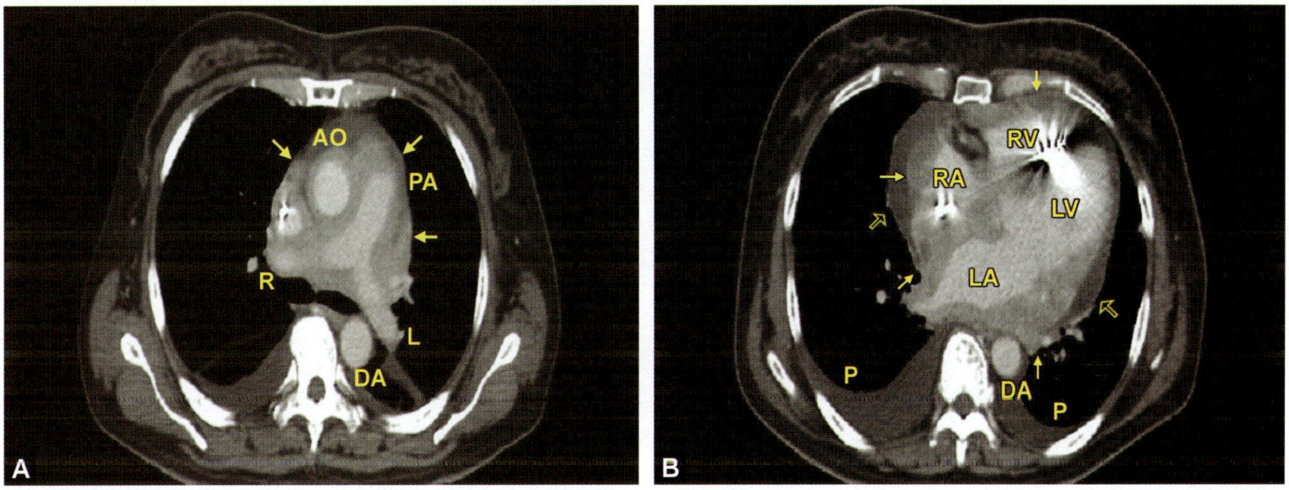

Figs. 197.3A and B: Computed tomography of the chest in cardiac lymphoma. (A) Arrows point to a mass surrounding the ascending aorta (AO), main pulmonary artery (PA), right pulmonary artery (R), and left pulmonary artery (L). Descending aorta (DA) is also seen. (B) Arrows show a mass infiltrating the free walls of the right atrium (RA) and right ventricle (RV), the interatrial septum, and the free walls of the left atrium (LA) and left ventricle (LV). Hollow arrows show a pericardial effusion. Bilateral pleural effusions (P) and the descending aorta (DA) are also seen.

MOVIE LEGENDS

637A: Arrows point to a mass infiltrating the interatrial septum (IAS) and right atrioventricular groove consistent with a tumor. Hollow arrow shows pericardial effusion. Arrowhead points to pacemaker lead in the right atrium (RA). Mitral valve (MV), tricuspid valve (TV), and right ventricle (RV) are shown.

637B: Arrows point to a mass encasing the aortic valve (AV) annulus and between left atrium (LA) and aorta (AO). The "Q" tip (Q) appears thickened. MV, TV, RA, and RV are shown.

638A: Lobular infiltration of the interatrial septum. Cropping the 3D dataset from back to front initially shows infiltrated tissue in the right atrioventricular groove (arrow) and causing lobulation and inhomogeneity of the interatrial septum (arrows). A hollow arrow points to the pericardial effusion. Further cropping in the same direction shows an increasingly lobulated septum and shows the uninvolved pacemaker lead (arrowhead) extending into RV.

638B: Ventricular septum. Cropping the 3D dataset from front to back initially shows the mass infiltrating the left ventricular (LV) free wall (arrow) and also involving the anterior ventricular septum (VS). Further cropping in the same direction reveals that the posterior portion of the ventricular septum is more involved (VS*) as compared to the anterior portion. Arrows also show involvement of RV wall and LA wall.

638C: Coronaries. Cropping the 3D dataset from the side initially reveals the lumen of the proximal right coronary artery (R) encased by infiltrated tissue. Further cropping one slice at a time in the same direction demonstrates the origin of the right coronary artery adjacent to the right coronary cusp and the origin of the left main coronary artery (L) adjacent to the left coronary cusp. Further cropping shows the lumen of the left main coronary artery (L) encased by infiltrated tissue, and further cropping shows infiltrated tissue (arrows) encasing the AV. There is no compression of the lumen of any of the coronary arteries visualized. The pacemaker lead (arrowhead) is shown in the RV.

638D: Rotation to assess the interatrial septum. Rotating between two perpendicular slices through the fossa ovalis (F) demonstrates relative sparing of this portion of the interatrial septum. Infiltrated tissue can be seen in the right atrioventricular groove and the interatrial septum (arrows).

638E1: Pulmonary artery and aorta. Cropping the 3D dataset from the side at an oblique angle demonstrates the thickened walls of the AO and pulmonary artery (PA) infiltrated with the mass (arrows). Further cropping through to the AV and pulmonic valve (PV) shows the extension of the infiltrated tissue along the vessels. The pacemaker lead is also seen (arrowhead).

638E2: Pulmonary artery. Multiplanar reconstruction (MPR) mode. PA is shown in short axis (left upper panel, green box) and in long axis (right upper panel, red box). As the green cropping plane is moved in the long axis view, encasement of the PA by the mass (arrows) can be seen in the corresponding short axis view.

638E3: Rotation to assess the pulmonary artery. Rotating between the long and short axis of the PA demonstrates the full extent of its encasement by the mass (arrows).

638F1: Left upper pulmonary vein. Cropping the 3D dataset from back to front shows the left upper pulmonary vein (LUP) and the left atrial appendage (LAA). Subsequent cropping from the side at an oblique angle shows a short-axis view of the LUP with bordering infiltrated tissue but no invasion of the lumen.

638F2: Left upper pulmonary vein. Multiplanar reconstruction (MPR) mode. In the green box (left upper panel), a long-axis view of the LUP, Q, and LAA can be seen. The blue line within the green box indicates the level at which the dataset was cropped to view the LAA in short axis (blue box, left lower panel). Four lobes of LAA can be seen with adjacent infiltrated tissue. The red line within the green box indicates the level at which the dataset was cropped to view the LUP in short axis (red box, right upper panel). Infiltrated tissue can be seen adjacent to but not invading the LUP lumen.

638G1: Right upper and lower pulmonary veins. Cropping the 3D dataset from the top shows infiltrated tissue (arrows) on each side of the right upper (RUP) and right lower (RLP) pulmonary veins, which join to form a common right pulmonary vein (RPV). LA, MV, AV, AO, LAA, superior vena cava (SVC), inferior vena cava (IVC), and RV outflow tract (RVOT) are also seen. Subsequent cropping from back to front at an oblique angle shows a short-axis view of the confluent RPV encased by infiltrated tissue but no lumen invasion. The pacemaker lead (arrowhead) and pericardial effusion (hollow arrow) are also seen.

638G2: Right upper and lower pulmonary veins. Cropping the 3D dataset from the top shows infiltrated tissue on each side of RUP and RLP. LA, MV, AV, AO, LAA, SVC, IVC, and RVOT are also seen. Subsequent cropping from the side shows tumor tissue (arrows) in the IAS and between the RA and the confluent RPV. The pericardial effusion (hollow arrow) and pacemaker lead (arrowhead) are also seen.

638H1: Superior and inferior vena cava. Cropping the 3D dataset from the top shows infiltrated tissue on each side of the RUP and RLP. The LA, MV, AV, AO, LAA, SVC, IVC, and RVOT are also seen. Further cropping from the top at an oblique angle shows the mass (arrows) surrounding the SVC and IVC. The TV, Eustachian valve (dotted arrow), RV, and pacemaker lead (arrowhead) are also seen. Subsequent cropping from the side shows infiltrated tissue (arrows) in the interatrial septum and the right atrioventricular groove, and the pericardial effusion is seen (hollow arrow).

638H2: Superior and inferior vena cava. The 3D dataset cropped at an oblique angle from the top shows the SVC, IVC, TV, Eustachian valve (dotted arrow), and RV. Cropping from back to front shows the SVC in short axis encased by infiltrated tissue.

638H3: Superior and inferior vena cava. The 3D dataset cropped at an oblique angle from the top shows SVC, IVC, TV, and RV. Cropping from the side shows the IVC in short axis with some adjacent infiltrated tissue. The Eustachian valve (dotted arrow) can be seen in long axis and en face.

638I: Mitral valve annulus. Cropping the 3D dataset from the top initially shows infiltrated tissue (arrow) surrounding the MV annulus. Further cropping in the same direction shows infiltrated tissue (arrow) lateral to the AV annulus, and further cropping shows infiltrated tissue around LV, RV, and PA.

638J: Mitral valve annulus. Cropping the 3D dataset from the bottom initially shows the LV and pacemaker lead (arrowhead) in the RV, further cropping in the same direction shows the AV and PA, and further cropping then shows the MV. Other abbreviations as in figures.

Source: This case is reproduced with permission from: Thind M, Hsiung MC, Gok G, Elsayed M, Joson M, Nanda NC. Incremental value of live/real time three-dimensional transesophageal echocardiography over the two-dimensional modality in the assessment of cardiac lymphoma. Echocardiography. 2015 Apr;32(4):671-6.

CASE 198

Daniel W Groves, Robert A Quaife, Amber D Khanna, Ernesto E Salcedo

LEFT ATRIAL MASS

A 65-year-old male presents with shortness of breath and chest discomfort. He is in atrial fibrillation with rapid ventricular response. His heart rate on presentation is approximately 150 beats per minute. He is started on heparin and esmolol drips, but quickly converts to sinus rhythm. He had a prior surgical resection of a bone cancer in his right hip over 10 years ago. A chest CT scan performed 3 years prior to presentation demonstrated multiple pulmonary nodules. A transthoracic echocardiogram and cardiac CT were performed during this admission.

1. **Based on the history and images provided, what is the patient's most likely diagnosis (Figs. 198.1 to 198.5 and 639 to 645)?**
   (a) Myxoma
   (b) Angiosarcoma
   (c) Left atrial thrombus
   (d) Metastatic chondrosarcoma

Ans. (d)

This patient has metastatic chondrosarcoma. Chondrosarcoma is a primary bone cancer that can metastasize to the lungs. In rare instances, these metastatic lesions can directly extend into the heart. From the history, he reports a prior surgical resection of a bone cancer and a prior chest CT showed multiple pulmonary nodules which are concerning for metastatic disease. On the transthoracic echocardiogram, there is a large, heterogenous echogenic mass seen in the left atrium that protrudes into the left ventricle during diastole causing obstruction of mitral flow. From the apical four chamber view, this mass appears to extend from the right pulmonary veins. The CT images demonstrate a large right hilar mass which has obliterated the right inferior pulmonary vein and eroded through the posterior left atrial wall. Angiosarcoma is a malignant primary cardiac tumor, but is typically right-sided and associated with a hemorrhagic pericardial effusion. Myxoma is a benign primary cardiac tumor and is most commonly located in the left atrium originating from the interatrial septum. However, a myxoma would typically be more echodense and would not have lung involvement as seen in this case. The images are not consistent with a left atrial thrombus.

2. **What is the mechanism of metastases in this patient?**
   (a) Direct extension
   (b) Hematogenous spread
   (c) Lymphatic spread

Ans. (a)

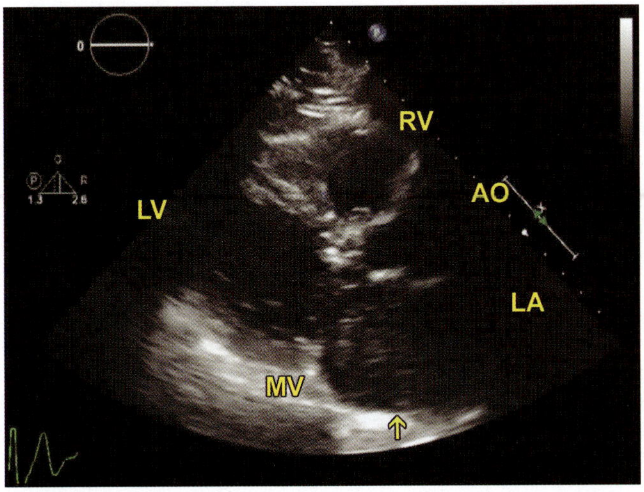

Fig. 198.1: Transthoracic parasternal long axis view. Arrow points to the large mass filling most of LA.

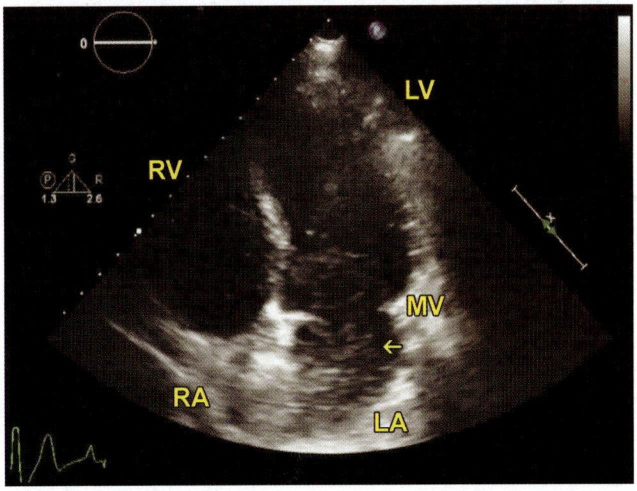

Fig. 198.2: Transthoracic apical 4 chamber view. Arrow points to mass protruding through MV.

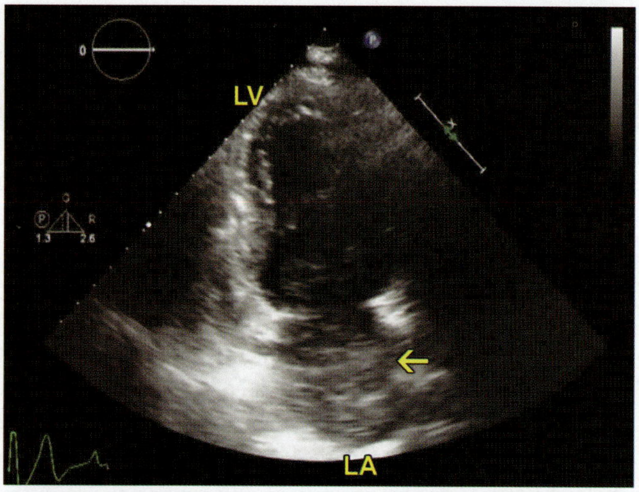

Fig. 198.3: Transthoracic apical 2 chamber view with similar findings as above. Arrow points to the mass.

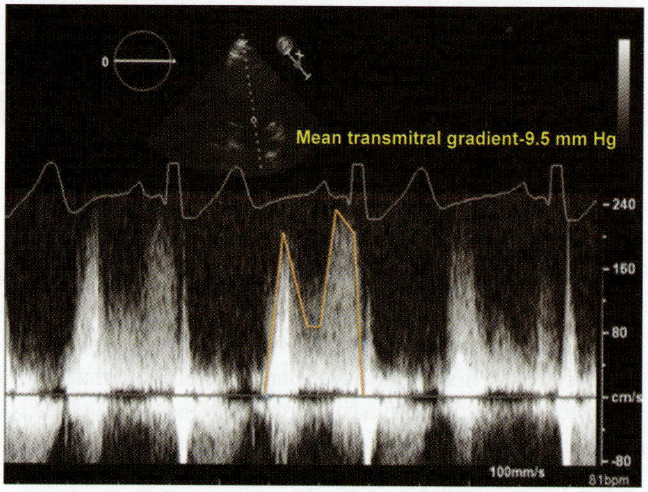

Fig. 198.4: Continuous wave Doppler showing mean pressure gradient of 9.5 mm Hg through the mitral valve.

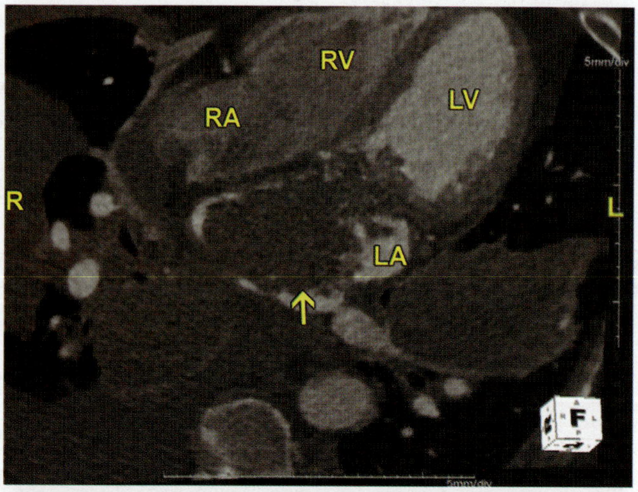

Fig. 198.5: Computed tomography (CT) with contrast. Arrow points to the mass occupying most of LA.

A. In rare cases, chrondrosarcoma lung metastases will directly invade the heart often through the pulmonary veins. Breast cancer can have hematogenous spread to the heart while lymphomas can have lymphatic spread to the heart.

MOVIE LEGENDS

639: Transthoracic parasternal long axis view. Arrow points to the large mass filling most of LA.

640: Transthoracic apical 4 chamber view. Arrow points to mass protruding through MV.

641: Transthoracic apical 2 chamber view with similar findings as above. Arrow points to the mass.

CASE 199

Inga Vaitenas, Nicholas Furiasse, Kameswari Maganti

A DUCK IN THE HEART?

A 56-year-old male with history of metastatic myxoid liposarcoma of the left thigh with pulmonary metastases underwent 4 cycles of chemotherapy followed by surgical resection of lung and lower extremity masses who remained asymptomatic and disease-free for the next 3.5 years. He was admitted with dyspnea and syncope due to an acute pulmonary embolism. A TTE demonstrated a 4 × 3 cm mass in the right ventricle (RV) (Fig. 199.1). He was treated with chemotherapy and radiation, and remained asymptomatic.

A follow-up echo (Fig. 199.2) performed 6 weeks following his treatment revealed RV enlargement with mildly depressed systolic function, a large well-circumscribed mass (8.2 × 3.4 cm) attached to mid interventricular septum beneath the tricuspid valve. It had a bi-lobed appearance with central echolucent areas that were felt to likely be consistent with necrotic areas. The mass was noted to protrude into the RV outflow tract (RVOT), resulting in intermittent RVOT obstruction and moderate tricuspid regurgitation. Septal flattening was also present in diastole, consistent with RV volume overload. Please see 642 and 643.

These findings were confirmed on CT chest that revealed no extracardiac spread (Fig. 199.3). The patient was referred to CT surgery, and underwent resection of the intracardiac tumor, limited septal myectomy and tricuspid valve repair (Fig. 199.4 644). Low and high power slides of the pathology are submitted in Figure 199.5. Four years later patient remains disease free with no cardiac involvement noted on surveillance echocardiograms.

DISCUSSION

Approximately 15–20% of primary cardiac tumors are malignant in nature. Sarcomas are the most common. Sarcomas are associated with rapid spread, with infiltration of myocardium causing obstruction to blood flow. Metastatic spread is often seen. Although complete resection is the treatment of choice, most patients develop recurrent disease with high rates of mortality even if their tumor can be completely resected.[1-3] Amongst the sarcomas, liposarcomas are rare. Cardiac myxoid liposarcoma is soft tissue tumor of limbs and mesentery in adults with rare cardiac involvement. They have an indolent course with favorable outcomes when

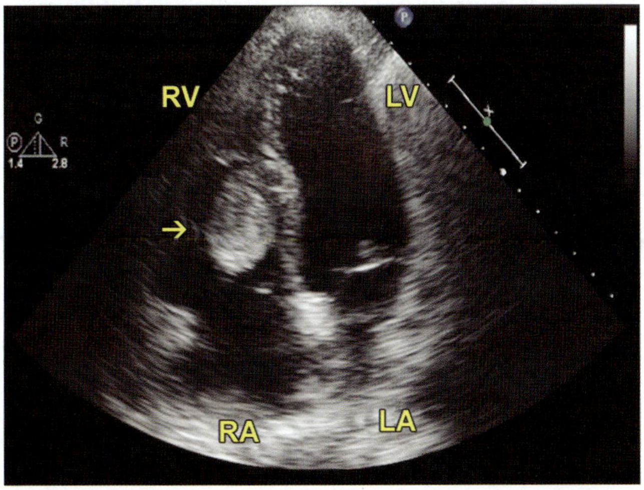

Fig. 199.1: A 4 x 3 cm, well circumscribed echodensity (arrow) is noted within the right ventricle with an attachment to the septum.

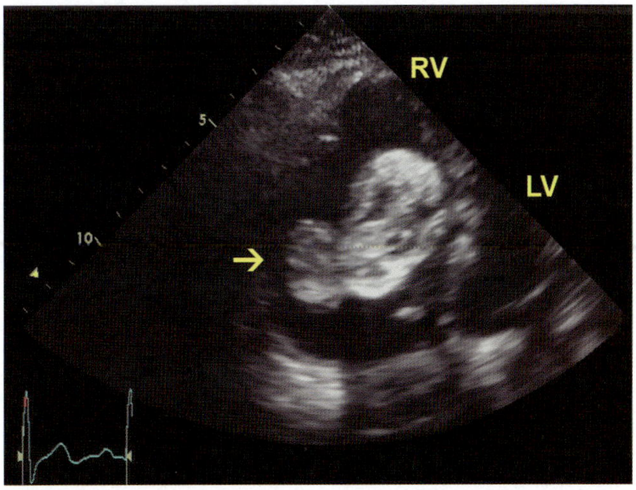

Fig. 199.2: RV enlargement with a large well-circumscribed mass (arrow, 8.2 x 3.4 cm) attached to mid interventricular septum beneath the tricuspid valve is seen. It has a bi-lobed appearance with central echolucent areas.

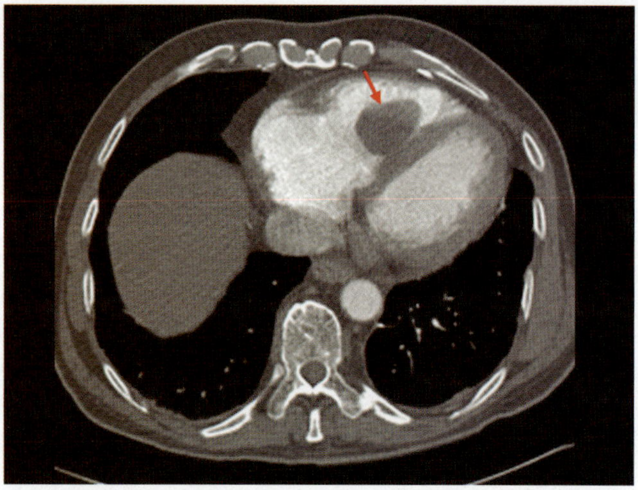

Fig. 199.3: CT chest that demonstrated the right ventricular neoplasm (arrow) with attachment to septum.

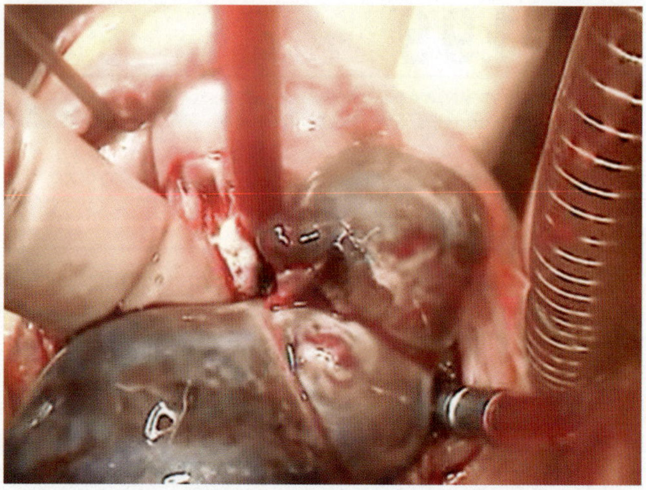

Fig. 199.4: Intraoperative image demonstrating the extent of the tumor and its proximity to the tricuspid valve by digital manipulation.

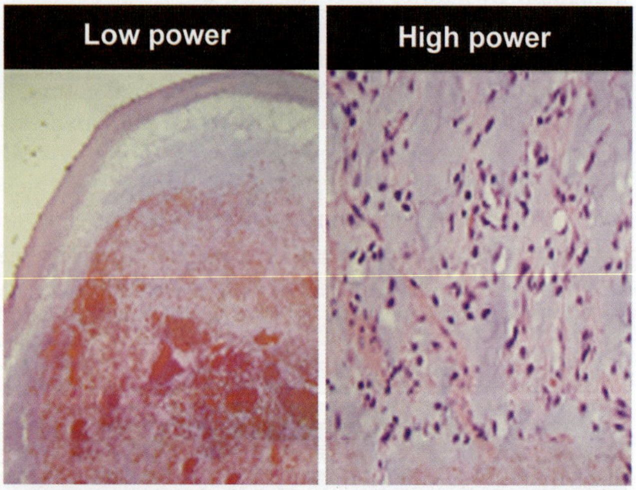

Fig. 199.5: Pathology slide showing the tumor under low power and high power.

appropriate surgical resection is undertaken. Adjunct chemotherapy and radiation therapy is utilized in select cases.[1,2] Prognosis depends upon the histologic grade. Primary cardiac sarcoma has a worse prognosis when compared to secondary tumors.[2-4]

1. **What normal anatomic structures in the right ventricle can mimic a cardiac mass?**
   (a) Large papillary muscles
   (b) Moderator band
   (c) Monitoring lines/Pacemaker wires
   (d) All of the above

Ans. (d)

Majority of the malignant tumors occur preferentially in the right side of the heart with the exception of leiomyosarcoma that is found in the left atrium. One should be able to distinguish the normal variants that can mimic cardiac tumors. The right ventricle is highly trabeculated with three large papillary muscles that can be hypertrophied and mistakes for a mass. The moderator band is a normal structure located in the right ventricular apex that connects the interventricular septum to the anterior papillary muscle. Sometimes the monitoring wires and pacemaker wires are difficult to visualize, and require multiple acoustic windows for interrogation.

2. **What is the most common malignant tumor of the heart?**
   (a) Left atrial myxoma
   (b) Fibroelastoma
   (c) Angiosarcoma
   (d) Metastates
   (e) Melanoma

Ans. (d)

Cardiac masses are rare entities that can be broadly categorized as either neoplastic or non-neoplastic. Neoplastic masses include benign and malignant tumors. In the heart, metastatic tumors are more common than primary malignant tumors. Whether incidentally found or diagnosed as a result of patients' symptoms, cardiac masses can be identified and further characterized by a range of cardiovascular imaging options. While echocardiography remains the first-line imaging modality, other modalities such as cardiac computed tomography and cardiac magnetic resonance imaging are increasingly used for furtherassessmentofcardiacmassestoidentifyextracardiac infiltration and also provide further tissue characterization.

PATHOLOGY

Tumor is partially encapsulated by endocardium and fibrous tissue. It is paucicellular with myxoid background and extensive hemorrhage.

There is cytologic atypia characterized by dark nuclei, pleomorphism and typical lipoblasts.

MOVIE LEGENDS

642: RV enlargement with a large well-circumscribed mass (8.2 × 3.4 cm) (arrow) attached to mid interventricular septum beneath the tricuspid valve is seen. It has a bi-lobed appearance with central echolucent areas.

643: The echodensity (arrow) was noted to protrude into the RV outflow tract (RVOT), resulting in intermittent RVOT obstruction and moderate tricuspid regurgitation.

644: Intraoperative movie.

REFERENCES

1. Pearlstone DB, Pisters PW, Bold RJ, et al. Patterns of recurrence in extremity liposarcoma: implications for staging and follow-up. Cancer. 1999;85:85–92.
2. Fiore M, Grosso F, Lo Vullo S, et al. Myxoid/round cell and pleomorphic liposarcomas: prognostic factors and survival in a series of patients treated at a single institution. Cancer. 2007;109:2522–31.
3. Hamidi M, Moody JS, Weigel TL, et al. Primary cardiac sarcoma. Ann Thorac Surg. 2010;90:176–81.
4. Maria D, Caterina S, Antonio B, et al. Jellyfish in the heart. Circulation. 2013;127(6):e443-5.

CASE 200

Mustafa Gökhan Vural, Murat Aksoy, Sabiye Sevinç, Saadet Demirtaş, Türker Pabuççu, Harun Kiliç, Ramazan Akdemir, Ersan Tatli, Nurgül Keser

AN UNUSUAL CASE OF RENAL CELL CARCINOMA WITH A DISTANT RIGHT VENTRICULAR METASTASIS AND WITHOUT VENA CAVA INFERIOR INVOLVEMENT

An unusual case of renal cell carcinoma with a distant right ventricular metastasis and without vena cava involvement in a 59-year-old man is reported.

The patient was admitted to our clinic with the complaints of dyspnea and fatigue. He had heart failure symptoms durting the last 6 months and was currently in New York Heart Association II-III. He also had low platelet values of 44500 showing severe thrombocytopenia.

The transthoracic echocardiogram done initially revealed a large mass originating from the apex of the RV. The 2.2 × 4.6 cm mobile mass was found to be extending through the RV outflow tract into the left main pulmonary artery (Figs. 200.1 to 200.3 and 645-647).

Systolic right ventricular pressure was elevated to 30 mm Hg and a pressure gradient of 19/8 mm Hg was recorded in RVOT.

3D transthoracic echocardiography gave us the precise localization of the mass being attached to the apex and protruding into the pulmonic valve (Figs. 200.4 and 200.5 and 648 and 649).

Computed tomography of the chest revealed a large mass in the RV apex attached to the endocardial surface with the dimensions of 45 × 30 mm, but no RA mass or IVC involvement was present.

The intense hypermetabolic activity of the apical mass in Positron emission tomography-computed tomography was thought to be due to the metastatic renal cell carcinoma. Besides, the low metabolic activity in a small portion of the tumor was suggestive of an attached thrombus or tumor embolus.

DISCUSSION

In renal cell carcinoma (RCC) which accounts for 2–3% of all adult malignancies[1] almost one-third of patients were found to have metastatic disease during initial diagnosis with the other 30% developing metastases at a later stage.[1,2]

The bone, liver, brain, lymphatic and lung are the most common sites of RCC metastases and cardiac metastases are reported to be rarer.[3]

Cardiac metastasis occurs as direct extension of the tumor into the inferior vena cava in 5–15% of patients[4] and growing into right heart chamber and right atrium in 1% of paients.[5]

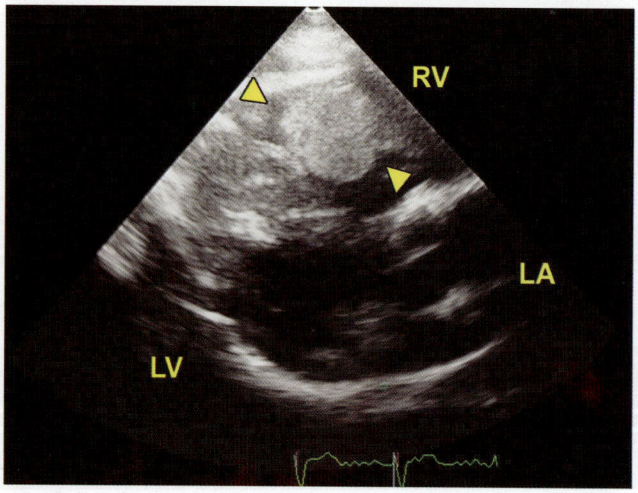

Fig. 200.1: The RV mass (arrowhead) originating from the apex and extending through RV outflow tract in 2D parasternal long-axis view.

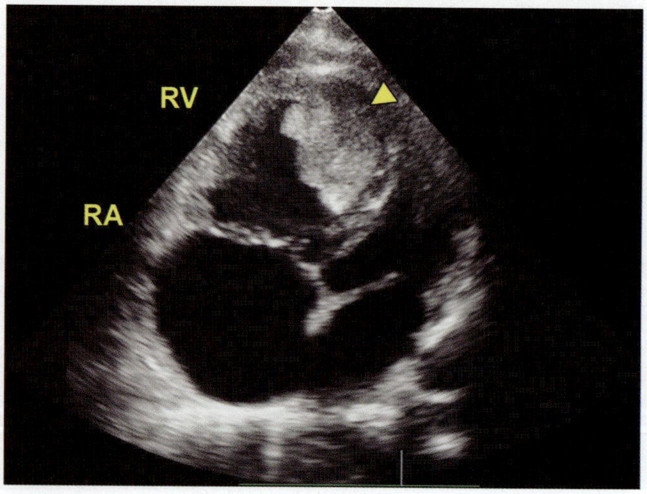

Fig. 200.2: The RV mass (arrowhead) originating from the apex in 2D apical 4-chamber view.

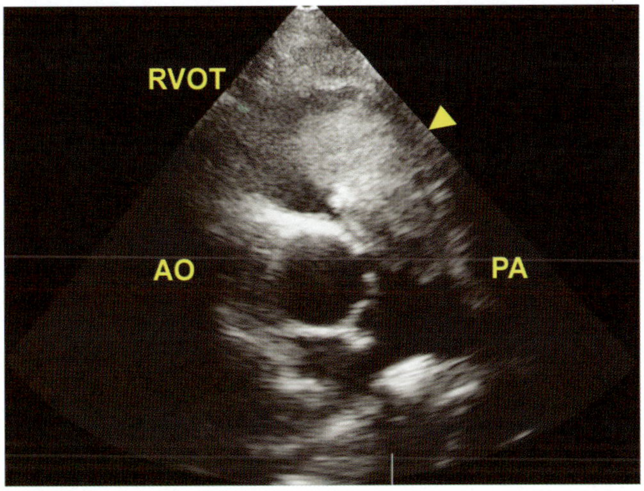

Fig. 200.3: The RV mass (arrowhead) extending through RV outflow tract into main pulmonary artery in 2D parasternal short axis view.

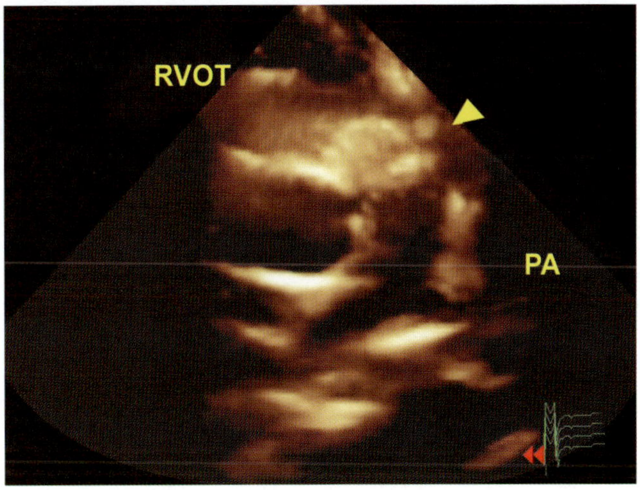

Fig. 200.4: The RV mass (arrowhead) extending through RV outflow tract into main pulmonary artery in 3D parasternal short axis view.

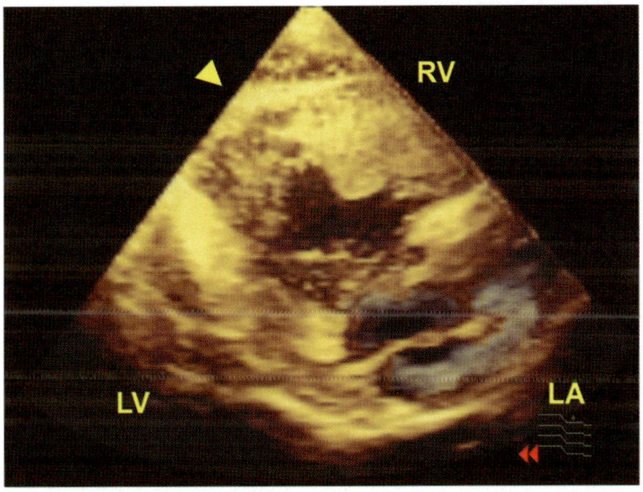

Fig. 200.5: Precise localization of the RV mass (arrowhead) in parasternal long axis view by 3D transthoracic echocardiography.

Right ventricular (RV) metastases sparing IVC or RA involvement have been reported three times which shows its rare appearance. They are also considered as metastatic stage IV RCC.[5]

Tumor cells may also disseminate to the heart by retrograde lymphatic or lymphohematogenous spread through the thoracic duct into the superior vena cava, or by the hematogenous spread of embolic cells which occurs in 10–20% of patients dying of systemic RCC.[1,6]

In patients with isolated disease and no involvement of IVC venous hematogenous pathway is claimed to be the primary mechanism while the other route[1] which is through the lymphatic vessels of the thorax with reversed lymphatic flow from metatatic nodes leading to metastatic RCC is reported to involve frequently left side of the heart.[1] Although in our patient the disease was found to be disseminated by PET CT the first pattern of spread is more compatible as there is no involvement of the left heart which occurs in disseminated disease.

Since CT or MRI gives additional information[1,7] we had CT and PET images of the patient which confirmed 3D echo findings and furthermore PET showed the attached thrombus.

Because secondary heart tumors are generally silent any kind of heart failure symptoms in patients with RCC should alert one to the possible presence of cardiac metastasis.

MOVIES 645 TO 649

REFERENCES

1. Bazine A, Fetohi M, Tanz R, et al. Cardiac Metastases of Renal Cell Carcinoma Revealed by Syncope: Diagnosis and Treatment Case reports in oncology Case Rep Oncol. 2014;7:560-64.
2. Custodio S, Joaqui A, Peixoto V, et al. Metastatic renal cell carcinoma:the importance of immunohistochemistry in differential diagnosis. Case Rep Oncol. 2012;5:30-34.
3. Bouzouita M, Ben Slamaa MR, Mohameda MOS, et al. Cardiac metastasis of renal cell carcinoma, a rare location. Prog Urol. 2011;21:492-94.

4. Sato T, Takeda A, Yamada S, et al. Metastatic renal cell carcinoma to right ventricle without vena caval involvement International Journal of Urology. 2008; 15:366-68.
5. Atik F, Navia JL, Krishnamurthi V, et al. Solitary massive right ventricular metastasis of renal cell carcinoma without inferior vena cava or right atrium involvement. J Card Surg. 2006;21:304-6.
6. Min JK, et al. A case of multiple metastatic renal cell carcinoma in an adult patient presenting with ventricular tachycardia Korean Circ J. 2005;35:341-4.
7. Alghamdi A, Tam J Cardiac metastasis from a renal cell carcinoma. Can J Cardiol. 2006;22:1231-32.

CASE 201

José Carlos Armendáriz Ferrari

UNUSUAL CHEST PAIN

The patient is a woman from the highlands of Peru (Junin), aged 31, previously perfectly healthy and without any relative or personal cardiac health issues. She was evaluated for thoracic pain related to effort. The patient previously went to the gym regularly 5 days a week. Thirty hours before being admitted to the hospital, the pain was accentuated and irradiated to her back and was associated with respiratory difficulties, sweating and palpitations.

Clinical Exam: BP: 110/70 mm Hg Pulse: 97 bpm SO_2 98%

Lungs: Normal to auscultation

Heart: Systolic murmur III/VI in the aortic area, with radiation to neck and apex.

1. **What is your diagnosis? (Figs. 201.1 and 201.2)**
   (a) Coronary artery disease
   (b) Cardiomyopathy
   (c) Pericardial disease
   (d) Acute aortic syndrome
   (e) None of the above
   (f) All are possible

Ans. (f)

Need more information specially images.

2. **Question by the surgeon: Is the interventricular septum involved? Is there any risk of producing a VSD while excising the cystic mass? (Figs. 201.3 to 201.7 and 650 to 658)**

Ans. There should be no risk.

3. **What is the best way to access the cyst?**

Ans. Transventricular approach

(Figs. 201.8 to 201.10). Figure 201.11 and 659 and 660 show post-surgery 2D TTEs demonstrating normal LV flow signals.

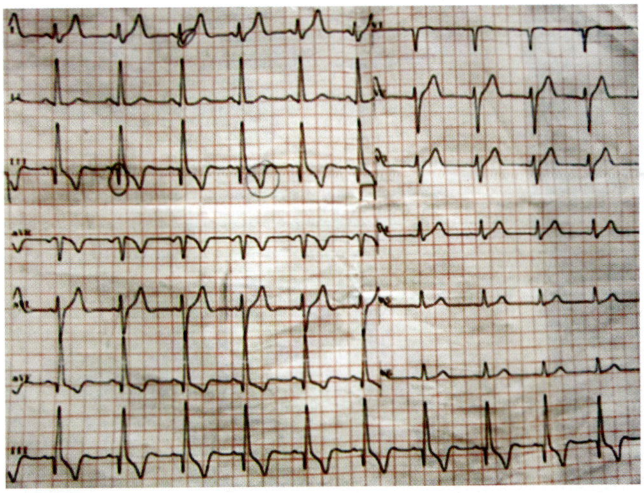

Fig. 201.1: EKG.

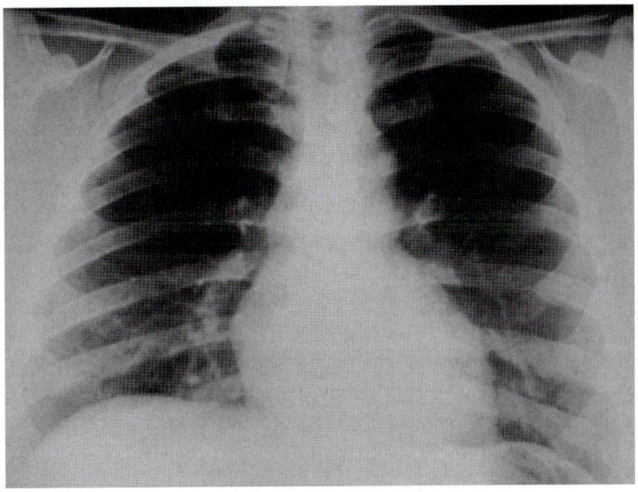

Fig. 201.2: Chest X-ray.

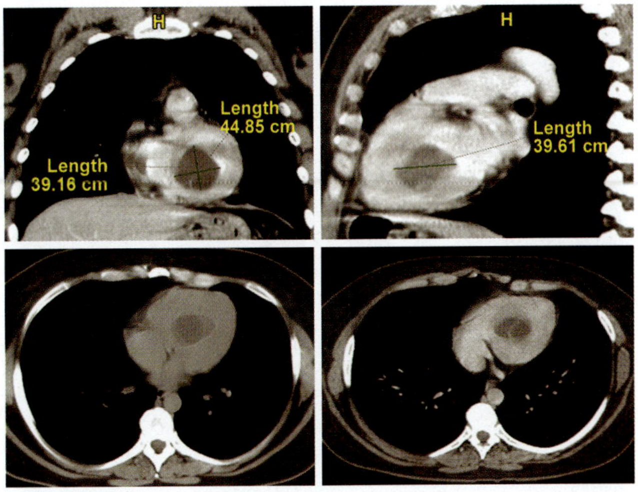

Fig. 201.3: CT scan. Shows hypodense image of ovoid shape, apparently trabeculated and located in the LV cavity.

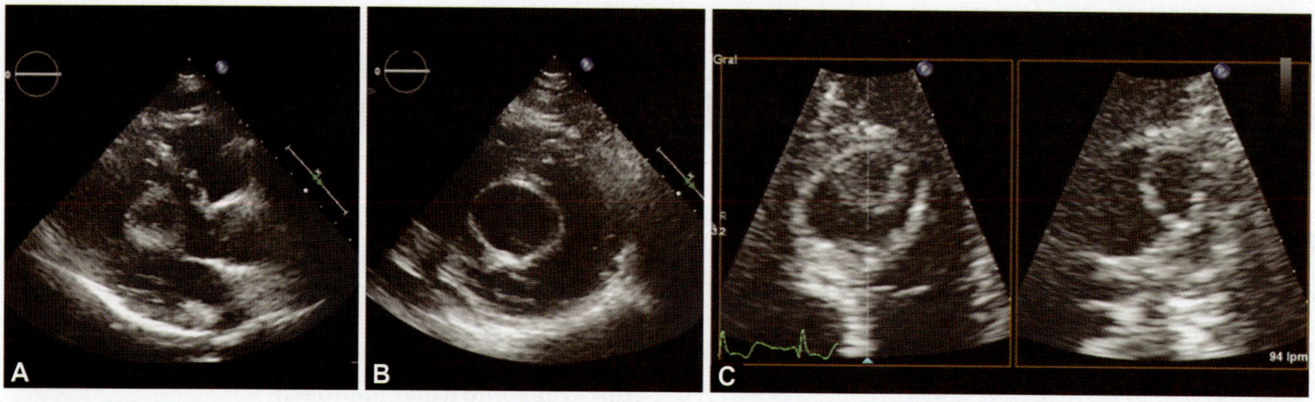

Figs. 201.4A to C: Two- dimensional echocardiography shows an ovoid structure (arrowhead in movies) in the LV cavity adherent to the interventricular septum (A and B). The mass is trabeculated (C).

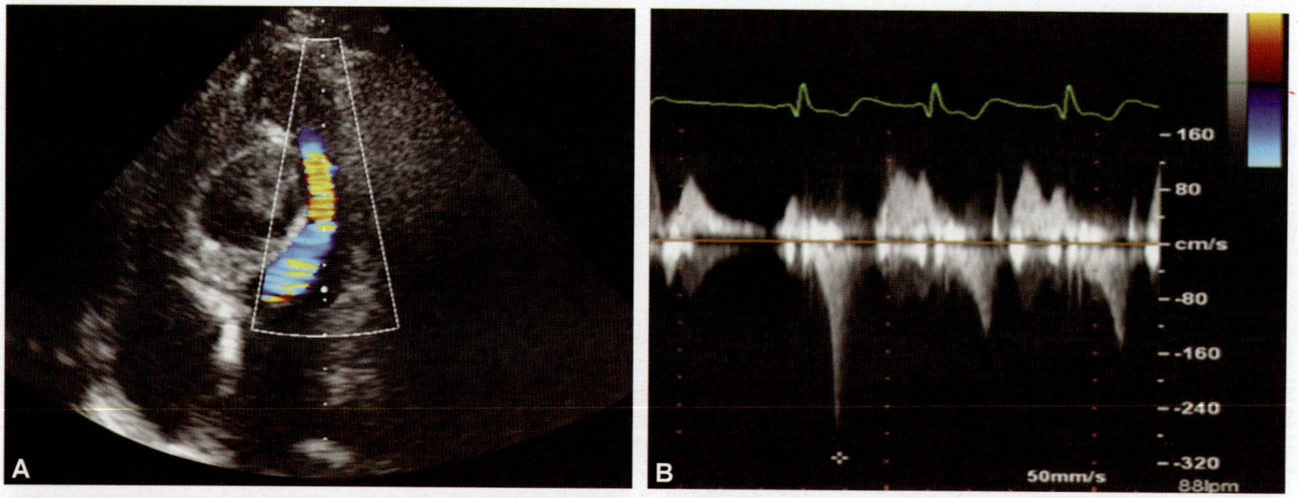

Figs. 201.5A and B: Doppler study. Color and CW Doppler shows turbulent flow at mid ventricular level (A). The continuous wave Doppler study shows a 40 mm Hg gradient at mid ventricular level. This is the origin of the murmur found on clinical exam (B).

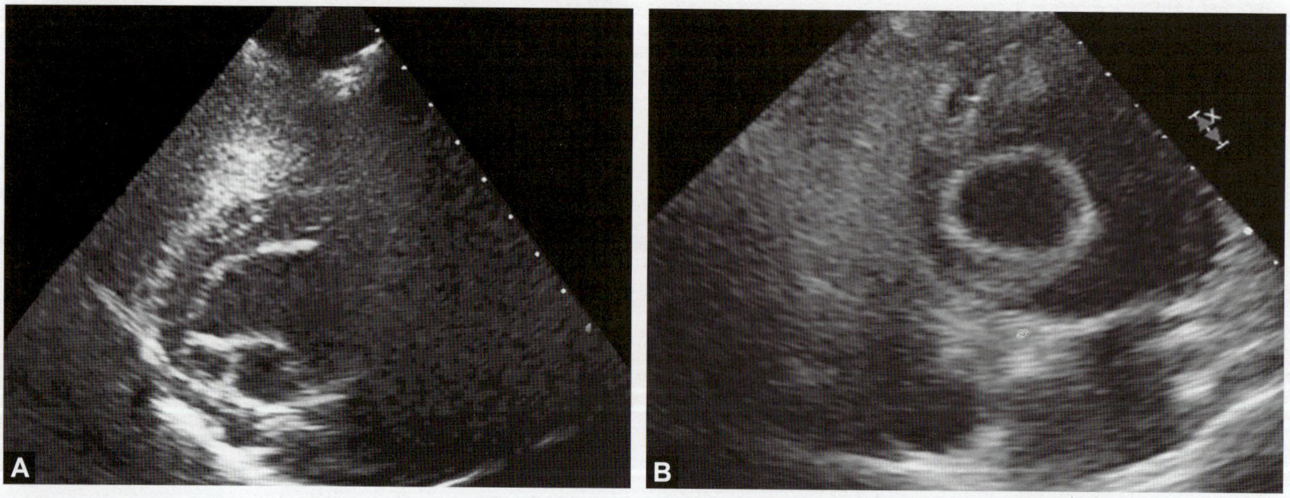

Figs. 201.6A and B: Saline contrast echo shows normal thickness of the interventricular septum: (A) Short axis); (B) Apical 4 chambers.

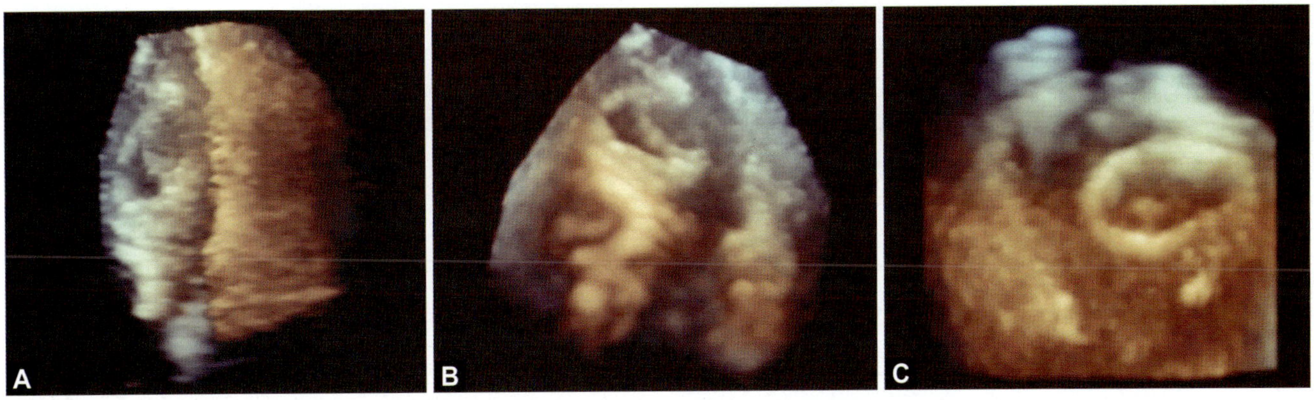

Figs. 201.7A to C: 3D echocardiography shows the trabeculated cyst in the interior of the interventricular septum. Because of the large size of the cyst, the best access would be transventricular (C). Transmitral approach would be more risky as the cyst is close to the MV and the subvalvular apparatus (B). (A) LV Apical view); (B) View from mitral plane; (C) View from apex.

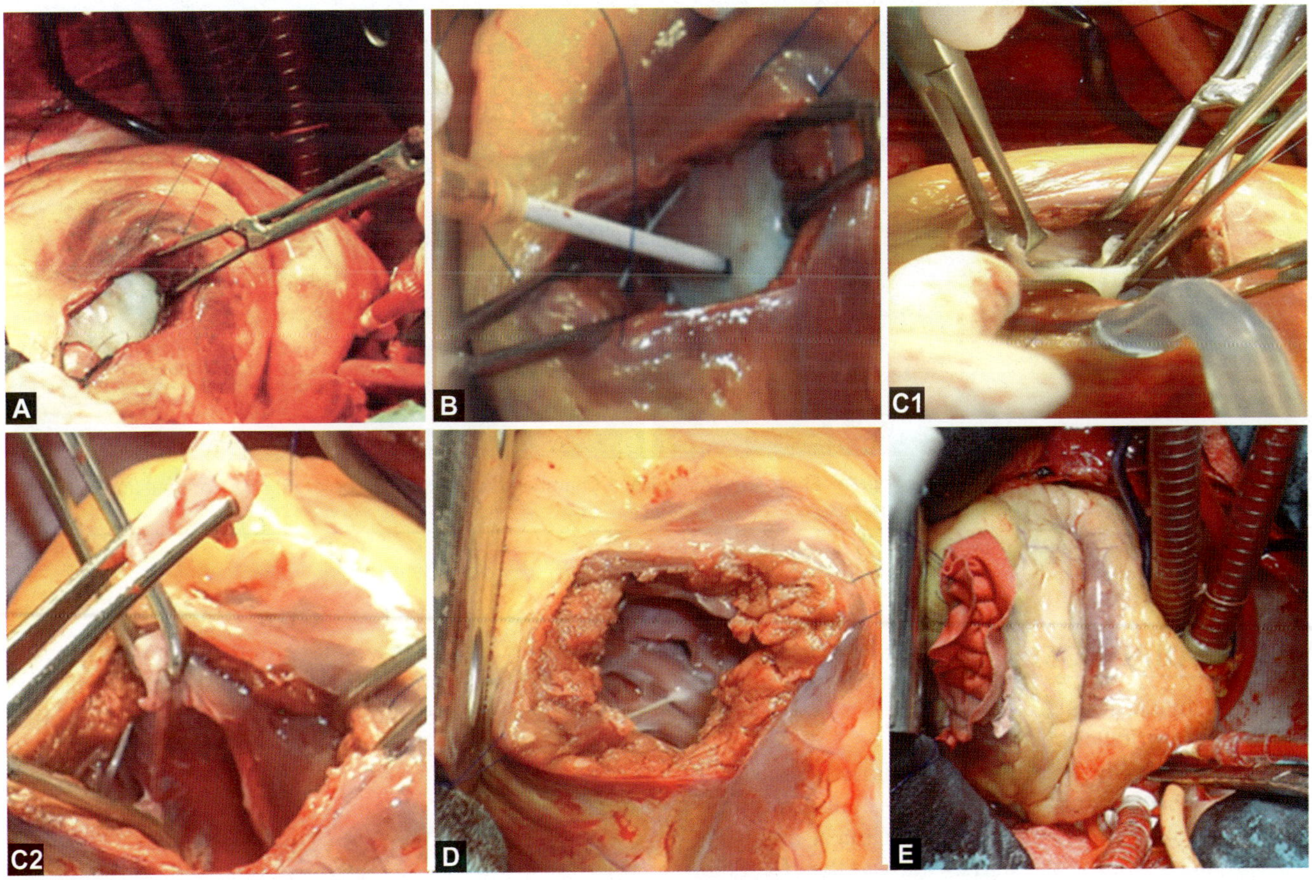

Figs. 201.8A to E: Show the surgical procedure using the transventricular approach to access the cyst (A). Puncture and drainage of the liquid content. The surgeon decided not to use liquid saline infusion due to the risk of compromising the cardiac conduction system (B). Dissection and removal of the cyst (C). Closure with stiches of the LV free wall (D and E).

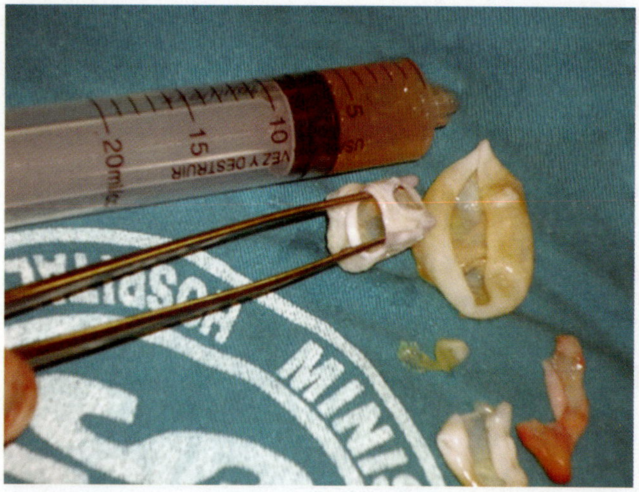

Fig. 201.9: Surgical specimen: all the structures of the cyst and its liquid content.

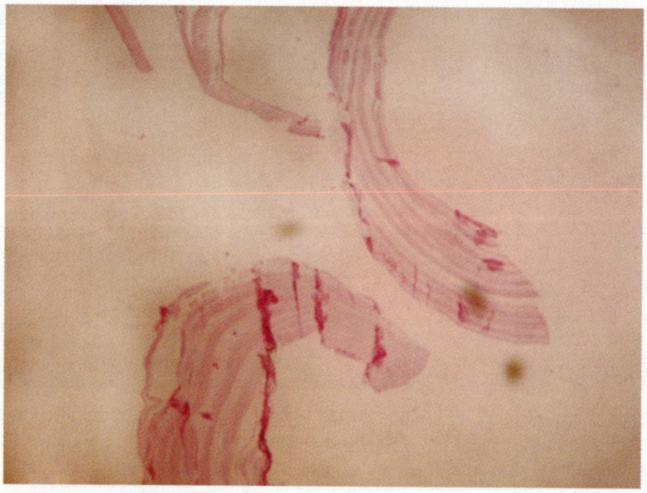

Fig. 201.10: Shows the anatomic—pathology study, anhistic membrane. No scolix found.

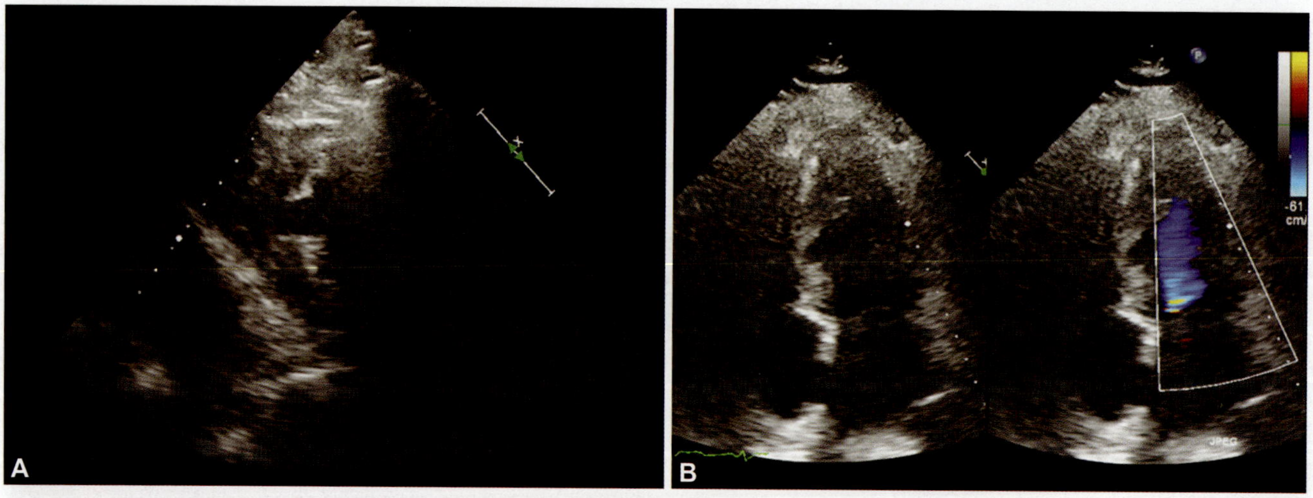

Figs. 201.11A and B: Post-surgical echocardiogram. Short Axis (A). Apical 4 Chamber 2D and color Doppler (B) show normal flow in the LV during systole. (A) Short axis; (B) Apical four chambers.

FINAL DIAGNOSIS

1. Cardiac hydatidosis
2. Mid left ventricular obstruction

Cardiac hydatidosis is a zoonosis caused by larvae of the echinococus granulosa (a parasite found in cattle). Cardiac involvement is unusual. The clinical manifestations are related to the size and location of the cyst. Echocardiography is a very useful tool for the diagnosis of cysts and other masses involving the heart. Surgery must be immediate once this condition has been diagnosed. The major risk is the rupture of the cyst, which may be fatal (anaphylaxis).

MOVIES 650 TO 660

CASE 202

Naveen Garg, Kanwal K Kapur

A RARE CASE OF PEDUNCULATED LV HEMANGIOMA EVALUATED BY 3D ECHOCARDIOGRAPHY AND COMPARED WITH MYXOMA

A 33-year-old male with no specific symptoms had undergone echocardiography, as a part of his medical examination. His ECG and chest X-rays (Figs. 202.1A and B) and other laboratory parameters were also normal. Transthoracic 2D echocardiography (Figs. 202.2A and B and 661A-D) using an i33-Philips ultrasound system revealed a large, mobile, smooth, oval, non-lobulated pedunculated mass in the left ventricle.

1. **What could be the possible differential diagnosis of this mass?**

This mass measured 3 × 5.2 cm and was attached to the interventricular septum by a pedicle of size 0.8 × 0.5 cm. Cropped 3D-TTE (Fig. 202.3 and 662A and B) as well as serial I-Slicing showed closely packed homogenous echolucent areas which were extending to the periphery (Figs. 202.4A and B and 663A and B).

2. **What these spaces reveal about the mass?**

Intraoperative transesophageal echocardiography (Fig. 202.5 and 664) confirmed the pre-operative TTE-findings. A complete resection of the LV tumor was performed using the transapical approach. On gross examination, the tumor was an oval shaped reddish brown mass of size 4 × 3.6 cm (Fig. 202.6).

3. **What could be the diagnosis?**

Histopathological evaluation with H&E staining showed multiple vascular spaces with thrombi as well as bulbous capillaries in an edematous stroma pathognomic of a cavernous hemangioma (Figs. 202.7A to C). Immunohistochemistry (IHC) with CD-31 (endothelial cell marker) confirmed the presence of endothelial cells.(Fig. 202.7D) The CALRETININ stain (marker for myxomas cells) was negative.

DISCUSSION

The usual sites of a hemangioma are right atrium, left ventricle, right ventricle, left atrium and pericardium, in that order. The highly mobile LV tumor seen on echocardiography gave a superficial impression of a myxoma. However, on 3D TTE careful cropping revealed densely packed small echolucent spaces which uniformly extended all the way to periphery. This feature indicated the presence of a hemangioma rather than a myxoma in which the echolucent spaces are sparse, of variable sizes and do not extend

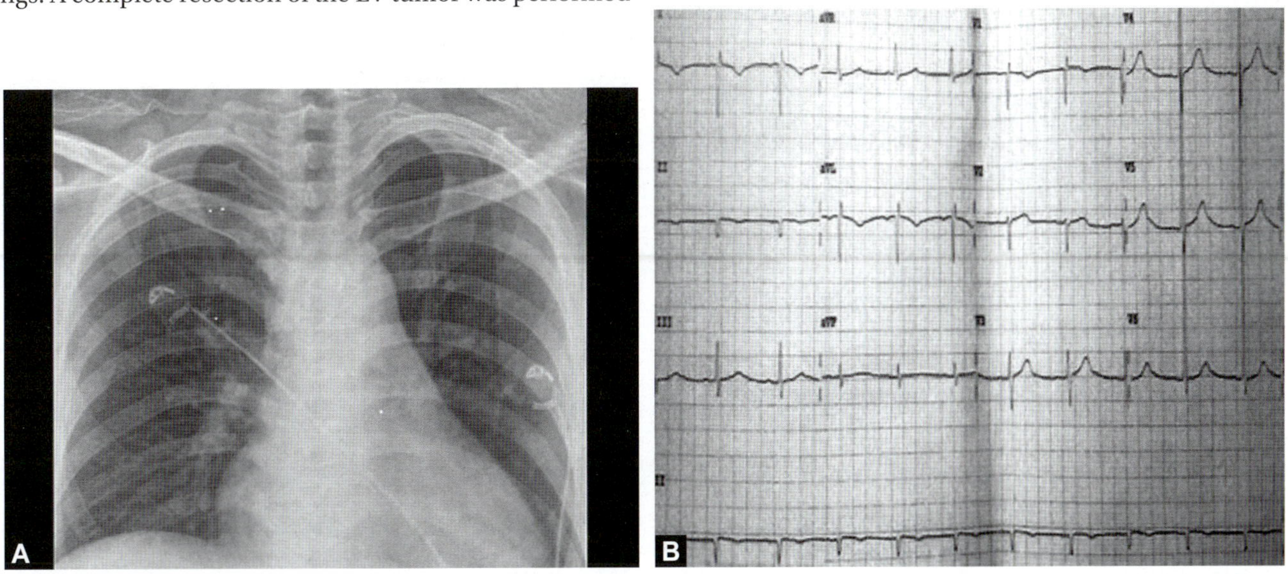

Figs. 202.1A and B: Chest X-ray and ECG.

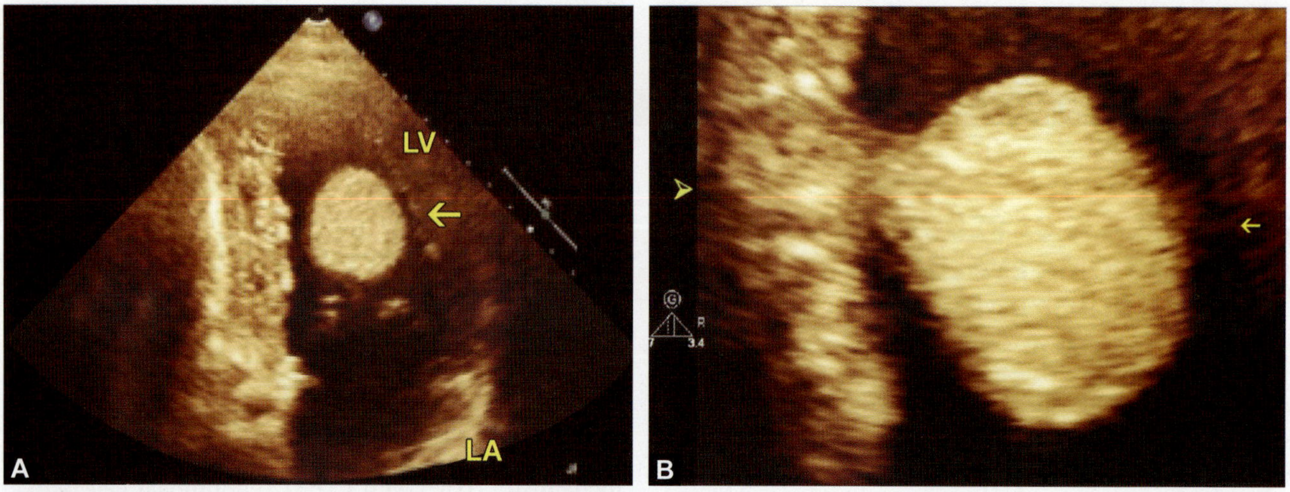

Figs. 202.2A and B: TTE showing a mass (arrow) in LV cavity (A) and zoomed view showing a pedicle (arrowhead) attached to the IVS (B).

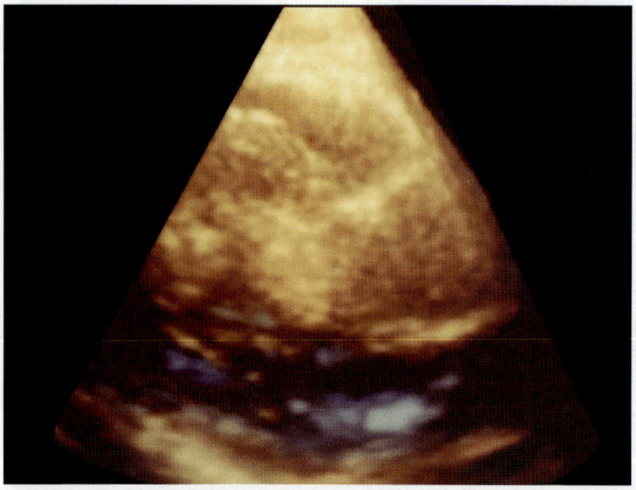

Fig. 202.3: 3D-TTE showing a mass in LV.

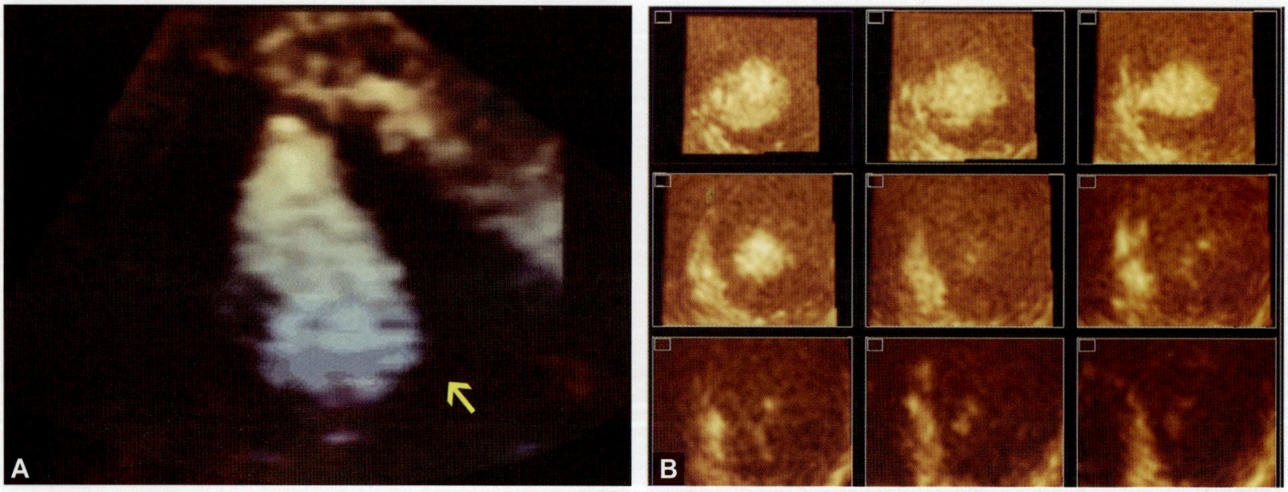

Figs. 202.4A and B: Zoomed view of the mass showing closely packed dense echolucent areas (arrow shows echolucent areas within the mass that are reaching to periphery) (A) and I-sliced view depicting echolucent areas extending to the periphery (B).

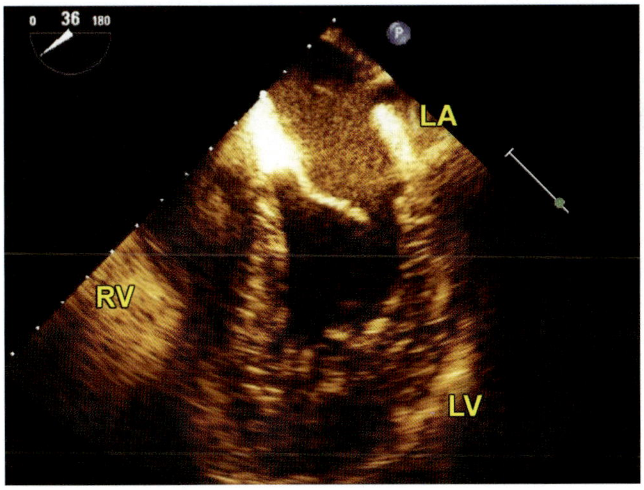

Fig. 202.5: Intraoperative TEE showing complete removal of the mass.

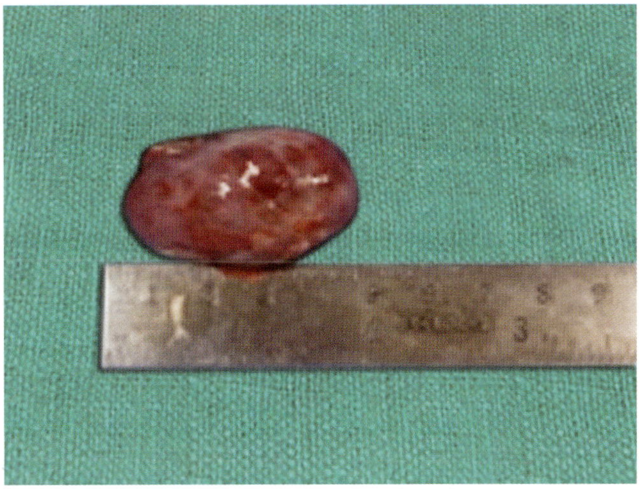

Fig. 202.6: Excised LV mass.

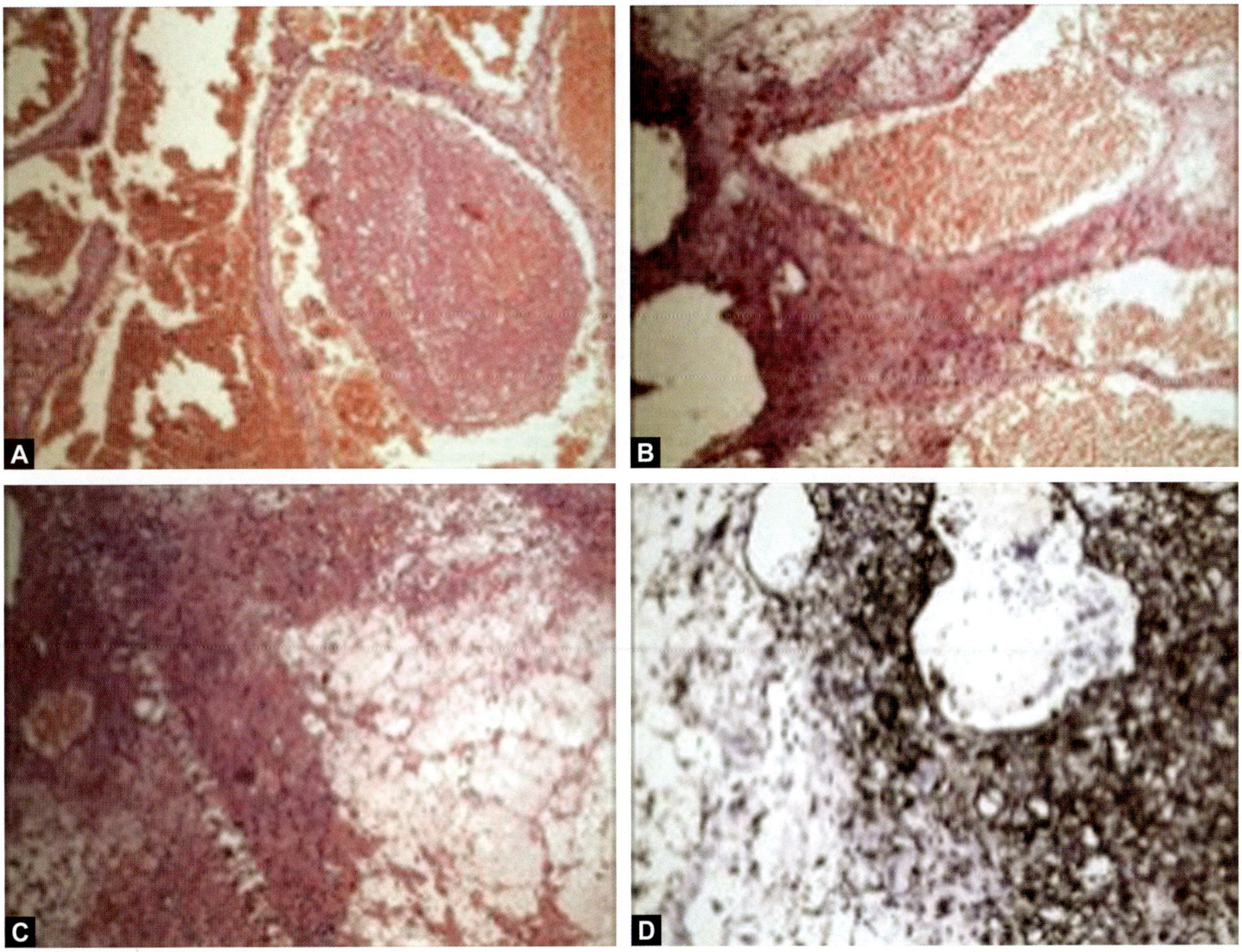

Figs. 202.7A to D: H & E strain depicting large bulbous cavernous spaces with thrombi in them. CD31 strain marks for endothelium (D).

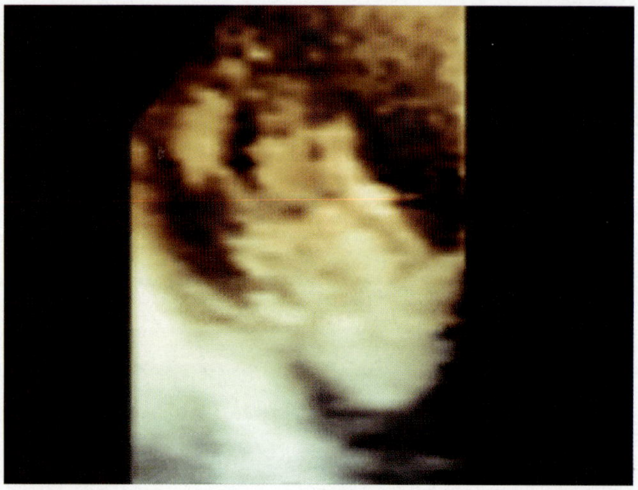

Fig. 202.8: Zoomed 3D view of a LA myxoma.

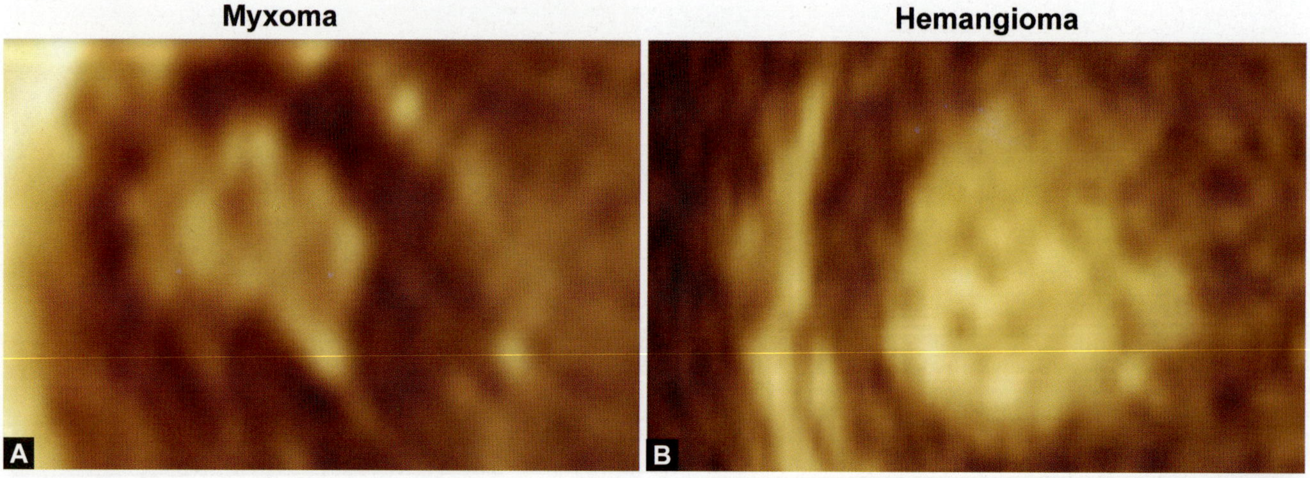

Figs. 202.9A and B: Cropped view of a myxoma versus a hemangioma. Myxoma shows large sparse echolucent areas while cropping of hemangioma reveals closely packed echolucent spaces involving the periphery also.

to the periphery. (Compare with a myxoma Figure 202.8 versus Figure 202.4 and 663A versus 665 and Figure 202.9 and 666A and B).

MOVIES 661A TO 666B

CASE 203

Mohamed Ayan, Mohsin Salih

MULTIPLE INTRACARDIAC MASSES PRESENTED WITH COMPLETE HEART BLOCK

A 77-year-old woman with history of recently diagnosed metastatic endometrial carcinosarcoma to the lung and brain presented to the emergency department complaining of severe weakness and dizziness. She was noted to be bradycardic and EKG demonstrated complete heart block with heart rate in the 50s. Lab work up showed urinary tract infection (UTI) with sepsis. 2D TTE demonstrated multiple mobile masses in the right and left ventricles (Fig. 203.1 and 667). Her ejection fraction was preserved.

1. Which of the following describes your diagnosis?
   (a) Multiple cardiac papillary fibroelastomas
   (b) Multiple cardiac myxomas
   (c) Multiple cardiac metastases
   (d) Multiple intracardiac thrombi

Ans. (c) Multiple cardiac metastases

The patient was found to have multiple cardiac metastases form endometrial carcinosarcoma. Given the extensiveness of her tumor and widespread metastatic burden including heart, lungs, and brain and her active infection, she was felt to be a very poor candidate for temporary/ permanent pacemaker. The patient elected to pursue comfort care via hospice.

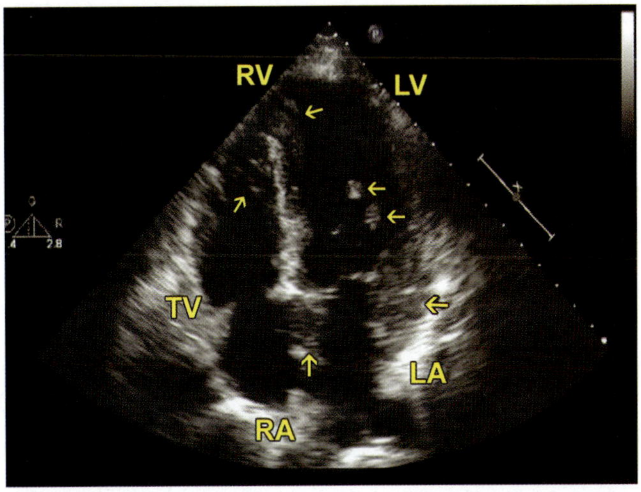

Fig. 203.1: TTE. Apical 4 chamber view showing multiple masses (arrows) in the right ventricle (RV) and left ventricle (LV).

MOVIE LEGEND

667: TTE. Apical 4 chamber view demonstrating a 3.3 cm × 1.6 cm mass extending from RV to LV through the apical septum; there was a pedunculated portion extending up to 2.0 cm within the LV cavity. There was a 3.0 cm × 2.7 cm mass noted in the RV free wall extending toward the septum and a mass measuring 2.2 cm × 1.7 cm in the atrial septum near the crux. Arrows point to the masses.

CASE 204

Roomi AU, Shah A, Siddiqui LI, Gupta N, Mohamed A, Nanda NC

The patient is a 24-year-old previously healthy female who presented with pain in the right thigh. X-ray revealed fracture of femur as well as a bone mass. She underwent surgery and the biopsy of bone mass was sent for histopathological examination. One week later she developed shortness of breath and was referred for a 2D TTE (Fig. 204.1, 668 and 669).

1. **What is the most likely diagnosis?**
    - (a) Thrombi
    - (b) Vegetations
    - (c) Metastases
    - (d) None of the above

Ans. (c)

This is a case of osteosarcoma confirmed by biopsy with metastases to the heart. 2D TTE showed large multiple mobile masses (arrow) in LVOT, LA and MV causing LVOT obstruction with a peak gradient of 50 mm Hg (Fig. 204.1). The tumor appeared to obstruct the MV also. The patient was placed on chemotherapy but died soon after from multiple organ failure.

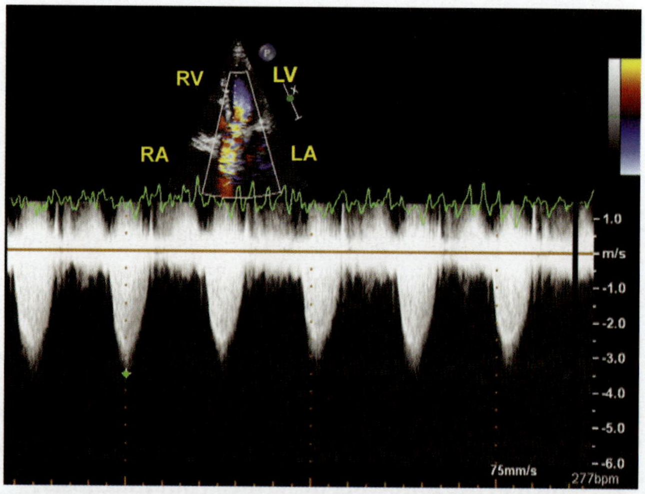

Fig. 204.1: Continuous wave Doppler interrogation of LVOT reveals a high gradient of 50 mm Hg.

MOVIES 668 AND 669

CASE 205

Leng Jiang

A 56-year-old female who presented to a local hospital for shortness of breath on exertion for 3 months with worsening (even at rest) over the past 3 weeks, and intermittent chest discomfort and fatigue.

- No HTN, DM, hyperlipidemia
- Ovarian carcinoma, s/p hysterectomy and bilateral salpingo-oophorectomy 6 years ago, followed by multiple courses of chemotherapy, and surgery for debulking 3 years ago, with chronic pleural effusion and right lower extremity lymphedema
- Cholecystectomy, 6 years ago
- Appendectomy, 12 years ago

Initial Work-up

- Echo: LVEF 50%, Mild RVE, PASP 50 mm Hg
- Nuclear cardiac scan: No ischemia, LVEF 47%
- Lung VQ scan: Low risk for PE
- CT: Negative for pulmonary emboli

Chest CT with Contrast

- No central or segmental pulmonary emboli (Fig. 205.7)
- 3D-CT shows normal pulmonary arteries (Fig. 205.8)

She was seen by a cardiologist there:

- An EKG suggesting an anterior MI, new from previous one (Figs. 205.9 and 205.10)
- Lab study: CK/MB normal; cTn-T 0.09 ng/mL
- Was started:
  - Aspirin 81 mg daily
  - Loaded with Plavix of 300 mg
  - Heparin drip
  - Lipitor 80 mg daily
- Was transferred to our medical center for further evaluation.

Physical exam

- T 97.5°F, HR 100 bpm, BP 95/38 mm Hg, O2 Sat 98 - 100% on 2 L of nasal cannula
- Cardiac: No JVD, RRR, Normal S1 and S2, No murmur or gallop
- Lungs: CTA, but breath sounds diminished bilaterally
- Abd: Soft, nontender, Liver not palpable, bowel sounds present
- Ext: chronic lymphedema in right leg

CXR: Bilateral pleural effusion - unchanged (Fig. 205.11)

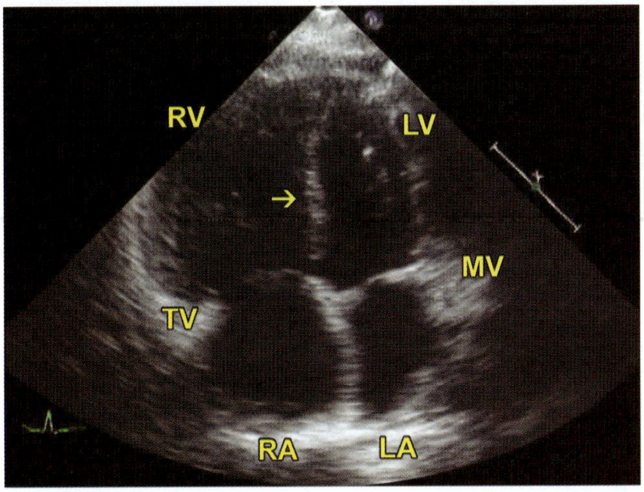

Fig. 205.1: Transthoracic apical 4 chamber view. Arrow points to interventricular septal flattening during systole and diastole. RV is significantly dilated.

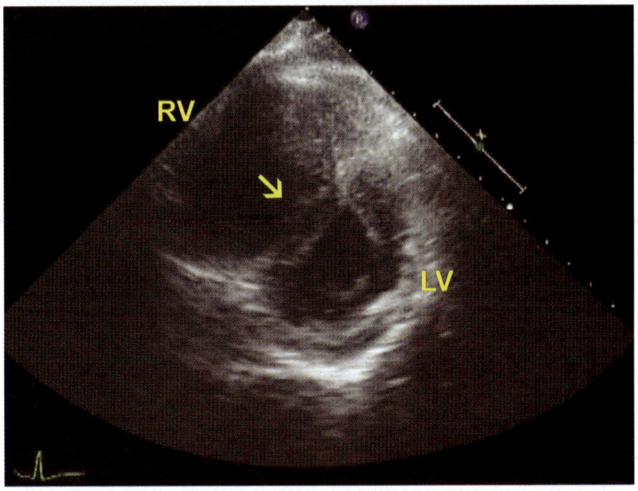

Fig. 205.2: Transthoracic short axis view. Arrow points to flattened interventricular septum.

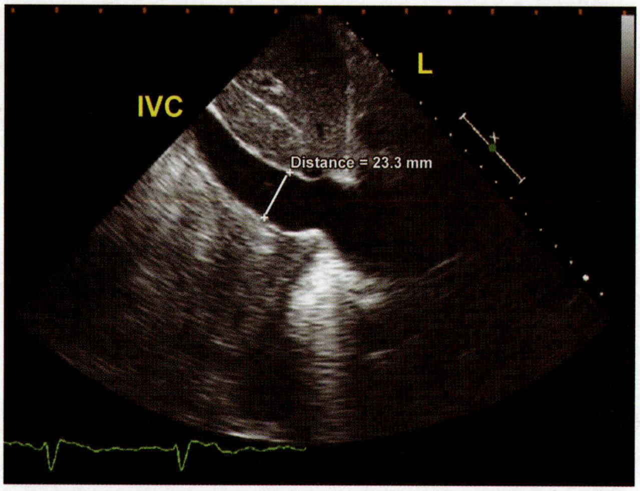

Fig. 205.3: Transthoracic subcostal view. Shows dilated IVC with diameter of 23.3 mm.

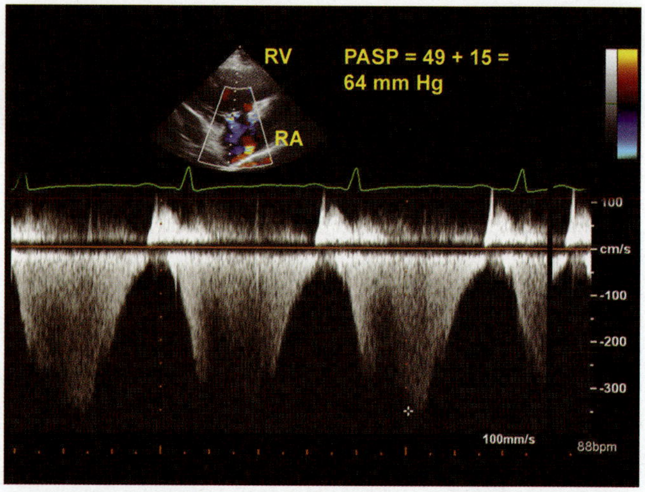

Fig. 205.4: Continuous wave Doppler of tricuspid regurgitation. Shows PASP of 64 mm Hg.

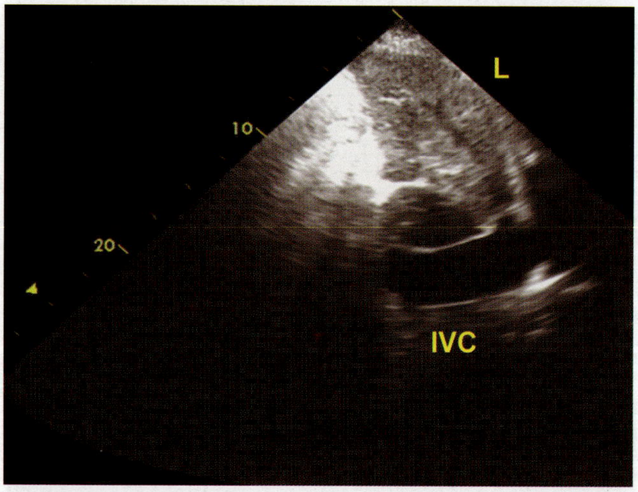

Fig. 205.5: Follow-up transthoracic echocardiography shows significant dilatation of IVC.

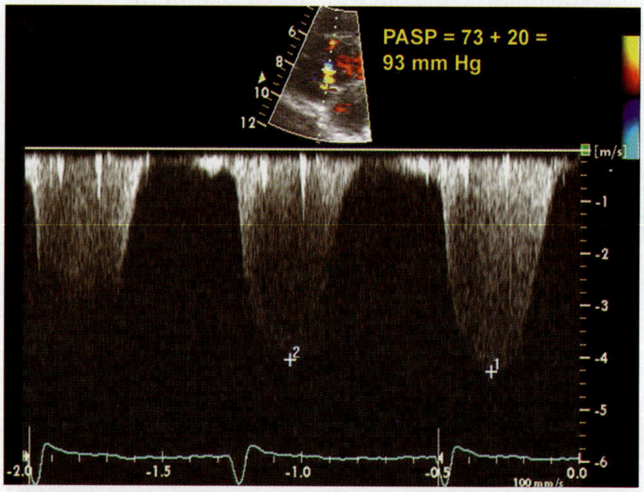

Fig. 205.6: Follow-up transthoracic echocardiography. Continuous wave Doppler of tricuspid regurgitation. PASP = 93 mm Hg.

Labs

- CBC: WBC 5.8 × 109/L, Hct 16.6/48.9%, Plt 159 × 109/L
- Na 140 mEq/L, K 3 mEq/L, BUN 26 mg/dL, Cr 1.1 mg/dL
- Lipids: NL, with LDL 105 mg/dL
- CPK 40 U/L, 50 U/L, cTn-T 0.6 ng/mL, 1.1 ng/mL
- Pro BNP: 1,788 pg/mL, 10,421 pg/mL
- INR 1.2, PTT 74.9 sec

You are called for consultation

1. **What would you recommend?**
   (a) Order a Dobutamine stress echo
   (b) Repeat a nuclear myocardial perfusion scan
   (c) Cardiac cath for NSTEMI
   (d) CTA to assess CAD
   (e) Repeat an echocardigram

Ans. (e)

F/U Echocardiogram

See Figures 205.1 to 205.6 and 670 and 671.

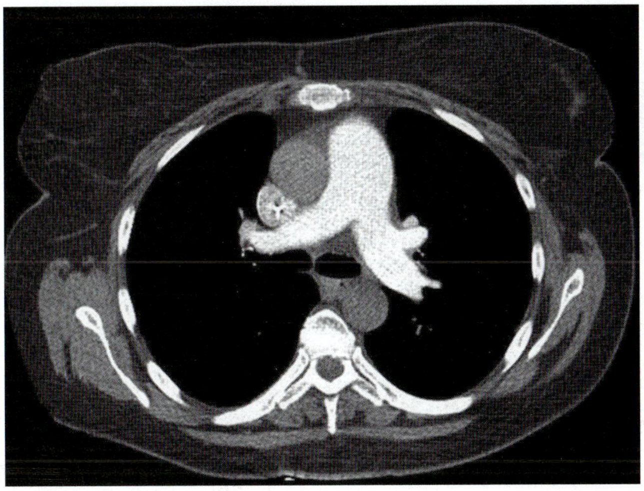

Fig. 205.7: Chest CT with contrast, showing no central or segmental pulmonary emboli.

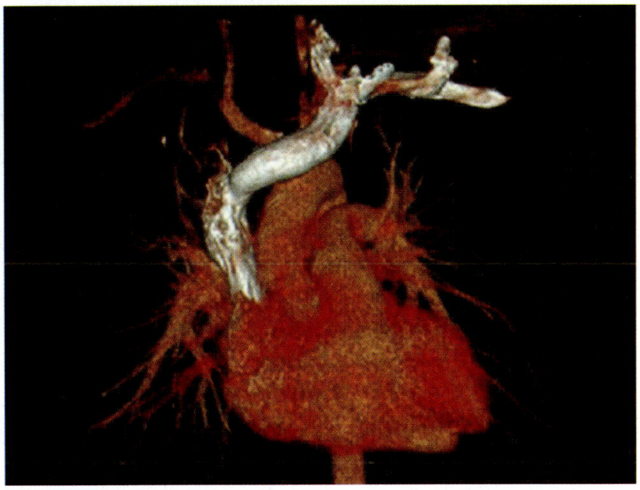

Fig. 205.8: 3D-CT showing normal pulmonary arteries.

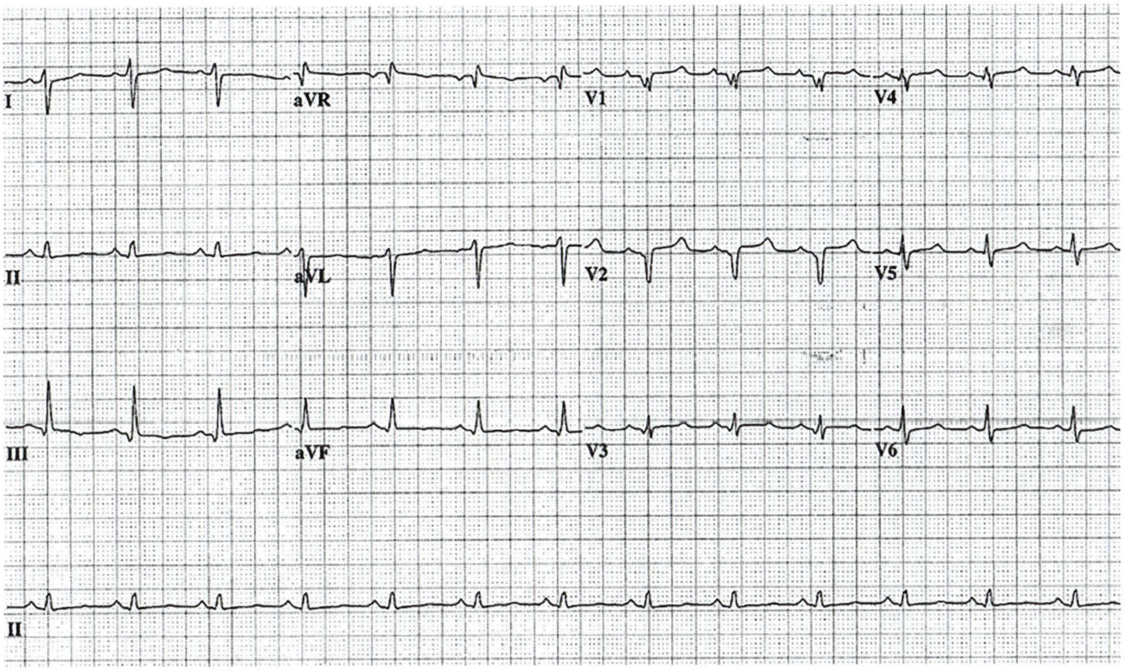

Fig. 205.9: EKG shows right axis deviation, poor R wave progression in the anterior leads.

The Echo Findings

- LV: Normal size, mild LVH, EF 50%
- The IVS: Marked flattening during systole and diastole c/w RV pressure/volume overload
- RV: Markedly dilated RV with RVH and markedly reduced systolic function
- RA: dilated
- Moderate TR, RVSP ≥ 64 mm Hg

Hospital Course

- *Cardiology consult:*
  - Does not think she needs a cardiac cath
  - Recommend pulmonary/oncology consults
- *Pulmonary consult*:
  - Reviewed outside studies (V/Q, CTA)
  - ABG: pH 7.54, P_aCO_2 34 mm Hg, P_aO_2 48 mm Hg, Bicarb 28 mEq/L, 0_2 Sat. 85%
  - Dx: PHTN of unclear etiology
  - Consider RHC +/- reversibility study

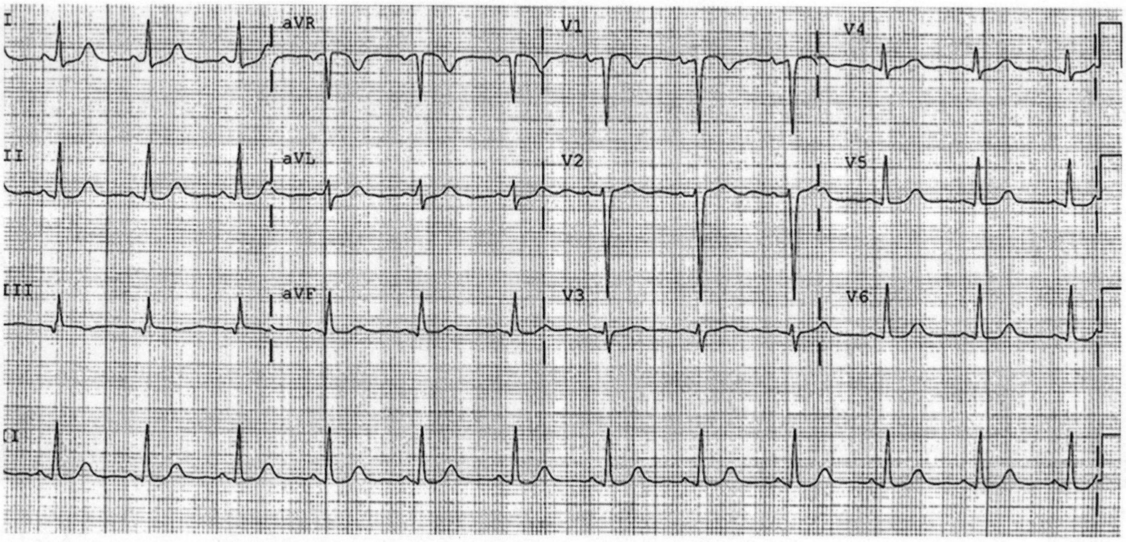

Fig. 205.10: Compared to the previous EKG (4 months ago), there was no right axis deviation.

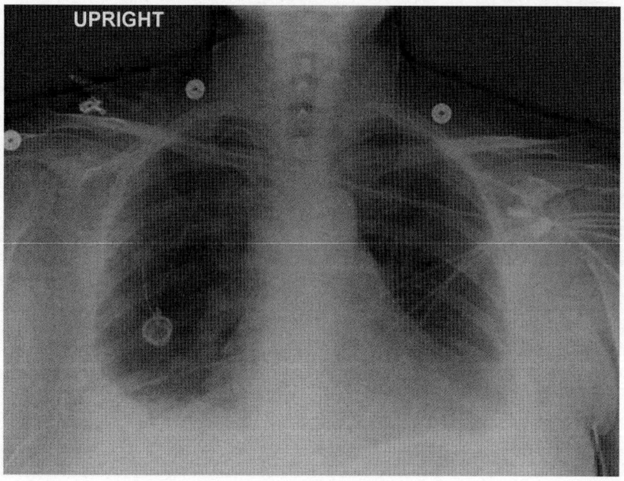

Fig. 205.11: CXR showing bilateral pleural effusion.

However, Before the RHC

- The patient developed hypotension with SBP of 70 mm Hg
- Pro-BNP 37,421 pg/mL
- BUN 52.2 mg/dL, Cr 2.1 mg/dL, K 5.3 mEq/L
- ABG: pH 7.27, P_aCO_2 37 mm Hg, P_aO_2 162 mm Hg, Bicarb 16 mEq/L
- Stat 2-D echo: PASP > 90 mm Hg
- The patient remained in shock with multiorgan failure, not responding to fluid replacement, Levophed and ventilation
- She developed PEA, failed to CPR on-off for 2 hours, and was finally pronounced dead.

Major Gross Autopsy Findings

- Cardiomegaly: marked RV dilatation, LV hypertrophy and mild coronary atherosclerotic disease. No evidence of gross pulmonary emboli.
- Fibrous adhesions were present in the chest, pelvis and abdomen, with diffuse metastatic mesenteric nodules.

Microscopic Examination

- Diffuse pulmonary vascular microtumor emboli, and thrombotic microangiopathy with marked arterial and arteriolar intimal thickening (Fig. 205.12).

Take Home Messages

- Elevated cTn indicates the presence but not the mechanism of myocardial injury; myocardial damage can occur from a variety of mechanisms other than acute ischemia. Diagnosis should be based on the clinical scenario
- Echo helps differential diagnosis
- Negative CT cannot rule out PE, as seen in this case—microtumor embolization

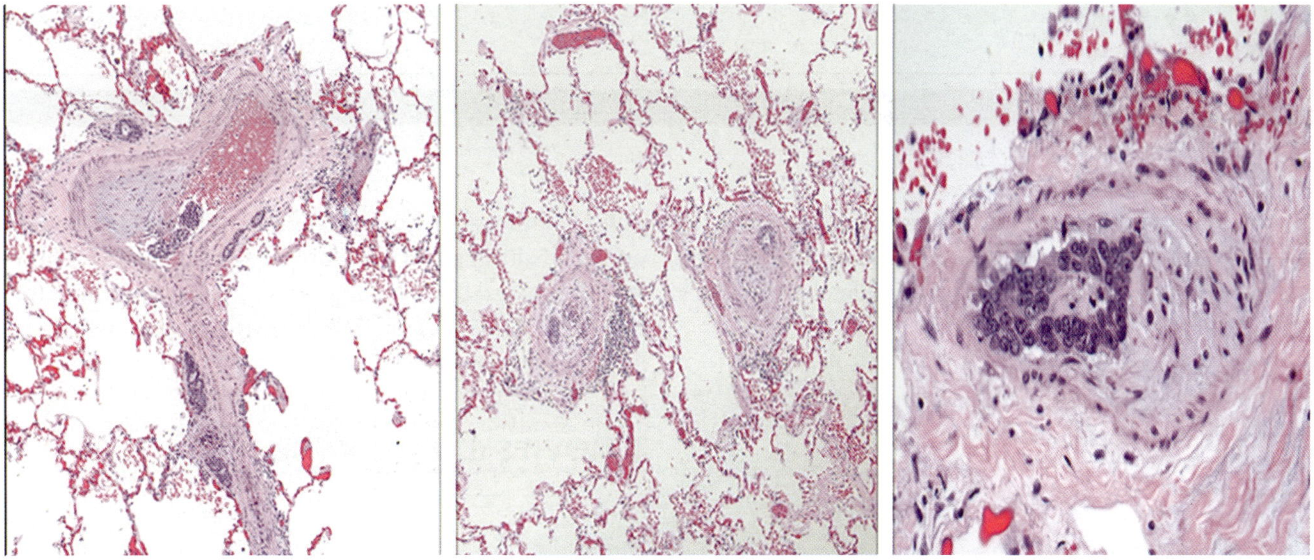

Fig. 205.12: Autopsy microscopic examination, showing diffuse pulmonary vascular microtumor emboli, and thrombotic microangiopathy with marked arterial and arteriolar intimal thickening.

MOVIE LEGENDS

670: Transthoracic apical 4 chamber view. Arrow points to interventricular septal flattening during systole and diastole. RV is significantly dilated.

671: Transthoracic short axis view. Arrow points to flattened interventricular septum.

CASE 206

Bulur S, Nanda NC

This is a male patient with lung carcinoma who was sent for an echocardiogram to assess LV function. 2D TTE showed normal LV and RV function and no valvular abnormalities (🎥 672-674).

1. **What do the echoes show?**
   (a) Small RA with obstructed flow
   (b) Small RA with no flow obstruction

Ans. (b)

Color Doppler shows essentially laminar flow signals with only mild aliasing and therefore no obstruction to RA flow. RA is narrowed by an enlarged liver (L) which shows multiple echo densities (asterisks) consistent with metastases from lung carcinoma.

MOVIES 672 TO 674 🎥

CASE 207*

Mohamed A, Elsayed M, Kalra R, Bulur S, Nanda NC, Arisha MJ, Elkaryoni A, Mohamed AH, Gupta N

The patient was a 54-year-old female with a medical history of systemic hypertension, mitral valve prolapse complicated by mild-to-moderate mitral regurgitation, and aortic root dilation, who presented to the cardiology clinic with palpitations causing chest discomfort. She did not have any dyspnea, paroxysmal nocturnal dyspnea, orthopnea, presyncope, or syncope. The patient was able to exercise intensely without any exacerbation of her symptoms. Examination was unremarkable with regular heart rate and rhythm and without a murmur or S3.

Electrocardiogram revealed the presence of sinus rhythm with a heart rate of 65 beats per minute and left-axis deviation. The patient also had chronic T-wave inversion in the anteroseptal leads, but this had improved compared to prior electrocardiograms.

2DTTE was performed and revealed normal left and right ventricular size, wall thickness, and function. There was mild tricuspid regurgitation with mild-to-moderate aortic regurgitation and mild mitral regurgitation. While undergoing 2DTTE, the echocardiography technologist detected a 3.5 × 3.4 cm mass with multiple echolucent areas consistent with cysts in the RA in the apical four-chamber view. Color Doppler revealed unobstructed flow in the RA.

1. **(Figures 207.1, 207.2A and 675). What could be the etiology of the mass (arrow) visualized in the apical four-chamber view?**
   (a) Myxoma
   (b) Thrombus
   (c) Some type of cystic lesion
   (d) All of the above
   (e) None of the above

Ans. (d)

The help of the echo attending cardiologist was sought. During examination by the attending cardiologist, meticulous angulation and rotation of the transducer from the apical four-chamber view demonstrated that the mass was, in fact, a dilated aortic root, which was impinging on the RA. The aortic root measured 40–43 mm and appeared clear with no evidence of dissection. The aortic valve was mildly thickened without stenosis (Figs. 207.2B to 207.2D and 676 to 678).

Cardiovascular magnetic resonance imaging was subsequently performed and showed the aortic aneurysm bulging inferiorly into the RA. No dissection was noted.

Coronary angiogram was normal. The patient was referred for surgery, and aortic valve-sparing aortic root replacement was performed 3 months after the echocardiogram was obtained. At the time of surgical exploration, the operating surgeon also noted an incidental finding of an old healed focal aortic dissection in the noncoronary cusp. The patient was discharged on the fifth postoperative day and noted to be asymptomatic when she was followed up in clinic 2 weeks later.

Our case demonstrates the importance of careful angulation and rotation of the transducer with off-axis imaging during all imaging views to prevent a misdiagnosis, which could have easily occurred in our case.

The mass appeared cystic most likely due to differing echo densities between the aortic wall, aortic lumen, and the aortic cusps.

Our case thus emphasizes the importance of not only using the standard planes when performing a 2DTTE but also using "in between" and off-axis views, especially when

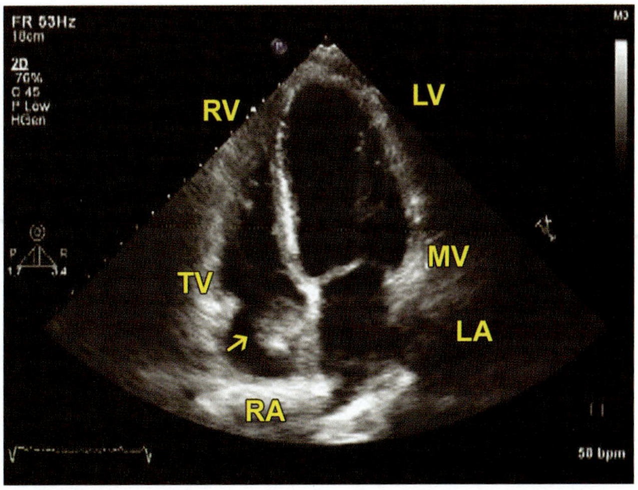

Fig. 207.1: 2DTTE. The arrow points to a mass in the right atrium (RA) imaged using the apical four-chamber view.

*This case is reproduced with permission from Mohamed A, Elsayed M, Kalra R, Bulur S, Nanda NC (2016). Aortic aneurysm mimicking a right atrial mass. Echocardiography, 33:1579-1580. doi:10. 1111/echo. 13329.

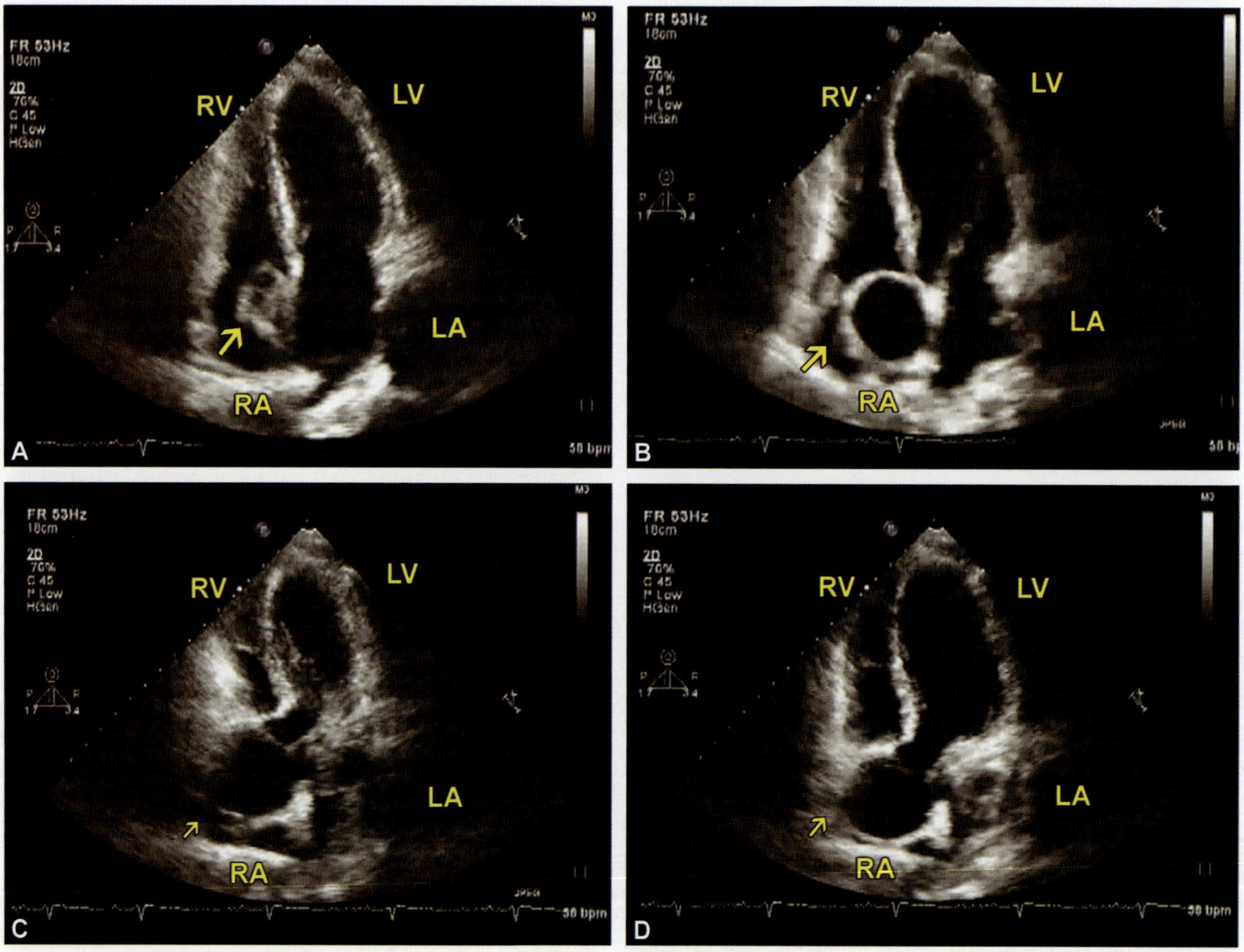

Figs. 207.2A to D: 2DTTE. A sequence showing, by suitable angulation, the cystic "mass" turning out to be a dilated aortic root (AO) communicating with the left ventricular outflow tract.

an unusual or abnormal intracardiac structure is encountered, otherwise an erroneous diagnosis could be made.

MOVIE LEGENDS

675: Shows the cystic mass in the RA imaged in the apical four-chamber view.

676: Shows the mass turning out to be a dilated AO with suitable transducer angulation.

677: Shows mild-to-moderate aortic regurgitation (AR) in the apical five-chamber view.

678A: Shows a dilated AO viewed in parasternal long-axis view.

678B: Depicts AR (arrow) in the same view.

678C: Subcostal view showing a cystic structure (arrow) in the RA (which ultimately turned out to be a dilated AO).

(DA: Descending thoracic aorta; L: Liver; LA: Left atrium; LV: Left ventricle; MR: Mitral regurgitation; MV: Mitral valve; RA: Right atrium; RV: Right ventricle; TV: Tricuspid valve).

CASE 208

Roomi AU, Elsayed M, Bulur S, Nanda NC

The patient is a 65-year-old female complaining of dyspnea on exertion and leg edema. She is a known case of hypertension (HTN) and hypothyroidism. Referred to echo lab to evaluate dyspnea (Figs. 208.1 and 208.2 and 679 and 680).

1. **What is the diagnosis?**
   (a) Cyst in stomach
   (b) Echolucent tumor below the LV
   (c) Hiatus hernia
   (d) Pericardial cyst

Ans. (c)

Any large echo-free space posterior to LV in the parasternal long or short axis view specially if located at the LV LA junction warrants an echo examination while drinking an aerated beverage. Hiatus hernia is diagnosed if bubble echoes appear in the space (stomach, S) as in this patient. This is an important procedure to perform to preclude other unnecessary costly investigations such as CT or MRI.

MOVIES 679 AND 680

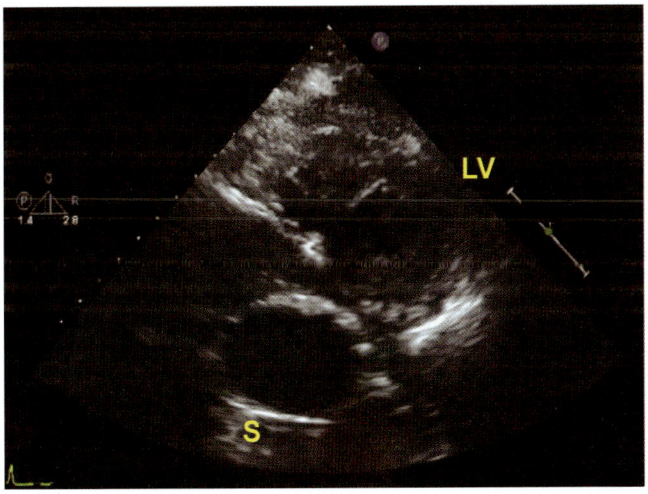

Fig. 208.1: A large echo-free bounded space (S) is noted behind the LV.

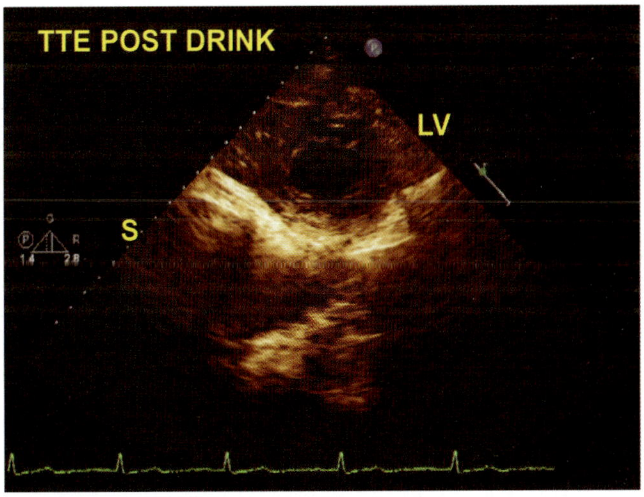

Fig. 208.2: Bubbles are visualized in the space (S) following ingestion of an aerated beverage, confirming it is the stomach.

CASE 209

Bulur S, Elsayed M, Alagic N, Uygur B, Turaga NSN, Chahwala JR, Adarna LG, Bhagatwala K, Nanda NC

Subcostal examination in an adult patient presenting with palpitations.

1. **What does the arrow point to in 681?**
   (a) Loculated ascites
   (b) Loculated pericardial effusion
   (c) Loculated right pleural effusion
   (d) Cysts in liver
   (e) Cystic tumor in liver

Ans. (d)

The finding is typical of liver cysts which may be associated with cysts in other organs such as the kidney.

MOVIE 681

SECTION 10

Congenital Heart Disease

CASE 210

Alagic N, Nanda NC

Bubble studies from 3 different adult patients are shown.

1. **What do the bubble studies show (682 to 684)?**
   (a) Two of the bubble studies most likely show interatrial shunt; in the remainder, the shunt level cannot be determined
   (b) At least one bubble study shows intrapulmonary shunt
   (c) All three bubble studies most likely show interatrial shunt
   (d) The level of the shunt cannot be determined by a 2D bubble study and 3D should have been done

Ans. (c)

Bubble studies in 682 and 683 show appearance of bubbles in LV/LA (arrow) within 3 beats of first appearance in the right heart consistent with interatrial shunt. In 684, it is not clear when the bubbles appeared in the left heart (arrow) but an atrial septal aneurysm is noted which makes interatrial shunt likely.

MOVIES 682 TO 684

CASE 211

Bulur S, Arisha MJ, Nanda NC

Right parasternal 2D TTE in a 57-year-old male is shown (Fig. 211.1 and 685).

1. **For this examination, the patient was placed in the:**
   (a) Right parasternal decubitus position at 90°
   (b) Right parasternal decubitus position at 60°
   (c) Right parasternal decubitus position at 30°

Ans. (a)

It is best to place the patient at 90°.

2. **The transducer is positioned:**
   (a) Very close to the sternum in the second right intercostal space
   (b) Very close to the sternum in the third right intercostal space
   (c) Very close to the sternum in the second to fifth right intercostal spaces

Ans. (c)

It is best to place the transducer close to the sternum and move it up and down the second to fifth or sixth intercostal spaces to find the SVC, interatrial septum (IAS), coronary sinus and IVC.

3. **Can you exclude a secundum ASD in this patient?**
   (a) Yes
   (b) No

Ans. (b)

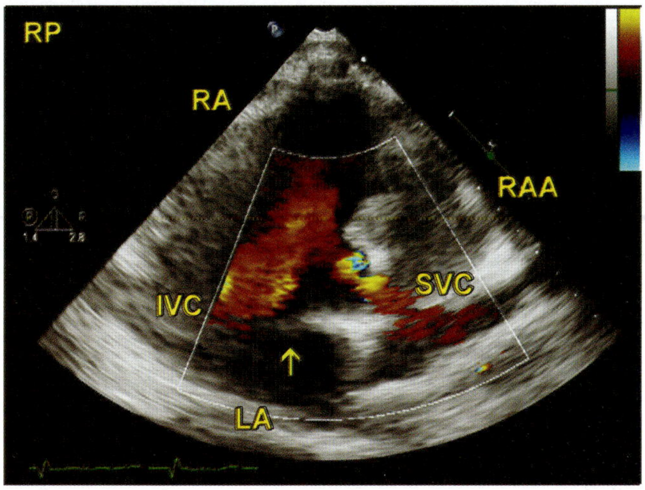

Fig. 211.1: Right parasternal examination. The arrow points to the interatrial septum. Flow signals are seen moving from SVC and IVC into the RA.

After finding the interatrial septum, one needs to angle and move the transducer in different directions to interrogate other parts of the septum with the color Doppler turned on because the ultrasonic beam may be imaging an intact portion of the atrial septum in a given view, thus missing an ASD. In this patient, no ASD could be found. Red flow signals can be seen in Figure 211.1 moving from the SVC and the IVC region into the RA.

Right parasternal 2D TTE in a 30-year-old female who is 28 weeks pregnant is demonstrated (Figs. 211.2A and B, 211.3, 211.4, 211.5A to D, 685, 686A and B, 687, 688 and 689A to C).

4. **The arrow shows:**
   (a) Two secundum ASDs with left to right shunt
   (b) PFO with left to right shunt
   (c) Sinus venosus ASD near the IVC with left to right shunt
   (d) Sinus venosus ASD near the SVC with left to right shunt
   (e) There is no ASD or PFO but it is an artifact which is seen when you examine from the right parasternal approach

Ans. (b)

This patient most likely has a PFO with left to right shunt since the defect is bound by septum primum (SP) and septum secundum (SS). Most PFOs result in right to left shunting, but in a certain number of patients, the shunt may be left to right because of local distortion of the IAS. Intact septum is seen superiorly next to SVC as well as inferiorly excluding a sinus venosus defect. This is a good view to diagnose PFO/ASD by color Doppler because the septum is oriented horizontally permitting parallel interrogation of the ultrasonic beam with ASD flow direction, as can be seen in this patient. In the apical 4-chamber view, the ultrasonic beam is perpendicular to the ASD flow direction making it difficult to recognize the shunt flow. Also, echo dropouts frequently occur in this view because of the curved nature of the IAS.

5. **What may be the additive value of 3D echo in this patient?**
   (a) No value at all because the shunt flow is clearly seen by 2D echo and size of the defect can also be measured. Also, 2D echo is useful in measuring shunt flow and the size of the RV which are very

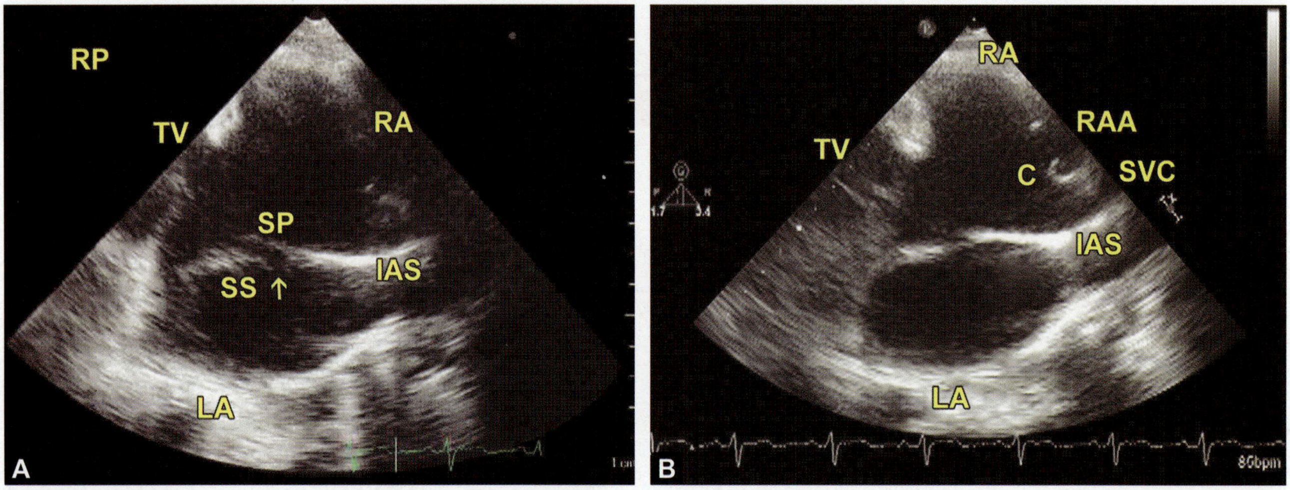

Figs. 211.2A and B: Right parasternal examination. (A) The arrow points to a patent foramen ovale (PFO) between the septum primum (SP) and the septum secundum (SS). (B) The crista terminalis (C) is well seen.

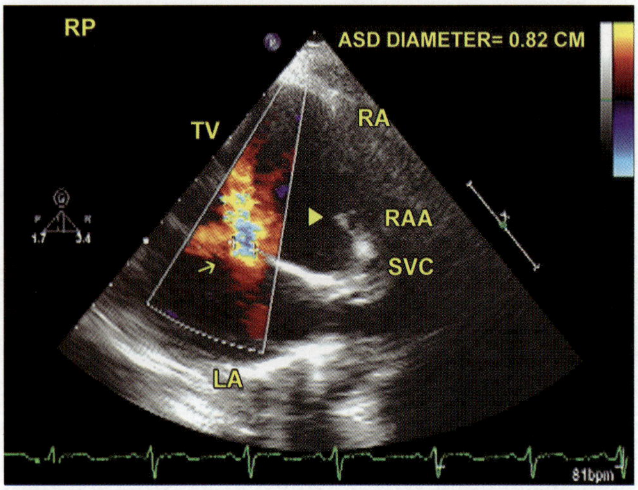

Fig. 211.3: Right parasternal (RP) examination. The arrow shows flow signals moving from the LA into the RA indicative of a PFO/secundum atrial septal defect (ASD). Arrowhead points to crista terminalis.

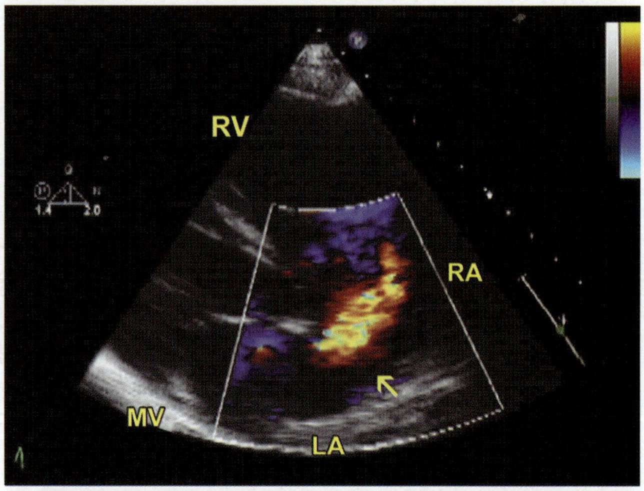

Fig. 211.4: Modified four-chamber view. Arrow shows flow signals moving from the LA into the RA indicative of a PFO/ASD.

important in deciding whether the ASD needs to be closed.

(b) Because the complete extent of IAS can be potentially studied by 3D echo, including enface view of the defect and shunt, more reliable measurements of the ASD size can be obtained by this technique. 3D echo may also be useful in excluding a second or third ASD which may be missed by 2D echo because at any given time, the latter shows only a thin slice of the IAS and not its full extent.

Ans. (b)

Although 2D echo is very useful in diagnosing and assessing chamber sizes, 3D echo provides additive value as described in b. The size of any defect or mass lesion by 3D echo has been shown to be more reliable than 2D techniques.

6. Which anatomic structures that are not generally visualized with standard 2D TTE in an adult may be imaged with right parasternal 2D TTE?

(a) SVC-RA junction
(b) Crista terminalis
(c) Right atrial appendage
(d) Ascending aorta
(e) TV

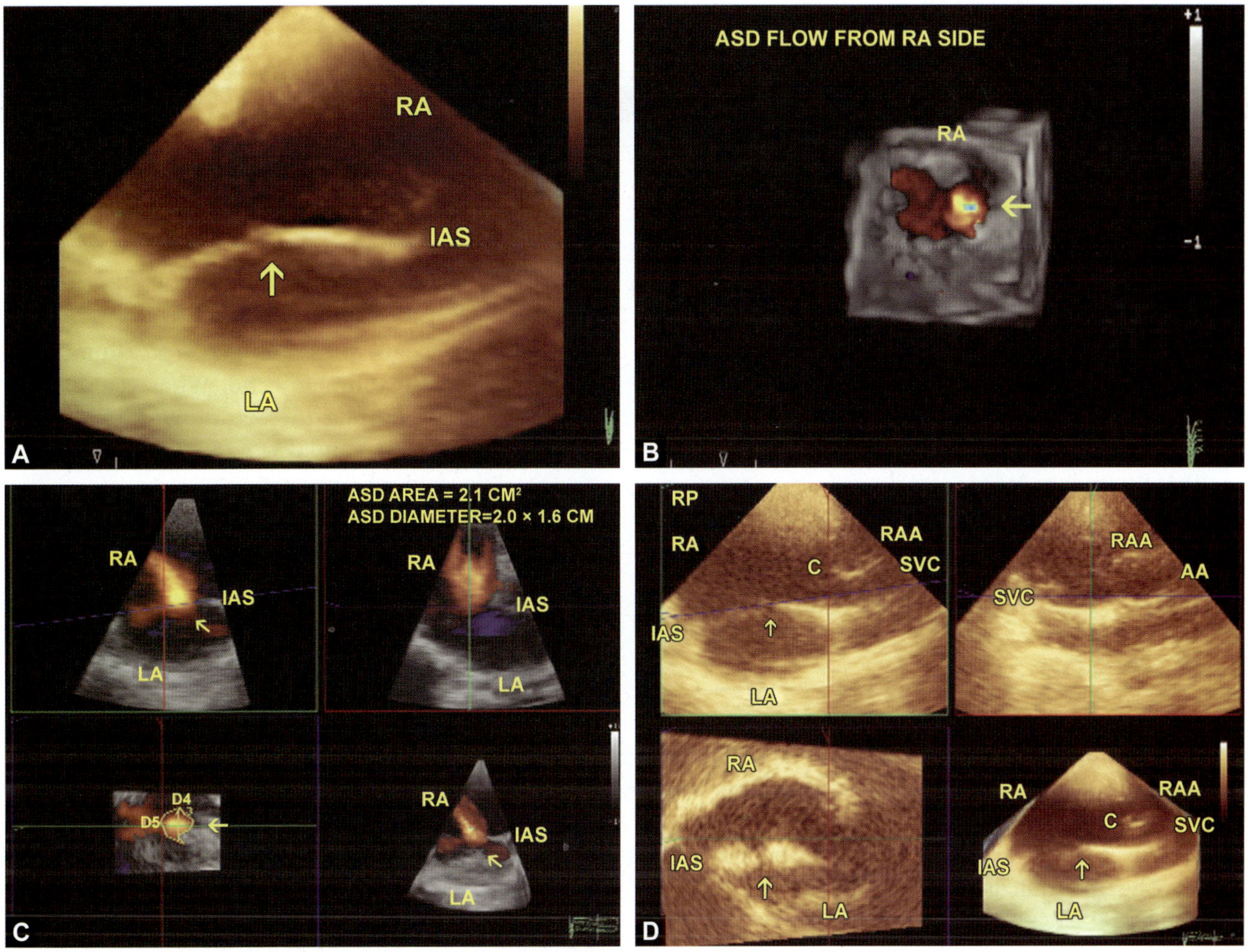

Figs. 211.5A to D: Right parasternal examination. 3DTTE. A. The B mode study shows a defect (arrow) between the septum primum and septum secundum. B, C. Multiplanar reconstruction. In B, color Doppler is utilized to view the defect en face from the RA side (arrow). In C, color Doppler is utilized to view the defect en face from the LA aspect (arrows). It measures 2.0 × 1.6 cm, area 2.1 cm^2. The crista terminalis is shown in D.

(f) All of the above
(g) Only 3 of the above
(h) Only 2 of the above

Ans. (f)

It is difficult to visualize SVC-RA junction, crista terminalis (C) and RAA in an adult during standard 2D TTE. Imaging of SVC-RA junction using the right parasternal approach permits visualization of sinus venosus ASD. Crista terminalis, vestigial tissue seen at the SVC-RA junction, is also well seen as well as the RAA by right parasternal 2D TTE. A large extent of ascending aorta (AA) is also well imaged by right parasternal 2D TTE but may also be seen using high left parasternal and suprasternal approaches.

MOVIES 685 TO 689

REFERENCE

1. Nanda NC, Abd-El Rahman SN, Khatri G, et al. Incremental value of three-dimensional echocardiography over transesophageal multiplane two-dimensional echocardiography in qualitative and quantitative assessment of cardiac masses and defects. Echocardiography. 1995;12: 619–28.

CASE 212

Susan T Laing, Beverly Smulevitz

This patient is a 54-year-old female, who presented with chest pain. She has no significant cardiac history. 2DTTE was performed, resulting in the discovery of a 1.5 cm atrial septal defect (ASD). The ASD was further delineated with a 2DTEE.

1. **In the image below, what type of defect is measured? (Fig. 212.1 and 690)**
   (a) Primum ASD
   (b) Secundum ASD
   (c) Sinus venosus ASD
   (d) Coronary sinus ASD

Ans. (b)

DISCUSSION

Atrial septal defect is one of the congenital anomalies that may remain undiagnosed until adulthood. It does not always have a distinct murmur and it may never cause symptoms.

The patient was sent to the cath lab for percutaneous closure of her ASD utilizing the Amplatzer device. The procedure was successful and she was transferred back to her room. Several hours after the procedure, she developed intermittent ventricular tachycardia and multiform PVCs. An emergent transthoracic echo was ordered.

2. **Below is a parasternal long-axis RV inflow view from the transthoracic echo. What is the arrow most likely pointing to? See moving image (Fig. 212.2 and 691A and B).**
   (a) Tricuspid valve vegetation
   (b) Tricuspid valve clot
   (c) Right atrial myxoma
   (d) Embolized amplatzer device

Ans. (d)

DISCUSSION

The Amplatzer device (arrow in Figs. 212.2 and 212.3) became detached from the atrial septum. In this image, it is in the right ventricle, having come from the right atrium and crossing through the tricuspid valve. In the 4th video clip, the device is seen bouncing around in the RV and some arrhythmia is evident.

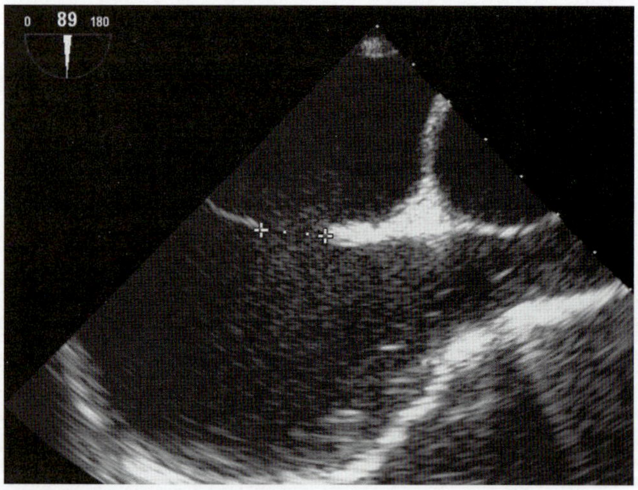

Fig. 212.1: Transesophageal echocardiogram of interatrial septum with measured atrial septal defect.

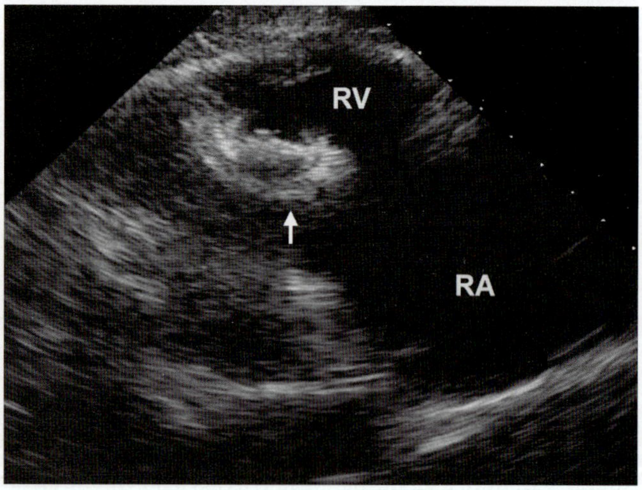

Fig. 212.2: Parasternal long axis view of the right-sided chambers showing an unusual mass (arrow) within the right ventricle.

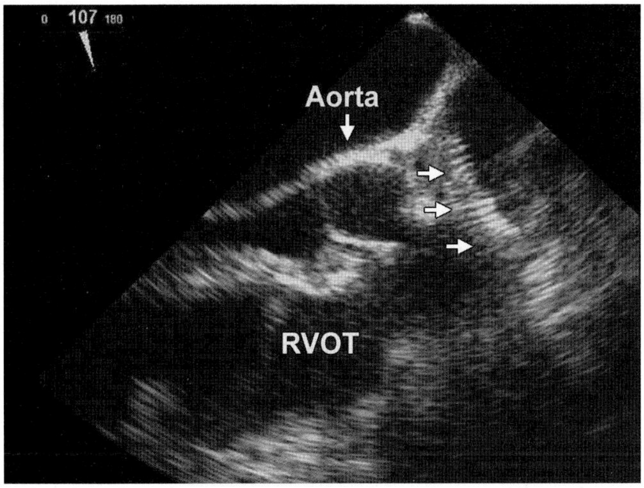

Fig. 212.3: Intraoperative transesophageal echocardiogram of the right ventricular outflow tract.

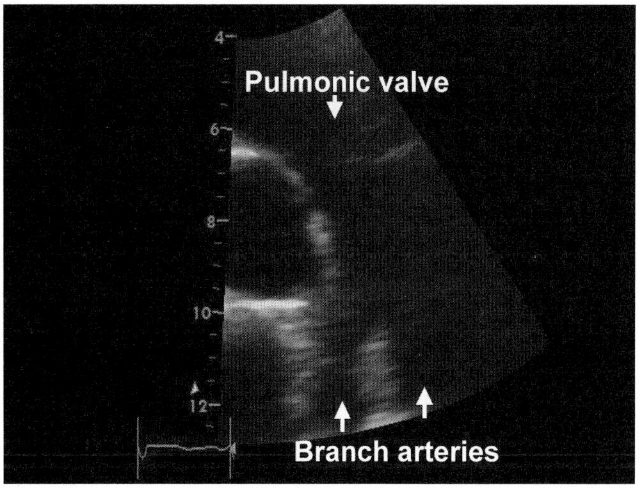

Fig. 212.4: Postoperative transthoracic echocardiogram of the pulmonary artery bifurcation.

This patient was emergently sent for surgery to retrieve the Amplatzer device and repair the ASD.

3. In the intraoperative TEE image below, what has happened to the device? (Fig. 212.3 and 692)

(a) It remains in the right ventricle
(b) It has crossed into the left ventricle
(c) It has crossed into the pulmonary artery
(d) It is in the right atrium.

Ans. (c)

The device is now in the pulmonary artery, just before the bifurcation.

DISCUSSION

The device came loose from the atrial septum, ending up in the right atrium. It then crossed the tricuspid valve into the right ventricle, finally ending up in the pulmonary artery, at the bifurcation. The embolized Amplatzer device was retrieved and the ASD was repaired with a bovine patch.

A short-axis view of the pulmonary artery the day after the Amplatzer device was surgically removed is shown in Fig. 212.4 and 693.

MOVIES 690 TO 693

CASE 213

Sudarshan Balla, Archana Vasudevan, Kul Aggarwal

A 61-year-old Caucasian male with no significant past medical history presented to his primary care physician with complaints of bilateral lower extremity edema and shortness of breath on exertion. There was no family history of coronary artery disease. In view of shortness of breath on exertion, an exercise stress echo was ordered by the primary care physician. He exercised for 6 minutes on Bruce protocol. Exercise stress echo was negative for inducible ischemia. However, the stress images were suggestive of right atrial and right ventricular enlargement. A bubble study was performed to detect intracardiac shunts. Bubble study was positive for an intracardiac shunt likely at the atrial level based on bubbles crossing over from right atrium to left atrium. In order to assess for the anatomic basis of the intracardiac shunt, a transesophageal echocardiogram (TEE) was performed. Repeat bubble study was performed during the transesophageal echocardiogram. Images are shown below (Fig. 213.1).

1. **Assuming you were the physician performing the transesophageal echocardiogram, what would you do as the next step?**
   (a) Complete the TEE and refer the patient for cardiac MRI/CT
   (b) Findings are suggestive of PFO
   (c) Findings are suggestive of secundum ASD
   (d) Findings are suggestive of pulmonary artriovenous malformation
   (e) Continue to look for the site of the shunt at the atrial level

Ans. (e)

2. **The most common associated anomaly with sinus venosus atrial septal defect is?**
   (a) Ventricular septal defect
   (b) Cleft mitral valve
   (c) Partial anomalous pulmonary venous return
   (d) Left sided SVC

Ans. (c)

DISCUSSION

The transesophageal echocardiogram diagnosed the presence of atrial septal defect - sinus venosus type (Figs. 213.2 and 213.3, 694). This was located in the superior portion of the septum close to the superior vena cava (SVC). Sinus venosus defects are the third most common type of atrial septal defects following ostium secundum and

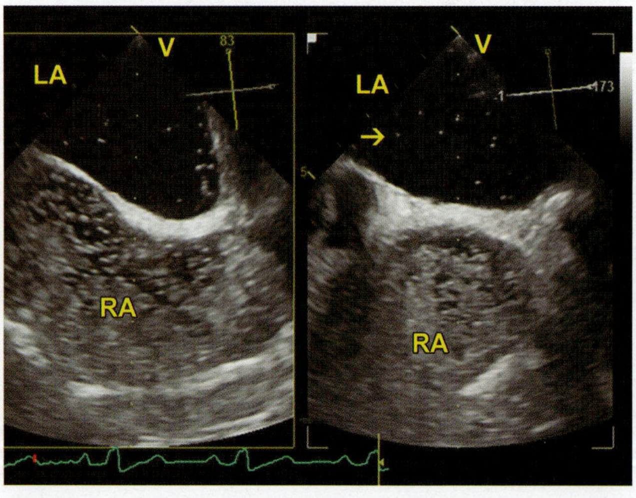

Fig. 213.1: TEE. Arrow points to bubbles in left atrium.

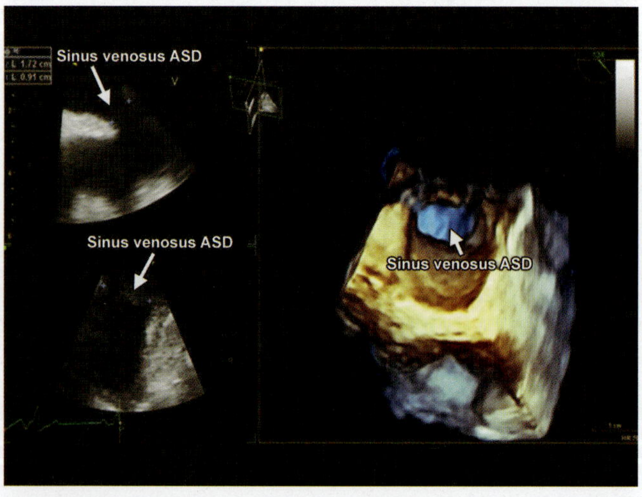

Fig. 213.2: Arrow shows the defect in two- and three-dimensional echocardiography.

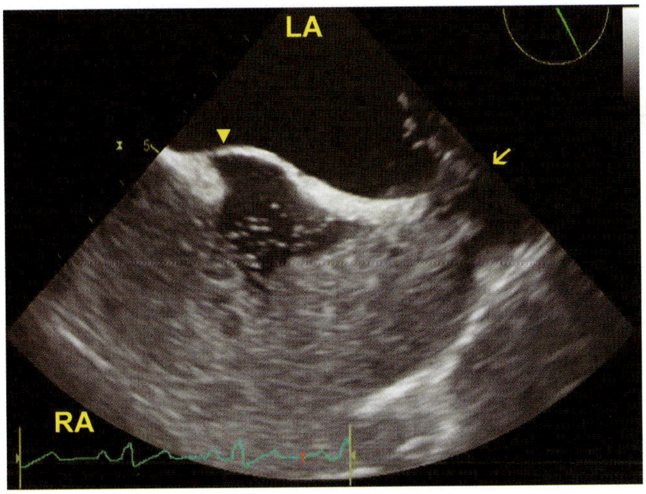

Fig. 213.3: TEE. Arrow points to sinus venosus defect and arrowhead to fossa ovalis in this figure and 694.

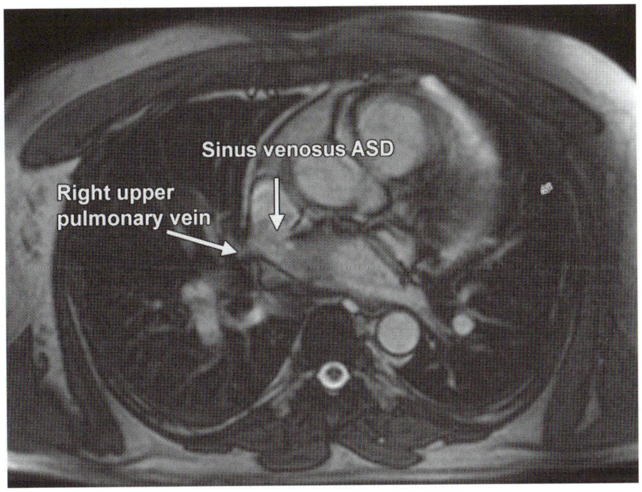

Fig. 213.4: Magnetic resonance imaging showing the defect and right upper pulmonary vein.

ostium primum types. In patients suspected of intracardiac shunts, transesophageal echocardiogram is an essential imaging modality for accurate anatomic diagnosis. At the time of transesophageal echocardiography, the entire interatrial septum should be visualized to confirm the anatomic location of the shunt. Ideally visualization of the interatrial septum using 3-D TEE can be helpful as was in this case. The most common associated anomaly in patients with the superior sinus venosus defect is partial anomalous pulmonary venous return (PAPVR). Most common PAPVR is anomalous drainage of right upper pulmonary vein into the right atrium, across the defect. Cardiac MRI was performed to assess drainage of all the other pulmonary veins prior to surgery. Cardiac MRI images revealed superior sinus venosus defect and anomalous drainage of the right upper pulmonary vein (Fig. 213.4). There were no other anomalous venous connections. Shortness of breath on exertion in middle-aged and elderly population is a nonspecific symptom and could be due to multiple cardiac and respiratory etiologies. This symptom is also an angina equivalent. Stress echo performed to assess for coronary artery disease gave the suggestion that the etiology of his symptoms is probably an atrial septal defect. The first suggestion of atrial septal defects can be evidence of right atrial and right ventricular enlargement on transthoracic echocardiogram as was in this case. Multimodality imaging with TEE supplemented with cardiac MRI resulted in accurate diagnosis. The patient underwent successful surgical correction of the defect. Postoperative course was complicated by atrial fibrillation and was treated with amiodarone. The patient is recovering well postoperatively and is actively participating in cardiac rehabilitation.

MOVIE 694

CASE 214

Gautam D, Choudhary R, Singhal G, Kotti K, Agarwal A, Elsayed M, Nanda NC

This is an 18-year-old male who presented with dyspnea on exertion. 2D TTE was done.

1. **What does the arrow in the parasternal (Fig. 214.1 and 695) and subcostal 4-chamber views (Fig. 214.2 and 696) point to?**
   (a) Secundum atrial septal defect (ASD)
   (b) Sinus venosus ASD
   (c) Ostium primum ASD
   (d) Atrioventricular septal defect

Ans. (b)

The defect is seen in the most superior part of the interatrial septum (IAS) with no intact septum between the defect and the atrial wall. A secundum defect, on the other hand, will show an intact septum on both sides of the defect. Ostium primum/atrioventricular septal defect would be noted in the inferior portion of the IAS with no intact septum between the defect and the atrioventricular valves.

2. **The coronary sinus (CS) in this patient is markedly dilated (Figs. 214.1, 214.2 and 695 and 696) because:**
   (a) Associated left-sided SVC is present
   (b) The right-sided chambers are huge
   (c) Both (a) and (b)

Ans. (a)

Both the RV and RA are enlarged but they are not huge which could have resulted in marked dilatation of the CS. Therefore, the most likely cause is a left-sided SVC which drains into the CS causing marked enlargement. Left-sided SVC may be associated in some patients with an absent right-sided SVC. In this patient, both left- and right-sided SVC were present. Left-sided SVC can be diagnosed by performing a bubble study using a left arm vein which will show opacification of the coronary sinus before the bubbles appear in the RV. Left-sided SVC may also be detected from the left supraclavicular transducer position.

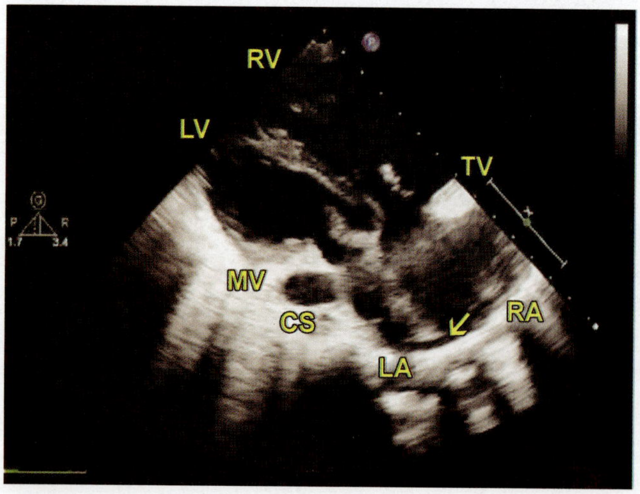

Fig. 214.1: The arrow in the left parasternal view demonstrates the sinus venosus ASD and an enlarged coronary sinus (CS).

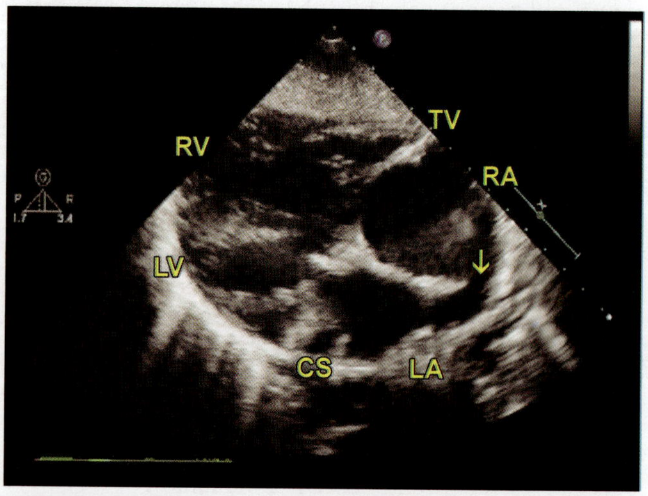

Fig. 214.2: Subcostal view also shows the sinus venosus defect (arrow) and an enlarged coronary sinus (CS).

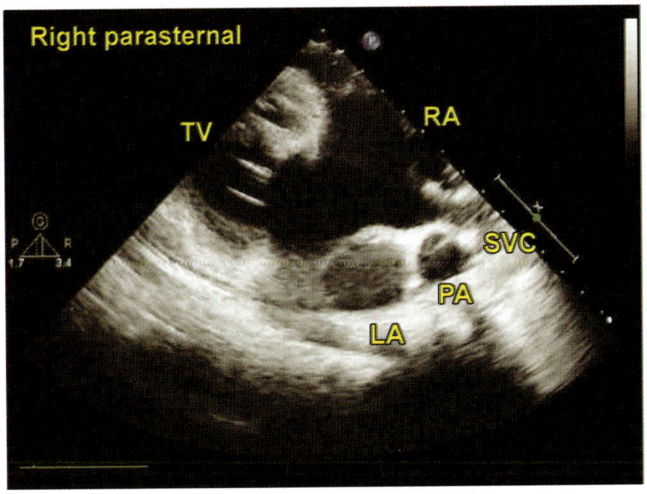

Fig. 214.3: Right parasternal examination. Initially, the atrial septum next to the SVC appeared intact but slight transducer angulation showed the sinus venosus defect which was subsequently confirmed by color Doppler.

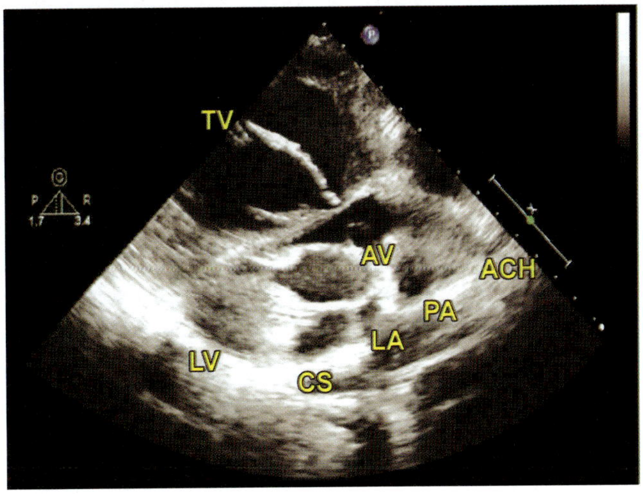

Fig. 214.4: Right parasternal examination. The ascending aorta and arch (ACH) are well imaged.

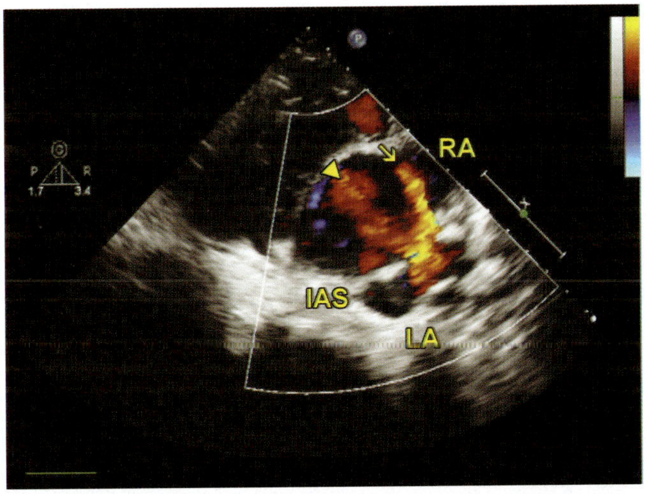

Fig. 214.5: Right parasternal approach. Two jets (arrowhead and arrow) are seen in the RA, one of which could be flow from an anomalous pulmonary vein and the other the sinus venosus shunt.

3. **How does right parasternal examination (Figs. 214.3 to 214.5 and 697 to 699) supplement routine left-sided parasternal approaches in the diagnosis of an ASD? Identify the incorrect answer.**
   (a) This approach is generally not utilized to find an ostium primum ASD
   (b) Secundum ASDs are well visualized
   (c) Sinus venosus ASDs involving both the superior (adjacent to SVC) and inferior (next to IVC) portions of the interatrial septum (IAS) are well detected with this approach.
   (d) Using this approach is a waste of valuable time.

Ans. (d)

This approach views not only the junction of the SVC with the IAS (Fig. 214.3 and 697) but also with slight transducer tilting the relationship of the IVC with the IAS. Also, the IAS is oriented horizontally facilitating detection of left to right shunt by color Doppler since the ultrasonic beam is parallel to shunt direction. It is important to tilt and slightly adjust the transducer to move away from the intact portion of the IAS (Fig. 214.3 and 697) and find the defect (Fig. 214.5 and 699). This approach is also useful to view and assess a long segment of the ascending aorta and sometimes the aortic arch (ACH) (Fig. 214.4 and 698). It is also important to place the patient in the 90 degree right lateral decubitus position to maximally displace the right lung laterally. The transducer is kept very close to the sternum on the right side and moved up and down the interspaces. A dilated right heart or enlargement of the ascending aorta tends to displace the right lung laterally (can be seen on a routine chest X-ray) facilitating right parasternal echo examination specially in an adult. The arrow and arrowhead in Figure 214.5 and 699 demonstrate two separate jets, one of which probably represents flow entering the right atrium from an anomalous right upper pulmonary vein, which is commonly associated with a sinus venosus ASD and the other is the shunt.

MOVIES 695 TO 699

CASE 215

Chahwala JR, Elsayed M, Alagic N, Uygur B, Turaga NSN, Adarna LG, Bulur S, Nanda NC

This is an adult patient who underwent anterior MV cleft repair and closure of partial atrioventricular septal defect in childhood. He presents with dyspnea on exertion. 2D TTE was done.

1. **What abnormalities are shown in 700 to 702?**
   (a) Mild MR
   (b) Moderate MR
   (c) Severe MR

Ans. (c)

MR jet occupies > 40% of LA in 702. 701 also shows severe MR since we need to take into account the red flow signals which are moving in the same phase as the blue signals (swirling MR). The arrows in movies 700 and 702 denote the site of previous failed MV repair. The patient was scheduled for re-repair of MR.

MOVIES 700 TO 702

CASE 216

Gyanendra K Sharma

VENTRICULAR SEPTAL DEFECT

A 35-year-old man was referred by a family medicine physician for evaluation of a heart murmur. The patient says that he always had a heart murmur. He does not have any history of shortness of breath, leg swelling or palpitations and denied having any history of endocarditis. On physical examination, pulse 72 beats per minute, blood pressure 145/70 mm Hg. He did not have jugular venous distention and pulmonary examination was unremarkable. Heart sounds were normal and the PMI was not displaced. A grade 3/6 systolic murmur was best heard in the left parasternal area. Transthoracic echocardiogram was performed to evaluate the heart murmur (Figs. 216.1, 216.3 and 703).

1. **Based on your review of images, what is the estimated right ventricular systolic pressure?**
   (a) Insufficient information to calculate
   (b) 15–20 mm Hg
   (c) 25–35 mm Hg
   (d) 40–50 mm Hg

Ans. (b)

In absence of aortic stenosis or LVOT obstruction, LV systolic blood pressure is equal to systemic systolic blood pressure. Therefore, the LV systolic pressure is 145 mm Hg. Pulse wave Doppler shows a gradient of 128 mm Hg between the LV and RV. Thus, RV systolic pressure is equal to 145–128 = 17 mm Hg.

2. **Which one of the following is true?**
   (a) VSD constitutes the most common type of congenital heart disease in adults.
   (b) Right ventricular enlargement is common due to left to right shunting.
   (c) Aortic regurgitation is most commonly seen in patients with supracristal VSD.
   (d) Inlet VSD can be closed by Amplatz device.
   (e) Most VSDs are associated with chromosomal abnormalities.

Ans. (c)

Because of location of supracristal VSD in close proximity to the aortic valve, it is more commonly associated with aortic regurgitation.

Bicuspid aortic valve is the most common congenital heart disease in adults. Left-sided chamber enlargement is more common with VSD while right-sided chamber enlargement is more often seen in patients with ASD. Inlet VSDs are generally due to an endocardial cushion defect and, therefore, may not be suitable for closure by an Amplatz device. Chromosomal abnormalities are not seen in the majority of patients with VSD. Tetralogy of Fallot is associated with chromosome 22 deletions.

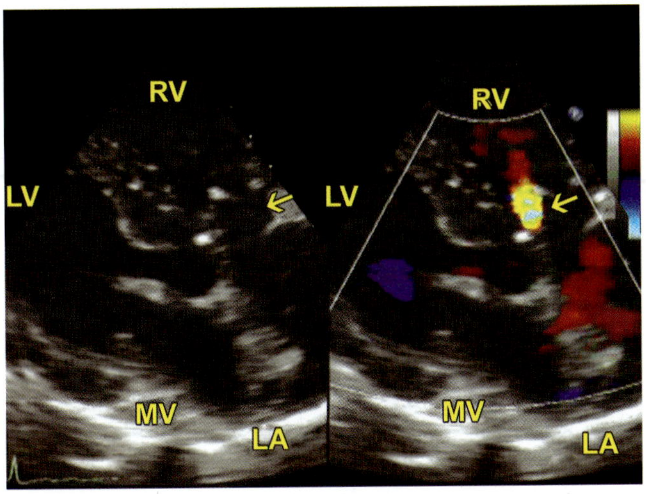

Fig. 216.1: Parasternal long axis view showing membranous VSD (arrow) below the aortic valve.

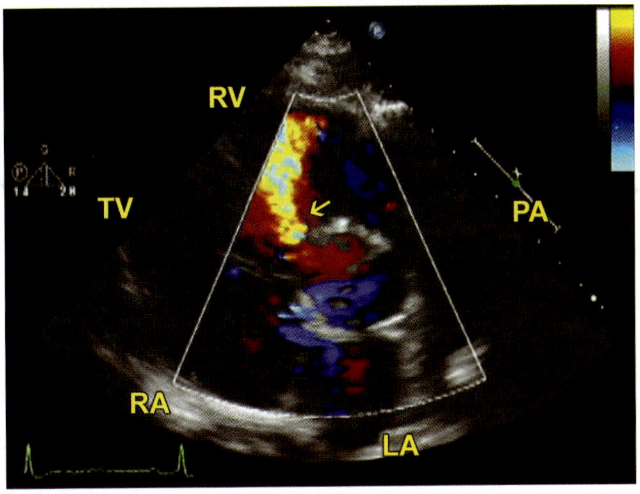

Fig. 216.2: Short axis view with color Doppler showing VSD (arrow).

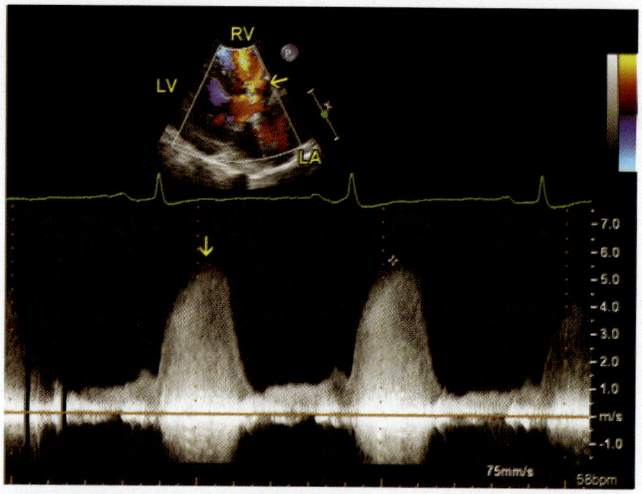

Fig. 216.3: Pulsed wave Doppler to show maximum VSD velocity (arrow). This is utilized to calculate LV-RV gradient.

3. **Which of the following is a true statement?**
   (a) This is the most common type of ventricular septal defect.
   (b) This patient should be referred for closure of VSD.
   (c) Most (> 90%) membranous and muscular VSDs close spontaneously by the age of two years.
   (d) Endocarditis prophylaxis is indicated before dental procedures.

Ans. (a)

A membranous ventricular septal defect is thought to be the most common type of VSD. It is seen in the parasternal short axis view at 10 degree position closer to the tricuspid valve as opposed to the supracristal VSD which is seen close to the pulmonary valve (Fig. 216.2 and 704). In the absence of symptoms or pulmonary hypertension, a small VSD does not require surgical closure. Most muscular VSDs close by the age of 3 years and membranous VSD by 6 years. A small VSD may remain asymptomatic for a long period of time. With current change in guidelines in the absence of history of endocarditis, there is no indication for endocarditis prophylaxis in this patient.

MOVIE LEGENDS

703: Parasternal long axis view 2-D and color Doppler show VSD (arrow).

704: Short axis color Doppler showing VSD (arrow) close to the tricuspid valve.

REFERENCE

1. Mary S Minette, David J Sahn. Congenital heart disease for the adult cardiologist; ventricular septal defects. Circulation. 2006;114:2190-97.

CASE 217

Naveen Garg, Kanwal K Kapur

A 40-year-old male with known diagnosis of VSD with h/o dyspnea on exertion underwent echocardiographic examination (Figs. 217.1 to 217.4 and 705A and B to 707A and B).

CALCULATIONS

Qp/Qs = in VSD Qp/Qs = RVOT flow/ LVOT flow

Flow = $(\text{diameter})^2 \times \text{VTI}$

Qp/Qs = $(0.785 \times 3.8 \times 3.8 \times 15.4)/(0.785 \times 2.5 \times 2.5 \times 21.8)$

$= 174/106.9 = 1.62$

PASP (PA Systolic Pressure) = $(\text{TR velocity})^2$ + RAP (calculated from IVC)

$= 78 + 15 = 93$ mm Hg

Mean PAP = $(\text{PR velocity})^2$ + RAP

$= 32 + 15 = 47$ mm Hg

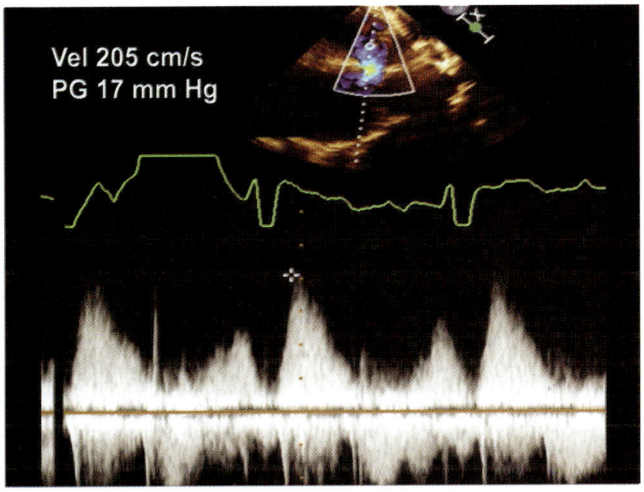

Fig. 217.1: VSD flow; VSD = 2.74 cm.

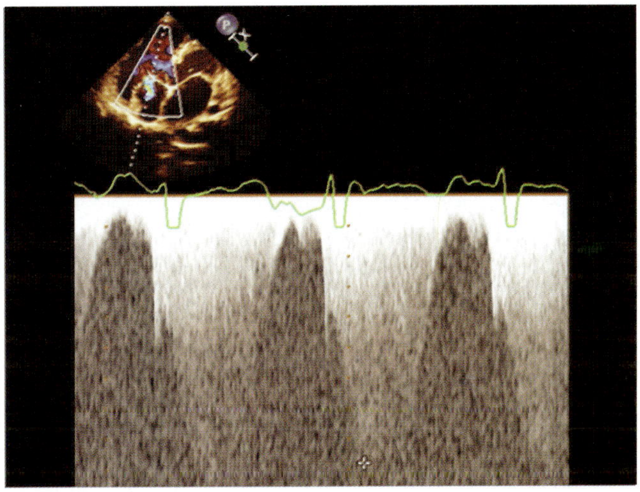

Fig. 217.2: TR jet.

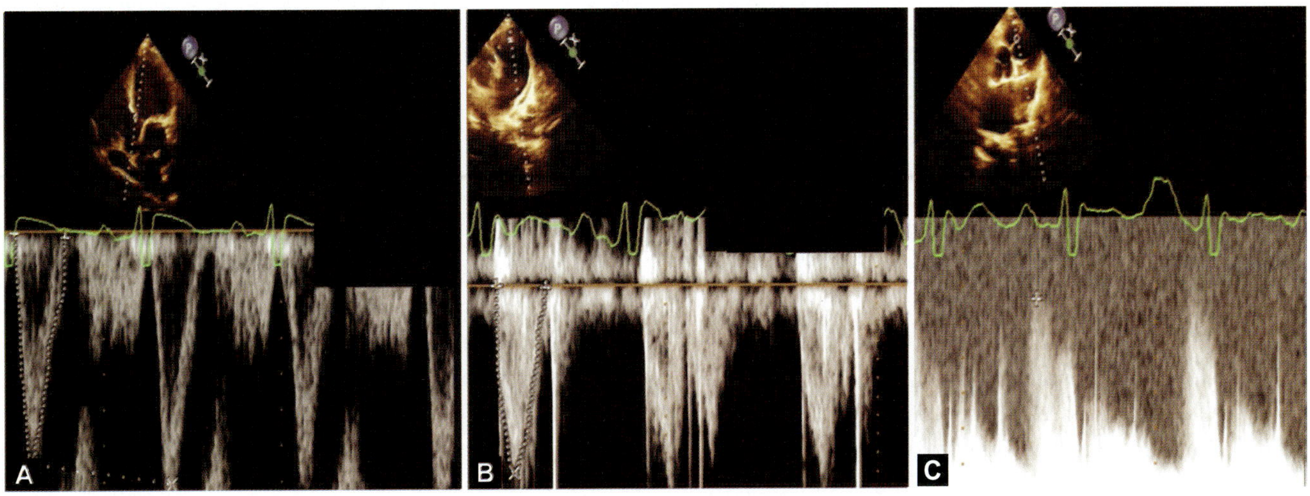

Figs. 217.3A to C: (A) LVOT; (B) RVOT; (C) PR velocity.

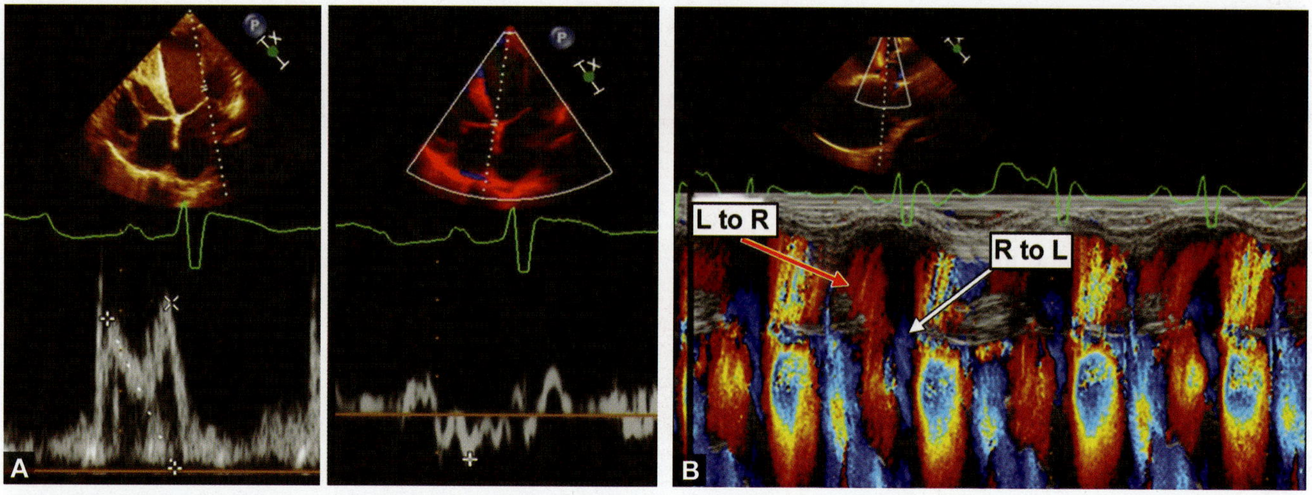

Figs. 217.4A and B: (A) E and e' mitral valve septal; (B) M-mode.

Table 217.1: Indices.	
LVOT	2.5 cm
RVOT	3.8 cm
LVOT VTI	21.8 cm
RVOT VTI	15.4 cm
TR JET Peak	441 cm/s PG = 78 mm Hg
IVC Diameter	1.5 cm
E and e'	76 and 5.3 cm/s
VSD	2.74 cm PG = 17 mm Hg
HR	90/min
PR Velocity	282 cm/s PG = 32 mm Hg

PA flow = RVOT flow × HR

= 174 × 90 = 15660 mL = 15.5 L/min

PCWP (Pulmonary Capillary Wedge Pressure) = 1.24 × E/e' + 1.9

= 1.24 × 76/5.3 + 1.9

= 19.68 mm Hg

PVR (Pulmonary Vascular Resistance) = (Mean PAP – PCWP)/PA Flow

= (47–19.68)/15.5

= 1.76 Wu

The patient was given oxygen for inhalation for 20 mins. Oxygen being a pulmonary arteriolar vasodilator causes a drop in the PA pressures and pulmonary vascular resistance. This indicates potential reactivity of pulmonary vasculature, could predict reversibility of the high PA pressures post VSD repair. The parameters were recalculated. The results were the following (Figs. 217.5A and B):

- Mean PAP = 27 +15 = 42 mm Hg
- RVOT flow = 0.785 × 3.8 × 3.8 × 21.7 = 245.97 mL (high RVOT flow)
- LVOT Flow = 0.785 × 2.5 × 2.5 × 19.7 = 96.65 mL
- PA FLOW = 245.97 × 87 = 21.6 L/min
- PVR O_2 = 42–19.68/21.6 = 1.04 Wu
- Qp/Qs = RVOT flow/ LVOT flow = 245.97/96.65 = 2.54

Thus, pre- and post-oxygen therapy indices were:

	Pre –O_2	*Pre –O_2*
RVOT SV	174 mL	245.97 mL
LVOT SV	106.9 mL	96.65 mL
PA flow	15.5 L/min	21.6 L/min
PVR	1.76 Wu	1.04 Wu
Mean PAP	47 mm Hg	42 mm Hg
Qp/Qs	1.62	2.54

Findings were consistent with cardiac catheterization—although there were discrepancies between the echo and the cardiac cath-derived parameters for shunt computation and PVR before and after oxygen study. Both studies, however, indicated a substantial fall in the PVR and a significant increase in the left to right shunt after 20 minutes of oxygen inhalation.

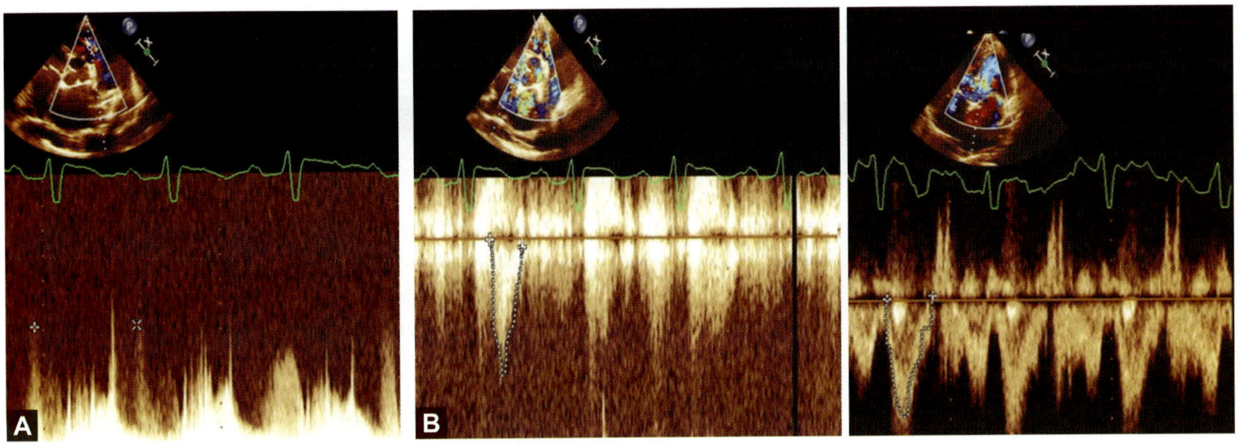

Figs. 217.5A and B: (A) PR velocity; (B) RVOT flow, LVOT flow.

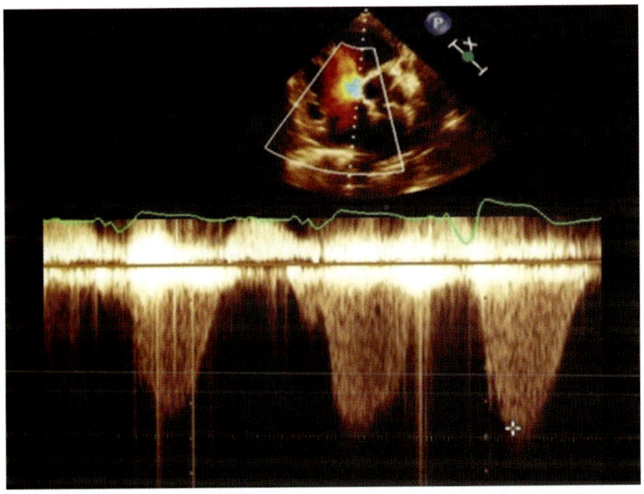

Fig. 217.6: TR jet post-repair (PASP = 23 + 15 = 38 mm Hg).

	Pre-O_2		Post-O_2	
	CATH	ECHO	CATH	ECHO
Qo/Qs	2.1	1.62	5.5	2.54
PVR	13.75	1.76	1.86	1.04

DISCUSSION

- Immediately after VSD repair (patient came off pump in good shape), PASP was 60 mm Hg and aortic systolic was 100 mm Hg
- In recovery room, PASP was 50 mm Hg
- Predischarge echo PASP using TR JET = 38 mm Hg (Fig. 217.6)
- However, LV was still large with estimated LVEF 34% (this reduced ejection fraction was probably due to a sudden reduction in the volume load after surgical closure of the VSD and this is likely to recover in the subsequent weeks) (🎥 708A and B).

EXCEPTIONAL FEATURES

- Large VSD in 40 years male with systemic level PASP with bidirectional shunt (Net Left to Right Shunt—Fig. 217.4-M-Mode) with volume-overloaded LV.
- Excellent results in immediate post-op period with dramatic fall of PASP and mean PAP to normal levels in first 48 hours.
- The drop in the LVEF is likely to be a temporary phenomenon owing to loss of volume load to LV.
- Although patients with moderate to large VSDs have been operated during adult life, the operative mortality in patients with systemic level PAH is extremely high.
- The best results in these group of patients are achieved when PASP < 65 mm Hg. Our patient has been a notable exception (systemic level PAH, high PVR and normal PA pressures after 10 days of VSD repair).

MOVIE LEGENDS 🎥

705A and B: PLAX view

706A and B: 4C view

707A and B: RVOT SAX (SAX-Aortic level)

708A and B: Post VSD Repair PLAX View

CASE 218

Kasprzak Jaroslaw

1. **Presented continuous Doppler flow pattern (Fig. 218.1, arrow) may be potentially due to:**
   (a) Tricuspid regurgitation
   (b) Atrial septal defect
   (c) Ventricular septal defect
   (d) Ruptured aneurysm of Valsalva
   (e) (A) and (C)

Ans. (e)

2. **Presented color Doppler finding (Fig. 218.2 and 709, arrow/left arrowhead) may result from:**
   (a) Tricuspid regurgitant flow
   (b) Atrial septal shunt
   (c) Atrioventricular septal shunt
   (d) (A) and (C)
   (e) All of the above

Ans. (d)

3. **Abnormal flow findings (arrow) in TEE view shown on Figs. 218.2, 218.3, 710 and 711 include:**
   (a) Shunt or regurgitant flow in the right atrium
   (b) Aortic regurgitation
   (c) Sinus venosus atrial septal defect or anomalous pulmonary venous/superior vena cava connection
   (d) All of the above
   (e) Either (A) or (B)

Ans. (e)

4. **Principal diagnosis of this abnormality (Figs. 218.3 and 218.4) is:**
   (a) Tricuspid regurgitation
   (b) Sinus venosus type atrial septal defect
   (c) Ventricular septal defect
   (d) Coronary - right ventricular fistula
   (e) Gerbode (atrioventricular septal) defect

Ans. (e)

5. **Based on preceding information including Figure 218.1 and assuming systolic blood pressure of 120 mm Hg, indicate the correct implication.**
   (a) Systolic right ventricular pressure is 18 mm Hg
   (b) Systolic pulmonary artery pressure is 102 mm Hg
   (c) Mean left ventricular-left atrial gradient is 18 mm Hg
   (d) Mean right ventricular-right atrial gradient is 18 mm Hg
   (e) None of the above
   (**LV - RA gradient 102 mm Hg, RAP 18 mm Hg)

Ans. (e)

Atrioventricular (Gerbode) Defect in a Mildly Symptomatic Adult

The Gerbode defect is a type of intracardiac left-to-right shunt lesion. The diagnosis is based on demonstrating

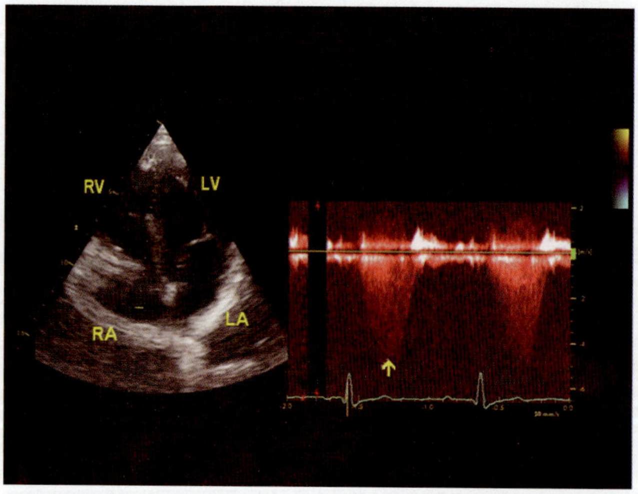

Fig. 218.1: Continuous wave Doppler sampled along the right side of cardiac septum, apical 4-chamber view. (LA: Left atrium; LV: Left ventricle; RA: Right atrium; RV: Right ventricle).

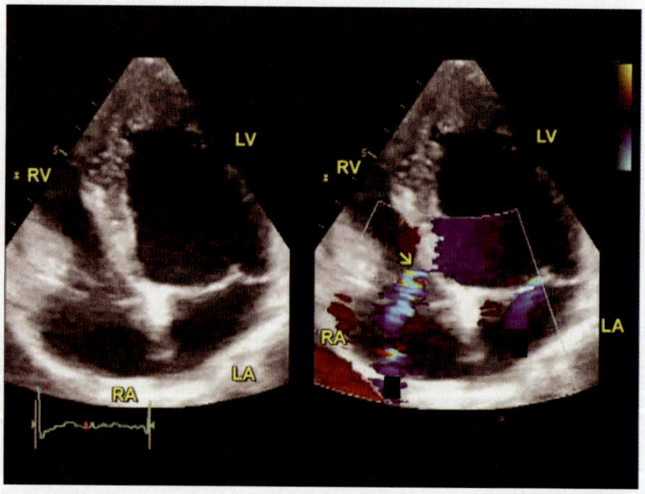

Fig. 218.2: Abnormal color Doppler finding, apical 4-chamber view. (LA: Left atrium; LV: Left ventricle; RA: Right atrium; RV: Right ventricle).

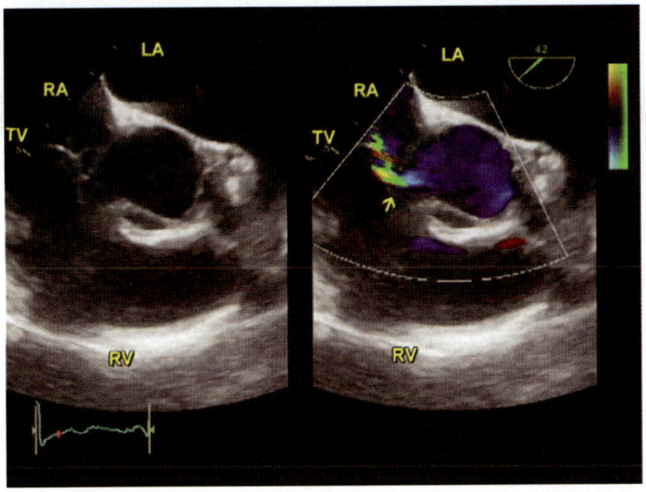

Fig. 218.3: Abnormal flow (arrow) in transesophageal study. (LA: Left atrium; LV: Left ventricle; RA: Right atrium; RV: Right ventricle; TV: Tricuspid valve).

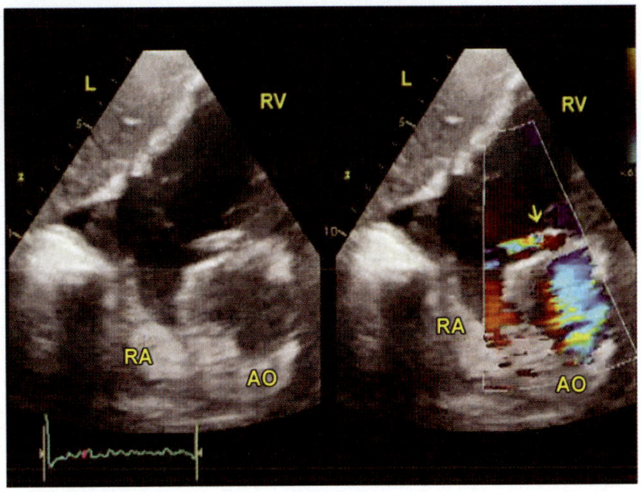

Fig. 218.4: Abnormal flow (arrow) seen in the subcostal view. (AO: Aorta; RA: Right atrium; RV: Right ventricle).

communication between the left ventricular and left atrial cavity. The defect is usually small, a few millimeters in diameter. The main imaging features include right atrial enlargement due to high-velocity blood shunt from the left ventricular to right atrial cavity.

This type of shunt lesion involves two main types of the pathology - direct atrioventricular septal defect (consistent with current definition of Gerbode defect) and indirect lesion—where the abnormal flow passes between the ventricles and further to the right atrium across basal perforations of septal tricuspid leaflet. The lesion may be acquired (e.g. after cardiac surgery, chest trauma or endocarditis[1,2]) or congenital, which is an uncommon congenital heart disease variety first described by Buhl in 1857. In the fifties, first successful surgical closures were reported[3] and the lesion was classified according to the first series of cases published by American surgeon, Frank Leven Albert Gerbode in 1958.[4] Estimated prevalence is around 1–2% among all types of ventricular septal defects undergoing surgery.[5]

Besides echocardiography, phase-contrast MRI is useful for localization of the shunt flow as well as its quantification (shunt volume and fraction). This is useful because precise imaging of atrioventricular septum, even using three-dimensional echocardiography is challenging due to proximity of tricuspid valve and its apparatus. Principal shunt visualization in four-chamber view (atrioventricular septum rather than outflow membranous septum) between the atrioventricular valves annuluses may support proper diagnosis. However, careful transthoracic and transesophageal imaging is usually sufficient for proper diagnosis as shown in our case. The main differential diagnoses are ventricular septal defect and tricuspid regurgitation. Treatment is surgical, usually with patch plasty; percutaneous closure is an alternative in select cases.

Right arrowhead in 710 points to MR.

MOVIES 709 TO 711

REFERENCES

1. Wasserman SM, Fann JI, Atwood JE, et al. Acquired left ventricular-right atrial communication: Gerbode-type defect. Echocardiography. 2002;19:67-72.
2. Battin M, Monro JL, Fong LV. Gerbode ventricular septal defect following endocarditis. Eur J Cardiothorac Surg. 1991;5(11):613-4.
3. Kirby CK, Johnson JJ, Zinsser HF. Successful closure of a left ventricular-right atrial shunt. Ann Surg. 1957;145:392.
4. Gerbode F, Hultgren H, Melrose D, et al. Syndrome of left ventricular-right atrial shunt: successful surgical repair of defect in five cases with observation of bradycardia on closure. Ann Surg. 1958;148:433-6.
5. Kelle AM, Young L, Kaushal S, et al. The Gerbode defect: the significance of a left ventricular to right atrial shunt. Cardiol Young. 2009; Suppl 2:96-9.

CASE 219

Ahmed MI, Gok G, Yuzbas B, Burkhart J, Escañuela MGA, Alli OO, Nanda NC

The patient was a 76-year-old male with progressive exertional dyspnea which developed 2 years ago. A restrictive VSD was found when he was a young man. A grade IV/VI holosystolic murmur and a soft diastolic murmur were noted in the left parasternal region during the current examination. There was no continuous murmur. Electrocardiogram was notable for atrial fibrillation, with a ventricular rate of 83, right axis deviation, and T-wave inversions in V1 and V2.

2D TTE was performed which initially demonstrated a turbulent color jet moving into the RV from the region of the AO-LV junction. A more meticulous examination showed two overlapping jets originating very close to each other which could be clearly separated by frame by frame examination of two-dimensional color Doppler images. Using color Doppler-guided continuous wave Doppler, one jet was noted to be continuous throughout systole and diastole consistent with sinus of Valsalva (SV) rupture into

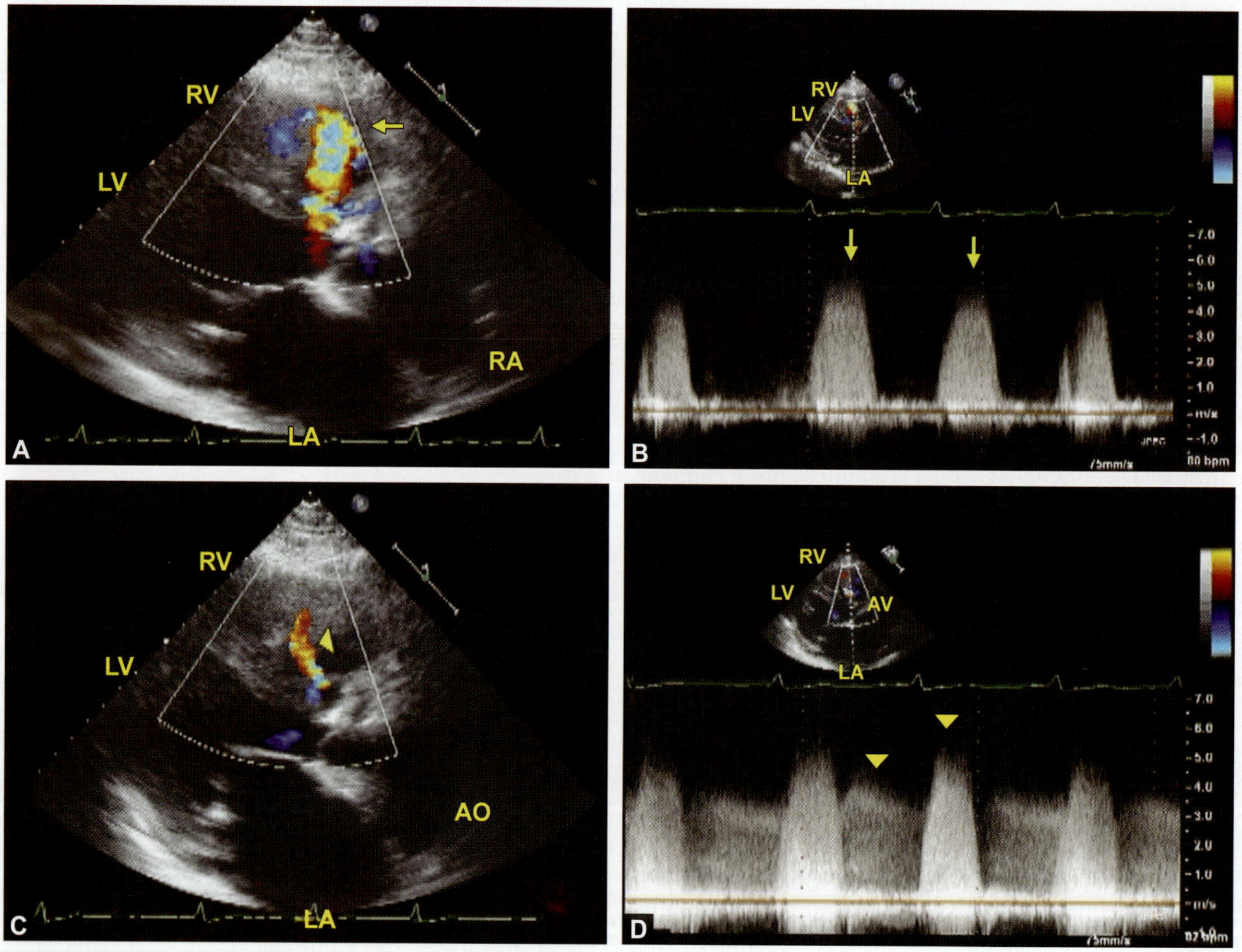

Figs. 219.1A to D: Two-dimensional transthoracic echocardiography. (A-D) Parasternal long axis views. (A,B) Color Doppler-guided continuous wave examination shows flow signals only in systole consistent with a ventricular septal defect (arrow). (C,D) Color Doppler-guided continuous wave examination shows flow signals throughout the cardiac cycle consistent with ruptured right sinus of Valsalva (arrowhead).

the RV, while the other was present only in systole consistent with a VSD, which was perimembranous in type (Figs. 219.1A to D, 712A to D). No aneurysm of right SV was found.

Percutaneous closure of the ruptured SV was attempted with a 4 mm Amplatzer septal occluder device under 3D TEE guidance. 2D and 3D TEE performed in the cardiac catheterization laboratory immediately after closure showed the occluder device in place with residual flow through the right SV into the RV but none through the VSD, most likely due to compression by the device occluder.

Rupture of a sinus of Valsalva without aneurysm formation (also known as sinus of Valsalva fistula or communication) and without any acquired trauma, infection, or degenerative disease is very rare. When SV rupture and VSD co-exist, especially when the VSD is an adjacent perimembranous type, the diagnosis may become very difficult by 2D TTE because the two jets may overlap as was noted in our patient. Only frame by frame viewing of the 2D color images and careful interrogation by continuous wave Doppler resulted in the correct diagnosis. We were able to delineate two different patterns of flow by continuous wave Doppler in practically the same location. One showed high velocity flow signals confined only to systole indicative of a VSD and the other demonstrated high velocity flow throughout the cardiac cycle pointing to a ruptured SV. Absence of low velocity diastolic flow signals through the VSD may suggest that the RV diastolic pressure was as high as the LV diastolic pressure presumably from rupture of the SV into the RV and this prevented left to right diastolic shunting into the RV. Despite the Doppler findings, a continuous murmur was not heard on clinical examination. The reason for this is not clear but it is possible the loud VSD murmur masked it to some extent.

MOVIE LEGENDS

712A and B: show flow signals from both VSD (arrow) and ruptured SV (arrowhead) which are overlapping and hence difficult to differentiate by both two-dimensional transthoracic (712A) and transesophageal echocardiography (712B).

712C: shows high velocity VSD flow practically confined to systole.

712D: shows continuous high velocity flow throughout the cardiac cycle from SV rupture. (AO: Aorta; AV: Aortic valve; LA: Left atrium; LV: Left ventricle; RA: Right atrium; RV: Right ventricle).

This case is reproduced with permission from Echocardiography. Ahmed MI, Gok G, Yuzbas B, Burkhart J, Amado Escañuela MG, Alli OO, et al. Incremental value of three-dimensional echocardiography over the two-dimensional technique in the assessment of combined sinus of valsalva rupture into the right ventricle and adjacent perimembranous ventricular septal defect. Echocardiography. 2014 Jul;31(6):779-82. PubMed PMID: 24931316.

CASE 220

Bulur S, Turaga NSN, Kalla A, Elsayed M, Alagic N, Uygur B, Chahwala JR, Adarna LG, Nanda NC

An 11-year-old female was referred to our institution for an evaluation of palpitations and chest pain. Physical examination revealed normal heart rate of 84 bpm with a blood pressure of 100/70 mm Hg; on cardiac auscultation, she was in regular rate and rhythm and no gallops or murmurs were heard. A 2D TTE showed normal biventricular function and size, normal left atrial size, and normal aortic diameter.

1. What is the diagnosis? (Figs. 220.1 to 220.4 and 713 to 716):

(a) Severe PR
(b) Aortopulmonary window
(c) Anomalous coronary artery arising from PA
(d) Patent ductus arteriosus (PDA)

Ans. (d)

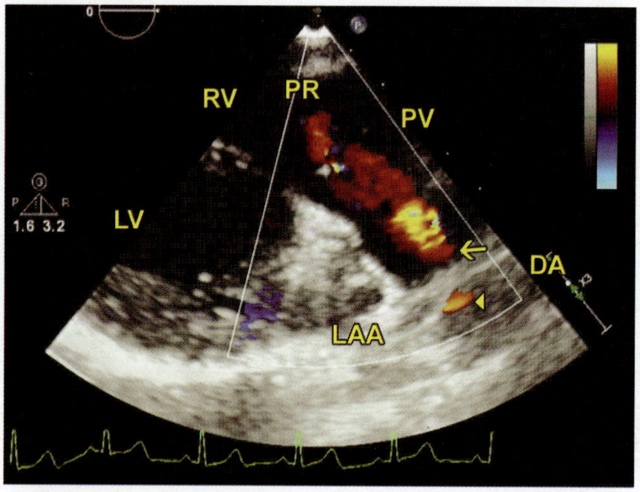

Fig. 220.1: LV-pulmonic plane. Arrow points to PDA.

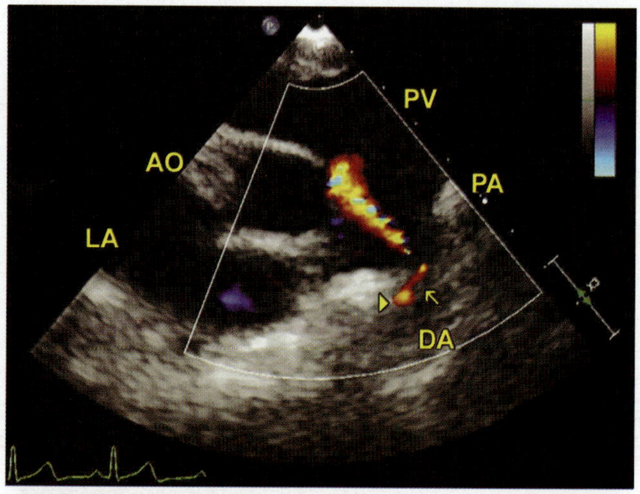

Fig. 220.2: LV-pulmonic plane. Complete length of the PDA (arrow) is visualized and measures 0.3 cm. Arrowhead points to flow acceleration in the thoracic descending aorta (DA).

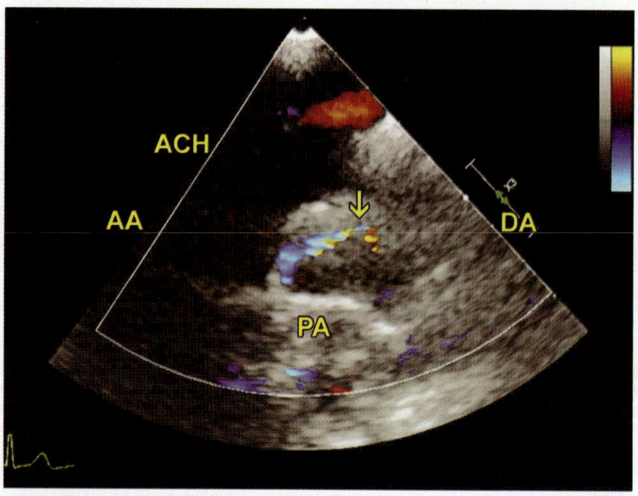

Fig. 220.3: Suprasternal examination. Arrow points to PDA flow signals moving into the pulmonary artery (PA).

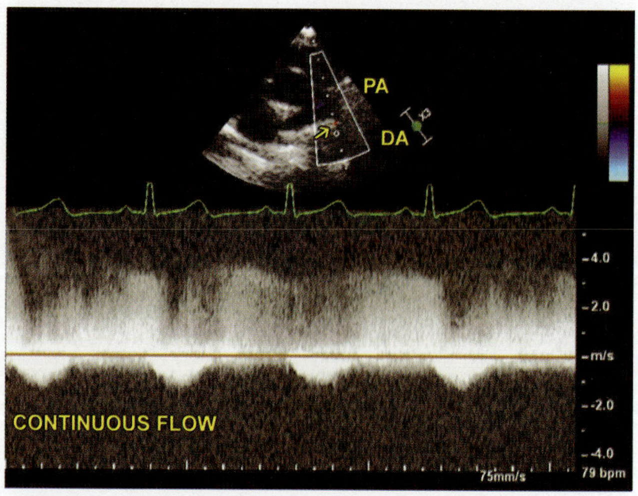

Fig. 220.4: Continuous wave Doppler shows high velocity signals throughout the cardiac cycle typical of PDA.

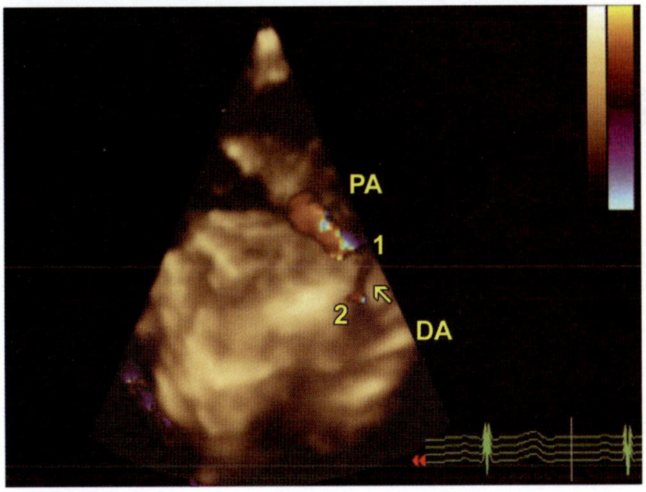

Fig. 220.5: 3DTTE. 1 and 2 represent the pulmonary and aortic connections of the PDA.

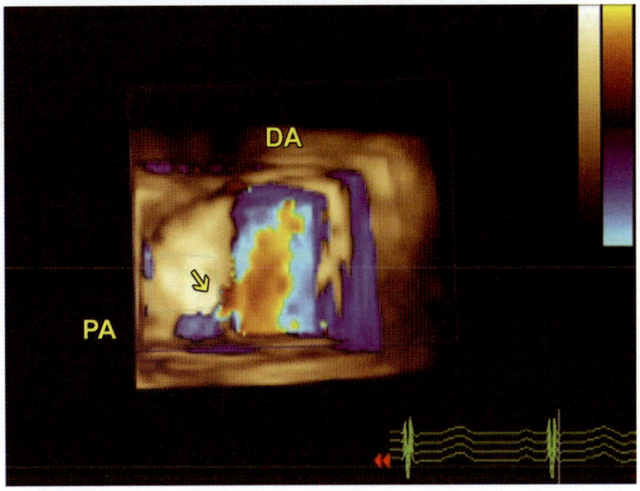

Fig. 220.6: 3DTTE. Visualization of PDA (arrow) by cropping from the top.

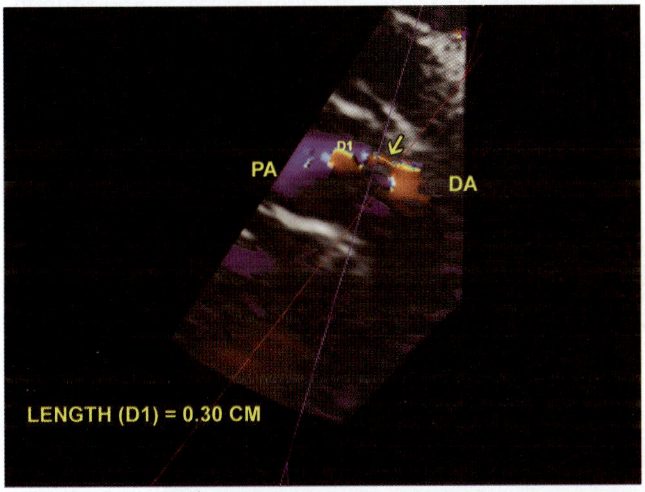

Fig. 220.7: 3DTTE. The length of the PDA (arrow) is 0.3 cm.

The arrow points to a jet arising from the DA and moving into the main PA typical of PDA. CW Doppler shows flow signals continuous throughout the cardiac cycle, also a finding in PDA. Arrowhead points to flow acceleration in DA. Mild PR is also noted.

2. **Which of the following views is/are not useful in detecting a PDA?**
   (a) AO short axis view
   (b) LV-PV plane
   (c) Suprasternal view
   (d) MV-PV plane
   (e) High left parasternal short-axis view
   (f) Subcostal RA-RV-apex-PA plane view
   (g) Right parasternal views

Ans. (g)

3. **What incremental value is provided by 3D TTE? Find the incorrect statement. (Figs. 220.5 to 220.7 and 717 to 720):**
   (a) No incremental value was provided
   (b) The entire length of PDA was well visualized by 3D TTE (denoted by #1 and #2 and arrow in Fig. 220.5) and measured 0.3 cm (Fig. 220.7) same as 2D TTE (Fig. 220.2).
   (c) Both the AO and PA ends of PDA can be visualized en face and measured only by 3D TTE.
   (d) Both (b) and (c) are useful when assessing the patient for percutaneous PDA closure.

Ans. (a)

The parents of the patient were told that the PDA was very small and it was decided not to close it.

MOVIES 713 TO 720

CASE 221

Murzilli Romina, Leo Laura Anna, Faletra Francesco

A 76-year-old female patient was admitted to our hospital complaining of dyspnea on exertion for the last 3 months (NYHA III). The patient had permanent atrial fibrillation (Average HR = 85 beats per minute). Blood pressure, respiratory rate, and breath sounds were normal, $SpO_2 = 96\%$ ($FiO_2 = 0.21$).

Transthoracic echocardiography (TTE) was performed.

1. **What do arrows show in TTE (Figs. 221.1A and B)?**
   (a) Pericardial effusion
   (b) Descending aorta aneurysm
   (c) Persistent left superior vena cava
   (d) Giant coronary sinus
   (e) Coronary anomaly

Ans. (e)

The patient has a coronary arteriovenous fistula (CAVF). Figures 221.1 and 221.2 and 🎥 721A and B show an aneurysmal dilatation (Aneu) of right coronary artery draining to coronary sinus (CS). Coronary computed tomography angiography (CCTA) confirms the diagnosis of coronary arteriovenous fistula showing an ectatic right coronary artery (RCA) with a distal saccular aneurysmal dilatation along the posterior interventricular sulcus draining to CS (arrow) (Fig. 221.3).

CAVF is a rare anomaly which consists of abnormal communication between a coronary artery and one of the cardiac chambers or vessels adjacent to the heart. CAVFs are present in 0.002% of the general population and are visualized in nearly 0.25% of patients undergoing catheterization.[1-5] Origin of the CAVF can be any of the three major coronary arteries. The majority of these fistulas arise from the right coronary arteries or the left anterior descending; the circumflex coronary artery is rarely involved. These fistulae most often drain into the right ventricle (41%), or into the right atrium (26%), pulmonary artery (17%), CS (7%), left atrium (5%), left ventricle (3%), or superior vena cava (1%). Congenital RCA–CS fistulae are uncommon.[1,4-6] Coronary angiography remains the most common method for detection of coronary fistulae. The diagnosis is also possible with CCTA and cardiac magnetic resonance. A markedly enlarged coronary artery can usually be detected also with echocardiography.

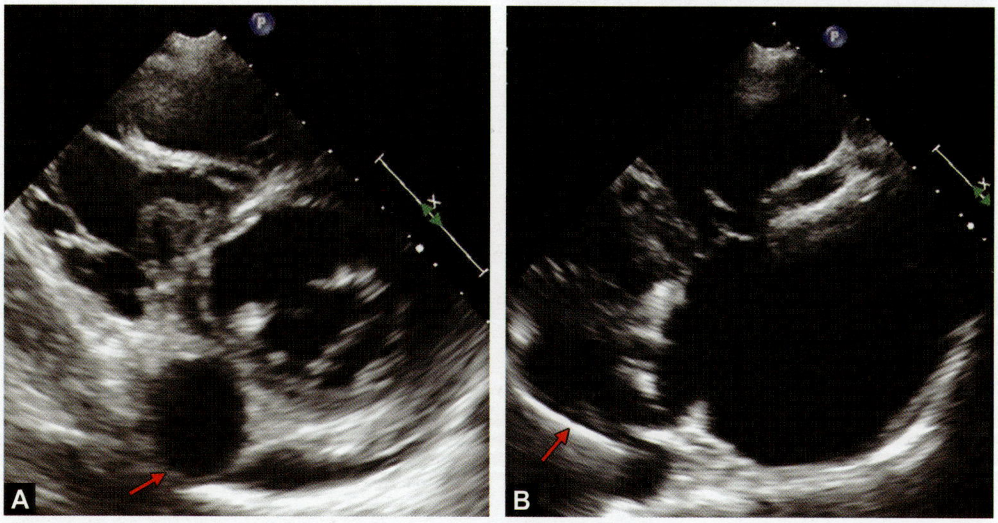

Figs. 221.1A and B: Transthoracic echocardiography. Parasternal short-axis view (A) and right ventricle inflow view (B).

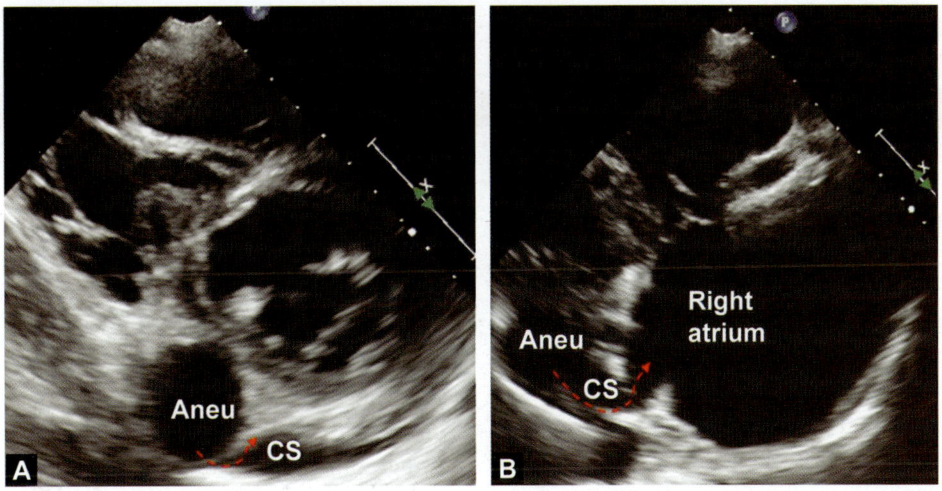

Figs. 221.2A and B: Transthoracic echocardiography. Parasternal short-axis view (A) and right ventricle inflow view (B) show a distal saccular aneurysmal dilatation (Aneu, A) of right coronary artery draining to coronary sinus (CS) (arrow).

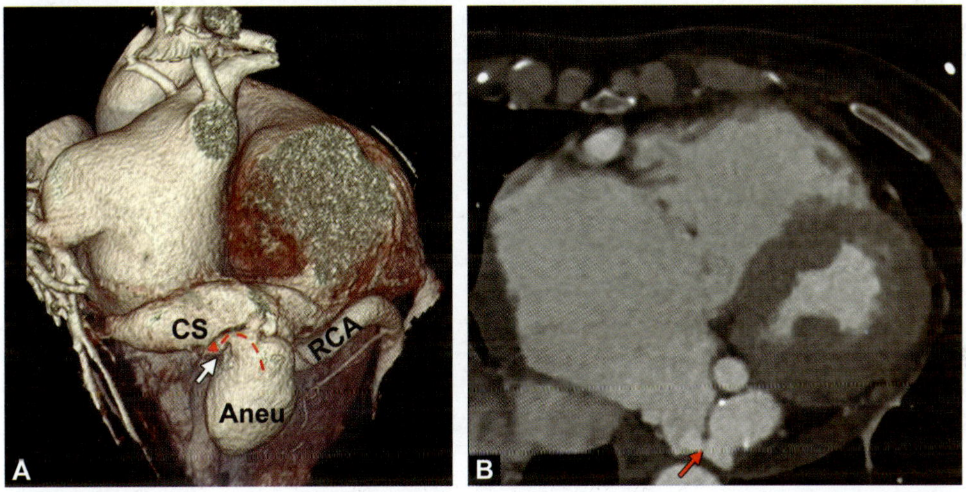

Figs. 221.3A and B: Coronary computed tomography angiography (CCTA). Volume-rendering image (A) and multiplanar reconstruction image (B) show an ectatic right coronary artery (RCA) with a distal saccular aneurysmal dilatation (Aneu) along the posterior interventricular sulcus draining to coronary sinus (CS) (arrow).

MOVIE LEGENDS

721A and B: Transthoracic echocardiography. Parasternal short-axis view (A) and right ventricle inflow view (B) show a distal saccular aneurysmal dilatation (Aneu, A) of right coronary artery draining to coronary sinus (CS) (arrow).

REFERENCES

1. Fernandes ED, Kadivar H, Hallman GL, Reul GJ, Ott DA, Cooley DA. Congenital malformations of the coronary arteries: the Texas Heart Institute experience. Ann Thorac Surg. 1992;54:732-40.
2. Olearchyk AS, Runk DM, Alavi M, Grosso MA. Congenital bilateral coronary-to-pulmonary artery fistulas. Ann Thorac Surg. 1997;64:233-35.
3. Urrutia-S CO, Falaschi G, Ott DA, Cooley DA. Surgical management of 56 patients with congenital coronary artery fistulas. Ann Thorac Surg. 1983;35:300-07.
4. Dodge-Khatami A, Mavroudis C, Backer CL. Congenital heart surgery nomenclature and database project: anomalies of the coronary arteries. Ann Thorac Surg. 2000;69:270-97.
5. Gowda RM, Vasavada BC, Khan IA. Coronary artery fistulas: clinical and therapeutic considerations. Int J Cardiol. 2006;107:7-10.
6. Levin DC, Fellows KE, Abrams HL. Hemodynamically significant primary anomalies of the coronary arteries. Angiographic aspects. Circulation. 1978;58:25-34.

CASE 222

Tao Yu Lee, Shoa-Lin Lin

ECHOCARDIOGRAPHIC DIAGNOSIS OF CORONARY ARTERY FISTULA

A congenital coronary artery fistula is an uncommon cardiac anomaly. The diagnosis of coronary artery fistula has been made in the past by cardiac catheterization. With recent advances in echocardiography, coronary artery fistula can be imaged noninvasively using two-dimensional transthoracic echocardiography (TTE). However, direct visualization of the entire coronary artery fistula from the precordium can be difficult. This report describes a patient with coronary artery fistula that was clearly diagnosed by multiplane transesophageal echocardiography (TEE) before cardiac catheterization.

The patient was a 23-year-old male student. He began having intermittent chest pain 2 months ago. The pain used to last for a few minutes at a time but became more frequent over the past 2 weeks. He sought medical attention and was referred to us. Physical examination at admission was essentially negative except for a grade 3/4 diastolic murmur over the apex with extension to left sternal border. Biochemistry data were all within normal limits. The electrocardiogram and maximal treadmill exercise test were both negative. 2D TTE was done and showed an abnormal diastolic blood flow draining into the LV cavity (Figs. 222.1, 222.2, 722 and 723). Multiplane TEE was next done and found a coronary artery fistula which arose from the right coronary artery and drained into the left ventricle (Figs. 222.3, 222.4A and B, 724 and 725). The whole outline of this tortuous and dilated right coronary artery fistula was also delineated on computed tomographic (CT) angiograms (Fig. 222.5). Cardiac catheterization confirmed the multiplane TEE findings (Fig. 222.6, 726 to 728). Surgical view of the fistula is shown in Figure 222.7. Thus, a carefully done multiplane TEE may be useful in the diagnosis of coronary artery fistulas. Arrows in figures and movie clips point to the dilated and tortuous fistula.

1. **A congenital coronary artery fistula is rare. Among unilateral coronary artery fistulas, approximately what percentage originate from the right coronary artery?**
   (a) 40%
   (b) 30%
   (c) 20%
   (d) <10%

Ans. (b)

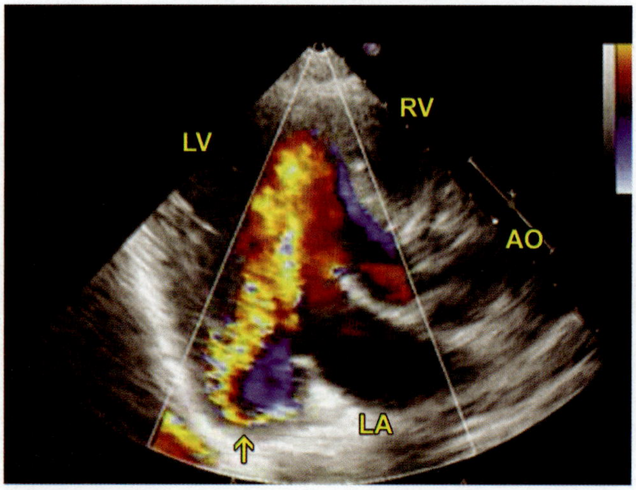

Fig. 222.1: TTE. A mosaic jet (arrow) from the posterior wall of the LV draining into LV was noted.

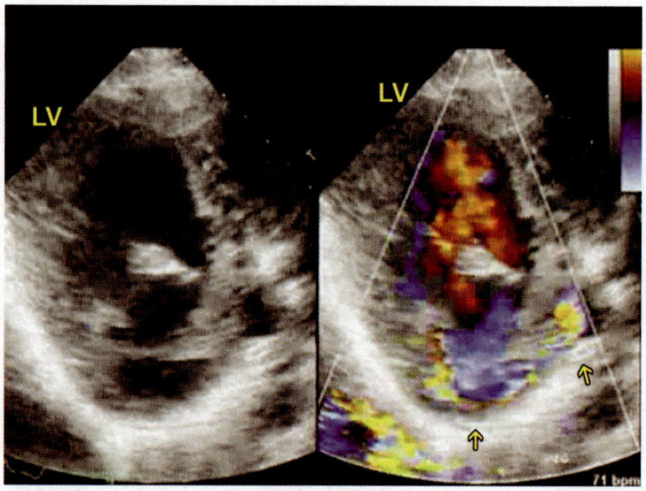

Fig. 222.2: TTE. A mosaic jet (arrows) from the basal posterior wall of the LV draining into LV cavity was noted.

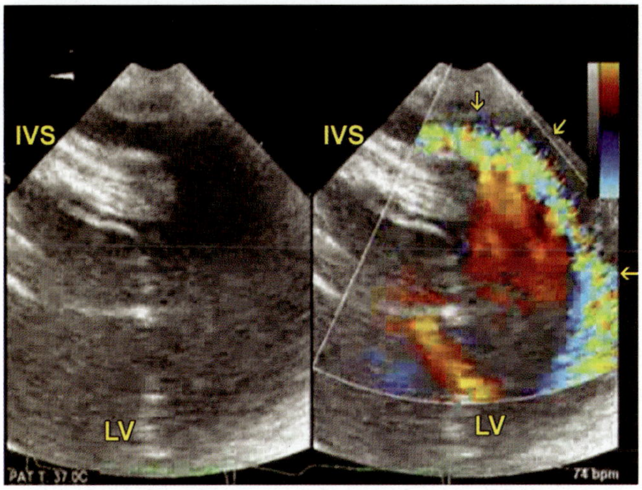

Fig. 222.3: Multiplane TEE with (right) and without (left) color flow images. A curved and dilated (diameter >1 cm) coronary artery fistula adjacent to the RA and AO was seen. Cut sections of the fistula (arrows) are shown. This curved coronary artery fistula encircled a round-shaped vessel, which eventually was found to be a part of the same coronary artery fistula.

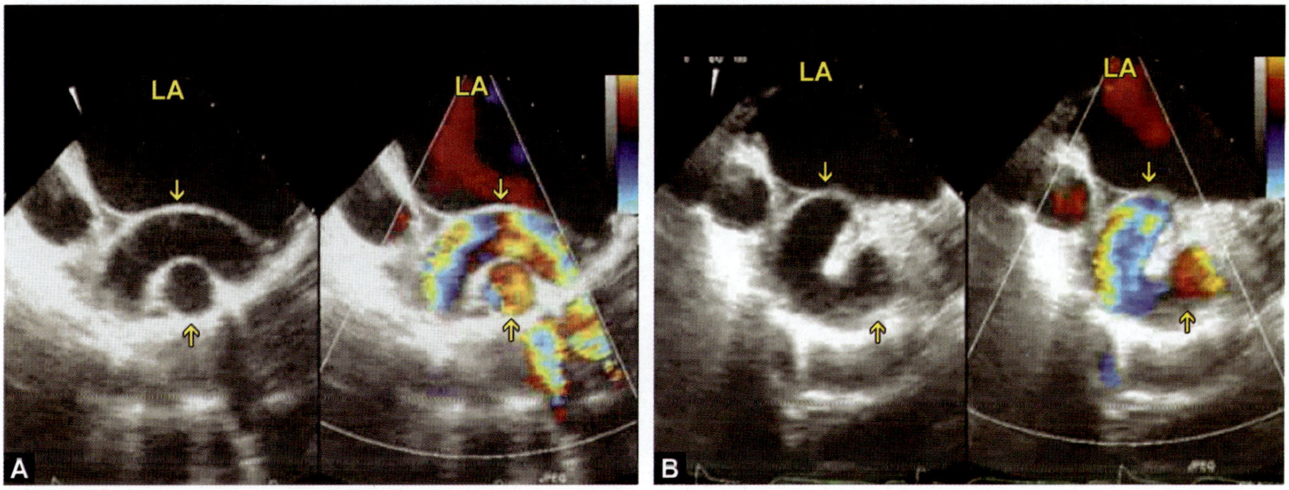

Figs. 222.4A and B: Multiplane TEE with (right) and without (left) color flow images. A curved and dilated (diameter > 1cm) coronary artery fistula adjacent to the RA and AO was seen. Cut sections of the fistula (arrows) are shown. This curved coronary artery fistula encircled a round-shaped vessel, which eventually was found to be a part of the same coronary artery fistula.

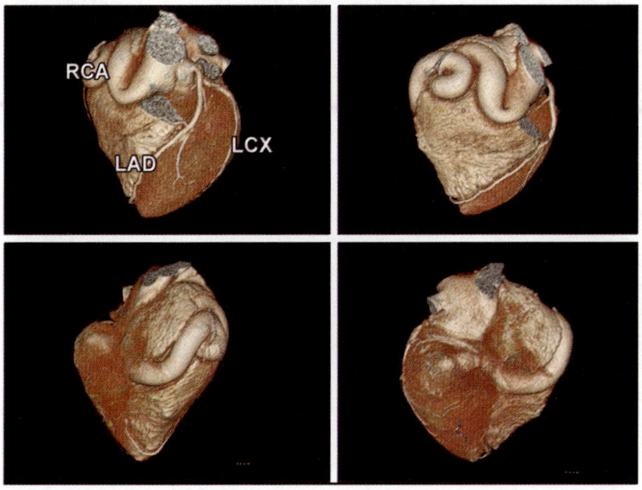

Fig. 222.5: Computed tomographic angiogram showing the tortuous and dilated right coronary artery fistula.

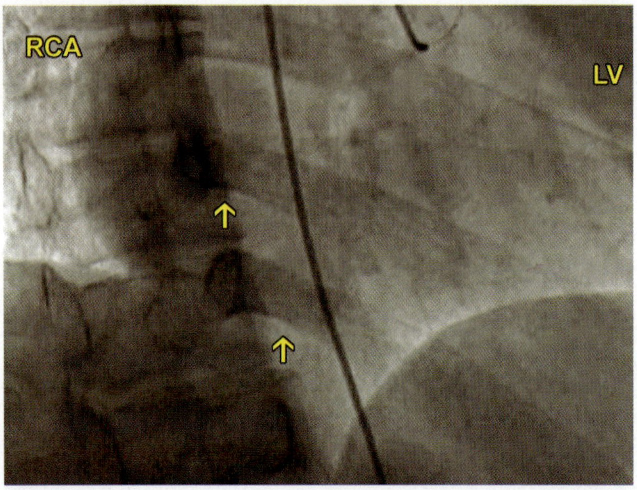

Fig. 222.6: Right coronary angiogram showing the tortuous and dilated right coronary artery fistula (arrows) draining into the LV.

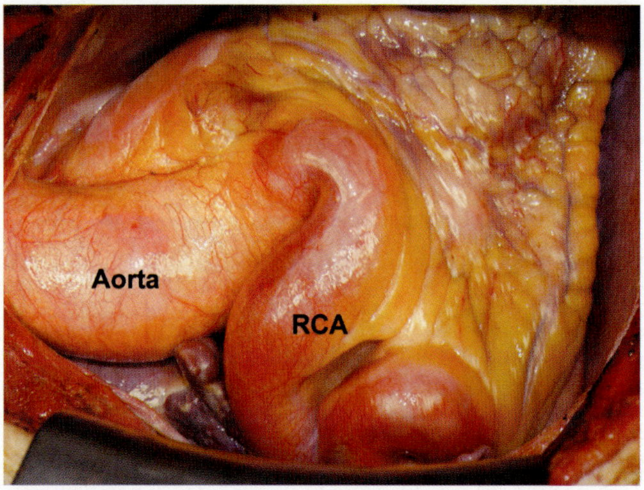

Fig. 222.7: Surgical view. The tortuous and dilated right coronary artery (RCA) fistula can be seen.

Comment: Among unilateral fistulas, LAD was the origin in 42% followed by RCA (31%), Cx (20%) and finally the left main trunk (7%). [*Source*: Page 272 of the review article: World J Cardiol 2011; 3(8): 267-277].

MOVIE LEGENDS

722 and 723: TTE. A mosaic jet (arrow) from the posterior wall of the LV draining into LV was noted.

724 and 725: Multiplane TEE with (right) and without (left) color flow images at 0, 64 and 180 degrees. A curved and dilated (diameter > 1 cm) coronary artery fistula adjacent to the RA and AO was seen. Cut sections of the fistula (arrows) are shown. This curved coronary artery fistula encircled a round shaped vessel, which eventually was found to be a part of the same coronary artery fistula.

726: Right coronary angiogram showing the tortuous and dilated right coronary artery fistula (arrows) draining into the LV.

727: The catheter was advanced in the mid portion of the fistula.

728: The catheter was advanced into the distal portion of the fistula and shows the contrast agent promptly draining into the left ventricle.

CASE 223

Jose Ricardo FP, Kishan Jasti, Robert WW Biederman, Rachel Hughes-Doichev

An 85-year-old Caucasian man with longstanding history of hypertension was transferred from an outside hospital for surgical evaluation of newly diagnosed severe mitral regurgitation. He presented initially with complaints of dyspnea and lower extremity swelling. Physical exam at presentation showed heart rate of 76 bpm, blood pressure 210/108 mm Hg, mild jugular venous distension, normally split S2, S4, and a soft diastolic murmur at the left sternal border with the patient leaning forward on expiration. Prior to transfer, a transthoracic echocardiogram (TTE) showed mildly dilated left ventricle with normal systolic function, normal right ventricle size and systolic function, and abnormal diastolic function (pseudonormal pattern), normal-sized left atrium, and what appeared to be moderate mitral regurgitation with a very eccentric jet (729).

Transesophageal echocardiogram showed abnormal systolic flow into the medial aspect of the left atrium (Figs. 223.2 to 223.4 and 730). There was no flow seen across the atrial septum via Doppler or agitated saline injection. Incidental findings were a bicuspid aortic valve with no significant stenosis but moderate eccentric aortic regurgitation and a small-moderate-sized circumferential pericardial effusion. After diuresis equivalent to a 10-pound weight loss, right heart catheterization showed mildly elevated pulmonary artery pressure (mean 30 mm Hg) and absence of oxygen saturation step-up between the right atrium and right ventricle or pulmonary artery. Left heart catheterization showed mild coronary artery disease.

1. **Based on the transthoracic echocardiogram which of the following is the most likely explanation for the abnormal systolic flow in the left atrium? (See Fig. 223.1 and 730)**
   (a) Eccentric mitral regurgitation.
   (b) Coronary sinus fistula.
   (c) Coronary artery to left atrium fistula.
   (d) Secundum atrial septal defect.

Ans. (b)

Coronary sinus fistula. The systolic jet was mistaken for mitral regurgitation on TTE at the referring hospital, but it is clear that the jet is arising from the medial aspect of the atrium and not from the mitral valve. Flow from a coronary

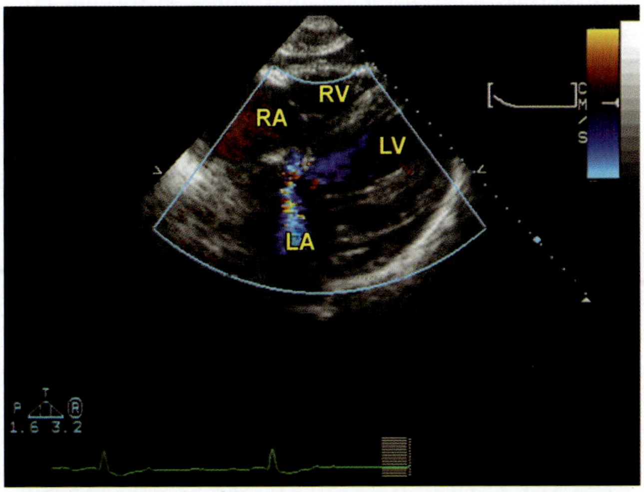

Fig. 223.1: Color Doppler flow image in transthoracic subcostal view revealing a jet that mimics mitral regurgitation. This jet actually represents the right to left shunt between the coronary sinus and left atrium.

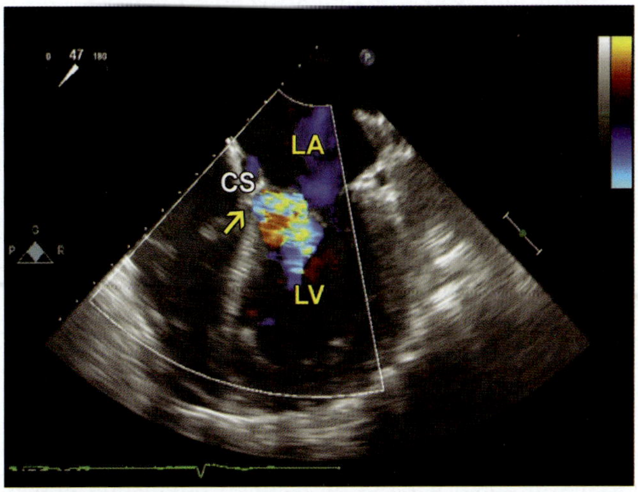

Fig. 223.2: Transesophageal four-chamber view demonstrating a fistulous connection (arrow) between the coronary sinus and left atrium. (CS: Coronary sinus; LA: Left atrium; LV: Left ventricle).

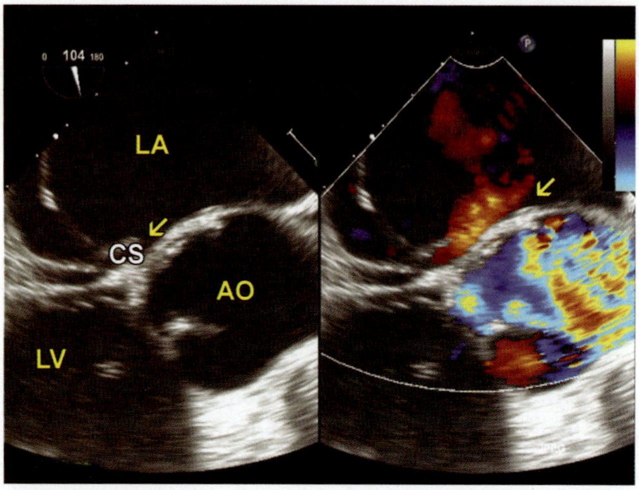

Fig. 223.3: Mid-esophageal aortic long axis view at 104° demonstrating a distinct channel (arrow) which lies adjacent to the junction between the mitral annulus and aortic root. (AO: Aorta; CS: Coronary sinus; LA: Left atrium; LV: Left ventricle).

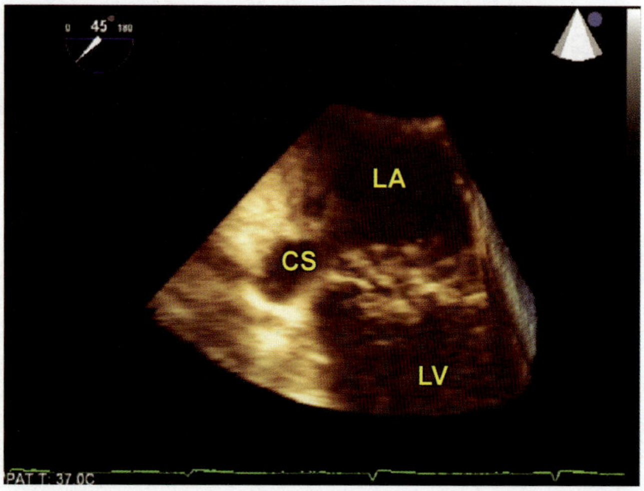

Fig. 223.4: A cropped three-dimensional transesophageal four chamber view showing the opening of the coronary sinus fistula into the left atrium. (CS: Coronary sinus; LA: Left atrium; LV: Left ventricle).

artery to atrial fistula, one type of cameral fistula, would be seen during diastole and not systole and would be seen on coronary angiography. A secundum atrial septal defect would more commonly present as a left to right shunt in the absence of significant pulmonary hypertension and would be demonstrated by agitated saline injection.

2. **Which is the least likely cause of a dilated coronary sinus?**
   (a) Recurrent pulmonary embolism
   (b) Anomalous pulmonary venous drainage
   (c) Right ventricular infarction
   (d) Persistent left superior vena cava
   (e) Aortic stenosis

Ans. (e)

An enlarged coronary sinus results from increased pressure or volume load in the right side of the heart which may occur in choices (a) to (d). Both recurrent pulmonary embolism and right ventricular infarction may cause increased right heart pressures. Both anomalous pulmonary venous drainage and persistent left superior vena cava may cause increased flow through the coronary sinus. Persistent left superior vena cava is the most common cause in patient without shunts. It occurs in about 0.5% of the general population and in 3 to 10% of patients with congenital heart disease.[1]

3. **How is a persistent left superior vena cava (SVC) usually diagnosed by echocardiography?**
   (a) Intravenous bolus injection of microspheres (ultrasound contrast agent).
   (b) Intravenous infusion of microspheres (ultrasound contrast agent).
   (c) Intravenous injection of agitated saline in the right arm.
   (d) Intravenous injection of agitated saline in the left arm.
   (e) Doppler imaging of coronary sinus to estimate flow.

Ans. (d)

Intravenous injection of agitated saline in the left arm. With agitated saline contrast injection in a left arm vein, bubbles will appear in the dilated coronary sinus before the right atrium and right ventricle if there is a persistent left SVC. This is best observed in the parasternal long axis view. Subsequent injection of agitated saline in the right arm will show opacification of the right atrium without appearance of bubbles in the coronary sinus. Use of lipid microspheres is approved only for use in patients with suboptimal echocardiograms to opacify the left ventricle and to improve the delineation of the left ventricular endocardial borders. It should not be used in patients with known or suspected right-to-left, bi-directional, or transient right-to-left cardiac shunts. This type of contrast agent can be administered by either continuous IV infusion or bolus, depending on the specific agent used. Doppler imaging of the coronary sinus is difficult because the coronary sinus is perpendicular to the transducer on the standard parasternal and apical 4-chamber view. It demonstrates flow but may not be reliable in determining the presence of a persistent left SVC.

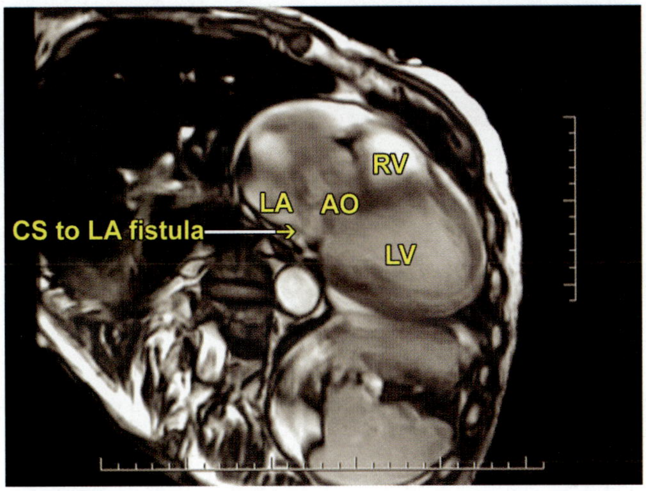

Fig. 223.5: Cardiac MRI revealing the fistulous communication between the left atrium and the coronary sinus. (AO: Aorta; CS: Coronary sinus; LA: Left atrium; LV: Left ventricle).

DISCUSSION

Cardiac MRI (Fig. 223.5) revealed a series of tributaries from the coronary sinus that entered the posterior left atrial wall and opened into the left atrium adjacent to the junction of the interatrial septum and the aorta. There was no evidence of persistent left superior vena cava or atrial septal defects.

Enlargement of the coronary sinus is one of four classification groups of coronary sinus anomalies. Mantini's classification, originally described in 1966, groups coronary sinus anomalies into four anatomic groups on the basis of: (1) enlargement of coronary sinus, (2) absence of coronary sinus, (3) atresia of the right atrial coronary sinus ostium and (4) hypoplasia of the coronary sinus.[2]

Patients with an enlarged coronary sinus may be further divided into two groups based on the absence or presence of a left to right shunt into the coronary sinus. Persistent left superior vena cava draining into the coronary sinus (right to right shunt) is the most common cause of enlarged coronary sinus among the group without any shunts. Anomalous communications between the left atrium (LA) or pulmonary venous system to the coronary sinus (low pressure shunts) or between the aorta and the coronary sinus (high pressure shunts) account for the left to right shunts into the coronary sinus.

Communication of the coronary sinus with the left atrium may be indirect through an anomalous channel which bridges the two structures[3] such as in our case or direct by way of an opening between the coronary sinus into the left atrial cavity as in unroofed coronary sinus[4,5] or left atrial-coronary sinus fenestration.[6]

In this patient, anomalous channels between the coronary sinus and left atrium were identified by cardiac MRI and predominantly showed a right to left shunt without significant hypoxemia or left atrial enlargement. This isolated defect appeared to have no functional significance and the patient's symptoms in this case were likely related to diastolic dysfunction from systemic hypertension.

Anomalies of the coronary sinus are rare but it is important to identify them as they are under recognized, can present as volume overload and may pose a challenge for electrophysiological procedures while navigating through the coronary sinus or during retrograde coronary sinus cardioplegia in open heart procedures and hence correct identification would limit further unnecessary diagnostic testing. The natural history of this under recognized defect remains unknown but with the advent of advanced imaging techniques, this defect will be more frequently observed.

MOVIE LEGENDS

729: Color Doppler flow in transthoracic subcostal view revealing a jet that mimics mitral regurgitation (arrow). This jet actually represents the right to left shunt between the coronary sinus and left atrium.

730: Transesophageal four-chamber view demonstrating a fistulous connection (arrow) between the coronary sinus and left atrium. CS, coronary sinus; LA, left atrium, LV left ventricle.

REFERENCES

1. Winter FS. Persistent left superior vena cava. Angiology. 1954;5:90-132.
2. Mantini E, Grondin CM, Lillehei WC, et al. Congenital anomalies involving the coronary sinus. Circulation. 1966;33:317-327.
3. Neuser H, Kerber S, Schumacher B. Fistulous communication between coronary sinus and left atrium. Circulation. 2002;106:e137-e138.
4. Adatia I, Gittenberger-de Groot AC. Unroofed coronary sinus and coronary sinus orifice atresia. J Am Coll Cardiol. 1995;25:947-53.
5. Rowe RD, Freedom RM, Culham JA. Left atrial to coronary sinus fenestration (partially unroofed coronary sinus). Br Heart J. 1981;46:63-8
6. Nath PH, Delaney DJ, Zollikofer C, Ben-Sacher G, et al. Coronary sinus-left atrial window. Radiology. 1980;135: 319-22.

CASE 224

Shelley Sarson, Sanjiv J Shah, Jyothy John Puthumana

Clinical History

A 35-year-old female with a history of pulmonary sarcoidosis and asthma presented with chest pain and anemia. Chest pain was non-pleuritic and was intermittent for 3 months. No prior cardiac history was elicited. Physical examination was within normal limits. There were no rubs, murmurs, or gallops appreciated. There were no physical exam findings suggestive of left or right heart failure.

An echocardiogram was ordered.

Transthoracic Echocardiogram Findings (Figs. 224.1 to 224.6)

- Normal left ventricular size, systolic function, wall thickness, and wall motion. Normal tissue Doppler velocities with normal diastolic function. Calculated biplane LV ejection fraction was 60%.
- A prominent membrane was noted dividing the left atrium into two chambers (Figs. 224.1 to 224.4 and 731 to 735). Because of the unusual angle of the flow across the membrane, an accurate gradient could not be calculated.
- The interatrial septum bows from left to right, consistent with increased LA pressure.
- There is no evidence of right-to-left shunting by agitated saline bubble contrast study x 3 (at rest, with cough and with Valsalva maneuver).
- Peak TR jet velocity and estimated right ventricular systolic pressure were within normal limits.

Other unique findings on echo included diastolic fluttering of the anterior and posterior mitral valve leaflets (Fig. 224.6).

1. **What is the pathology? (Fig. 224.1 and 731)**
   (a) Mitral stenosis
   (b) LA myxoma
   (c) Cor triatriatum sinistrum
   (d) Eustachian valve in the left atrium

Ans. (c)

An extremely rare congenital anomaly where the left atrium is divided into two compartments by a membrane. The proximal chamber is the accessory LA and pulmonary venous chamber, while the chamber closest to the mitral valve is considered the true LA, which contains the interatrial septum.[2]

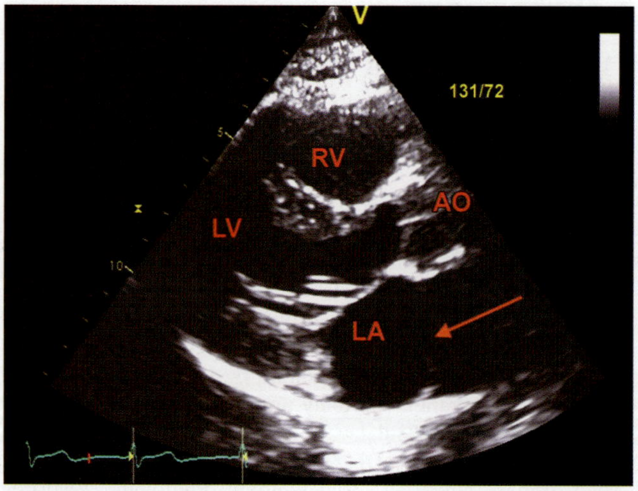

Fig. 224.1: Parasternal long-axis view demonstrating a membrane in the left atrium (arrow).

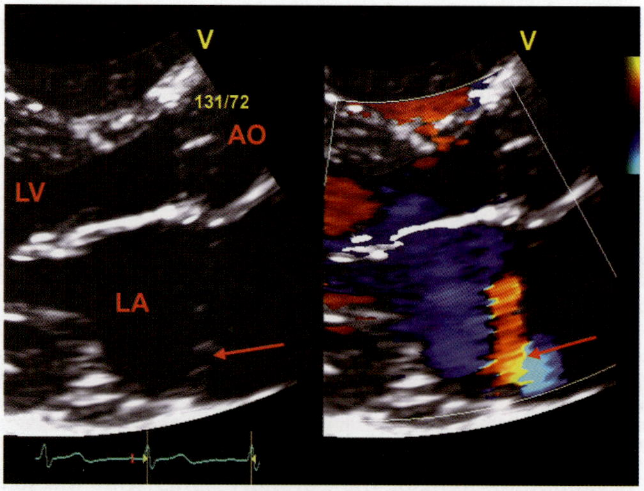

Fig. 224.2: Parasternal long-axis view with color flow Doppler showing turbulence at the location of the membrane (arrow).

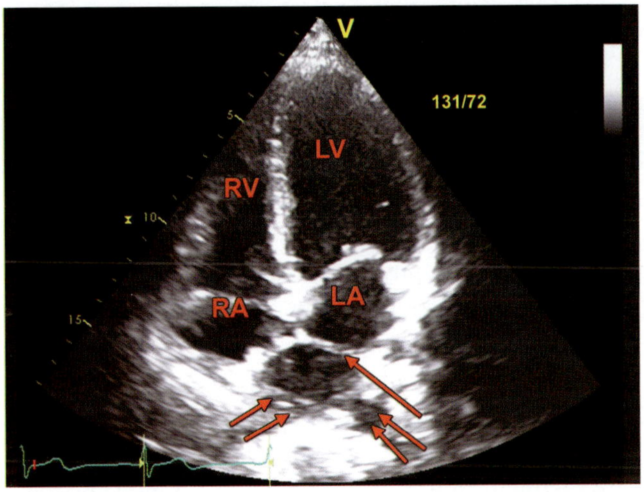

Fig. 224.3: Apical 4-chamber view showing the membrane dividing the left atrium into two chambers (arrow). Note the pulmonary veins draining into the proximal chamber (double arrow).

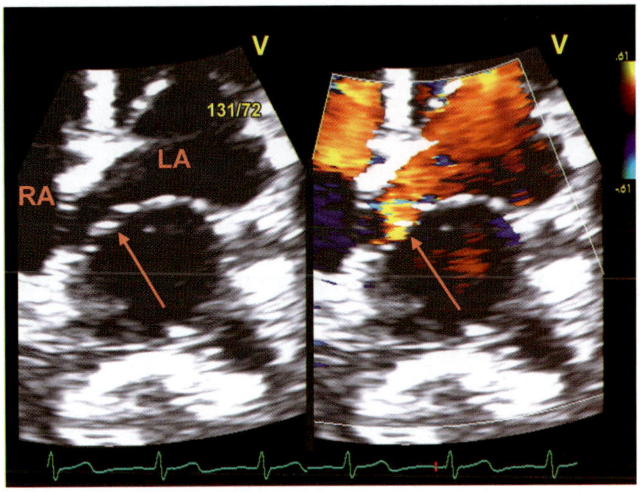

Fig. 224.4: Apical 4-chamber view of the membrane in the left atrium with color flow Doppler demonstrating flow across the membrane with some turbulence (arrow).

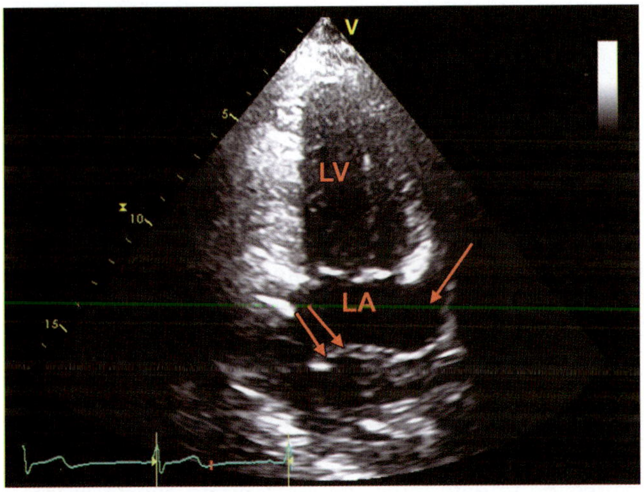

Fig. 224.5: Apical 2-chamber viewing demonstrating the left atrial appendage (arrow) arising from the lower chamber. This helps differentiate CTS from supravalvular mitral stenosis. Double arrow shows the membrane.

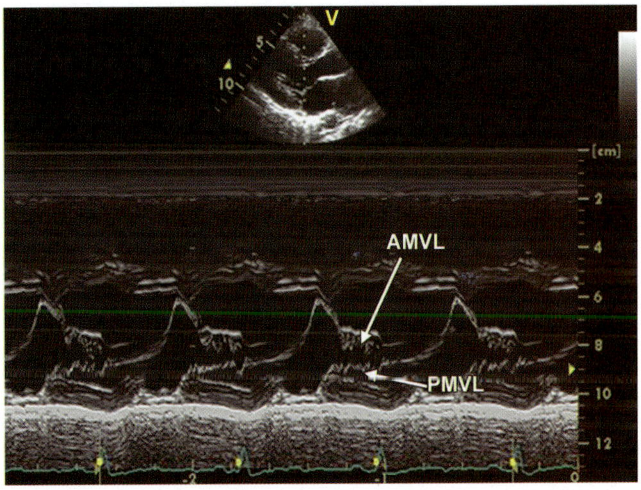

Fig. 224.6: M-mode tracing of the mitral valve demonstrating diastolic flutter of the anterior and posterior mitral valve leaflets.

2. **What is/are secondary findings associated with cor triatriatum sinistrum?**
   (a) Anomalous pulmonary venous drainage
   (b) ASD/PFO
   (c) (a) and (b)
   (d) Systolic flow reversal in the pulmonary veins

Ans. (c)

In the adult, cor triatriatum can be an isolated finding but has also been associated with ostium secundum atrial septal defect, dilated coronary sinus due to persistent left superior vena cava, bicuspid aortic valve, and anomalous pulmonary venous drainage. Bubble study should be performed to evaluate for shunting and persistent left superior vena cava.[3]

3. **If clinically significant, patient will present with symptoms suggestive of:**
   (a) Mitral stenosis
   (b) Mitral regurgitation

(c) Pulmonic regurgitation
(d) Atrial septal defect

Ans. (a)

In adult patients, a heart murmur may be detected. In most cases, the opening in the membrane is severely restricted, producing symptoms similar to mitral stenosis with or without pulmonary hypertension.[2]

4. **If a patient with cor triatriatum presents with clinically significant shortness of breath, what would you see on echocardiography?**
   (a) Increased E/e'
   (b) Increased pulmonary artery systolic pressure
   (c) LV systolic dysfunction
   (d) Increased left ventricular outflow tract VTI

Ans. (b)

An elevation in the pulmonary venous pressure related to elevated gradients across the membrane can lead to an increase in the pulmonary artery pressure.[3]

DISCUSSION

Cor triatriatum sinistrum (CTS) is a rare congenital heart defect that is estimated to occur in ~0.4% of all patients referred for echocardiography.[1] In severe cases, the abnormality is evident in infancy. In less severe cases, the diagnosis of this defect is often incidental later in life.

CTS should be distinguished from a supramitral membrane which is inferior to the left atrial appendage as opposed to being superior to the appendage, in the case of CTS (Fig. 224.5). The separating membrane in CTS is often characterized by one or more small openings allowing communication between the two chambers of the left atrium. CTS can be classified into three groups: Group I patients have no opening in their membrane, Group II patients have one or more small openings, and Group III have a wide opening in the separating membrane. Individuals in Group III patients are likely to survive to late adulthood and often present with few or no symptoms of this disease. Our patient falls into Group III.

Symptoms are related to the degree of obstruction across the membrane and may range from mild shortness of breath on exertion to heart failure with pulmonary congestion. Generally, patients with an opening greater than 1 cm in diameter have no or minimal symptoms. In patients with a smaller opening, the presentation of CTS may mimic that of mitral stenosis.[2] The presentation may include symptoms of pulmonary congestion, pulmonary arterial hypertension,[3] and obstruction of pulmonary venous return. Cor triatriatum sinistrum may present as an isolated finding or it may co-exist with a number of other cardiac lesions, most frequently with atrial septal defect, patent ductus arteriosus, and anomalous pulmonary venous drainage.

The findings on physical exam also depend upon the degree of obstruction. If the membrane significantly obstructs flow, auscultation can reveal a diastolic rumble that is similar to that of mitral stenosis. A loud P2 may be present in the setting of pulmonary hypertension. S1 is normal and there is no opening snap. This is in contrast with rheumatic mitral stenosis where S1 is loud and there is usually an opening snap.

Because the range in severity of symptoms in CTS, treatment options are variable. For patients who are diagnosed much later in life who have less severe obstruction, surgery may not be needed unless symptoms are present.[4] In the presence of dyspnea and signs of pulmonary congestion, diuretics (for preload reduction) is used to relieve symptoms. However, surgery to remove the membrane is the definitive course of therapy. Other complications of CTS that may require treatment include an increased risk of thromboembolic events due to stagnation of flow in the accessory atrial chamber and electrical and mechanical remodeling of the myocardial tissue leading to atrial arrhythmias.[5] In the presence of atrial fibrillation, the membrane can make catheter manipulation during electrophysiologic pulmonary vein ablation more difficult.[6]

Our patient is currently undergoing further diagnostic testing to determine the appropriate course of treatment.

Sonographer Tips

When imaging the left atrium, always inspect the chamber carefully. When a membrane is seen, thoroughly evaluate for two separate chambers. Use color Doppler to identify the presence and number of openings (i.e. single vs. fenestrated openings) in this membrane. Measure the size of the opening by bi-plane 2D or 3D imaging. Use spectral [PW] Doppler to measure presence of any gradient across this membrane. Use M-mode to interrogate the mitral valve to evaluate for any diastolic fluttering of the atrial aspect of the mitral valve leaflets.

MOVIES 731 TO 735

REFERENCES

1. Kadner A, Meszaros K, Mueller C, et al. Cor triatriatum sinister. Multimed Man Cardiothorac Surg. 2014;2014. Doi:10.1093/mmcts/mmu005.
2. Slight RD, Nzewi OC, Buell R, Mankad PS. Cor triatriatum sinister presenting in the adult as mitral stenosis: an analysis of factors which may be relevant in late presentation. Heart Lung Circ. 2005;14(1):8-12.
3. Howe MJ, Thomas MP, Agarwal PP, Bach DS, Rubenfire M. Cor triatriatum: a reversible cause of severe pulmonary hypertension. Can J Cardiol. 2015;31(4):548e1-548e3. http://dx.doi.org/10.1016/j.cjca.2014.11.009.
4. Modi KA, Annamali S, Ernest K, et al. Diagnosis and surgical correction of cor triatriatum in an adult: combined use of transesophageal and contrast echocardiography, and a review of literature. Echocardiography. 2006;23: 506-9.
5. Siniorakis E, Arvanitakis S, Pantelis N, et al. Left atrium in cor triatriatum: arrhythmogenesis and thrombogenesis leading to stroke [Letter]. Int J Cardiol. 2013;17:0167-5273.
6. Ker J. Cor triatriatum sinister presenting with adult onset atrial fibrillation—another rare cause for a common clinical problem. [Letter]. Int J Cardiol. 2013;167:e12-e13.

CASE 225

Daniel W Groves, Amber D Khanna, Robert A Quaife, Ernesto E Salcedo

A 50-year-old male with no significant past medical history presents to the emergency room with 3 days of worsening dyspnea on exertion and orthopnea. He has not seen a physician in over 20 years. In the emergency room, he is in atrial fibrillation with rapid ventricular response. On admission, his blood pressure is 158/72 mm Hg and heart rate 134 beats per minute. He is started on a beta-blocker and heparin drip and converts into sinus rhythm overnight. He underwent a transthoracic echocardiogram (Figs. 225.1, 225.2, 736 and 737) the following morning. During his admission, he also underwent a transesophageal echocardiogram (Figs. 225.3 to 225.6 and 738 to 741B) and cardiac CT (Fig. 225.7). Figure 225.4 and 741A represent three-dimensional TEE.

1. **Based on the provided images, what is the patient's diagnosis?**
   (a) Shone syndrome
   (b) Cor triatriatum sinister
   (c) Cor triatriatum dexter
   (d) Pericardial cyst

Ans. (b)

This patient has cor triatriatum sinister. In cor triatriatum sinister, a fibromuscular membrane develops due to failure of common pulmonary vein resorption and divides the left atrium into a proximal and distal chamber. In cor triatriatum dexter, a membrane divides the right atrium into two chambers. Shone syndrome consists of left-sided defects including supramitral ring, parachute mitral valve, subvalvular aortic stenosis, and coarctation of the aorta. There is no evidence of parachute mitral valve, subvalvular aortic stenosis, or coarctation. A supramitral ring excludes the left atrial appendage unlike the membrane seen in this case. A pericardial cyst is a benign anomaly that is most commonly located adjacent to the right atrium.

2. **The pulmonary veins and left atrial appendage are typically associated with which left atrial chamber in this condition:**
   (a) Pulmonary veins and the left atrial appendage are associated with the proximal left atrial chamber.
   (b) Pulmonary veins are associated with the proximal left atrial chamber and the left atrial appendage is associated with the distal left atrial chamber.

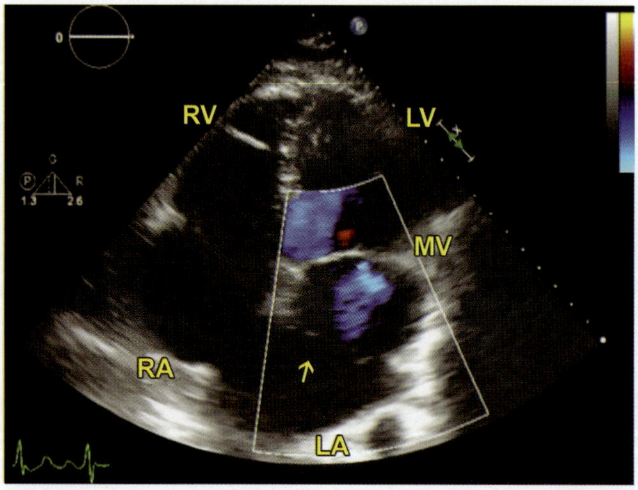

Fig. 225.1: Transthoracic apical 4-chamber view. Arrow points to a linear echodensity in the left atrium.

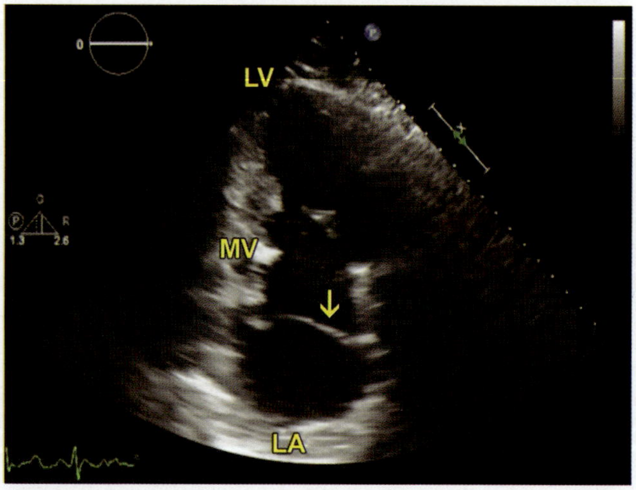

Fig. 225.2: Transthoracic apical 2-chamber view. Arrow points to a linear echodensity in the left atrium.

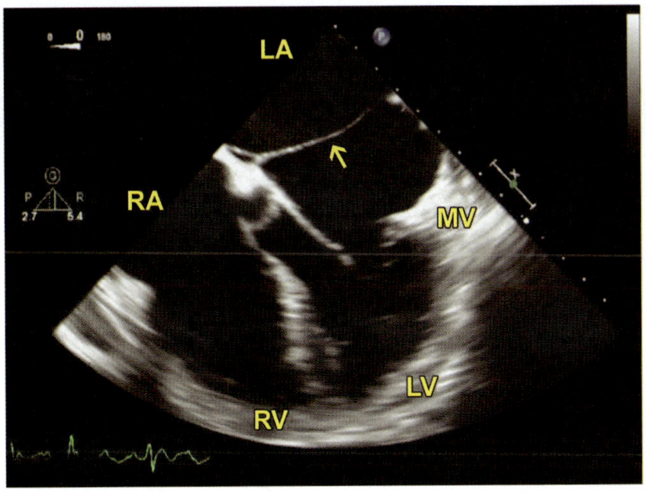

Fig. 225.3: Transesophageal 4-chamber view. Arrow points to a linear echodensity in the left atrium.

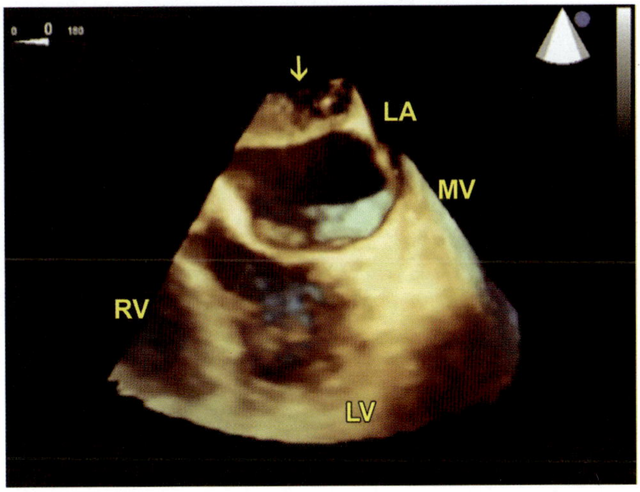

Fig. 225.4: Transesophageal echocardiogram 4-chamber 3D image. Arrow points to a linear echodensity within the left atrium.

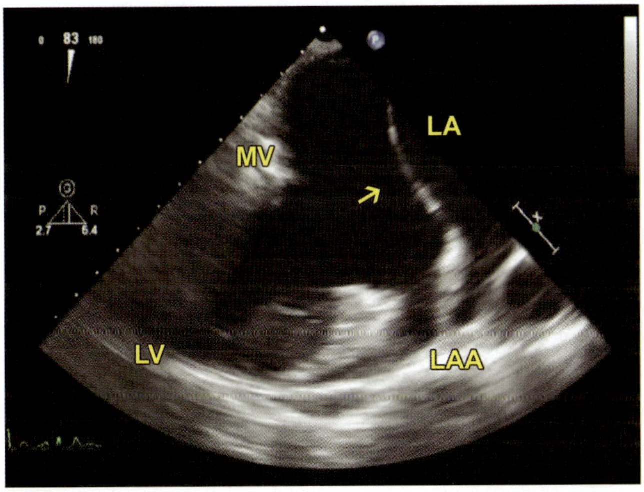

Fig. 225.5: Transesophageal 2-chamber view. Arrow points to a linear echodensity in the left atrium.

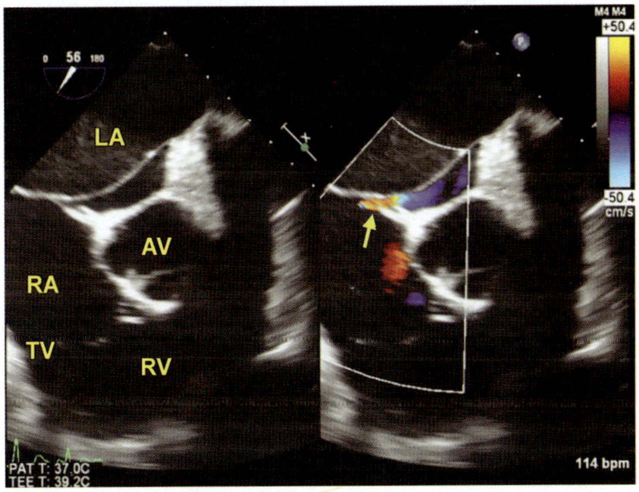

Fig. 225.6: Transesophageal aortic valve short-axis view. Arrow points to a patent foramen ovale.

(c) Pulmonary veins and the left atrial appendage are associated with the distal left atrial chamber.
(d) Pulmonary veins are associated with the distal chamber and the left atrial appendage is associated with the proximal left atrial chamber.

Ans. (b)

In cor triatriatum sinister, the pulmonary veins are associated with the proximal left atrial chamber (as seen in Figure 225.7) and the left atrial appendage is associated with the distal left atrial chamber (as seen in Figure 225.5). There can be partial anomalous pulmonary venous drainage in this condition, so a CT scan may be helpful.

3. **Based on the aortic valve short-axis transesophageal echocardiographic view, (Fig. 225.6) what additional diagnosis is present?**
   (a) Pulmonary vein stenosis
   (b) Supracristal ventricular septal defect
   (c) Patent foramen ovale
   (d) Membranous ventricular septal defect

Ans. (c)

There is a patent foramen ovale with left-to-right shunt seen on color Doppler imaging (arrow in Fig. 225.6). The patent foramen ovale is associated with the distal left atrial chamber. Pulmonary veins are not visualized in this view. In an aortic valve short-axis transesophageal view,

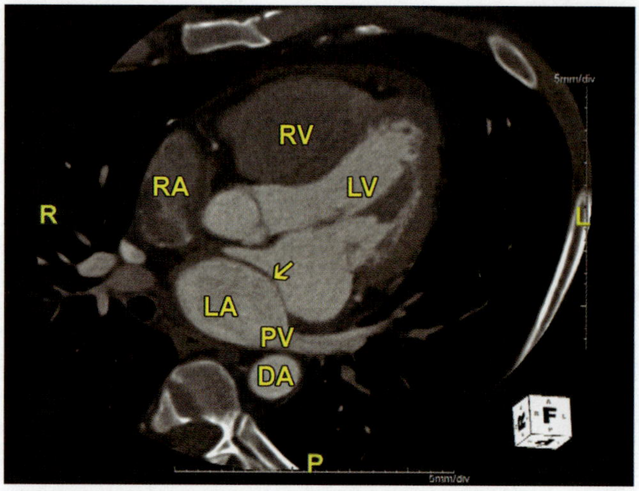

Fig. 225.7: Cardiac computed tomography. Arrow points to a linear structure within the left atrium.

supracristal and membranous ventricular septal defects would typically be seen at approximately 4 and 8 o'clock, respectively.

MOVIE LEGENDS

736: 2D TTE. Apical 4-chamber view. Arrow points to a linear echodensity in the left atrium. Arrowhead points to mitral regurgitation.

737: 2D TTE. Apical 2-chamber view. Arrow points to a linear echodensity in the left atrium

738: 2D TEE. 2-chamber view. Arrow points to a linear echodensity in the left atrium.

739: 2D TEE. 4-chamber view. Arrow points to a linear echodensity in the left atrium.

740: 2D TEE. 4-chamber view, color Doppler shows mitral regurgitation and a linear echodensity in the left atrium (arrow).

741A: 3D TEE. Arrow points to a linear echodensity in the left atrium.

741B: 2D TEE. Aortic short-axis view. Arrow points to a patent foramen ovale with left to right shunt seen on color Doppler imaging .

CASE 226

Armin Baraktain, Ahmed Abuzaid, Aiman Smer

A 54-year-old female presented with progressive dyspnea on exertion. On physical examination she was found to have a grade 3/6 systolic ejection murmur at the left sternal border with no radiation or thrill. Dynamic auscultation revealed attenuated murmur intensity with Valsalva maneuver. Transthoracic echocardiogram (TTE) showed mild left ventricular hypertrophy and normal LV systolic function. The continuous wave (CW) Doppler of the aortic valve revealed maximum pressure gradient of 91 mm Hg and mean pressure gradient of 37 mm Hg. Color Doppler revealed a mosaic pattern indicative of turbulent flow in the LV outflow tract. Two-dimensional (2D) echocardiogram showed morphologically normal tri-leaflet aortic valve with normal excursion of the leaflets. Neither systolic anterior motion of the mitral valve nor hypertrophic cardiomyopathy was found. Transesophageal echocardiography (TEE) was done as illustrated (Figs. 226.1, 226.2, 742 and 743).

1. **Which of the following describes your diagnosis?**
   (a) Subaortic membrane
   (b) Valvular aortic stenosis
   (c) Hypertrophic cardiomyopathy (HOCM)
   (d) Supravalvular aortic stenosis

Ans. (a)

Transesophageal echocardiography shows a thin subaortic membrane arising from the interventricular septum just proximal to the junction of the aortic root with the septum and mild aortic regurgitation. The lesion, however, is often suspected on TTE when CW Doppler reveals high gradients and color Doppler shows mosaic pattern in the outflow tract indicative of turbulent and high subaortic flow velocities. Careful high-pulse repetition-frequency Doppler allows localization of the level of obstruction by detection of the site of maximum velocities. Absence of systolic anterior motion of the mitral valve, mitral regurgitation, and septal hypertrophy help differentiate subvalvular membrane from causes of dynamic LVOT obstruction such as HOCM. Surgical resection of the membrane with or without myectomy is the definitive treatment of the subaortic AS. Indications for surgery include symptoms, high pressure gradients, and development of significant aortic regurgitation. Coronary angiography was unremarkable. She subsequently underwent successful surgical resection of the subaortic membrane.

MOVIE LEGENDS

742 and 743: Transesophaugeal echocardiography, transgastric long axis view showing the subaortic membrane (arrow).

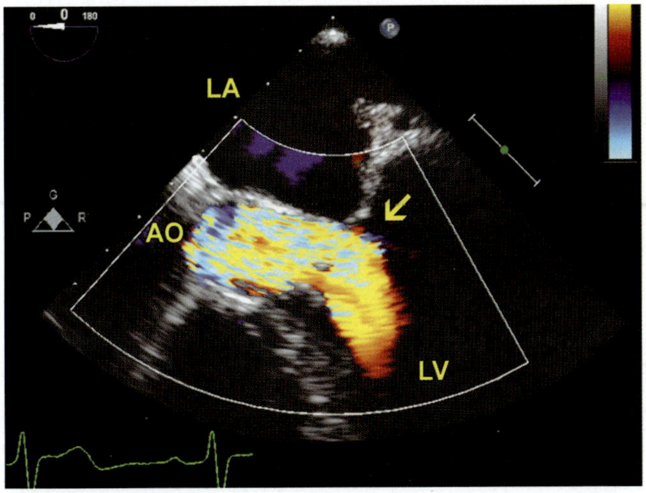

Fig. 226.1: Transesophageal echocardiography with color Doppler showing mosaic turbulent outflow at the subaortic level (arrow) indicative of obstructive physiology.

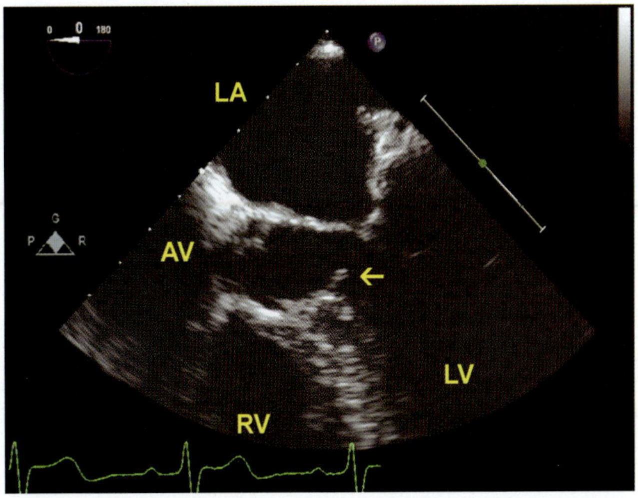

Fig. 226.2: Transesophageal echocardiography showing the subaortic membrane (arrow) arising from the interventricular septum just proximal to the junction of the aortic root with the septum.

CASE 227

Saurabh Sharma, Aman Amanullah

DISCRETE SUBAORTIC AND AORTIC STENOSIS

A 54-year-old female with history of hypertension, presented with symptoms of progressive dyspnea on exertion and lower extremity edema since past 1 month. An echocardiogram performed at outside facility reported to depict severe aortic stenosis. Coronary angiogram demonstrated normal coronaries. She was sent to a tertiary care center for aortic valve replacement. On physical exam, heart rate was 86/min and blood pressure of 136/82 mm Hg. A 3/6 intensity, harsh "shrieking" systolic ejection type murmur was heard at the mid-left sternal border associated with a thrill palpable at the same site. The transthoracic echocardiogram findings are shown in Figure 227.1 and 744. The transesophageal echocardiogram is shown in 745.

1. **What is the most likely diagnosis?**
   (a) Aortic stenosis
   (b) Subaortic stenosis
   (c) Hypertrophic cardiomyopathy (Septal hypertrophy)
   (d) Subaortic membrane
   (e) All of the above

Ans. (e)

The term "subaortic stenosis" includes a variety of obstructions of the left ventricular outflow tract (LVOT), ranging from a short (discrete) subvalvular membrane to long, tunnel-like narrowing. Discrete subaortic membranes are rare congenital abnormalities that can also be found in adults and are the most common reason of subaortic stenosis. It may present as an isolated abnormality or may accompany other congenital abnormalities such as ventricular septal defects (14.9%) and bicuspid aortic valve (2.2%) and coarctation of aorta (12.7%). The prevalence of discrete subvalvular membrane in adults has been reported as 6.5%.[1]

This is an interesting case of concurrent presence of LVOT obstruction due to septal hypertrophy causing tunnel like narrowing of LVOT, subaortic membrane (* in 745); and aortic stenosis. The Figures clearly show turbulence across the LVOT (arrow in 744) with increased peak velocity (by CW Doppler) of almost 6 meters/second (arrow in Fig. 227.1). The transesophageal echocardiogram (Figs. 227.2, 227.3 and 745) shows tunnel-like narrowing of the LVOT, septal hypertrophy and a discrete subaortic membrane. Patient underwent surgery that involved aortic valve replacement using a 21 mm Edwards pericardial bioprosthesis, resection of the subaortic membrane and septal myomectomy.

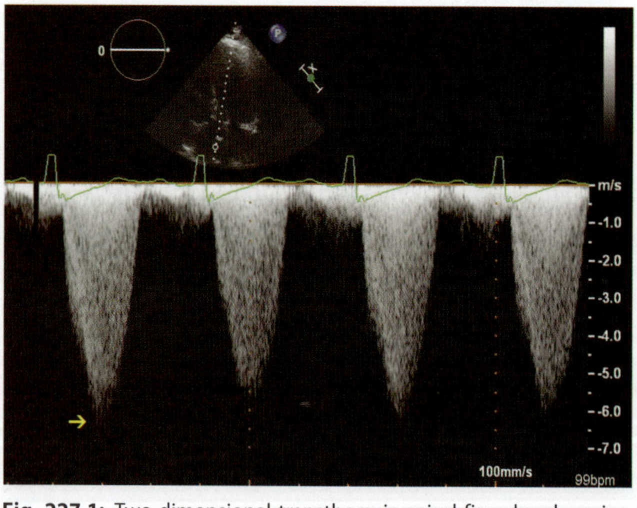

Fig. 227.1: Two dimensional transthoracic apical five chamber view with continuous wave Doppler flow across aortic valve.

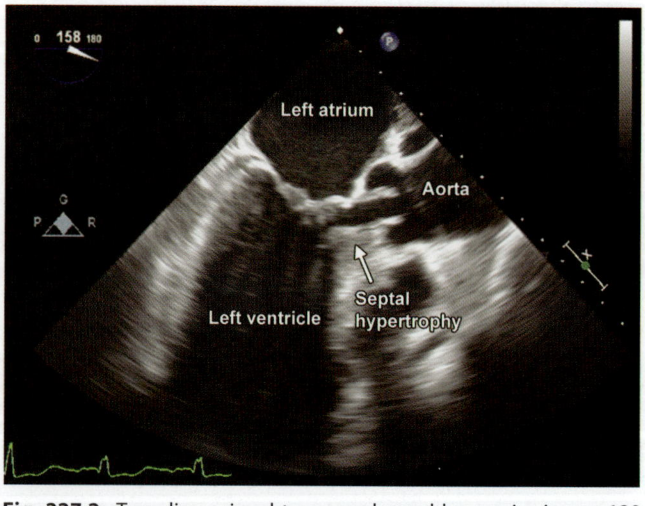

Fig. 227.2: Two dimensional transesophageal long axis view at 120 degrees.

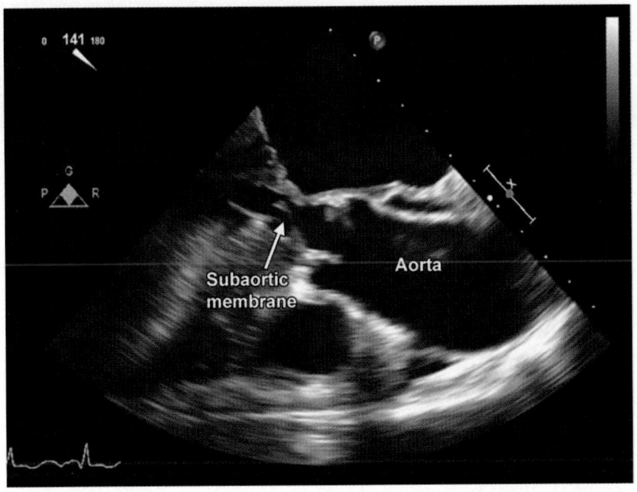

Fig. 227.3: Two dimensional transesophageal long axis view at 120 degrees.

MOVIES 744 AND 745

REFERENCE

1. Oliver JM, Gonzalez A, Gallego P, et al. Discrete subaortic stenosis in adults: increased prevalence and slow rate of progression of the obstruction and aortic regurgitation. J Am Coll Cardiol. 2001;38:835-42.

CASE 228

Arnav Kumar, Masood Ahmad

TRANSTHORACIC 3D ECHOCARDIOGRAPHY IN ASSESSMENT OF STENTED COARCTATION OF AORTA

A 30-year-old female presents with symptoms of dizziness and fatigue for several months. Her medical history is significant for coarctation of the aorta for which she underwent surgical repair at the age of 5 years, followed by balloon angioplasty with stenting of the coarctation at ages 15 and 18 years. On physical examination, her blood pressure is 131/80 mm Hg in the right arm, 130/82 mm Hg in the left arm, with an ankle-brachial index of 1.02 and 0.99, respectively. On cardiac examination she is in sinus rhythm with grade 2/6 systolic ejection murmur at the left sternal border, and has preserved peripheral pulses with no delays. Figure 228.1 and 746 (live/real time three dimensional echocardiogram, suprasternal view) shows the ascending aorta (AA), aortic arch (AR), descending aorta (DA), and descending aorta stent (arrow). Figure 228.2 and 747 (real time three-dimensional multiplanar views) demonstrates the descending aorta stent (arrow) in three orthogonal planes simultaneously. Longitudinal and cross sectional views at multiple levels of the stent are shown (arrows, 1–9).

1. **Which one of the following views in transthoracic echocardiogram is optimal for visualizing and diagnosing the complications of coarctation of aorta in adult patients?**
   (a) Suprasternal view
   (b) Right parasternal view
   (c) Left parasternal view
   (d) Subcostal view

Ans. (a)

Coarctation of aorta, a relatively common condition is the result of localized narrowing of the descending aorta near the origin of the ductus arteriosus. Echocardiographic detection of coarctation requires both an index of suspicion and careful recording of the descending aorta from the suprasternal window. The origins of the carotid and subclavian arteries serve as landmarks when localizing the juxtaductal area. The location of the left subclavian artery relative to the coarctation is an important factor in surgical management. If an area of stenosis is suspected, care should be taken to ensure proper beam alignment.

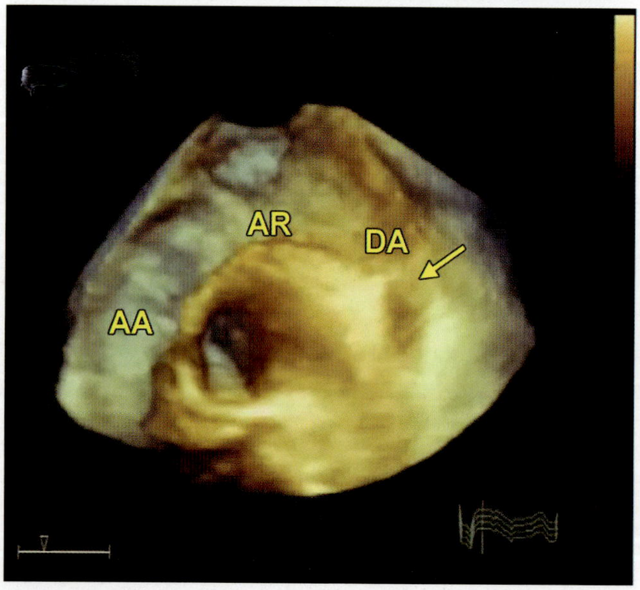

Fig. 228.1: Three dimensional echocardiogram, suprasternel view, (AA: Ascending aorta; AR: Aortic arch; DA: Descending aorta stent [arrow]).

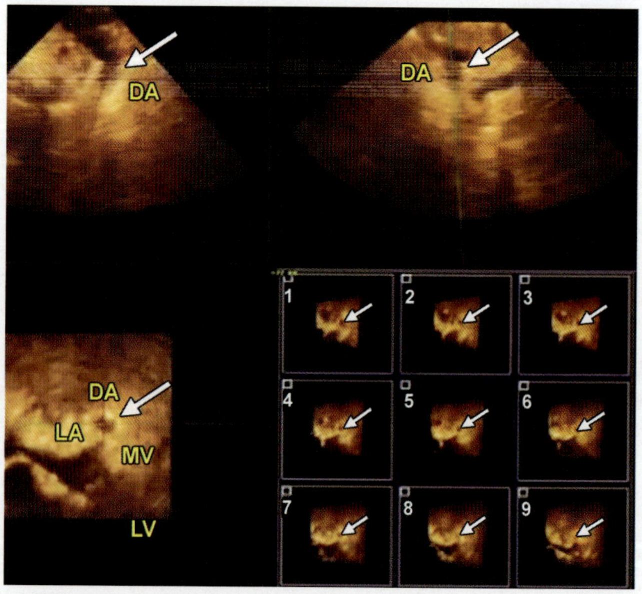

Fig. 228.2: Three dimensional multiplanar views with arrows pointing to descending aorta start, (DA: Descending aorta; LA: Left atrium; MV: Mitral valve; LV: Left ventricle).

In this video (🎥 746), full volume real time three-dimensional image is captured from the suprasternal window and demonstrates the ascending aorta (AA), aortic arch (AR), descending aorta (DA), and stented area of coarctation (arrow).[1] 🎥 747 shows multiplanar views with longitudinal and cross sectional views of the coarctation stent enabling measurements of the aorta and the stent at multiple levels by alignment of the cropping planes along the stented portion of the descending aorta.[1] Three-dimensional echocardiography enables direct visualization of the stent from the inside at its narrowest point. Complications including restenosis of the stent, aneurysm, dissection, and endarteritis can be detected.

2. What cardiac abnormalities are commonly associated with coarctation of aorta?

(a) Bicuspid aortic valve
(b) Ventricular septal defect (VSD)
(c) Mitral tegurgitation (MR)
(d) Patent ductus arteriosus (PDA)
(e) All of the above

Ans. (e)

In a large case series of 1892 patients with coarctation of aorta, only 7% of cases did not have any cardiac anomaly other than a bicuspid aortic valve. Cardiac anomalies include bicuspid aortic valve, atrial septal defect, patent ductus, mitral regurgitation, aortic stenosis, and transposition of great vessels.[2]

3. What coexistent cardiac anomaly can lead to missed diagnosis of coarctation of aorta by transthoracic echocardiogram?

(a) Large patent ductus arteriosus (PDA)
(b) Ventricular septal defect (VSD)
(c) Atrial septal defect (ASD)
(d) Transposition of great arteries (TGA)

Ans. (a)

Doppler examination for coarctation is unreliable in the presence of a large PDA. Instead, one must rely on anatomic (2D) demonstration of the narrowed aortic lumen beyond the origin of the left subclavian artery.

Although Doppler imaging is sensitive for the detection of coarctation, false-negative results can occur in the presence of a patent ductus arteriosus. Left-to-right runoff of blood flow through the ductus reduces the jet velocity through the coarctation and leads to an underestimation of the pressure gradient. This can also occur in the presence of well-developed collaterals. In such cases, the Doppler gradient will lead to an underestimation of the actual severity of obstruction.

4. What findings listed below indicate severe coarctation of aorta in adults?

(a) High-velocity turbulent jet at the level of obstruction on color Doppler images
(b) Persistence of flow signal in diastole confirmed by continuous wave Doppler imaging
(c) Severe upper extremity systolic hypertension
(d) Claudication in lower extremities
(e) All of the above

Ans. (e)

A pressure gradient throughout the cardiac cycle indicates a more severe form of obstruction compared with a pressure gradient that is confined to systole. The presence of a diastolic gradient is confirmed by continuous wave Doppler imaging. The persistence of the jet throughout diastole is an indicator of significant obstruction. Continuous wave Doppler can estimate the severity of coarctation based upon the maximal flow velocity across the narrow area, by measuring the pressure gradient across the coarctation with appropriate correction for velocity proximal to the site of coarctation.

To estimate the peak pressure gradient, the Bernoulli equation can be used. When this equation is applied to aortic coarctation, however, it may be inappropriate to ignore the proximal aortic flow velocity. As a general rule, if this proximal velocity is less than 1.5 m/sec, it can be ignored and the simplified equation can be used. If it is greater than 1.5 m/sec, the expanded Bernoulli equation is necessary. Expanded Bernoulli equation: $[4(v_2^2 - v_1^2)]$ = corrected maximum instantaneous gradient, where v_2 = maximum coarctation velocity and v_1 = velocity proximal to the obstruction.

5. All of the following information can be provided by three-dimensional echocardiographic visualization of a stented coractation *except*:

(a) Cross-sectional area of the stent at multiple levels
(b) Longitudinal view of the coarctation segment
(c) Patency by lumen size
(d) Cross-sectional views of aorta proximal and distal to the stent
(e) Flow gradient across the coarctation

Ans. (e)

MOVIES 746 AND 747

REFERENCES

1. Almomani A, Modi S, Ahmad M. Real time three-dimensional transthoracic echocardiography in assessment of stented coarctation of aorta: a case-based presentation. Echocardiography. 2014;31:E310-4.
2. Keane JF, Flyer DC. Coarctation of the aorta. In: Nadas' Pediatric Cardiology, 2nd ed, Keane JF, Lock JE, Fyler DC (Eds), Saunders Elsevier, Philadelphia, 2006. p. 627.

CASE 229

Claudia Carolina Cajas-Morales, Nilda Espinola-Zavaleta, Jose Antonio Arias-Godinez, Juan Francisco Fritche-Salazar, Nydia Avila-Vanzzini, Maria Eugenia Ruiz-Esparza, Angel Romero-Cardenas, Maria del Sol Ordaz

ABSENT PULMONARY VALVE SYNDROME

A 23-year-old man presented to our institution with a history of dyspnea on exertion and palpitations since childhood. Physical examination revealed systolic murmur in pulmonary focus II/IV with vertical irradiation and holodiastolic murmur in pulmonary focus III/IV, with presence of low parasternal upwelling. A transthoracic echocardiogram was performed and the images are shown below (Figs. 229.1A and B and 748 and 749).

1. **What is the diagnosis (Figs. 229.1A and B and 748 to 750)?**
   (a) Double pulmonary valve lesion
   (b) Aorto-pulmonary fistula
   (c) Absent pulmonary valve syndrome
   (d) Tetralogy of Fallot with absent pulmonary valve

Ans. (d)

Absent pulmonary valve syndrome is a congenital lesion that was first described in 1847 by Cheevers.[1] This syndrome is associated with microdeletion of chromosome 22q11 in 25% of cases and it has been reported to occur in 3–6% of cases of tetralogy of Fallot. This syndrome is associated with conotruncal malformation with abnormal division of truncus arteriosus and therefore, the pulmonary annulus is hypoplastic, the pulmonary valve is rudimentary and aneurysmal dilatation of pulmonary artery and its branches is observed. In 90% of cases it is associated with other malformations and it is more common in men than women with a ratio of 4:1.[1,2] In the movies, to and fro flow through the area of absent pulmonary valve (PV) is labeled as pulmonary regurgitation (PR). Figures 229.1A and B shows color M-mode and CW Doppler flows through the area of absent PV in systole and diastole.

MOVIE LEGENDS

748: Parasternal long axis view with color Doppler. A perimembranous ventricular septal defect is observed with aortic overriding.

749: Parasternal short axis view with color Doppler at the level of the great arteries. Both systolic and diastolic turbulence is observed in the region of pulmonary valve.

750: Subcostal view at the level of the great arteries with color Doppler showing both systolic and diastolic turbulence in the region of pulmonary valve.

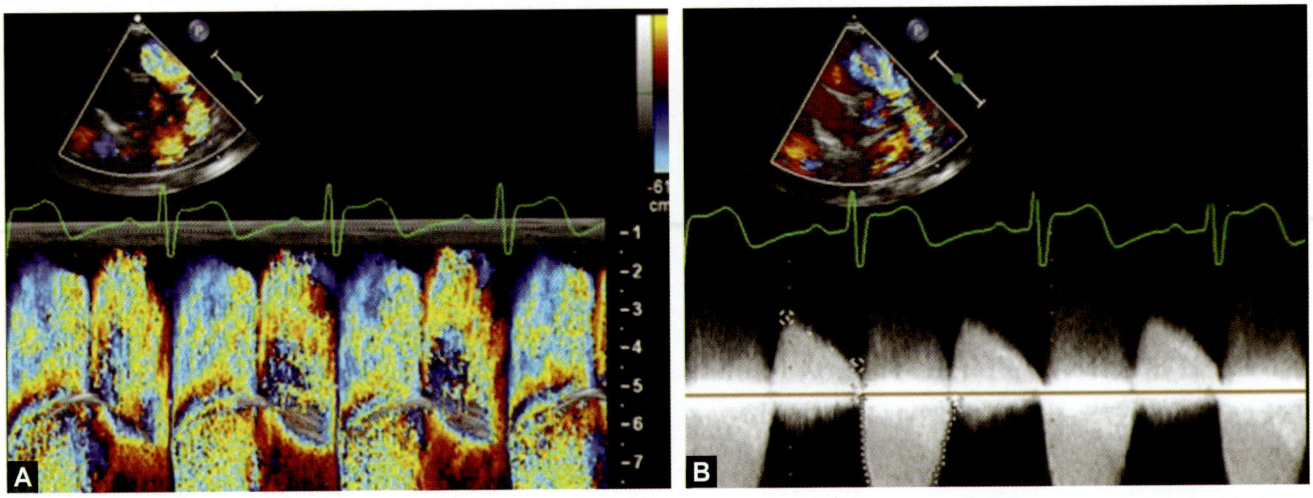

Figs. 229.1A and B: (A) Short axis view at the level of great arteries with color Doppler and M-mode showing systolic and diastolic turbulence at the level of pulmonary valve. (B) With continuous wave Doppler at the level of pulmonary valve, both severe stenosis and regurgitation are visualized.

REFERENCES

1. Philip S, Varghese M, Manohar K, et al. Absent pulmonary valve syndrome: prenatal cardiac ultrasound diagnosis with autopsy correlation. Eur J Echocardiogr. 2011;12:E44.
2. Brown JW, Ruzmetov M, Vijay P, et al. Surgical treatment of absent pulmonary valve syndrome associated with bronchial obstruction. Ann Thoracic Surg. 2006;82:2221-6.

CASE 230

Ramdas G Pai

A 56-year-old female. Systolic murmur left upper sternal border (Fig. 230.1).

1. **What is the likely cause of this murmur?**
   (a) Ventricular septal defect
   (b) Mitral regurgitation
   (c) Aortic stenosis
   (d) Pulmonary stenosis

Ans. (d)

Note that the signal is ejection systolic rather than holosystolic suggesting origin at LV or RV outflow and forward flow in late diastole with atrial systole is diagnostic of pulmonary stenosis. Because of low PA pressure, right atrial systole can generate a forward flow. In aortic stenosis, left atrial systole cannot overcome the high aortic pressure.

2. **Where is the obstruction?**
   (a) Right ventricular infundibulum
   (b) Pulmonary valve
   (c) Neither

Ans. (a)

The obstruction is subvalvular and can be detected by noticing the onset of turbulence below the pulmonary valve in parasternal short axis view (arrow in Fig. 230.2 and 751), RV outflow long axis view and subcostal short axis view (Fig. 230.3 and 752, arrow). The subcostal short axis or RV outflow view from RV apex (by tilting the probe anteriorly) gives the best view to obtain spectral Doppler of RVOT obstruction.

MOVIES 751 AND 752

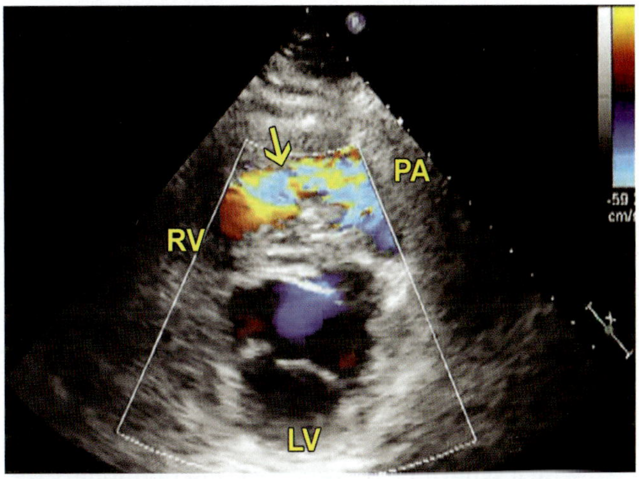

Fig. 230.2: Color flow Doppler interrogation of the right ventricular outflow tract from parasternal short axis view (systolic frame shown).

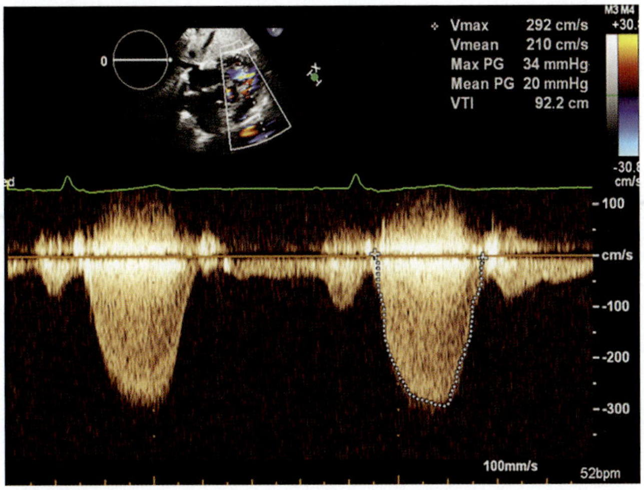

Fig. 230.1: Continuous wave Doppler signal interrogating the right ventricular outflow tract.

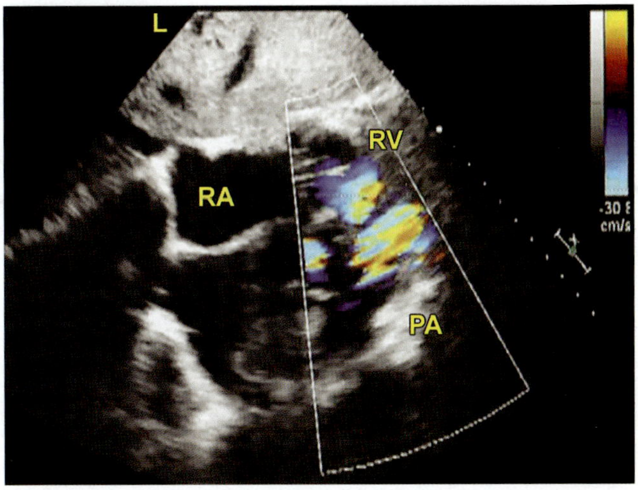

Fig. 230.3: Subcostal short axis view showing flow acceleration in right ventricular outflow tract.

CASE 231

Sangeeta Shah

A 25-year-old female presented with a history of murmur since childhood. She was followed by her pediatric cardiologist until 18 years old. Currently she has dyspnea on exertion two flights of stairs.

Vitals: Pulse rate = 70–80 bpm; Pulse oximetry 98%; Blood pressure: 130/70 mm Hg. CVS: III/VI mid systolic ejection murmur left sternal border. Lungs: Clear. Extremities: no LE edema. An echocardiogram was ordered (Figs. 231.1, 231.2, 753 and 754).

1. **What is the systolic pulmonary artery pressure (Figs. 231.1 and 231.2)?**
   (a) 38 mm Hg + RAP
   (b) 31 mm Hg + RAP
   (c) 10 mm Hg
   (d) 69 mm Hg

Ans. (c)

The tricuspid valve gradient reflects the RV systolic pressure not the pulmonary artery pressure in **pulmonary stenosis**. Pulmonary artery pressures = (TR systolic gradient + estimated RAP) - Pulmonary valve systolic gradient

2. **Which syndrome is associated with pulmonary stenosis?**
   (a) Down's syndrome
   (b) Turner's syndrome
   (c) Noonan's syndrome
   (d) Marfan' s syndrome

Ans. (c)

Noonan's syndrome has constellation of signs and symptoms including short stature, webbed neck, hypertelorism, low-set ears and hairline, hyperelastic skin and chest deformities. Indications for intervention - valvuloplasty.[1]

Asymptomatic: Peak systolic gradient of 60 mm Hg through the pulmonary valve.[1]

Symptomatic: Peak systolic gradient of 50 mm Hg through the pulmonary valve.[1]

MOVIE LEGENDS

753: Parasternal long axis view with normal RV size, Normal LV size and function.

754: Parasternal long short axis view showing systolic doming (arrow) of the pulmonary valve.

REFERENCE

1. ACC/AHA. 2008 Guidelines for the Management of Adults with Congenital Heart Disease. JACC. 2008;52:143-263.

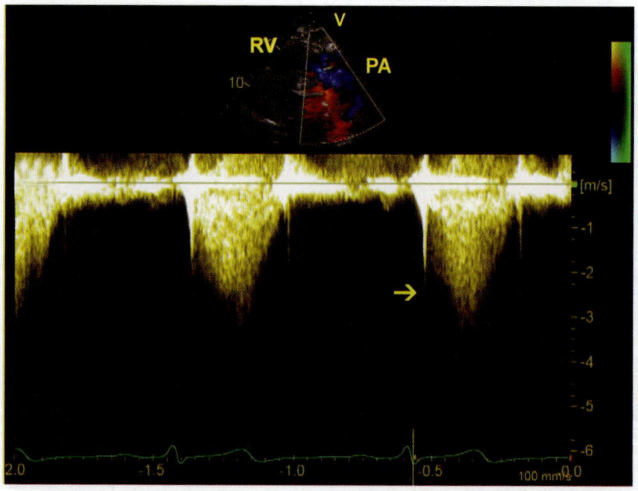

Fig. 231.1: Continuous wave Doppler through the pulmonary valve measures 2.5 m/sec (arrow).

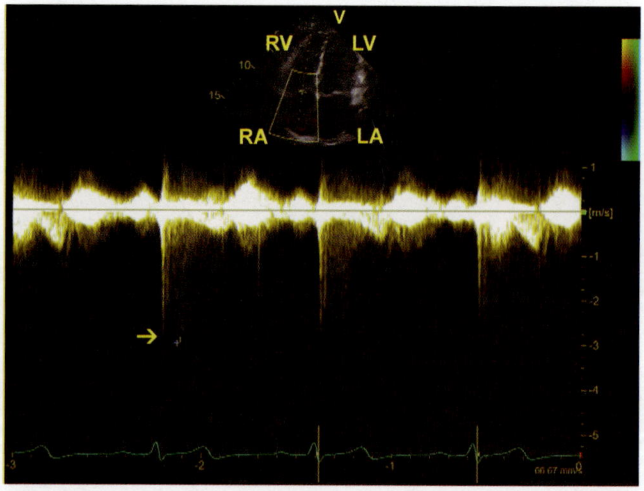

Fig. 231.2: Peak tricuspid regurgitation velocity = 3.1 m/sec (arrow).

CASE 232

Sozzi B Fabiola, Iacuzio Laura

Quadricuspid aortic valve is a rare congenital heart anomaly and rare cause of valve failure. Often, it is an incidental finding at transesophageal echo, surgery or post-mortem examination.[1,2]

A 36-year-old woman presented with symptoms of progressive dyspnea during exertion. On physical examination her blood pressure was 170/60 mm Hg and a diastolic murmur of grade 4/6 was heard at the left parasternal border. ECG displayed sinus rhythm with high QRS voltage and ST-T configuration consistent with left ventricular hypertrophy. Chest X-ray was normal. Transthoracic echocardiography demonstrated severe aortic regurgitation. The aortic valve ring diameter was normal (23 mm) as well the transvalvular peak velocity, suggesting a normal pressure gradient across the aortic valve.

A cardiac RMN performed in order to better assess the aortic valve anatomy displayed a quadricuspid aortic valve (755). Three cusps were of equal size and one cusp was larger (Fig. 232.1 in diastole and Fig. 232.2 in systole). The valve malformation was associated with severe aortic regurgitation; regurgitant fraction was 45%.

The regurgitation was huge and central, related to incomplete juxtaposition of the four cusps with a decrease in mobility of the leaflets and incomplete closure during diastole.

Left ventricle was moderately enlarged (EDVI and ESVI: 104 and 37 mL/m^2), with normal systolic function (EF 65%). No valsalva (36 mm) or aortic root (38 mm) dilatation was associated (756 and 757).

Quadricuspid aortic valve is difficult to identify using transthoracic echocardiography because of the anatomical features. In this case, the RMN shows its superiority in the anatomical asset.

A valvular surgery replacement was performed with a biological prosthesis (Perimount Magna n°23). The postoperative course was uneventfully and the patient was discharged home on 6th postoperative day.

1. **What is the morphology of the aortic valve?**
   (a) Normal
   (b) Bicuspid
   (c) Quadricuspid
   (d) Unclear

Ans. (c)

2. **At cardiac RMN, how would you characterize the left ventricle considering its volumes and function?**
   (a) Normal volumes and normal function

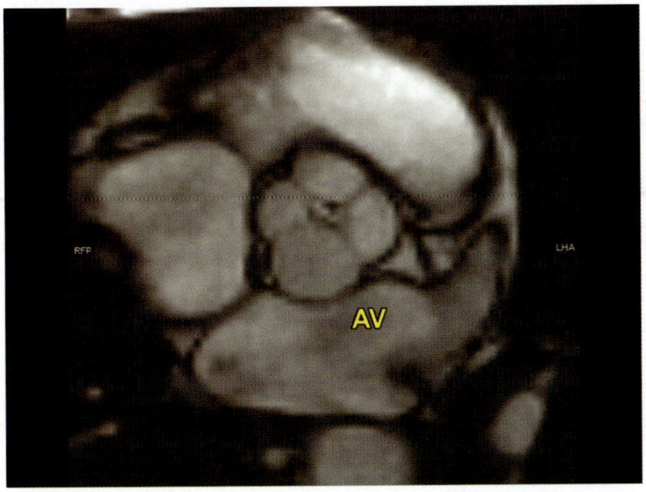

Fig. 232.1: Cine aortic valve (SSFP sequence). Aortic valve in diastole. Three cusps were of equal size and one cusp was larger.

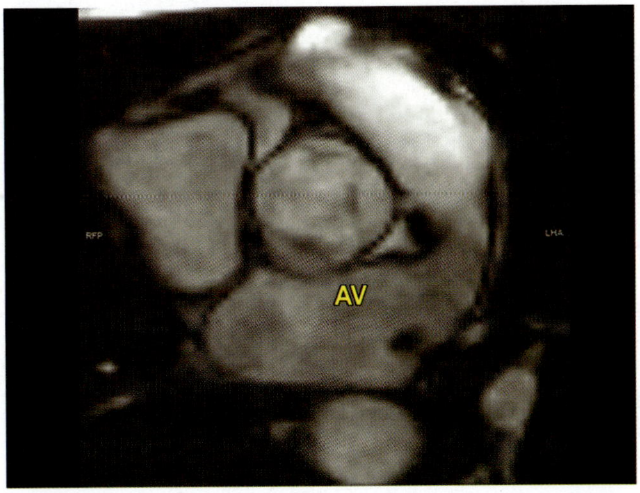

Fig. 232.2: Cine aortic valve (SSFP sequence). Aortic valve in systole.

(b) Dilated left ventricle with normal function
(c) Dilated left ventricle with reduced function

Ans. (b)

3. **How do the aortic cusps and the regurgitant jet appear in this view?**
   (a) Normal cusps with a central jet
   (b) Thickened cusps with an eccentric jet
   (c) Thickened cusps with a central jet

Ans. (c)

MOVIE LEGENDS

755: Cine aortic valve (SSFP sequence): quadricuspid valve dynamics during the cardiac cycle with one asymetric cusp and central regurgitation orifice.

756: Cine 4 chamber view (SSFP sequence) showing a moderately enlarged left ventricle with preserved systolic function. At cardiac RMN the end-diastolic and end-systolic left ventricular volumes were respectively: 104 and 37 mL/m^2. The ejection fraction was: 65%

757: LVOT view (SSFP sequence) showing aortic regurgitation with a central jet and no dilatation of the aortic root and sinuses of valsalva.

REFERENCES

1. Cooke JC, Dupuche DR, Gay TJ. Quadricuspid Aortic Valve. Echocardiography. 2000;17:699.
2. Schulze MR, Strasser RH. Uni-, bi-, tri-, and quadricuspid aortic valves. N Engl J Med. 2006;355(12):1262.

CASE 233

Roomi AU, Elsayed M, Bulur S, Arisha MJ, Nanda NC

EBSTEIN'S ANOMALY

The patient was a 39-year-old female complaining of chest discomfort and palpitations with no significant medical history. ECG showed normal sinus rhythm with RBBB. 2D TTE was done (Figs. 233.1 to 233.3 and 758 to 760).

1. **In Ebstein's anomaly all the following statements may be true *except*:**
   (a) Atrialization of RV is present.
   (b) In most cases the septal TV leaflet does not originate normally but its true attachment is further down the ventricular septum.
   (c) In almost all cases the septal TV leaflet originates normally but the proximal portion is tethered completely or partially to the ventricular septum displaying an apparent downward displacement of the attachment point. 759 shows only partial attachment of the septal TV leaflet to the proximal ventricular septum producing a bubble-like appearance (arrowhead).
   (d) RV function is related to the size of non-atrialized portion of RV.
   (e) PFO may be present
   (f) The posterior (inferior) TV leaflet is also commonly involved and shows tethering to RV wall.
   (g) The anterior TV leaflet is elongated and sail like producing a diastolic sound which may be mistaken for opening snap of mitral stenosis

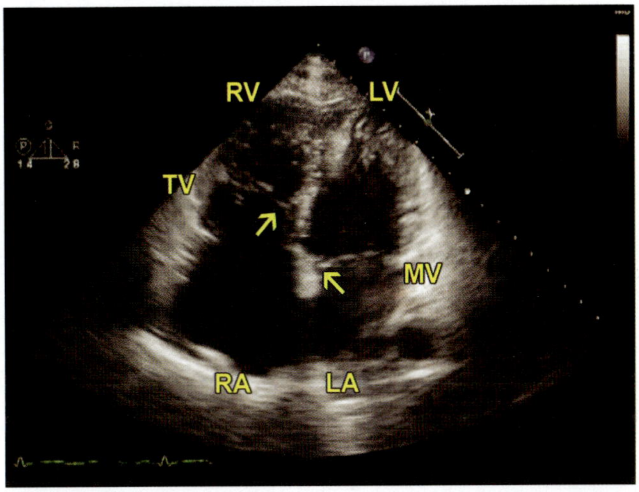

Fig. 233.2: Apical 4-chamber view. Shows apparent downward displacement of the septal TV (left arrow) attachment as compared to MV attachment (right arrow). The LV apex appears heavily trabeculated raising the possibility of associated LV noncompaction.

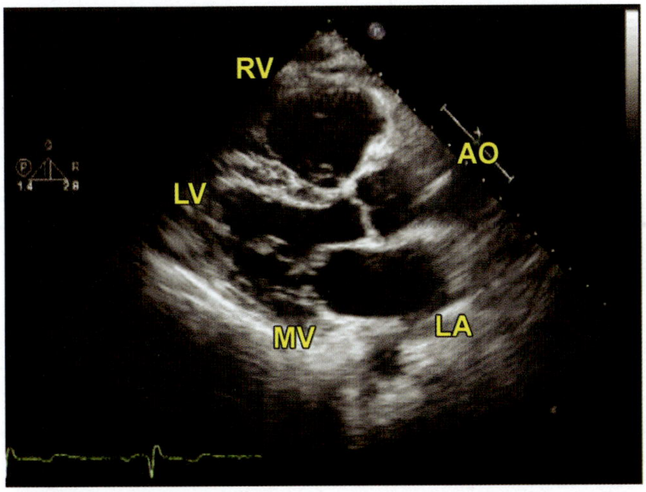

Fig. 233.1: Parasternal long axis view. Unremarkable except mild thickening and prolapse of AV.

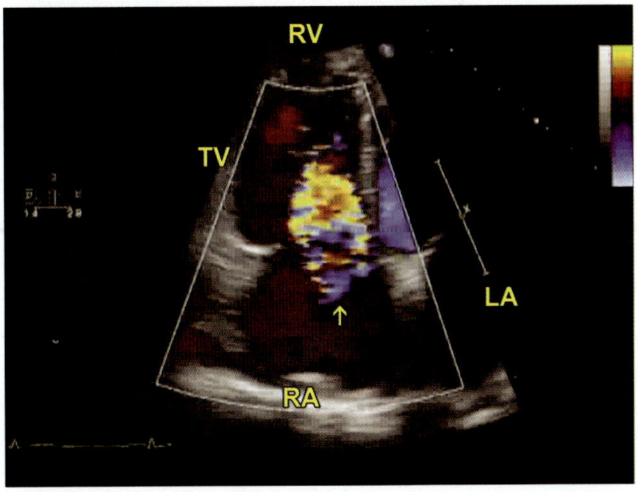

Fig. 233.3: Apical 4-chamber view. Color Doppler shows significant TR (arrow).

(h) TV closure is markedly delayed as compared to MV closure and this is best seen on M-mode.

Ans. (b)

MOVIE LEGENDS

758: Parasternal long axis view. Unremarkable except mild thickening and prolapse of AV.

759: Apical 4-chamber view. Shows apparent downward displacement of the septal TV leaflet attachment as compared to MV attachment. Arrow shows a bubble-like appearance produced by partial attachment of the septal TV leaflet to the proximal interventricular septum.

760: Apical 4-chamber view. Color Doppler shows significant TR (arrow).

CASE 234

Vidya Nadig, Anurag Sahu, Vincent L Sorrell

YOUNG ADULT WITH CYANOTIC CONGENITAL HEART DISEASE

A 25-year-old woman with history of congenital heart disease presented with dyspnea and cyanosis. She was found to have an oxygen saturation of low 90s. The ECG and ECHO performed at admission are shown (Fig. 234.1 and 761).

1. **Based upon the history, ECG, and ECHO findings, the most likely diagnosis is which of the following?**
   (a) Ebstein's anomaly
   (b) Arrhythmogenic right ventricular dysplasia
   (c) L-TGA (congenitally corrected transposition of the great arteries)
   (d) Double outlet right ventricle
   (e) Tricuspid atresia

Ans. (a)

Ebstein's anomaly is a congenital heart defect that is characterized by a failure of delamination of the tricuspid valve leaflets. This results in adhesion of the septal and posterior leaflets to the right ventricle, leading to anterior displacement of the functional annulus. There is varying degree of "atrialization" of the right ventricle with displacement of the septal leaflet. The anterior leaflet is the largest and often described as "sail-like". In this case, the displacement is marked and may not be as severe in other cases. A displacement index of >8 mm/m^2 is diagnostic of Ebstein's anomaly. Images in 761–763 also suggest the paradoxical septal motion seen in Ebstein's with volume overload related to severe tricuspid regurgitation.

2. **Which of the following associated pathologies are known to occur with this disease and can be demonstrated in 762–764?**
   (a) Atrial septal defect (or PFO) and ventricular septal defect
   (b) Atrial septal defect and LV noncompaction
   (c) Tricuspid regurgitation and aortic coarctation
   (d) Cleft mitral valve and pulmonic stenosis
   (e) Sub-aortic VSD and focal RV aneurysm

Ans. (b)

Atrial septal defects or PFO are the most commonly associated defects seen in Ebstein's anomaly. Up to 80% of patients with Ebstein's anomaly will have this association.

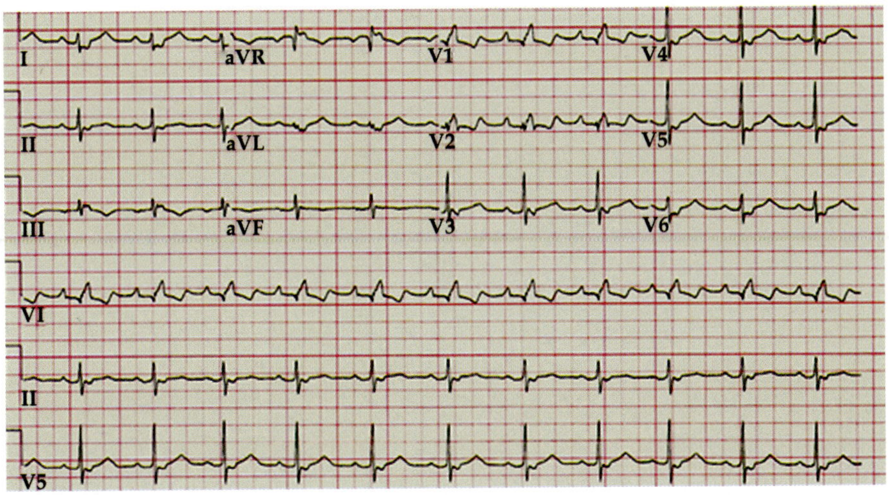

Fig. 234.1: ECG on admission.

Other less commonly associated structural defects include coarctation of the aorta, ventricular noncompaction, ventricular septal defect, and mitral valve prolapse.

3. **The patient underwent a cardiopulmonary exercise test prior to discharge and had a V02 of 14 mL/kg/min. Which of the following is considered an appropriate indication to recommend complex congenital heart surgery to repair this condition?**
   (a) Cyanosis alone is an indication
   (b) RV volume >150 mL/m^2
   (c) Lower extremity edema and right heart failure
   (d) Qp/Qs ratio >2:1
   (e) All the above

Ans. (a)

Indications for surgery include cyanosis, paradoxical embolism, refractory arrhythmia, and heart failure (ACC/AHA 2008 guidelines). There are no randomized trials comparing medical therapy to surgery. The ACC/AHA guidelines also suggest early surgery at expert centers for tricuspid valve repair. Cardiopulmonary exercise testing may also be useful in discriminating between highly functional patients and those who have their symptoms unmasked. This patient was referred for surgery due to the presence of cyanosis, NYHA functional class 3 heart failure symptoms and poor performance on a CPX study.

MOVIE LEGENDS

761: Apical 4-chamber view. Illustrates the displacement and failure of delamination of the septal leaflet of the tricuspid valve, with the rudimentary septal leaflet seen best in the short axis view.

762: Illustrates LV noncompaction with a noncompaction index of 4.0. A ratio of greater than 2.3 (noncompacted/compacted myocardial ratio) is diagnostic of LV noncompaction.

763: An in-plane velocity encoded cine imaging sequence that demonstrates right to left shunting across the patent foramen ovale (faint "black" flow noted at mid septum).

764: A LV short axis view that demonstrates the sail-like anterior RV leaflet and the diastolic septal flattening seen in RV volume overload.

CASE 235

Megan Y Kamath, Rachel Hughes-Doichev

DYSPNEA AND A MASS IN THE HEART LEADING TO A DIAGNOSIS OF A RARE CONGENITAL HEART DEFECT

Case Description

A 21-year-old female with no known past medical history presented to an outside hospital for evaluation of a 3-month history of progressive shortness of breath and productive cough. During this time, she had been treated at a local clinic with antibiotics for presumed bronchitis. She admitted to progressive fatigue, orthopnea, and peripheral edema, which was initially attributed to side effects of the antibiotics. She denied chest pain, palpitations, pre-syncope, or syncope. At the outside facility, she underwent a CT chest to assess for pulmonary embolus and this revealed a mass in the left atrium. Transthoracic echocardiogram and magnetic resonance imaging were performed (Figs. 235.1 to 235.4, 765 to 767).

1. **Based on the echocardiographic findings in Figures 235.1 and 235.2, the most likely diagnosis is:**
   (a) ARVD
   (b) VSD
   (c) Left atrial myxoma
   (d) Ebstein's anomaly

Ans. (d)

Ebstein's anomaly is a congenital heart defect with an incidence of 1 in 200,000 births. In Ebstein's anomaly there is malformation of the tricuspid valve and failure of the normal delamination process of the tricuspid leaflets resulting in "atrialization" of the right ventricle usually due to an apically displaced insertion site of the septal and posterior leaflets and displaced tricuspid annulus. There have been multiple variants and classification systems described, but the most common criteria used for diagnosis is to have an apically displaced septal and posterior tricuspid leaflet at least 8 mm/m^2 relative to the mitral valve.[2] The diagnosis is generally made by echocardiography, in particular the apical 4-chamber view.[3]

2. **All of the following are echocardiographic findings of Ebstein's anomaly *except* for:**
   (a) Apical displacement of the septal/posterior tricuspid valve leaflet

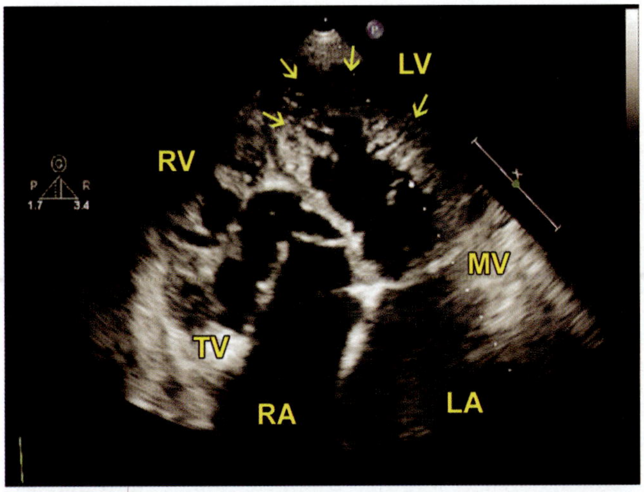

Fig. 235.1: Apical 4-chamber view shows significant apparent displacement of the attachment of the septal tricuspid valve leaflet as compared to the anterior mitral leaflet. Arrows point to multiple trabeculations in the left ventricle consistent with noncompaction.

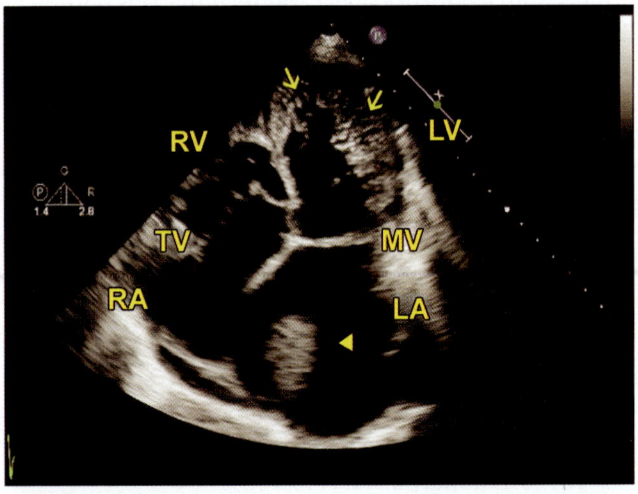

Fig. 235.2: Apical 4-chamber view. Arrowhead shows a large mass in the left atrium.

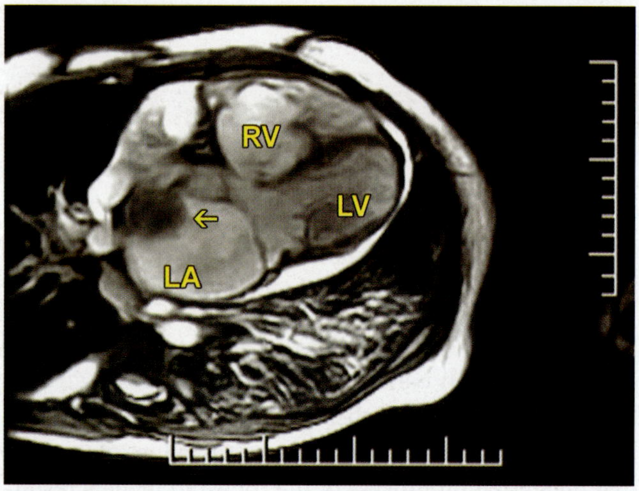

Fig. 235.3: Magnetic resonance imaging (MRI). Arrow shows a large mass in the left atrium.

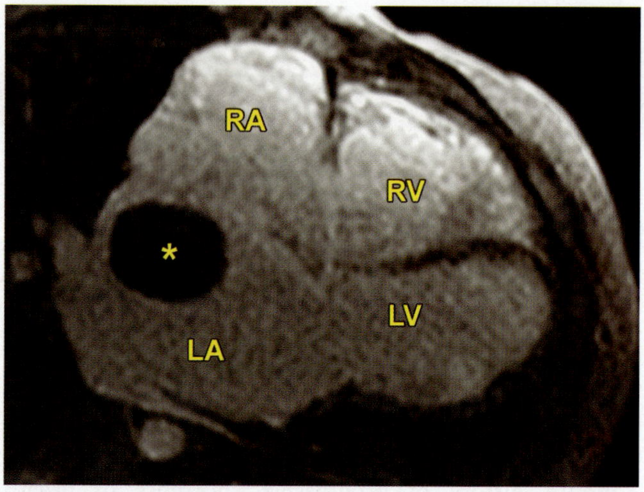

Fig. 235.4: Magnetic resonance imaging (MRI). Asterisk shows a large mass in the left atrium.

(b) Hypertrophy of the right ventricle
(c) Thinning of the right ventricle on the atrial side of the tricuspid valve
(d) Muscular ventricular septal defect
(e) McConnell's sign (right ventricular hypokinesis with sparing of the RV apex)
(f) Answers (d) and (e)

Ans. (f)

In Ebstein's anomaly, a portion of the right ventricle sits above the plane of the tricuspid valve due to the apical displacement of the insertion site of the septal and posterior leaflets from failure of leaflet delamination. This portion of the right ventricle may become thinned, and other regions of the right ventricle may have variable hypertrophy as a result. Though left sided defects may be seen in association with Ebstein's, muscular ventricular septal defect is not specifically associated with it. RV hypokinesis with sparing of the RV apex (McConnell's sign) is a finding that is generally thought to have a high specificity for acute pulmonary embolus and is thought to occur due to the circumferential fibers of the RV apex contracting in concert with the left ventricular apical fibers. This finding is not associated with Ebstein's anomaly.

3. What is the most common cardiac abnormality associated with Ebstein's anomaly?

(a) Pulmonary atresia
(b) Mitral valve prolapse
(c) Left ventricular noncompaction
(d) Atrial septal defect
(e) Coarctation of the aorta

Ans. (d)

An interatrial shunt is found in 80–94% of patients with Ebstein's anomaly.[1] Mitral valve prolapse, bicuspid aortic valve, coarctation of the aorta, and pulmonary atresia can also been seen less frequently. Left ventricular dysplasia in a pattern mimicking left ventricular noncompaction has been noted in up to 18% of patients with Ebstein's anomaly in one series.[4]

Left Ventricular Noncompaction

When noncompaction of the left ventricle is seen in conjunction with Ebstein's anomaly, clinical presentation can be variable: ranging from asymptomatic, as initially was the case with our patients ventricular arrhythmias, heart failure, thromboembolism, and sudden cardiac death.[4] Prognosis for patients is determined by the degree and progression of symptoms; some studies have suggested with regular monitoring prognosis may be improved with earlier initiation of medical therapy and consideration for advanced mechanical support and heart transplantation.[5] This patient's symptoms while initially mild, progressed rapidly to cardiogenic shock and biventricular heart failure despite aggressive intervention, highlighting the importance of considering congenital heart disease in the differential diagnosis for an adult patient who presents with insidious onset exertional dyspnea, fatigue, and palpitations. In patients with complex congenital heart disease, management must be both individualized. Intervention is generally performed early and aggressively to achieve the most optimal outcomes.

4. According to the 2008 ACC/AHA congenital heart disease guidelines, indications for surgical repair of Ebstein's anomaly beyond infancy include which of the following:

(a) Cyanosis
(b) Progressive cardiomegaly
(c) Evidence of progressive RV dilation and reduced RV function
(d) All of the above

Ans. (d)

KEY POINTS

1. Per the Jenni criteria, LV noncompaction can only be diagnosed after all other congenital defects have been excluded.[6,7]
2. Echocardiographic diagnosis of Ebstein's anomaly is confirmed by apparent apical displacement of the septal tricuspid leaflet by >8 mm/m^2 compared to the position of the mitral valve, enlarged right ventricular volume, and low velocity tricuspid regurgitation.
3. Patients with Ebstein's anomaly are at high risk for arrhythmias and pre-excitation secondary to the presence of one or more accessory conduction pathways often as a result of right atrial enlargement and coexisting atrial septal defects.
4. Clinical presentation of Ebstein's anomaly is variable from neonate to adult. It can be associated with multiple cardiac defects including atrial septal defect, patent foramen ovale, left ventricular noncompaction and right ventricular outflow tract obstruction.
5. In patients who have both Ebstein's anomaly and left ventricular noncompaction, the dysplasia of the left ventricular myocardium can lead to both systolic and diastolic dysfunction as well as predispose to the development of ventricular arrhythmias.
6. Surgical repair for Ebstein's anomaly is either done with tricuspid valve repair or replacement and is done when patients have symptoms, severe tricuspid regurgitation, evidence of right ventricular dysfunction and/or failure, or arrhythmias.

MOVIE LEGENDS

765: Apical 4-chamber view shows significant apparent displacement of the attachment of the septal tricuspid valve leaflet as compared to the anterior mitral leaflet. Arrows point to multiple trabeculations in the left ventricle consistent with noncompaction.

766: Apical 4-chamber view. Arrowhead shows a large mass in the left atrium.

767: Magnetic resonance imaging (MRI). Arrow shows a large mass in the left atrium.

REFERENCES

1. Attenhofer Jost CH, Connolly HM, Dearani JA, et al. Ebstein's anomaly. Circulation. 2007; 115(2):277-85.
2. Paranon J, Acar S. Ebstein's anomaly of the tricuspid valve: from fetus to adult: congenital heart disease. Heart. 2008; 94(2):237-43.
3. Dearani JA, Danielson GK. Congenital heart surgery nomenclature and database project: Ebstein's Anomaly and tricuspid valve disease. Ann Thorac Surg. 2000;69:S106.
4. Attenhofer Jost CH, Connolly HM, O'Leary PW, et al. Left heart lesions in patients with Ebstein anomaly. Mayo Clin Proc. 2005;80:361-68.
5. Bagur RH, Lederlin M, Montandon M, et al. Ebstein anomaly associated with left ventricular noncompaction. Circulation. 2008;118:e662-4.
6. Jenni R, Oechslin E, Schneider J, Attenhofer Jost C, Kaufmann PA. Echocardiographic and pathoanatomical characteristics of isolated left ventricular non-compaction: a step toward classification as a distinct cardiomyopathy. Heart. 2001;86:666-71.
7. Arbustini et al. Left Ventricular Noncompaction: A Distinct Genetic Cardiomyopathy? J Am Coll Cardiology. 2016; 68(9):949-66.

CASE 236

Alagic N, Elsayed M, Uygur B, Turaga NSN, Chahwala JR, Adarna LG, Bulur S, Nanda NC

Another adult patient from our Echo Laboratory showing Ebstein's anomaly with apparent displacement of the septal TV leaflet toward the RV apex and multiple trabeculations (arrows) in LV apex consistent with noncompaction (768 to 770).

MOVIES 768 TO 770

CASE 237

Susan T Laing, Beverly Smulevitz

This patient is a 55-year-old male who was born with dextro-transposition of the great arteries (d-TGA) and a large ventricular septal defect (VSD). He had a surgical procedure for his transposition at age 18. He has a history of atrial flutter, congestive heart failure, Eisenmenger's syndrome, nonischemic cardiomyopathy, diabetes and pulmonary hypertension. He has shortness of breath and is on home oxygen. 2DTTE and 3DTTE done.

1. **Looking at the images below, what is the type of repair he most likely had at age 18? (Figs. 237.1, 237.2 to 771, 774, 774 is 3DTTE)**
   (a) Fontan lateral tunnel
   (b) Heart transplant
   (c) Mustard procedure
   (d) Arterial switch procedure
   (e) Nanda repair

Ans. (c)

This patient had a Mustard procedure (atrial switch) performed when he was 18 years old. The images show the pulmonary venous baffle. This baffle directs the flow from the left atrial pulmonary veins to the anatomic tricuspid valve so that oxygenated blood can be pumped out of the right ventricle through the aorta.

2. **What direction is the blood flowing across the VSD in the 2D color image below? (Fig. 237.3 and 775).**
   A. Sub-pulmonic ventricle to sub-aortic ventricle
   B. Systemic circuit ventricle to Pulmonary circuit ventricle
   C. Anatomic RV to anatomic LV
   D. Bidirectional flow

Ans. (a)

With the atrial switch procedure, the ventricle to great artery connections are left intact. Instead the atrial septum is removed and baffles are created so that the left atrial inflow goes to the anatomic right heart while the right atrial inflow is directed to the anatomic left heart. The right ventricle becomes the systemic ventricle while the left becomes the pulmonary venous ventricle. This is a physiologic correction of the D-TGA. This patient has severe pulmonary hypertension.

3. **In the 3D image below, the arrow is pointing at what structure? (Fig. 237.4, 776 and 777. Figures 237.4 and 776 are 3DTTE)**
   (a) Calcified MV chord

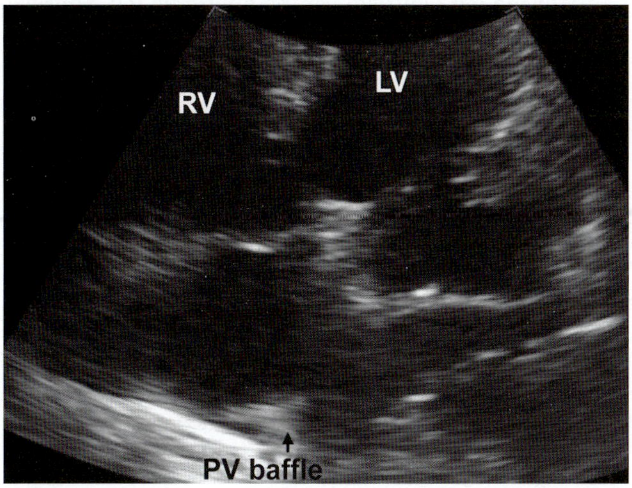

Fig. 237.1: Transthoracic 4-chamber view with focus on the tricuspid valve.

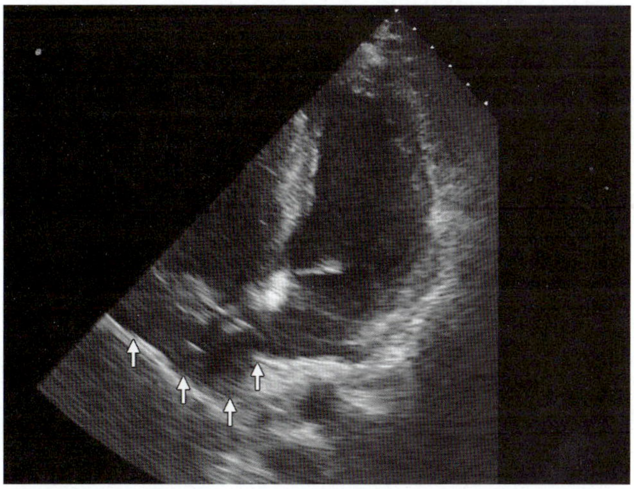

Fig. 237.2: Transthoracic 4-chamber view with focus on the mitral valve.

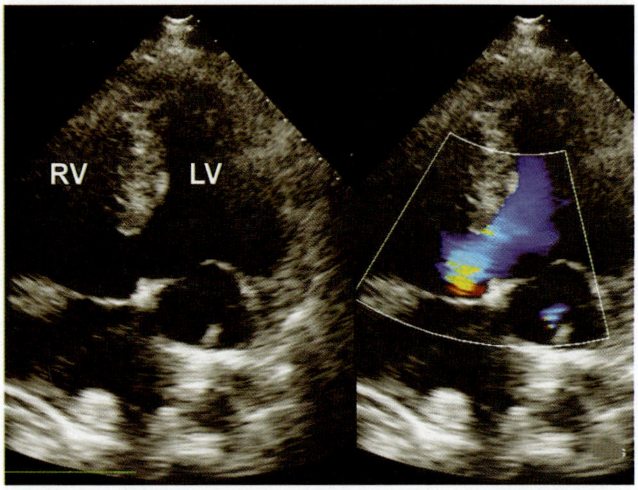

Fig. 237.3: Transthoracic apical 4-chamber view with color Doppler.

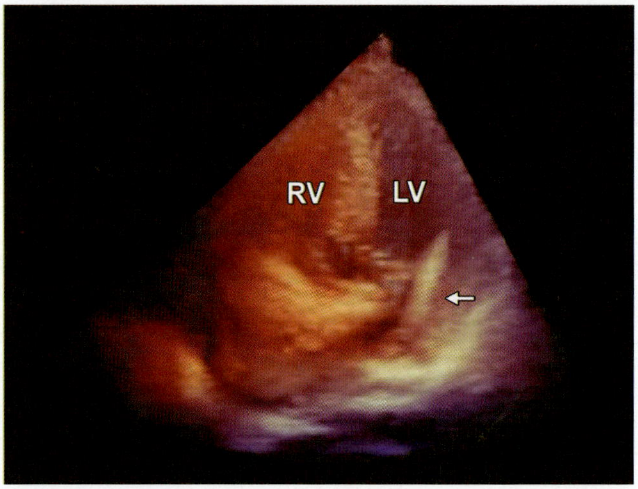

Fig. 237.4: 3D transthoracic 4-chamber view.

(b) Flail MV
(c) Left atrial thrombus
(d) Pacemaker wire
(e) Calcified mitral annulus

Ans. (d)

This patient has an AICD. The pacemaker wire was placed in the anatomic left ventricle because it is the sub-pulmonic ventricle.

4. **What is represented in the atrial area (arrows) in Figure 237.2 and 772?**
   A. Fontan origin
   B. Caval baffle
   C. Venous baffle
   D. Transplant suture lines

Ans. (b)

The caval baffle directs the inflow of the inferior vena cava and superior vena cava to the anatomic mitral valve so that it can enter the anatomic left ventricle and flow through the pulmonary artery.

5. **In Eisenmenger's syndrome, blood flow is usually described as flowing from right to left. In this complicated patient, how might the flow be described?**
   A. Anatomic left ventricle to anatomic right ventricle
   B. Pulmonary circuit ventricle to systemic circuit ventricle
   C. Sub-pulmonic ventricle to sub-aortic ventricle
   D. All of the above

Ans. (d)

Terminology in transposition of the great arteries, and with the atrial switch procedure can be confusing. After the atria are "switched", the left ventricle functions as the right ventricle, while the right ventricle functions as the left. The name of the left ventricle can be anatomic left ventricle, pulmonary venous ventricle, or sub-pulmonic ventricle. All are correct, but sub-pulmonic is probably the least confusing. For the right ventricle, its names are anatomic right ventricle, systemic ventricle and sub-aortic ventricle.

MOVIES 771 TO 777

CASE 238

Ahmad S Omran

TRANSPOSITION OF THE GREAT ARTERIES (D-TGA) WITH PREVIOUS MUSTARD/SENNING OPERATION

This 27-year-old woman with 35-week first time pregnancy presented to our center with acute pulmonary edema. Initial working diagnosis by ER physician was acute massive pulmonary embolism. The patient had a history of cardiac surgery in childhood in another center but no reports were available at the time of ER presentation. Transthoracic echocardiography (TTE) which was done in the ER was re-reviewed by a senior echocardiographer at the bedside. This changed the initial diagnosis and patient's management. In parasternal long-axis view (Fig. 238.1A and 778), severely dilated right ventricle (RV) was noted with reduced function. Left ventricle (LV) was small with normal contraction. Two great arteries were noted in this view positioned parallel to each other with the aorta arising from the RV and pulmonary artery from the LV. Slight tilting of the transducer, which is a necessary maneuver to establish the diagnosis of the transposition of the great arteries, visualized bifurcation of the main pulmonary artery (Fig. 238.1B). In the parasternal short axis view, the position of the 2 great arteries was better visualized with the aorta located anterior and to the right of the pulmonary artery indicative of transposition of the great arteries (D-TGA). In the short axis view, RV (systemic ventricle) function was reduced with EF about 30–40%, which explained the presentation of the patient with acute pulmonary edema (Figs. 238.2A and B, 779-781). Obtaining more detailed TTE views established the diagnosis of D-TGA with a previous Mustard/Senning operation and normally functioning atrial baffles with no leaks 782-784). The patient was diuresed and her pulmonary edema improved. Two days later, the patient delivered (by Cesarean section) a normal healthy baby. She was discharged home three days later in good general condition.

Follow-up visit after 2 month showed she was doing fine. TTE at follow-up study showed her systemic ventricular function was moderately reduced with EF about 30–40%. Her systemic A-V valve (tricuspid valve) showed severe tricuspid regurgitation (TR). SVC-IVC and pulmonary

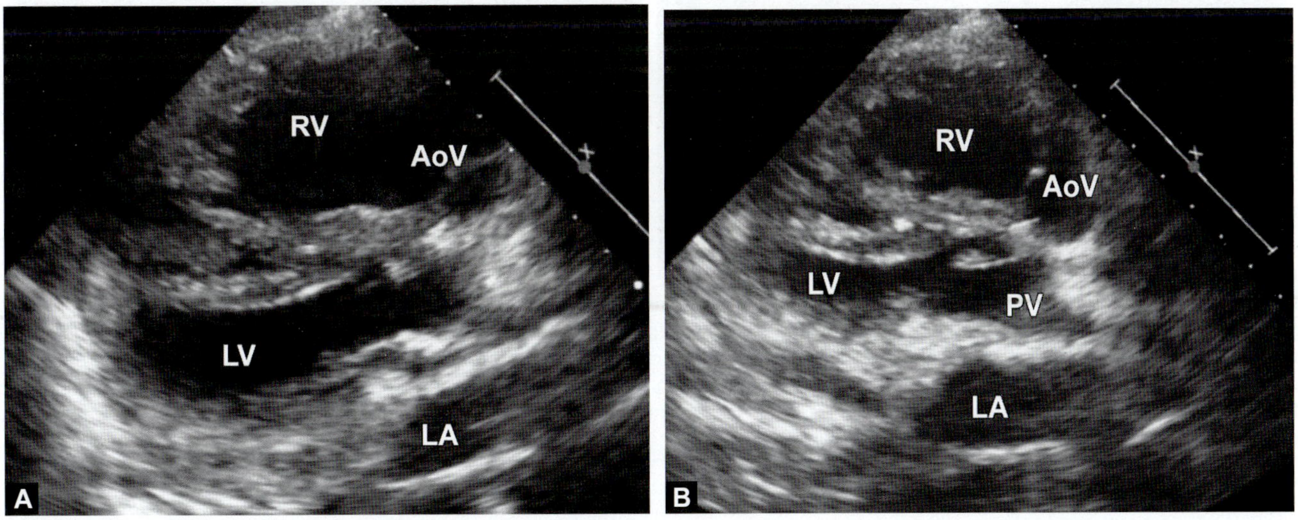

Figs. 238.1A and B: Transthoracic echocardiography (TTE). (A) Parasternal long-axis view showing a dilated RV and small LV. Two great arteries are running parallel to each other with the aorta arising from the RV and the pulmonary artery from the LV. (B) Previous view with slight tilting of the transducer toward the base of the heart, visualized the bifurcation of the main pulmonary artery. This maneuver is necessary to establish the diagnosis of the transposition of the great arteries (D-TGA and L-TGA). (RV: Right ventricle; LV: Left ventricle; LA: Left atrium; RA: Right atrium; AoV: Aortic valve; PV: Pulmonic valve).

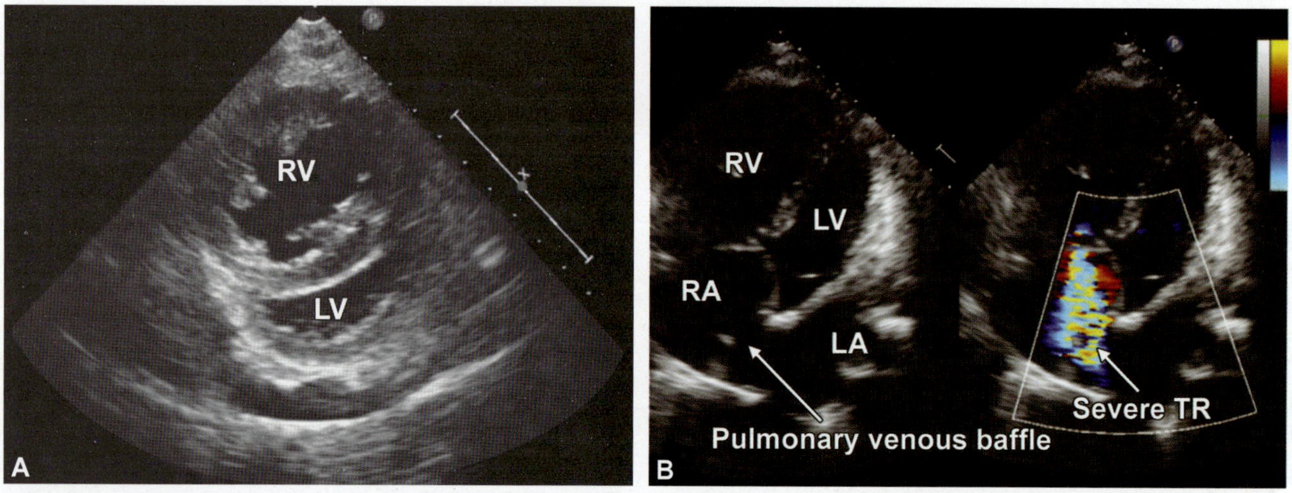

Figs. 238.2A and B: Transthoracic echocardiography (TTE). (A) Parasternal short-axis view showing a dilated (donut-shaped) RV with a thick wall, functioning as a systemic ventricle. LV is banana-shaped with a thin wall consistent with a functional venous ventricle. (B) Pulmonary venous baffle is shown directing oxygenated blood from pulmonary veins toward the right atrium. Severe tricuspid regurgitation (TR) is noted draining backward into the pulmonary baffle, which resulted in pulmonary congestion and pulmonary edema. (RV: Right ventricle; LV: Left ventricle; LA: Left atrium; RA: Right atrium).

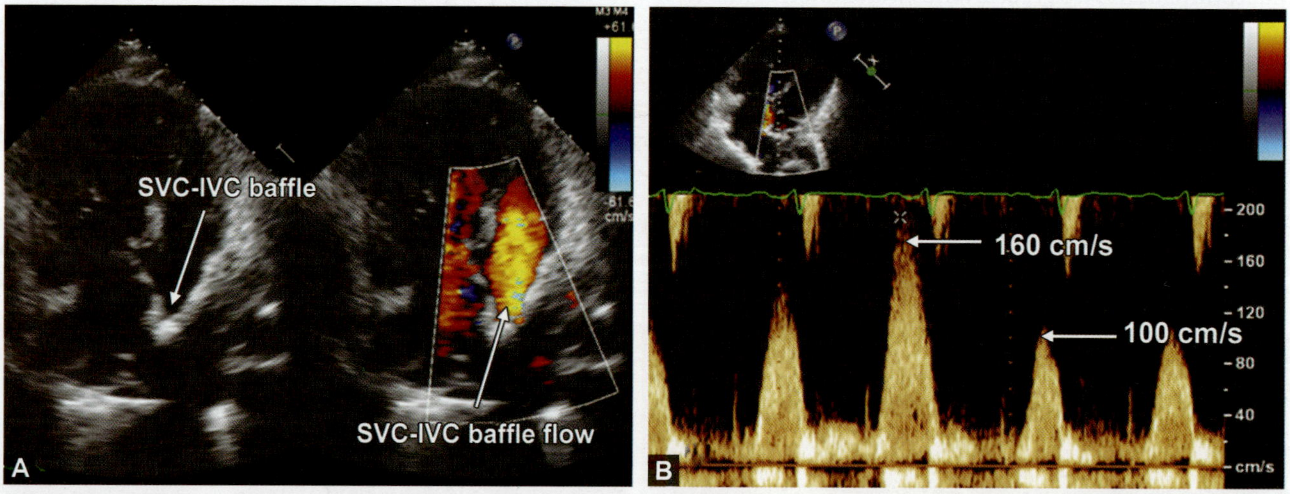

Figs. 238.3A and B: Transthoracic echocardiography (TTE) for assessment of SVC-IVC baffle. (A) Apical view with anterior angulation showing SVC-IVC baffle flow. Mild Doppler turbulence is seen. (B) Peak flow velocity by pulsed wave Doppler is 160 cm/s which is of at the upper limit normal for baffle flow. Baffle obstruction and kinking are recognized complications of the Mustard/Senning operation and may present with clinical manifestations. SVC-IVC baffle obstruction is more common in Mustard operation and may present with upper extremity edema and facial plethora. Pulmonary venous baffle obstruction is more common in Senning operation and may manifest with symptoms of reactive airway disease. (SVC: Superior vena cava; IVC: Inferior vena cava).

baffles were patent with laminar flows and acceptable velocities (Figs. 238.3A and B). Agitated saline contrast study was performed via a left arm vein, which showed no signs of IVC-SVC baffle leak (785). The patient was referred to our adult congenital heart disease clinic for further follow-up and counseling for future pregnancy.[1,2]

1. Pregnancy in all of the following adult congenital heart disease is high risk *except*:

(a) Severe pulmonary hypertension (Eisenmenger patients and others)
(b) Aortic root dilatation in Marfan's and similar syndromes
(c) Cyanosis (oxygen saturation is less than 90%)
(d) Poor systemic ventricular function (EF less than 40%)

Ans. (c)

MOVIE LEGENDS

778: Parasternal long-axis view showing a dilated RV, small LV and two parallel great arteries.

779: Parasternal short-axis view showing aortic valve anterior to the pulmonic valve.

780: Parasternal short-axis view showing dilated donut-shaped RV (functioning as a systemic ventricle) and banana-shaped LV (functioning as a venous ventricle). RV EF is estimated at 30–40%.

781: Apical 4-chamber view showing systemic ventricle (RV) with severe dilatation and severe RVH.

782: Apical 4-chamber view showing pulmonary venous baffle draining oxygenated blood from pulmonary vein in to the right atrium (atrial switch).

783: Apical 4-chamber view showing severe systemic A-V valve (morphologic TV) regurgitation. Regurgitant flow is seen moving backward inside the pulmonary baffle.

784: SVC-IVC baffle is visualized in this movie with mild turbulent flow. This baffle collects non-oxygenated blood from IVC and SVC and directs it to the LV to be pumped to the lungs and be oxygenated.

785: SVC-IVC baffle leak is uncommon but should be assessed at every long-term follow up visit of the patient. In this movie agitated saline contrast was injected in the left arm vein which opacified the left atrium and ventricle but no bubbles were seen in the right atrium or right ventricle. SVC-IVC baffle leak may present with mild cyanosis.

REFERENCE

1. Baumgartner H, Bonhoeffer P, De Groot NM, et al. ESC guidelines for the management of grown-up congenital heart disease. Eur Heart J. 2010;31(23):2915-57.

CASE 239

Salomon Rivera-Peralta, Nilda Espinola-Zavaleta, Hugo Rodriguez-Zanella, Jose Antonio Arias-Godinez, Maria Eugenia Ruiz-Esparza, Nydia Avila-Vanzzini, Juan Francisco Fritche-Salazar, Angel Romero-Cardenas

A 30-year-old man with a history of cyanosis since childhood presented to the outpatient clinic with shortness of breath and fatigue. In childhood the patient underwent a Blalock-Taussig shunt. Physical examination revealed cyanosis, clubbing of fingers and an apical systolic murmur. No diastolic murmur was heard. TTE was done.

1. **What is the diagnosis (Fig. 239.1 and 786)?**
   (a) Single ventricle
   (b) Tricuspid atresia
   (c) Tetralogy of Fallot
   (d) Hypoplastic right ventricle

Ans. (b)

2. **What other defects are associated with this lesion (Fig. 239.2 and 787)?**
   (a) Aortic stenosis
   (b) Pulmonary trunk aneurysm
   (c) Aortopulmonary window
   (d) Transposition of great arteries

Ans. (d)

Classical tricuspid atresia represents lack of tricuspid valve formation. Instead there is solid tissue between the right-sided chambers. The atrial septal defect (ASD) is an obligatory lesion to unload the blocked right atrium and allows mixing of blood from the right and left atria. Once the blood flows from the right atrium to the left atrium, the heart's left side must pump blood both to the rest of the body and to the lungs.

The most frequent associated heart defects are pulmonary valve stenosis and tansposition of the great arteries (TGA). Up to 20% of the patients have TGA. Tricuspid atresia is classified in 3 groups: type I: normally related great arteries, type II: D-transposition of the great arteries and type III with LTGA.[1,2]

Tricuspid atresia is uncommon in adult patients. In our adult patient the Blalock-Taussig shunt was closed and this caused deterioration of his New York functional class.

Abbreviations in figures and movies: TA, Tricuspid atresia; RA, Right atrium; RV, Right ventricle; VS, Ventricular septum; LA, Left atrium; LV, Left ventricle; LAA, Left atrial

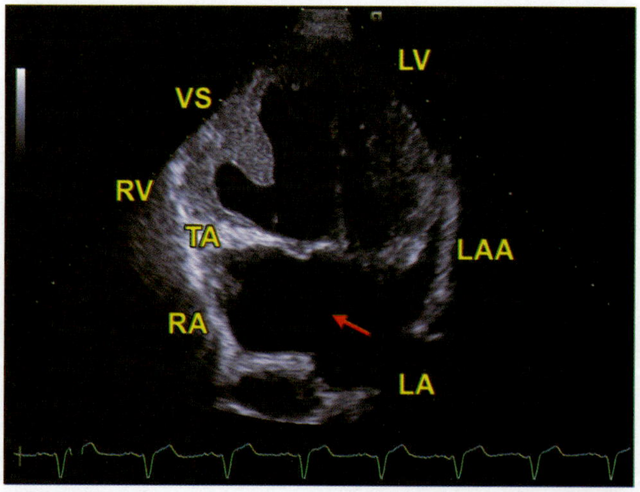

Fig. 239.1: Apical four-chamber view showing absence of right atrioventricular connection with atrial and ventricular septal defects. In the left atrium (LA), the let atrial appendage is seen. Arrow points to ASD.

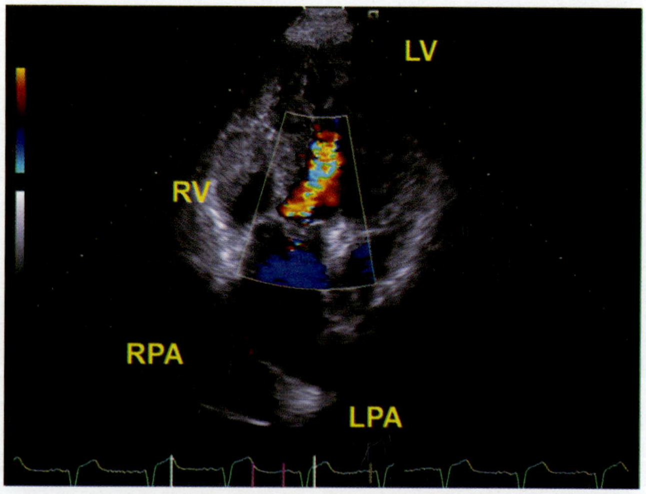

Fig. 239.2: Apical five chamber view. The vessel arising from the left ventricle is the pulmonary artery, because it bifurcates into its two branches (LPA and RPA). Pulmonary regurgitation was also noted. The pulmonary artery arises rightward and posterior to the aorta (D-transposition of great arteries).

appendage, RPA, Right pulmonary artery; LPA, Left pulmonary artery, PR, Pulmonary regurgitation; ASD, Atrial septal defect.

MOVIE LEGENDS

786: Apical four-chamber view showing absence of right atrioventricular connection with atrial and ventricular septal defects. The left atrial appendage is seen.

787: Apical five-chamber view. The vessel arising from the left ventricle is the pulmonary artery, because it bifurcates into its two branches. Pulmonary regurgitation was also noted. The pulmonary artery arises rightward and posterior to the aorta (D-transposition of great arteries).

REFERENCES

1. Tandon R, Edwards JE. Tricuspid atresia. A re-evaluation and classification. J Thorac Cardiovasc Surg. 1974;67:530-42.
2. Weinberg PM. Anatomy of tricuspid atresia and its relevance to currents forms of surgical therapy. Ann Thorac Surg. 1980;29:306-11.

CASE 240

Ahmad S Omran

CONGENITALLY CORRECTED TRANSPOSITION OF THE GREAT ARTERIES (L-TGA), TRICUSPID VALVE REPLACEMENT

This 23-year-old man presented to our center with progressive shortness of breath for the last 6 months. His past medical history was unremarkable. Transthoracic echocardiography (TTE) was done which showed findings of congenitally corrected transposition of the great arteries (L-TGA) with severe systemic A-V valve (tricuspid valve) regurgitation (Figs. 240.1A and B, 240.2A). No associated anomalies like ventricular septal defect (VSD) or pulmonary stenosis (PS) were noted. The mitral valve appeared normal. Systemic ventricular function (morphologic right ventricle) was reduced with RV EF about 30–35%. ECG showed no evidence of complete heart block or tachyarrhythmia. Transesophageal echocardiography (TEE) was performed which confirmed the diagnosis of L-TGA with apparent apical displacement of the tricuspid valve attachment (Fig. 240.2B and 788). Detailed 3D TEE assessment of the left sided A-V valve (TV) was performed which showed a trileaflet valve with 2 large cusps and one very small cusp. Morphology of the TV was thus a mixed configuration of the tricuspid and mitral valves (789–795). Due to severe TR and reduced systemic ventricular function, a decision was made to intervene surgically .

Surgical exploration of the tricuspid valve was performed via a left atriotomy (Figs. 240.3A and B). The tricuspid valve was found to be unrepairable and hence it was replaced with a mechanical valve (796). He was discharged home a week later in good general condition. Follow up visit after 5 years showed him doing fine with good functional capacity. TTE at follow-up showed a normally functioning mechanical systemic valve and a LVEF of about 35–40% (797).

Levo-transposition of the great arteries (L-TGA) is a rare form of congenital heart disease with a published incidence ranging from 0.02 to 0.07 per 1000 live births, accounting for less than 1 percent of congenital heart disease.[1] In patients with L-TGA, cardiac physiology is corrected, but the anatomy is not corrected (i.e. persistent

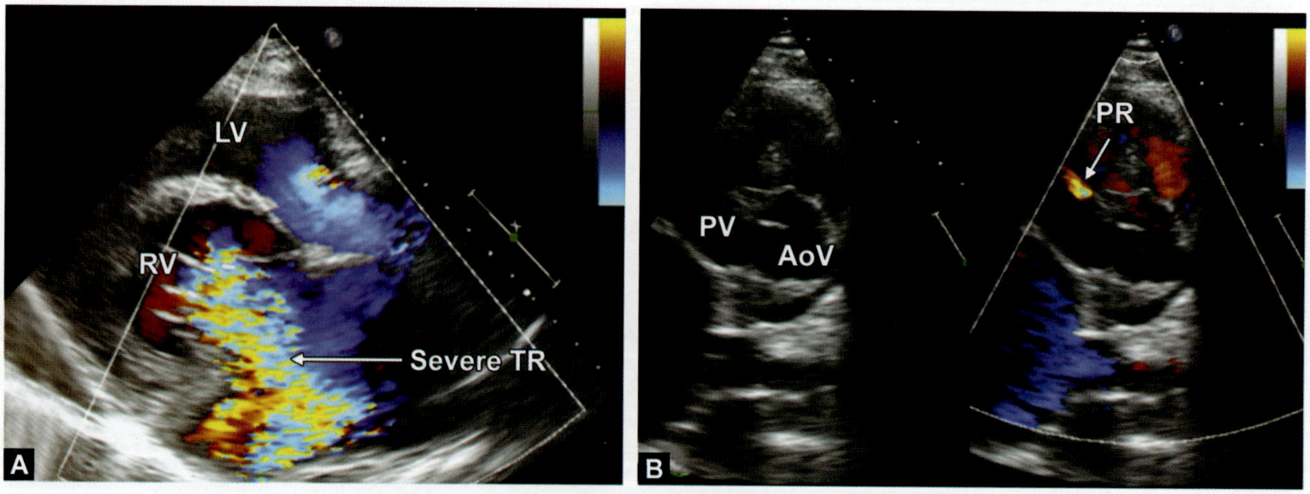

Figs. 240.1A and B: Transthoracic echocardiography (TTE). (A) Parasternal long-axis view showing a small LV at the top of the image and dilated RV at the bottom. Severe TR is seen. (B) Parasternal short-axis view of the great arteries showing aortic valve (AoV) located slightly anterior and to the left of the pulmonic valve (PV). There is a trace pulmonary regurgitation. (RV: Right ventricle; LV: Left ventricle; AoV: Aortic valve; PV: Pulmonic valve; PR: Pulmonary regurgitation).

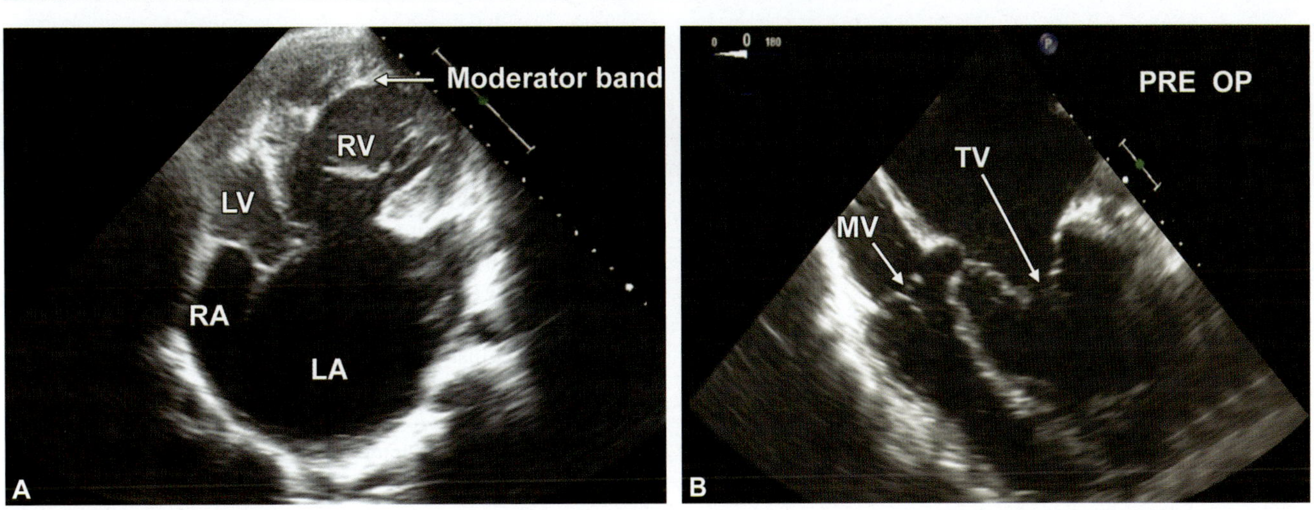

Figs. 240.2A and B: Transthoracic and transesophageal echocardiography (TTE and TEE). (A) TTE. Apical 4-chamber view showing morphologic right ventricle (RV) on the left side and morphologic left ventricle on the right side (LV). RV is dilated with hypertrabeculation and moderator band. Morphologic tricuspid valve (TV) is always connected to the RV and is working in this patient as a systemic A-V valve. Tricuspid valve shows apparent apical displacement. (B) TEE. Apical 4-chamber view showing same anatomy as TTE. Parasternal short-axis view showing a dilated (donut-shaped) RV with thick wall as a functionally systemic ventricle. LV is banana-shaped with a thin wall consistent with a venous ventricle. (LA: Left atrium; RA: Right atrium).

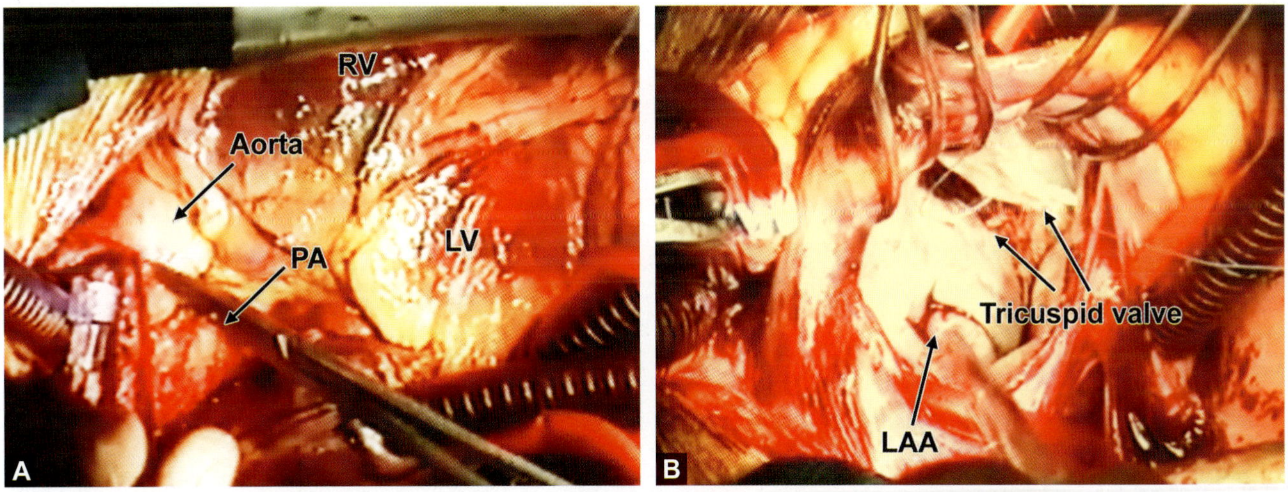

Figs. 240.3A and B: Surgical exploration. (A) Morphology of the heart prior to cardiopulmonary bypass. Aorta and pulmonary arteries are positioned side by side with aorta to the left and slightly anterior to the pulmonary artery. Aorta is connected to the right ventricle (RV) which is located anteriorly and on the left side of the chest. (B) Surgical inspection of the tricuspid valve through the left atrium shows 2 large leaflets and one very small cusp. Tricuspid valve was not repairable and had to be replaced by a mechanical valve.

atrioventricular and ventriculoarterial discordance). Another cardiac lesion is present in most cases of L-TGA (>90%). The associated lesion(s) generally determines the signs and symptoms at the time of presentation. Ventricular septal defect, pulmonary stenosis, tricuspid valve abnormalities, mitral valve abnormalities, and conduction abnormalities are the most common associated anomalies. Surgical management of patients includes tricuspid valve replacement, VSD or PS correction, pulmonary artery banding and double switch operation, and finally heart transplantation may need to be considered.[2]

1. **In echocardiographic assessment of patients with L-TGA all of the followings are correct *except*:**
   (a) An Ebstein-like malformation of the tricuspid valve has been reported in 20–50% of patients with L-TGA
   (b) Left ventricular outflow obstruction is the most common associated anomaly
   (c) VSD is seen in 70–80% of patients with L-TGA
   (d) Mitral valve abnormalities are less common than tricuspid valve but still can be seen in 50% of cases in autopsy series

Ans. (b)

MOVIE LEGENDS

788: Apical 4-chamber view showing severe TR.
789: 3D TEE full volume acquisition showing relationship of all 4 valves with each other in this case of L-TGA.
790: 3D TEE full volume acquisition of the tricuspid valve in surgical view.
791: 3D TEE full volume acquisition of the tricuspid valve from RV perspective.
792: 3D TEE full volume acquisition of the tricuspid valve with the color suppressed.
793: 3D TEE full volume acquisition showing severe TR.
794: 3D TEE full volume acquisition of the tricuspid valve in echo view (not surgical view). Aortic valve is located at the bottom of the image.
795: Same acquisition of previous movie viewing the tricuspid valve from RV side.
796: Tricuspid valve replacement with a mechanical valve.
797: Latest TEE at 5-year follow-up showed LV EF about 35–40%.

REFERENCES

1. Ferencz C, Rubin JD, McCarter RJ, et al. Congenital heart disease: prevalence at live birth. The Baltimore-Washington Infant Study. Am J Epidemiol. 1985;12:31.
2. Graham TP Jr., Bernard YD, Mellen BG, et al. Long-term outcome in congenitally corrected transposition of the great arteries: a multi-institutional study. J Am Coll Cardiol. 2000;36:255.

CASE 241

Mohamed Morsy, Patricia Rodriguez Lozano, Luba Frank, Shreyas Modi, Masood Ahmad

A 31-year-old African-American male with known uncorrected Tetralogy of Fallot and longstanding hypertension presented with gradually worsening dyspnea over a period of 6 months. His functional capacity on presentation was New York Heart Association (NYHA) class IV. At the time of hospitalization he also had an episode of syncope. Vital signs showed sinus tachycardia (103/minute), normal blood pressure (110/70 mm Hg), tachypnea (24/minute), and oxygen saturation of 83% to 88% which corrected to 92% by 100% oxygen via nonrebreather mask. Physical examination demonstrated clubbing in his fingers. There was no jugular venous distention, and cardiac examination revealed a 4/6 ejection systolic murmur in the second right intercostal space.

Electrocardiogram showed sinus tachycardia, right axis deviation, and right ventricular hypertrophy. Chest X-ray demonstrated cardiomegaly.

A 2-dimensional transthoracic echocardiogram was performed and the findings included a normal left ventricular size and function, a large nonrestrictive sub-aortic ventricular septal defect (VSD), and an overriding aorta without discrete flow across the VSD reflecting a balanced shunt. The right ventricle was moderately dilated, severely hypertrophied, and with mildly reduced systolic function. There was severe subpulmonic hypertrophy of the right ventricular outflow tract (RVOT) with mosaic color flow suggesting subpulmonic stenosis. Pulmonic valve appeared thickened and dystrophic with preserved systolic excursion. There was a peak systolic gradient of at least 81 mm Hg across the RVOT indicating a predominantly subpulmonic stenosis. Mild to moderate tricuspid regurgitation was present with right ventricular systolic pressure (RVSP) estimated at 100 mm Hg. The findings were consistent with Tetralogy of Fallot with a large subaortic VSD, and severe RVOT obstruction with a high RVSP (Figs. 241.1A to D and 241.2, 798 and 799). These findings were confirmed by a transesophageal echocardiogram (Figs. 241.3A to D, 800–802).

Cardiac magnetic resonance images (MRI) showed a dilated and a severely hypertrophied right ventricle involving the RVOT with significant narrowing. A large subaortic VSD was identified at the level of both outflow tracts measuring approximately 2.5 cm. There was no jet identified through the defect, likely due to its large size, bidirectional flow, or balanced flow. The aorta was overriding the VSD and received biventricular flow. The RVOT was markedly narrowed, measuring approximately 11 mm, with a high velocity jet of at least 250–300 cm/s. Pulmonary valve leaflets were thickened with limited mobility. Pulmonary trunk (PA) measured approximately 2.6 cm, right pulmonary artery measured 1.7 cm proximally and the left pulmonary artery measured 2.3 cm. The constellation of findings were compatible with unrepaired Tetralogy of Fallot (Figs. 241.4A and B).

Right heart catheterization was performed and showed a mean right atrial pressure of 9 mm Hg, RV 96/9 mm Hg, PA 16/9 mm Hg (mean PA 13 mm Hg), mean pulmonary capillary wedge pressure of 5 mm Hg, cardiac output by Fick 4.34 L/min and by Thermal 4.2 L/min with corresponding cardiac indices of 2.26 and 2.2 L/min/m^2, and a transpulmonary gradient of 8 mm Hg with pulmonary vascular resistance of 2 Woods Units. Percent oxygen saturations were 91 in aorta, 55 in superior vena cava, and 64 in right atrium and right ventricle. Pulmonary artery could not be sampled.

Patient underwent successful surgical repair of the VSD, RVOT and the tricuspid valve. Pulmonary valve was replaced with a porcine valve and the aortic valve was reimplanted.

1. **All of the following are features of Tetralogy of Fallot *except*:**
   - (a) Right ventricular hypertrophy
   - (b) Ventricular septal defect
   - (c) Overriding aorta
   - (d) Pulmonic stenosis due to anterior deviation of the infundibular septum
   - (e) Pulmonic stenosis due to posterior deviation of the infundibular septum

Ans. (e)

Choices (a), (b), (c), (d) and (e) are correct. Pulmonic stenosis in Tetralogy of Fallot is due to anterior deviation of the infundibular septum and not as a result of posterior deviation.[1]

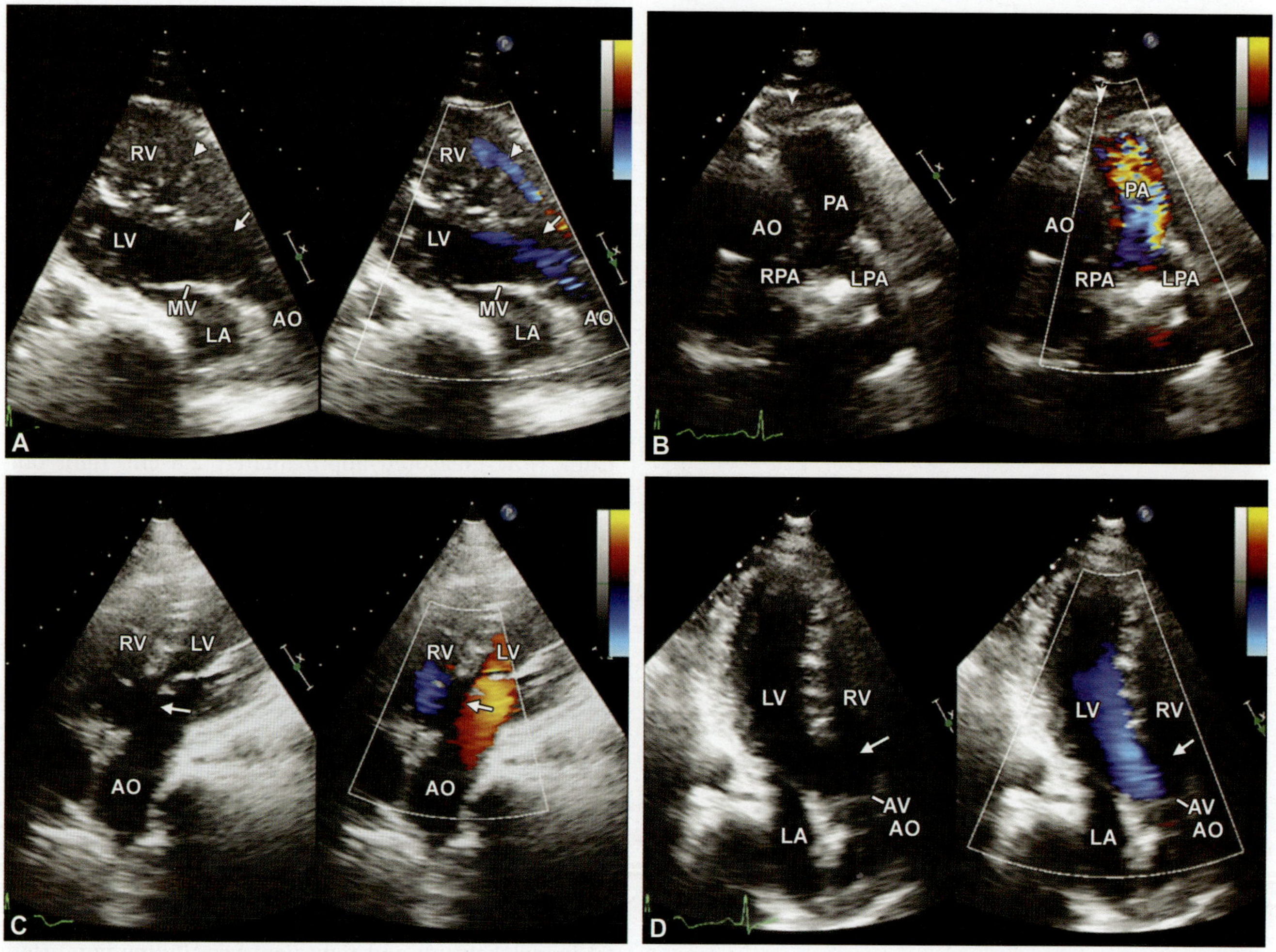

Figs. 241.1A to D: Transthoracic echocardiogram showing parasternal long-axis view (A), short-axis (B), modified apical 4 chamber (C) and apical 3 chamber (D) views with and without color flow. (RV: Right ventricle; LV: Left ventricle; AO: Aorta; PA: Pulmonary artery; RPA: Right pulmonary artery; LPA: Left pulmonary artery; LA: Left atrium; MV: Mitral valve; AV: Aortic valve). Arrows point to the subaortic VSD in A, C, and D. Arrowheads point to the hypertrophied right ventricular outflow tract with subpulmonic stenosis in A and B.

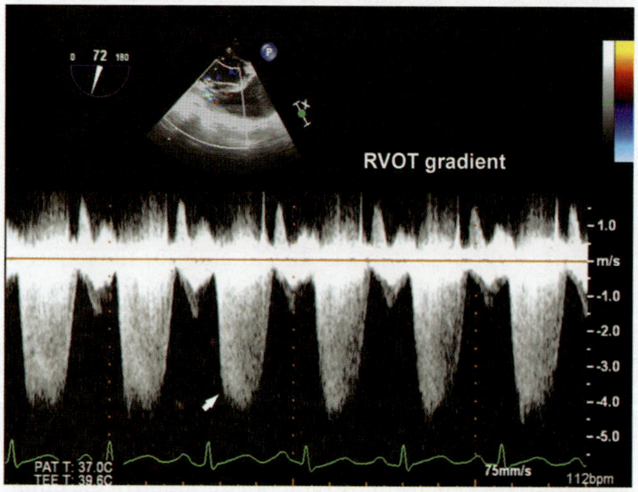

Fig. 241.2: Continuous wave Doppler across the right ventricular outflow tract with a systolic gradient of 81 mm Hg (arrow).

2. **All of the following are anomalies associated with Tetralogy of Fallot *except*:**
   (a) Right aortic arch
   (b) Atrial septal defect
   (c) Absent tricuspid valve
   (d) Coronary anomalies

Ans. (c)

Choices (a), (b) and (d) are correct. Tetralogy is rarely associated with absent pulmonic valve. However, absent tricuspid valve is not an anomaly associated with Tetralogy.[1]

3. **A major long-term post-operative complication of Tetralogy of Fallot is:**
   (a) Pulmonic insufficiency
   (b) Tricuspid insufficiency
   (c) Aortic insufficiency
   (d) Mitral insufficiency

Ans. (a)

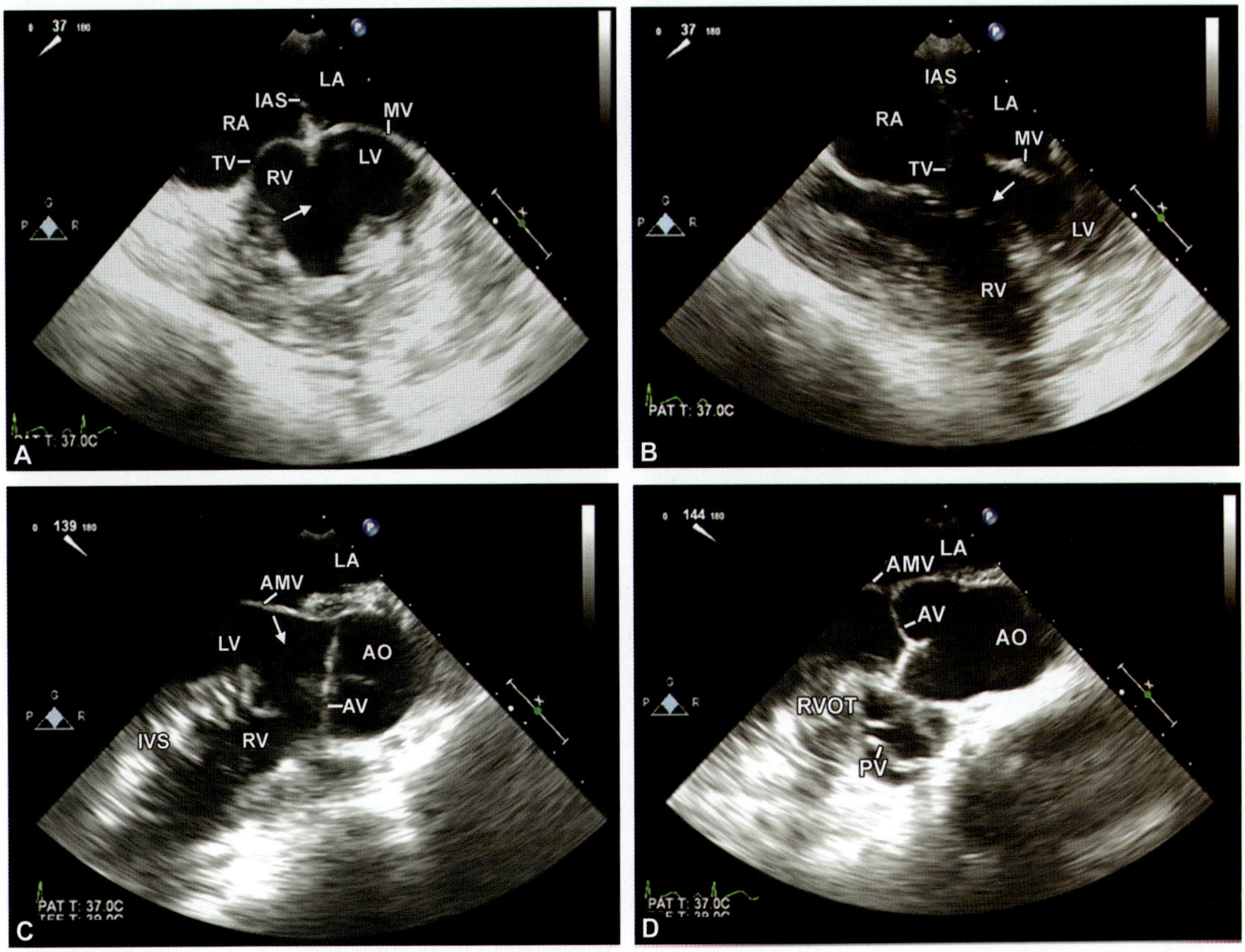

Figs. 241.3A to D: Transesophageal echocardiogram showing midesophageal short-axis views in systole (A) and diastole (B) and long-axis views in (C) and (D). (RA: Right atrium; LA: Left atrium; IAS: Inter-atrial septum; TV: Tricuspid valve; MV: Mitral valve; AV: Aortic valve; RV: Right ventricle; LV: Left ventricle; LA: Left atrium; IVS: Inter-ventricular septum; AO: Aortic valve; AMV: Anterior mitral valve; RVOT: Right ventricular outflow tract; PV: Pulmonic valve). Arrows point to the subaortic VSD.

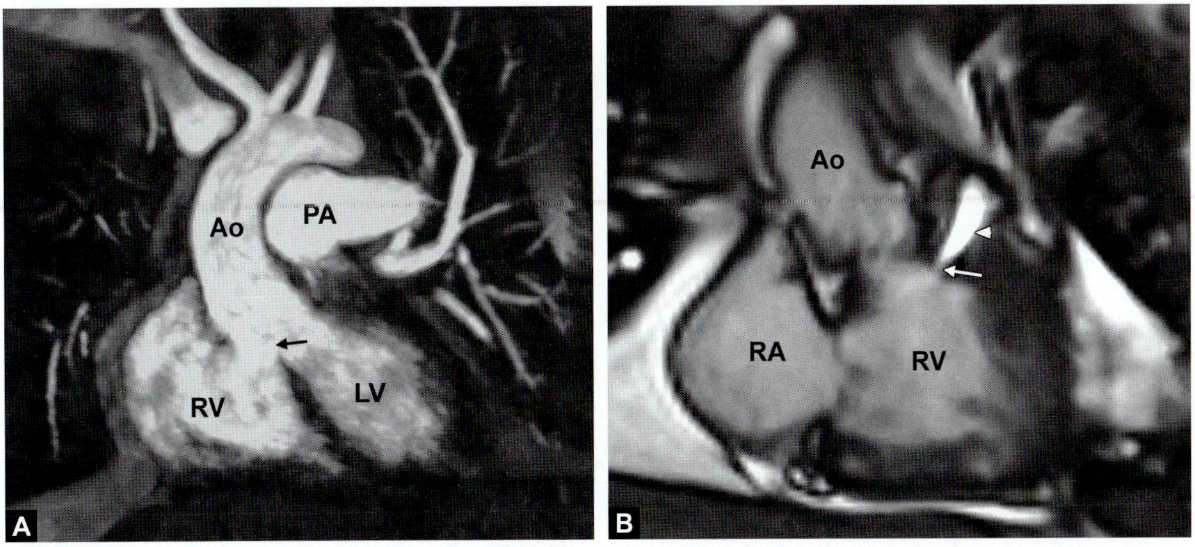

Figs. 241.4A and B: Cardiac magnetic resonance images (MRI). Coronal maximum intensity projection (A) and Coronal steady state free precession (B) views. (RV: Right ventricle; LV: Left ventricle; RA: Right atrium; AO: Aorta; PA: Pulmonary artery). Arrow points to the subaortic VSD in A and subpulmonic stenosis in B. Arrowhead shows a high velocity jet across the right ventricular outflow tract.

Choices (b to d) are not correct. Severe pulmonic insufficiency with progressive right ventricular failure are major long term issues in patients with surgically corrected Tetralogy of Fallot.[1]

4. Congenital heart defects following maternal rubella include all of the following *except*:

(a) Patent ductus arteriosus
(b) Pulmonic stenosis
(c) Tetralogy of Fallot
(d) Tricuspid atresia
(e) Atrial septal defect

Ans. (d)

Choices (a), (b), (c) and (e) are correct. Tetralogy of Fallot may occur in patients with maternal rubella syndrome. Tricuspid atresia is not known to be associated with maternal rubella.[1]

MOVIE LEGENDS

798: Transthoracic echocardiogram, parasternal long-axis view showing subaortic VSD and the hypertrophic RV outflow tract. Movie starts with a labeled still frame shown in Figure 241.1A.

799: Transthoracic echocardiogram, modified apical 3 chamber view showing the subaortic VSD. Movie starts with a labeled still frame shown in Figure 241.1D.

800: Transesophageal echocardiogram, midesophageal short axis views of the subaortic VSD. Movie starts with labeled still frames shown in Figures 241.3A and B.

801: Transesophageal echocardiogram, long-axis views of the subaortic VSD. Movie starts with a labeled still frame shown in Figure 241.3C.

802: Transesophageal echocardiogram, long-axis view of the right ventricular outflow tract and the pulmonic valve. Movie starts with a labeled still frame shown in Figure 241.3D.

REFERENCE

1. Villafañe J, Feinstein JA, Jenkins KJ, et al. Hot topics in tetralogy of fallot. Journal of American College of Cardiology (JACC). 2013;62(23):2155-66.

CASE 242

Hugo Zanella, Nilda Espinola-Zavaleta, Salomon Rivera-Peralta, Jose Antonio Arias-Godinez, Nydia Avila-Vanzzini, Maria Eugenia Ruiz-Esparza, Juan Francisco Fritche

A 24-year-old female came to the emergency department of our institution because of light headedness and dizziness. She had history of congenital heart disease corrected surgically when she was 2-year-old. After surgery she was asymptomatic till now.

On physical examination the vital signs were normal and a loud diastolic murmur was best heard at the left upper sternal border. Chest X-ray showed cardiomegaly. An echocardiogram was performed and the images are shown below.

1. **Which abnormalities are identified in this parasternal long-axis view (Fig. 242.1)?**
   (a) Flail mitral valve
   (b) Left ventricular enlargement and hypertrophy
   (c) Left atrial enlargement and mitral valve disease
   (d) Increased echogenicity in the interventricular septum

Ans. (d) (Fig. 242.1)

This patient had right ventricular enlargement with right ventricular outflow tract diameter of 40 mm and the ventricular septum showed increased echogenicity corresponding to surgical closure by patch (red arrow).

2. **What is the most likely cause of the murmur heard at the left upper sternal border?**
   (a) Aortic regurgitation
   (b) Residual ventricular septal defect
   (c) Pulmonary regurgitation
   (d) Tricuspid stenosis

Ans. (c) (Fig. 242.2, 803 and 804)

Patients with tetralogy of Fallot (ToF) who had been surgically repaired often present with pulmonary regurgitation (PR) during late follow-up. The presence of severe PR heralds a worse prognosis due to its impact on right ventricular volume eventually causing right ventricular dysfunction. This patient subset has an increased risk of heart failure, arrhythmia and sudden death.[1,2]

The echocardiogram revealed a dilated right ventricle (RV) with normal right ventricular function (TAPSE 22 mm, Tricuspid S' wave 11 cm/s, RVFAC 40%, RVEF by 3D echo 46%). Free PR is shown in the short-axis view at the level of great vessels.

On close examination a unicuspid pulmonary valve was identified, which was clearly defined by 3D views of the pulmonary valve (arrow, Figs. 242.3 and 242.4, 805 and 806).

2. **How should this patient be managed?**
   (a) Medical treatment
   (b) Follow-up until patient becomes symptomatic

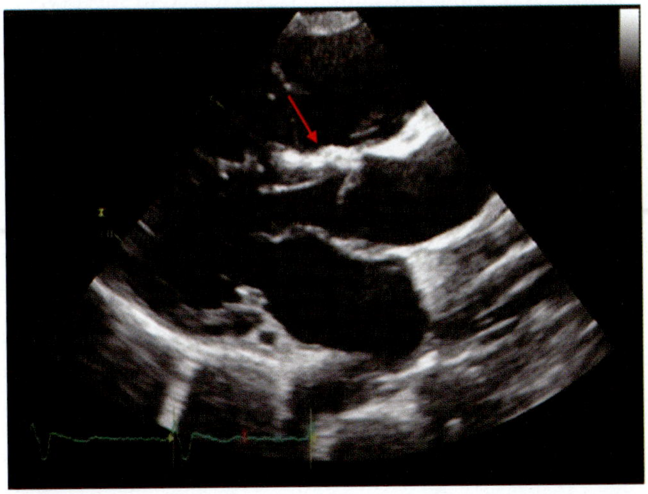

Fig. 242.1: Parasternal long axis view showing an increased echogenicity (red arrow) in the site of surgical closure of ventricular septal defect by patch.

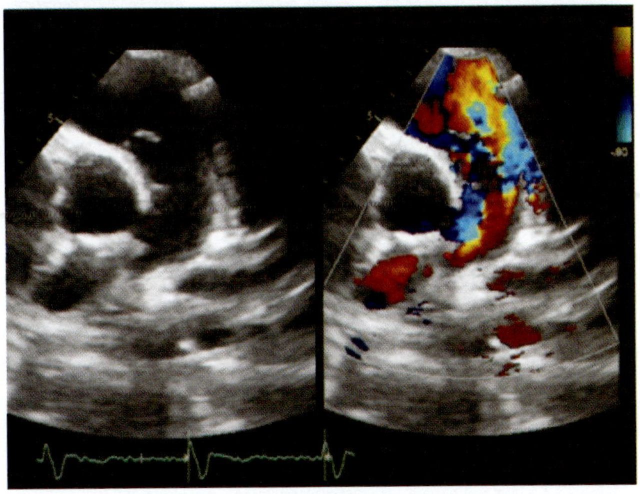

Fig. 242.2: Parasternal short axis bidimensional and color flow views at the level of great arteries with severe pulmonary regurgitation.

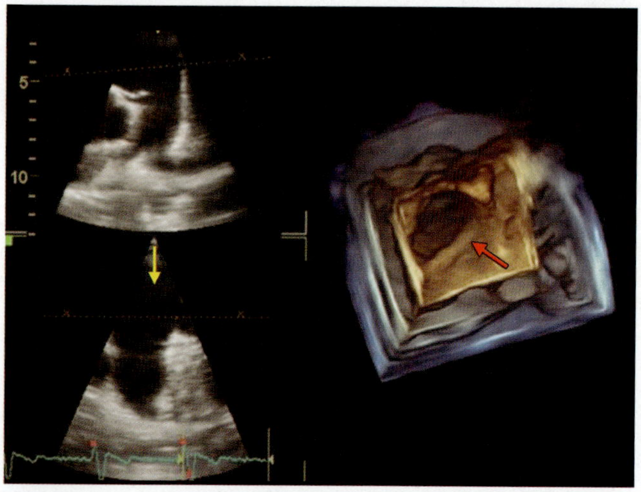

Fig. 242.3: A unicuspid pulmonary valve was found by 3D TTE view of the pulmonary valve (red arrow).

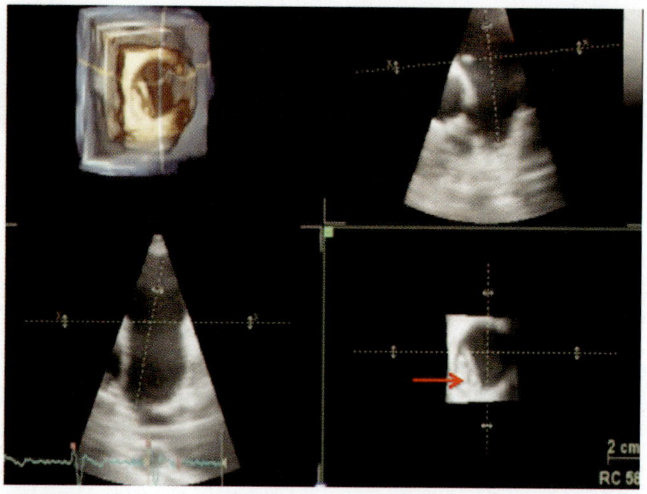

Fig. 242.4: The red arrow shows a unicuspid pulmonary valve clearly defined by 3D TTE.

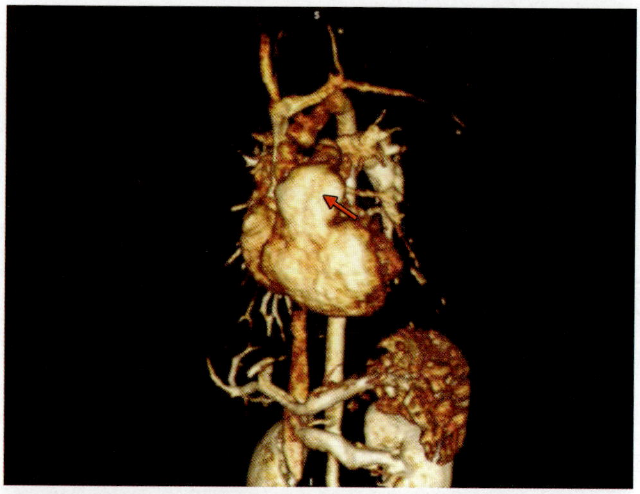

Fig. 242.5: CMRI showed pulmonary artery dilation (red wrrow).

(c) RV volumes should be evaluated by cardiac magnetic resonance imaging (CMRI)
(d) Patient should be referred for pulmonary valve replacement

Ans. (c)

Pulmonary regurgitation is not uncommon in operated patients with ToF. Their prognostic implications have been previously defined, however the optimal time for surgical correction in these patients is controversial. Current guidelines recommend surgery in asymptomatic patients with progressive RV dilation in order to prevent irreversible RV dysfunction. Pulmonary valve replacement (PVR) in patients with RV end-systolic volume (ESV) <80 mL/m^2 SC has been associated with RV normalization in contrast to patients with RV ESV > 95 mL/m^2 SC, who are at increased risk for RV dilation, dysfunction and adverse clinical outcome.[3] This suggests that the optimal time for PVR is triggered by increasing RV volume with a cut off of 80 mL/m^2 SC. This study measured RV volumes using CMRI, but the cost and availability of this technique forced us to explore the role of 3D echocardiography. However, thresholds are not yet interchangeable because 3D echocardiography underestimates RV volumes when compared to CMRI.

CMRI was performed, angiographic sequence showed pulmonary artery dilation (red arrow, Fig. 242.5). Right ventricular volumes were quantified, ESV was 90 mL/m^2 SC and RVEF 40%. The patient was referred to surgery.

MOVIES 803 TO 806

REFERENCES

1. Gatzoulis MA, Balaji S, Webber SA, et al. Risk factors for arrhythmia and sudden cardiac death late after repair of tetralogy of Fallot: a multicentre study. Lancet. 2000;356: 975-81.
2. Knauth AL, Gauvreau K, Powell AJ, et al. Ventricular size and function assessed by cardiac MRI predict major adverse clinical outcomes late after tetralogy of Fallot repair. Heart. 2008;94:211-16.
3. Bokma JP, Winter MM, Oosterhof T, Vliegen HW, et al. Preoperative thresholds for mid to late haemodynamic and clinical outcomes after pulmonary valve replacement in tetralogy of Fallot. Eur Heart J. 2015 Oct 27. pii: ehv550. [Epub ahead of print]

CASE 243

Leo Laura Anna, Murzilli Romina, Faletra Francesco

A 62-year-old woman with systolic heart murmur was referred to our institution to perform transesophageal echocardiography (TEE) for refining the diagnosis before surgery. 2D transthoracic echocardiography showed mitral valve prolapse (P2) with severe regurgitation.

1. **2D/3D TEE shows (Figs. 243.1A to C and 807):**
   (a) Mitral valve prolapse and paravalvular abscess
   (b) Mitral valve prolapse and suspected coronary anomaly
   (c) Rare congenital mitral valve anomaly
   (d) Rare congenital aortic valve anomaly
   (e) Other

Ans. (b)

2D/3D TEE shows mitral valve prolapse (P2 and P3, Figs. 243.1A and C 807) with severe regurgitation and suspected abnormal origin of a coronary artery with retroaortic course (Figs. 243.1A to C, arrow at the level of mitral-aortic continuity). Coronary angiography confirmed the abnormal origin of the circumflex coronary artery from the right sinus of Valsalva (Fig. 243.2 and 808).

Coronary artery anomalies have been identified in 0.6 to 1.5% of coronary angiograms.[1,2] An anomalous origin of the left circumflex coronary artery (LCX) from the proximal right coronary artery (RCA) or right sinus of Valsalva is a relatively common anatomical variation. It was first described by Antopol and Kugel in 1933[3] and is the most common congenital coronary variant, with prevalence at coronary angiography of 0.18–0.67%.[2,4-7] It is usually considered "benign"[8,9] since it is not known to predispose individuals to sudden cardiac death. However, due to the acute angulation of its origin from the aorta and its posterior retroaortic course, some have proposed an increase in coronary artery disease (CAD) in these aberrant vessels.[10]

Recognition and adequate visualization of the coronary anomaly with angiography are essential for proper patient management, especially in patients undergoing evaluation for percutaneous coronary intervention, coronary artery surgery or prosthetic valve replacement.[11]

However, the 3-dimensional course of a coronary anomaly is difficult to delineate by angiography, but non-invasive diagnostic modalities may be helpful. Multislice computed tomography (MSCT) allows accurate and non-invasive detection of coronary artery anomalies, displaying origin, size, course and relationship with surrounding structures (Fig. 243.3).[12,13]

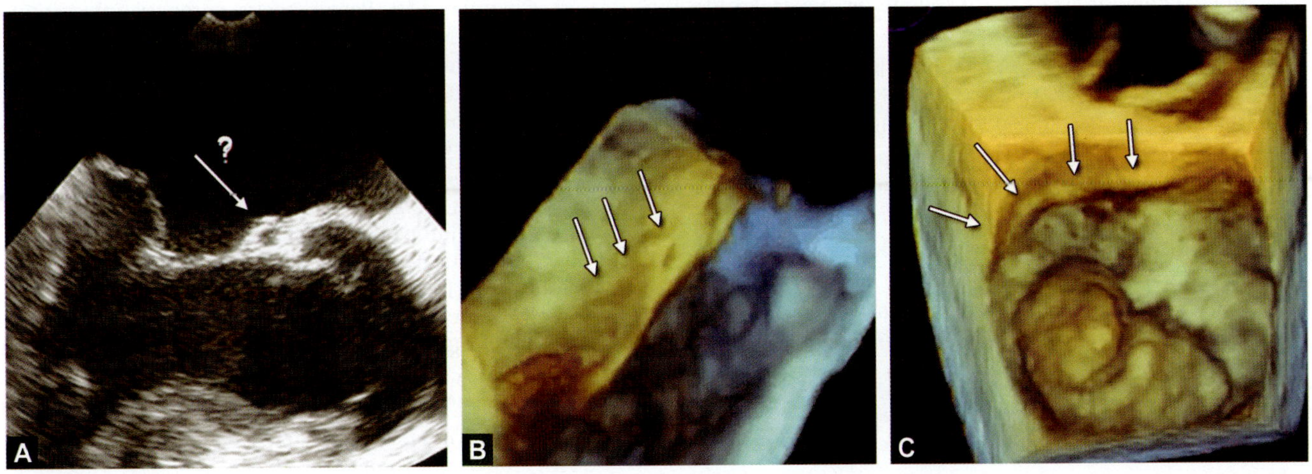

Figs. 243.1A to C: Transesophageal echocardiography, 2D long axis view (A), 3D long axis (B) and short axis view (C). It shows mitral valve prolapse (P2-P3) and suspected abnormal origin of a coronary artery with retroaortic course (arrows).

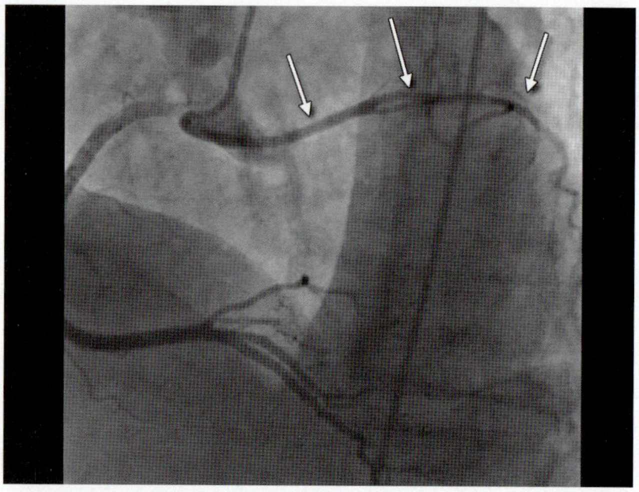

Fig. 243.2: Coronary angiography shows abnormal origin of circumflex coronary artery (arrows) from the right sinus of Valsalva.

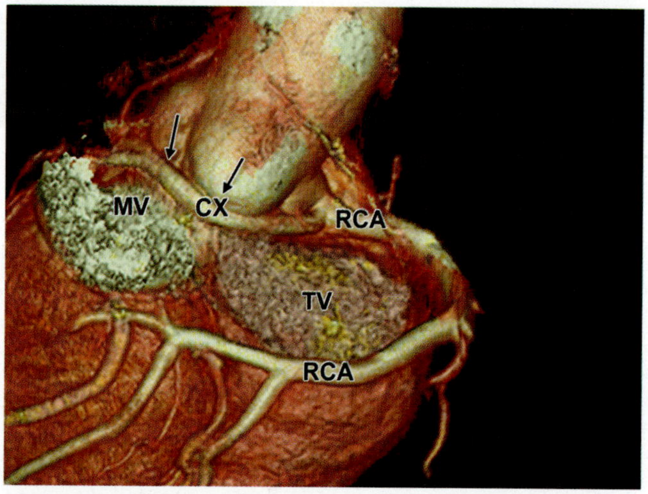

Fig. 243.3: Coronary computed tomography angiography with abnormal origin of circumflex coronary artery (CX) from right coronary artery (RCA), with retroaortic course. Mitral valve (MV). Tricuspid valve (TV).

MOVIE LEGENDS

807 and 808: 2D transesophageal echocardiography long axis view (807) with mitral prolapse (arrowhead) and suspected abnormal origin of circumflex coronary artery (arrow) confirmed by coronary angiography (808).

REFERENCES

1. Yamanaka O, Hobbs RE. Coronary artery anomalies in 126,595 patients undergoing coronary arteriography. Cathet Cardiovasc Diagn. 1990;21:28-40.
2. Wilkins CE, Betancourt B, Mathur VS, et al. Coronary artery anomalies: a review of more than 10,000 patients from the Clayton Cardiovascular Laboratories. Tex Heart Inst J. 1988;15:166-73.
3. Antopol W, Kugel MA. Anomalous origin of the left circumflex coronary artery. Am Heart J. 1933;8:802-6.
4. Harry L, Page HL, Engel HJ, Campbell WB, Thomas CS. Anomalous origin of the left circumflex coronary artery: recognition, angiographic demonstration and clinical significance. Circulation. 1974;50(4):768-73.
5. Click RL, Holmes DR, Vlietstra RE, Kosinski AS, Kronmal RA. Anomalous coronary arteries: location, degree of atherosclerosis and effect on survival—a report from the coronary artery surgery study. J Am Coll Cardiol. 1989;13(3): 531-7.
6. Liberthson RR, Dinsmore RE, Bharati S, et al. Aberrant coronary artery origin from the aorta: diagnosis and clinical significance. Circulation. 1974;50(4):774-9.
7. Kardos A, Babai L, Rudas L, et al. Epidemiology of congenital coronary anomalies: a coronary arteriography study on a central European population. Cathet Cardiovasc Diagn. 1997;42(3):270-5.
8. Samarendra P, Kumari S, Hafeez M, Vasavada BC, Sacchi TJ. Anomalous circumflex coronary artery: benign or predisposed to selective atherosclerosis. Angiology. 2001; 52(8):521-6.
9. Mohsen GA, Mohsin KG, Forsberg M, Miller E, Taniuchi M, Klein JPA: Anomalous left circumflex artery from the right coronary cusp: a benign variant? J Invasive Cardiol. 2013;25(6):284-87.
10. West N EJ, McKenna CJ, Ormerod O, Forfar JC, Banning AP, Channon KM. Percutaneous coronary intervention with stent deployment in anomalously-arising left circumflex coronary arteries. Catheter Cardiovasc Interv. 2006;68(6):882-90.
11. Hendiri T, Alibegovic J, Bonvini RF, Camenzind E. Successful angioplasty of an occluded aberrant coronary artery: a rare cause of acute myocardial infarction. Acute Card Care. 2006;8:125-7.
12. Angelini P. Coronary anomalies. Incidence, pathophysiology, and clinical relevance. Circulation. 2002;105:2449-54.
13. Kim SY, Seo JB, Do KH, et al. Coronary artery anomalies: classification and ECG-gated multidetector row CT findings with angiographic correlation. Radiographics. 2006; 26:317-33.

CASE 244

Arisha MJ, Mohamed AH, Elkaryoni A, Barssoum K, Mohamed A, Ibrahim D, Tageldin M, Gupta N, Nanda NC

The patient is a 66-year-old asymptomatic female with a pansystolic murmur audible in the left parasternal region. 2DTTE was done.

1. **What is the aortic short axis view (809) consistent with?**
   (a) Perimembranous VSD
   (b) Turbulent flow signals in the RV
   (c) Normal RV flow in a patient with hyperkinetic RV
   (d) I know the answer but I do not want to tell anybody

Ans. (b)

Turbulent flow signals (arrow) are seen some distance away from the TV. Hence, they are not due to a perimembranous VSD which would be adjacent to the TV. The etiology of these signals is not clear but they could be emanating from a VSD located in another part of the VS not visualized in this view.

2. **What does 810 demonstrate (modified four-chamber view)?**
   (a) Trabecular (muscular) VSD with L to R shunt
   (b) VS rupture with tremendous flow into the RV
   (c) The flow signals represent a color Doppler artifact and not a true VSD
   (d) Do not show me complicated congenital heart disease cases, they make me nervous.

Ans. (a)

The defect with L to R shunt (arrow) is clearly seen in the muscular or trabecular portion of the VS. 811A is an apical four-chamber view which does not show the defect emphasizing the need to meticulously interrogate non-standard off axis views also. In addition, the color Doppler should be turned on during examination, otherwise a small VSD like in this patient can be missed (see left panel without color Doppler in 810). Color Doppler-guided continuous wave Doppler (811B) shows very high velocity systolic signals suggesting that the PA systolic pressure is not high in this elderly patient with a small restrictive VSD.

MOVIES 809 TO 811

CASE 245

Aditi Naniwadekar, Olayinka Afolabi-Brown, Aman Amanullah

ECHOCARDIOGRAPHIC DIAGNOSIS OF A RARE CARDIAC ANOMALY

A 55-year-old female with past medical history of hypertension presented to the hospital with complaints of fever, productive cough, shortness of breath (SOB), and chest pain for 5 days. On physical examination, she was hypoxic with an oxygen saturation of 80% on room air and febrile with a temperature of 38.3°C. Her blood pressure was 100/70 mm Hg with a heart rate of 100/min and respiratory rate of 30/min.

Cardiovascular exam revealed normal 1st and 2nd heart sounds and without a murmur or gallop. There was no evidence of jugular venous distension or lower extremity edema. Lung exam revealed bilateral rhonchi.

The chest X-ray and electrocardiogram at the time of presentation are shown in Figures 245.1 and 245.2 respectively.

Echocardiography was performed after 1 week of treatment for pneumonia because of persistent hypoxemia (Figs. 245.3 to 245.5 and 812 to 815).

1. What is the most likely diagnosis?

(a) Patent ductus arteriosus
(b) Right ventricular pseudoaneurysm
(c) Sinus of valsalva aneurysm
(d) Anomalous origin of the right coronary artery from the pulmonary artery (ARCAPA)

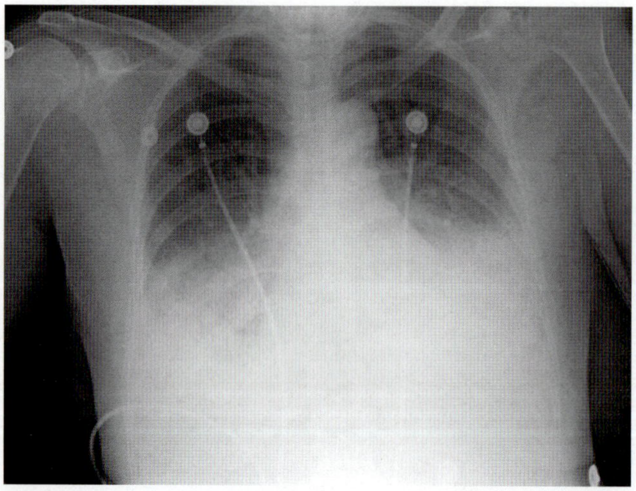

Fig. 245.1: Chest X-ray showing pulmonary edema and bilateral pleural effusions suggestive of congestive heart failure.

Ans. (d)

Coronary arteries normally arise from the sinuses of Valsalva of the aorta. The incidence of abnormal aortic origin of the coronary arteries has been reported to be approximately 0.64% of births.[1] Four variations of this condition have been described: origin of the left coronary artery from the pulmonary artery (ALCAPA), origin of the right coronary artery from the pulmonary artery (ARCAPA), origin of an accessory coronary artery from the pulmonary artery, and origin of the entire coronary circulation from the pulmonary artery.[2] First described in 1852, anomalous right coronary artery from the pulmonary artery (ARCAPA) has a reported incidence of only 0.002%. The true prevalence of ARCAPA is likely underestimated, as most patients are asymptomatic. Only 25–30% cases of ARCAPA are associated with structural heart defects. The most common associated cardiac defects reported were tetralogy of Fallot and aortopulmonary window, followed by aortic stenosis, septal defects and aortic coarctation.[3]

Typical echocardiographic findings in ARCAPA include:

a. Intercoronary collaterals within the ventricular septum and free wall visualized by color-flow Doppler imaging
b. Dilated left and right coronary arteries
c. Anomalous origin of the right coronary artery (RCA), with retrograde flow from the RCA into the main pulmonary artery.

Pathophysiology of ARCAPA is well-established. It is well tolerated in the neonatal period as high neonatal pulmonary vascular resistance allows forward perfusion of the abnormal coronary artery from the pulmonary artery. Once the pulmonary vascular resistance falls after birth, the fully oxygenated blood arrives in the anomalous coronary, via collateral vessels from the normally arising coronary. The pulmonary trunk steals this oxygenated blood which results in chronic myocardial ischemia. The degree of collateralization determines outcome as adequate collateralization may maintain adequate myocardial perfusion. Ventricular dilatation and dysfunction may result from the chronic left to right shunt and from

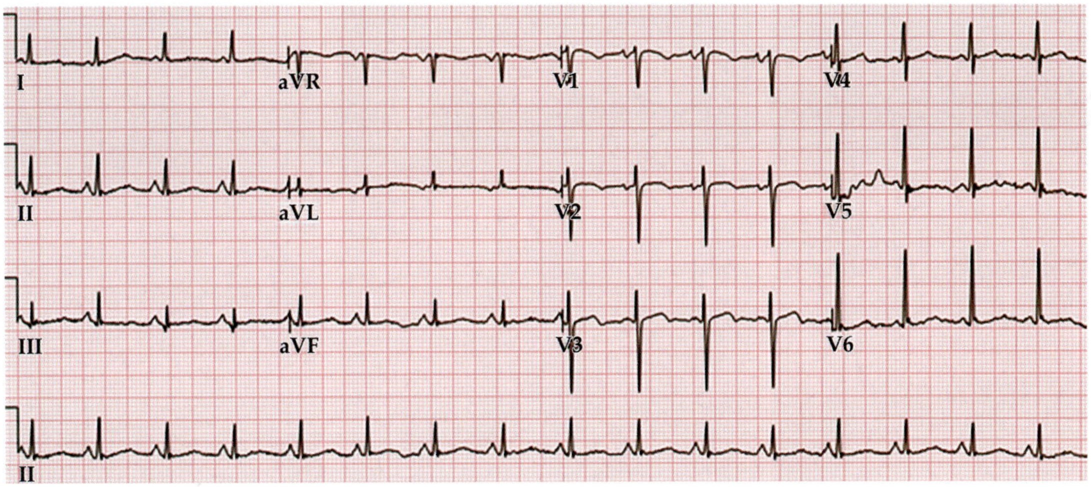

Fig. 245.2: Electrocardiogram showing sinus tachycardia and non-specific ST and T wave abnormalities.

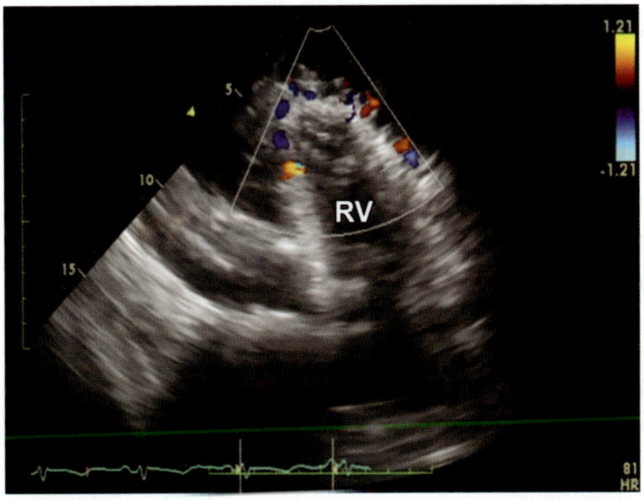

Fig. 245.3: 2D echocardiogram—Right ventricular inflow view demonstrating multiple abnormal color flow Doppler signals around the right ventricular free wall and apex exhibiting the typical "Christmas tree" pattern described with ARCAPA. Right ventricle (RV).

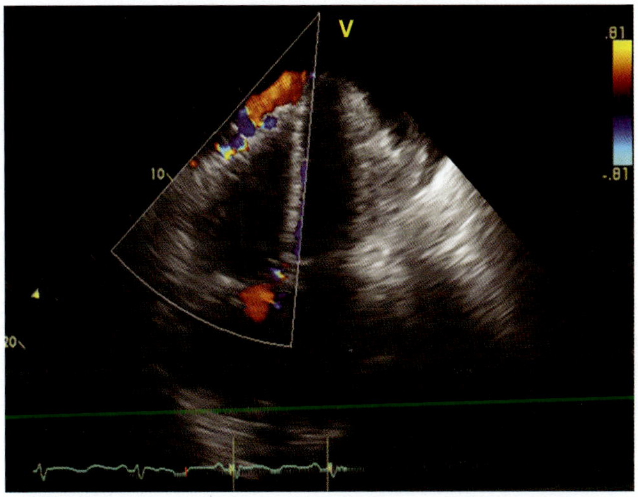

Fig. 245.4: 2D echocardiogram—Apical four-chamber view demonstrating abnormal color flow Doppler signals around the right ventricular free wall and apex.

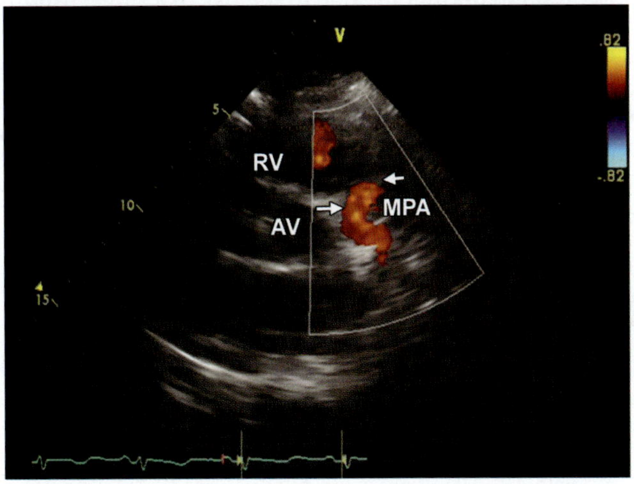

Fig. 245.5: 2D echocardiogram—Parasternal short-axis view at the level of the aortic valve (AV) demonstrating an abnormal reverse color flow jet (large arrow) into the pulmonary artery (MPA) just above the level of the valve leaflets (small arrow). This represents reversed flow in the anomalous coronary artery at its origin from the pulmonary artery. Right ventricle (RV).

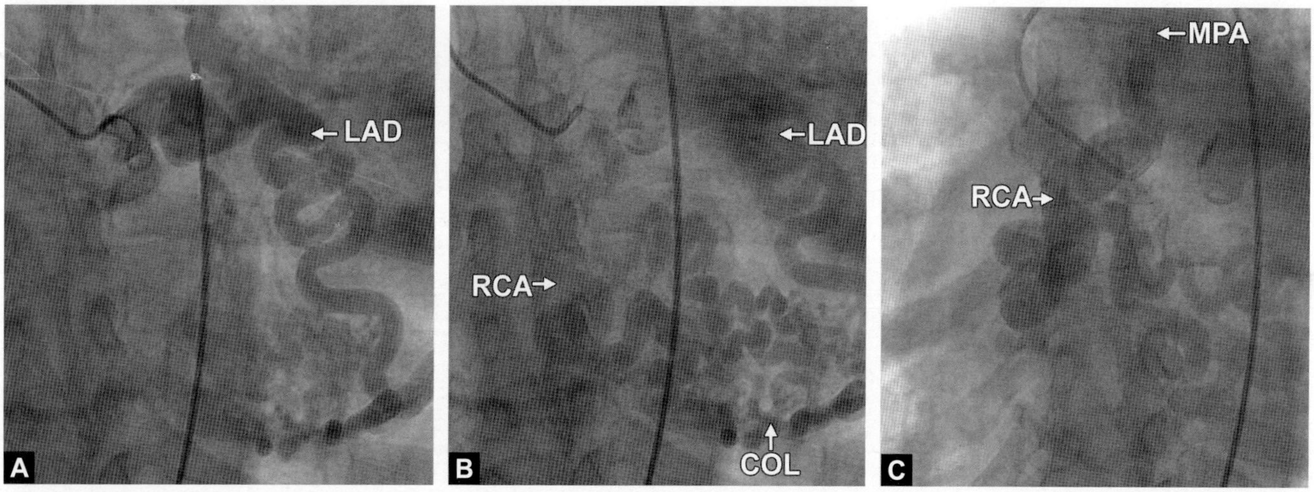

Figs. 245.6A to C: Three successive frames from a selective injection of the left coronary artery demonstrating filling of the left anterior descending (LAD) A. with subsequent opacification of extensive collaterals (COL) around the right ventricular free wall and apex B. with final reconstitution of the right coronary artery (RCA) which empties into the main pulmonary artery (MPA) C.

myocardial ischemia.[4] Patients with ARCAPA are usually asymptomatic and the diagnosis is typically made during evaluation of a murmur. Less commonly they may present with chest pain, SOB, or sudden death.

Although transthoracic echocardiography is an essential tool for the diagnosis of ARCAPA, the location of the right coronary artery ostium is always difficult to detect in adults by transthoracic two-dimensional (2D) imaging because of a low spatial resolution with poor penetration through the chest wall.

The findings in ARCAPA are usually confirmed by angiography with selective left coronary artery angiography demonstrating filling of the RCA through collaterals and subsequent filling of the pulmonary artery (PA). In our case, the right coronary artery (RCA) arose from the PA and filled in retrograde fashion via extensive left to right collaterals around the right ventricular free wall and apex (Figs. 245.6A to C). Cardiac computed tomography and cardiovascular magnetic resonance also provide detailed anatomic information of origin, course, and relationship of the anomalous coronary artery.

2. **What is the management strategy of choice in patients with ARCAPA?**
   (a) Treatment with dual antiplatelet agents
   (b) Surgical reimplantation of the anomalous coronary artery to the aorta
   (c) Serial echocardiography every 6 months till development of symptoms
   (d) Implantation of intracardiac defibrillator to decrease the risk of sudden cardiac death

Ans. (b)

Due to the potential risk of sudden cardiac death in patients with ARCAPA, surgical treatment is recommended as definitive therapy even for asymptomatic patients. The preferred technique is to establish a double-ostium coronary system by translocation of the aberrant vessel to the aortic root. This method decreases myocardial ischemia by providing relief from coronary steal and also decreases the risk of sudden cardiac death. In addition, it can prevent further dilatation and enlargement of the coronary artery, which in turn reduces the size of the shunt. Ligation of the RCA at its origin and coronary artery bypass grafting (CABG) with a saphenous vein graft or radial artery is also described. Simple ligation of the coronary system is not the standard therapy due to the risk of a single ostium coronary system.[5]

Follow-up with ARCAPA after surgical treatment is not well described in the literature. It is important that these patients are followed up long-term on a regular basis to evaluate their ventricular function and the patency of the reimplanted vessel.

MOVIE LEGENDS

812: 2D echocardiogram—Right ventricular inflow view demonstrating multiple abnormal color flow Doppler signals (arrows) around the right ventricular free wall and apex exhibiting the typical "Christmas tree" pattern described with ARCAPA. Right ventricle (RV).

813: 2D echocardiogram—Apical four-chamber view demonstrating abnormal color flow Doppler signals (arrows) around the right ventricular free wall and apex.

814: 2D echocardiogram—Parasternal short-axis view at the level of the aortic valve demonstrating an abnormal reverse color flow jet (arrow) into the pulmonary artery just above the level of the valve leaflets. This represents reversed flow in the anomalous coronary artery at its origin from the pulmonary artery. Arrowhead points to PR.

815: Coronary angiogram.

REFERENCES

1. Kimbiris D, Iskandrian AS, Segal BL, et al. Anomalous aortic origin of coronary arteries. Circulation. 1978;58:606-15.
2. Yamanaka O, Hobbs R. Coronary artery anomalies in 126,595 patients undergoing coronary arteriography. Cathet Cardiovasc Diagn. 1990;21:28-40.
3. Williams IA, Gersony WM, Hellenbrand WE. Anomalous right coronary artery arising from the pulmonary artery: A report of 7 cases and a review of the literature. Am Heart J 2006;152:1004.e9-1004.e17.
4. Mintz GS, Iskandrian AS, Bemis CE, et al. Myocardial ischemia in anomalous origin of the right coronary artery from the pulmonary trunk. Proof of a coronary steal. Am J Cardiol. 1983;51: 610-12.
5. Modi H, Ariyachaipanich A, Dia M. Anomalous origin of right coronary artery from pulmonary artery and severe mitral regurgitation due to myxomatous mitral valve disease: a case report and literature review. J Invasive Cardiol. 2010;22:e49-E55.

CASE 246

Roomi AU, Elsayed M, Bulur S, Nanda NC

A 26-year-old male with average height and built presented with acute coronary syndrome. No previous medical history. No history of smoking or substance abuse. Hemodynamically stable.

Cath findings: Isolated fusiform coronary aneurysm in the proximal LAD.

Biopsy report: Destruction of arterial wall, primarily involving the media with no evidence of inflammatory cells.

1. The differential diagnosis of the large bounded space seen lateral to LV and aortic root includes all of the following *except* (Figs. 246.1 to 246.4 and 816 to 819):

(a) Left main coronary aneurysm
(b) LAD aneurysm
(c) Double aortic root
(d) Left coronary artery/cameral fistula

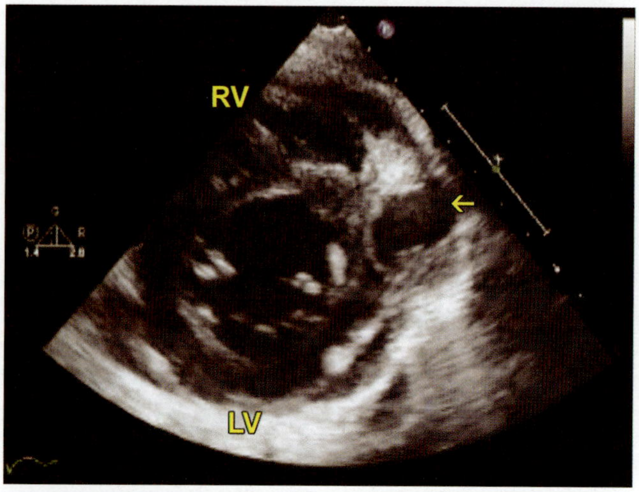

Fig. 246.1: 2D TTE. Arrow shows enlarged bounded space laterally.

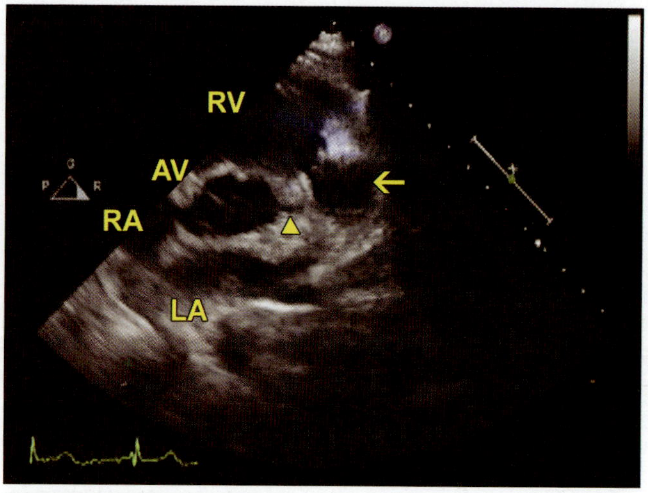

Fig. 246.2: 2DTTE. Arrow shows a bounded space distal to the proximal left main coronary artery (arrowhead).

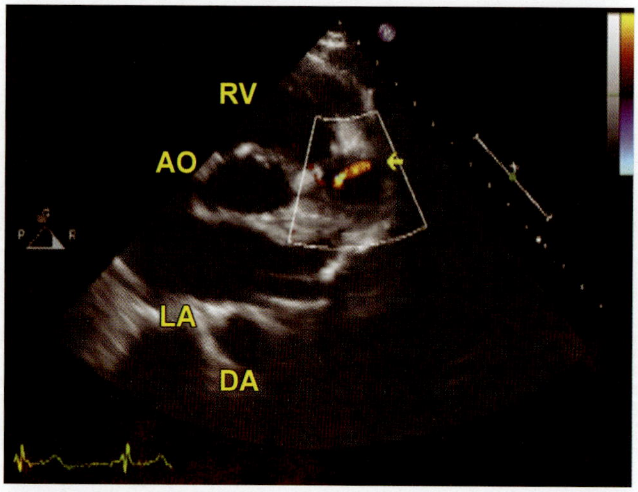

Fig. 246.3: 2DTTE. Color Doppler demonstrates flow signals in the space (arrow) predominantly in diastole.

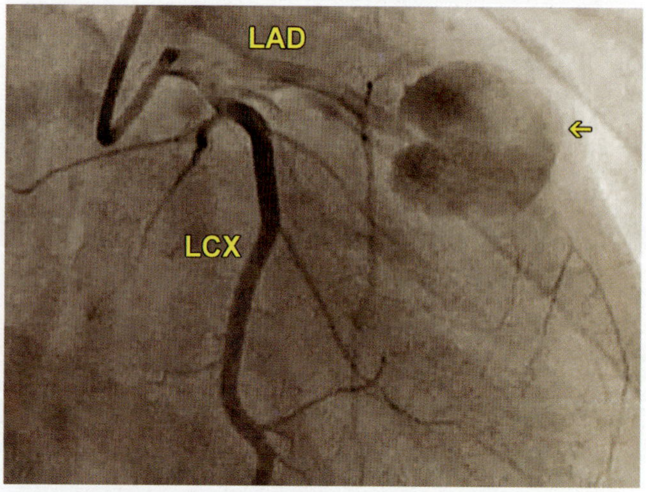

Fig. 246.4: Coronary angiography shows LAD aneurysm (arrow).

Ans. (c)

Left coronary artery/cameral fistula will show much more prominent and extensive color flow signals in the bounded space. Also, a thorough echo examination may show the fistula entering a cardiac chamber or coronary sinus.

MOVIE LEGENDS

816: 2DTTE. Arrow shows enlarged bounded space laterally.
817: 2DTTE. Arrow shows a bounded space distal to the proximal left main coronary artery.
818: 2DTTE. Color Doppler demonstrates flow signals in the space (arrow) predominantly in diastole.
819: Coronary angiography shows LAD aneurysm.

CASE 247

Roomi AU, Elsayed M, Bulur S, Adarna LG, Alagic N, Uygur B, Turaga NSN, Chahwala JR, Nanda NC

LEFT SIDED SVC

The patient is a 29-year-old female with history of palpitations and atypical chest pain. No significant history of any medical illness. Normal EKG. 2DTTE was done (Figs. 247.1 to 247.3 and 820 and 821).

1. **All of the following would be in the differential diagnosis of a markedly dilated coronary sinus (CS) *except*:**
   (a) Left sided SVC
   (b) Marked right heart enlargement
   (c) Lymphatics at the junction of LV and LA
   (d) Coronary artery fistula draining into CS

Ans. (c)

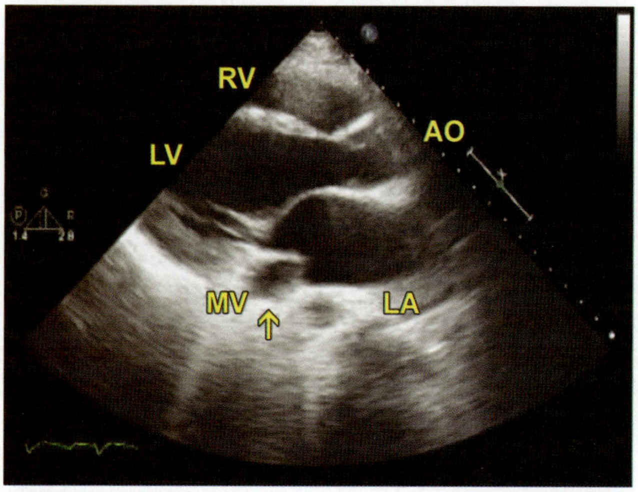

Fig. 247.1: 2DTTE. Arrow shows a dilated CS suggestive of left sided SVC. RV is not dilated and no turbulent flow signals were noted in the CS. These findings would go against the diagnosis of marked right heart enlargement or a fistula draining into the coronary sinus.

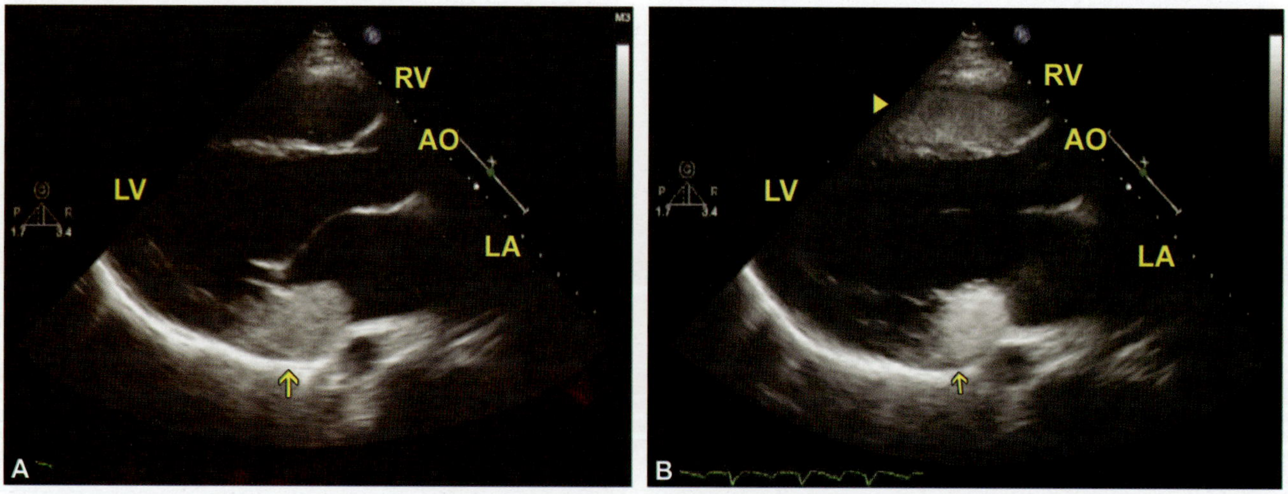

Figs. 247.2A and B: 2DTTE. Arrow shows bubbles filling first the CS and then the RV (arrowhead), from a left arm vein injection typical of left sided SVC which is connected to the CS.

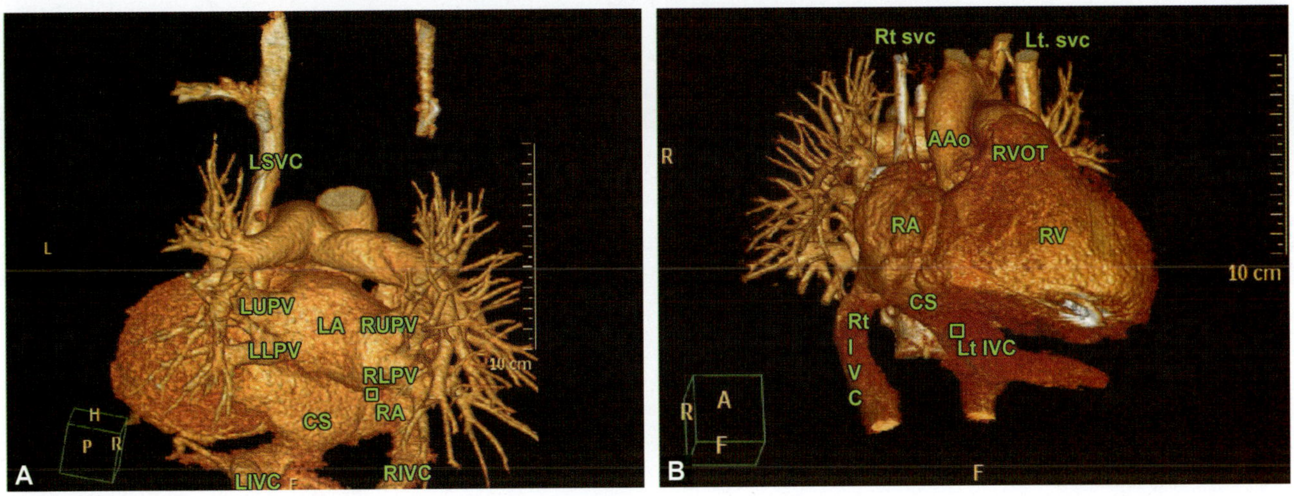

Figs. 247.3A and B: CT scan from the same patient shows a left sided SVC.

Another case from our Echo Laboratory showing first filling of the dilated coronary sinus (CS) and then the RV from a left arm venous injection typical of left sided SVC. 822 and 823.

MOVIES 820 TO 823

SECTION 11

Miscellaneous

CASE 248

Alagic N, Chahwala JR, Adarna LG, Bhagatwala K, Uygur B, Turaga NSN, Elsayed M, Bulur S, Arisha MJ, Nanda NC

M-mode echoes from different patients are shown (Figs. 248.1 to 248.4 and 824A and B, 825 A to E, 826 A and B and 827).

1. **What does the M-mode show (Fig. 248.4)?**
    (a) Normal AV motion
    (b) Posterior LA wall contraction
    (c) Abnormal LV contraction
    (d) A and B
    (e) A, B and C

Ans. (d)

In addition to normal AV motion producing a typical box-like appearance, the contraction of posterior LA wall during atrial systole is also visualized (arrow). LA wall contraction will not occur near the entrance of pulmonary veins.

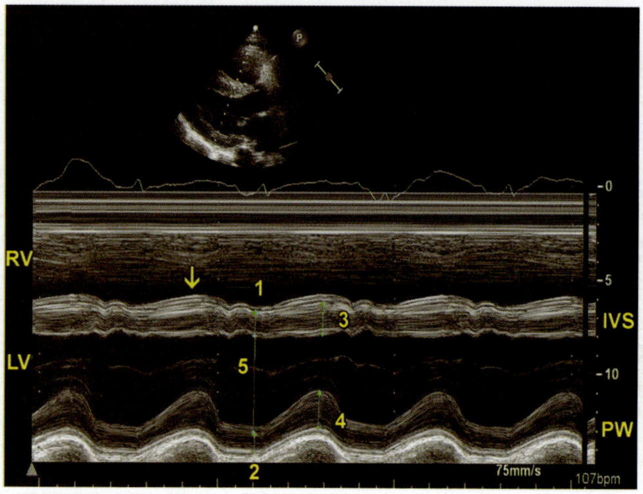

Fig. 248.1: Normal 2D TTE directed M-mode LV measurements. Arrow points to right side of interventricular septum which should be excluded when measuring IVS thickness. 1: end diastolic septal thickness taken at the beginning of QRS complex of the EKG; 2: PW (inferolateral wall) thickness taken at the beginning of QRS complex of the EKG; 3: end systolic thickness of IVS taken at the end of T-wave of EKG (ideally when the LV is maximally contracted); 4: end diastolic thickness of PW (inferolateral wall) taken at the end of T-wave of EKG (ideally when the LV is maximally contracted); 5: LV end diastolic dimensions. Unlike in this M-mode, it is best to take these measurements at the tip of the MV rather than at chordal level as done in this patient for greater inter-observer accuracy. Chordae have a finite length and the measurements can vary depending on whether they are taken at the proximal or distal chordal level. The aorta should be kept as horizontal as possible.

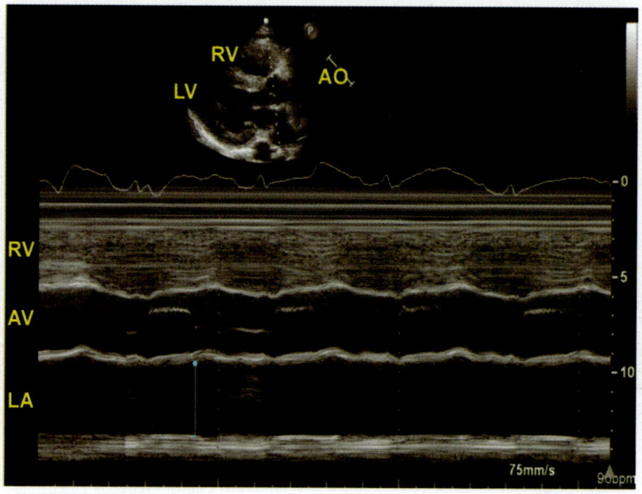

Fig. 248.2: 2D-directed M-mode measurement of LA (taken at end systole).

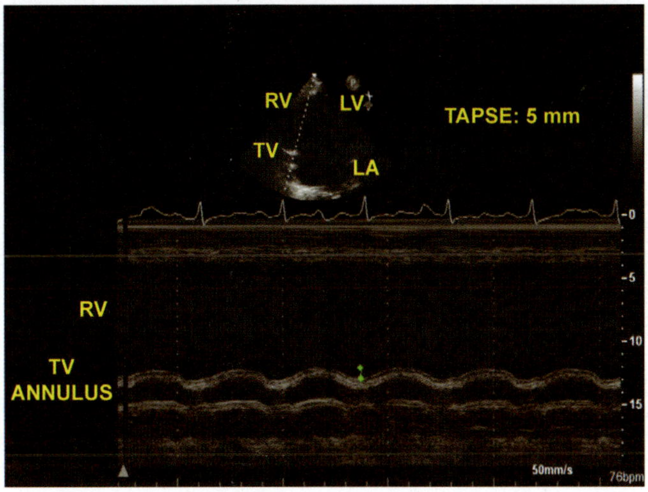

Fig. 248.3: Tricuspid annular plane systolic excursion (TAPSE). M-mode cursor interrogates the TV lateral annulus. TAPSE is abnormally low at 5 mm (normal > 16 mm).

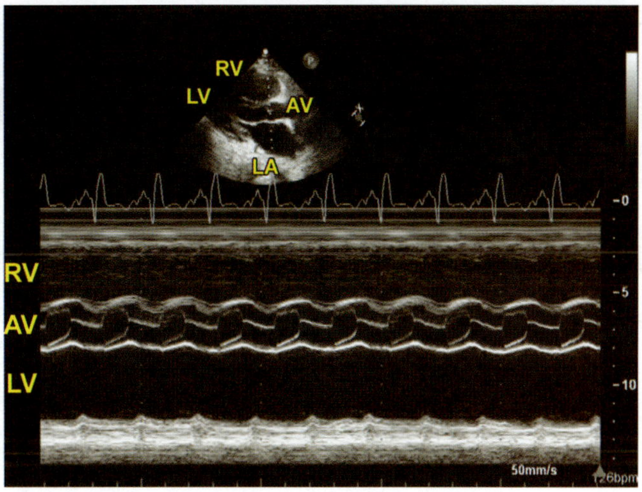

Fig. 248.4: M-mode examination of the AV.

MOVIE LEGENDS

824A. Normal MV nomenclature. The anterior MV leaflet is well seen. The posterior MV leaflet is not well recorded but it moves in opposite direction to the anterior leaflet. The B point is not recorded normally. It becomes prominent when the left-sided filling pressure is increased or when there is first-degree AV block with prolonged PR interval as in this patient (arrows). IVS : interventricular septum; PW : posterior (inferolateral) LV wall.

824B. MS. The mitral E-F slope is very flat, there is no A wave, the posterior MV leaflet moves in the same direction as the anterior leaflet and the valve is thickened (multiple linear echoes).

825A. MV. Atrial flutter. Arrows show the flutter waves.

825B. MV. Atrial flutter-fibrillation. Arrowheads show the waves.

825C. LV. Arrow shows normal septal thickening in systole. The PW (inferolateral) wall also moves well.

825D. LV. Arrow shows abnormal systolic anterior motion of the interventricular septum.

825E. LV. Shows hypertrophy. The PW (inferolateral) is flattened.

826A. Shows diminished stroke volume with an ectopic (arrow). The size of AV box is much reduced as compared to the previous normal sinus beat.

826B. Discrete subaortic stenosis. Shows early systolic preclosure (arrow) of AV with the closing movement same amplitude as the opening movement.

827. Tricuspid annular plane systolic excursion (TAPSE). This represents M-mode motion of the lateral TV annulus. Normal values are above 1.6 cm.

CASE 249

Nanda NC, Bulur S

The patient is a 51-year-old male undergoing chemotherapy for multiple myeloma. 2D TTE parasternal long-axis view is shown.

1. **How is the VS thickness measured on 2D TTE?**
   (a) Only the left side of VS/IVS should be measured at the level of MV tip in the parasternal long-axis view. Measurement should be perfor med when the LV is maximally dilated in end-diastole but in practice, it is easier to do it at the beginning of QRS complex of ECG.
   (b) The maximal thickness of VS should be measured at the level of the MV tip, other details as in A.
   (c) The maximal thickness of VS should be measured at the level of MV chordae/papillary muscles, other details as in A.

Ans. (a)

In this patient, a linear echo clearly separates the left and right sides of VS. Hence, it is easier to measure the left side of VS (828, arrow and 2 dots). An erroneous diagnosis of VS hypertrophy may be made if the measurement also includes the right side of VS. VS or PW (inferolateral wall) thickness > 1.0 cm represents hypertrophy.

MOVIE 828

CASE 250

Bulur S, Nanda NC

The patient is a 42-year-old male referred for echocardiogram prior to noncardiac surgery.

1. **What does the arrow point to in Figures 250.1A and B and 🎥 829?**
   (a) MV chordae tendinae
   (b) LV papillary muscle

Ans. (b)

Both the chordae and papillary muscle are adjacent to LV PW (inferolateral wall) and, therefore, one needs to be careful not to include them when measuring PW thickness.

2. **What is wrong with Figure 250.1A?**
   (a) The right side of the VS is not included when measuring its thickness.
   (b) Measurements are taken at the tip of the MV.
   (c) Measurements are taken at the beginning of QRS complex of ECG.
   (d) Chordal thickness is not included when measuring PW thickness in end-diastole.

Ans. (b)

Clearly measurements are taken at the level of papillary muscle and not at the MV tip. In addition, the LV end-systolic measurement in Figure 250.1B should have excluded the chord and papillary muscle.

MOVIE 829 🎥

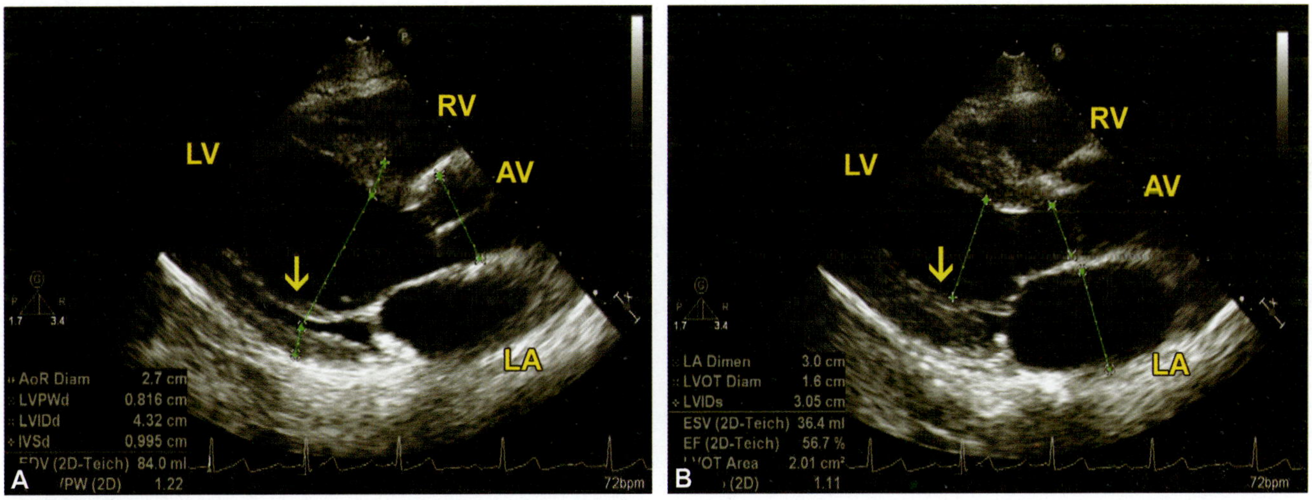

Figs. 250.1A and B: LV measurements using 2DTTE.

CASE 251

Adarna LG, Elsayed M, Alagic N, Uygur B, Turaga NSN, Chahwala JR, Bhagatwala K, Taher A, Mohamed A, Gupta N, Bulur S, Arisha MJ, Nanda NC

Normal cardiac structures and imaging planes not routinely acquired are shown (830 to 832) from three different patients.

MOVIE LEGENDS

830. AO short axis view showing a clear LAA without any thrombus.
831. Main pulmonary artery (MPA) and its bifurcation into right (RPA) and left (LPA) branches.
832. Right parasternal approach demonstrating a large extent of atrial septum.

CASE 252

Mohamed A, Gupta N, Elsayed M, Nanda NC

The patient is a 53-year-old male complaining of shortness of breath, who was referred for treadmill exercise echocardiography.

1. **How were these views obtained (Figs. 252.1, 252.2, 833 and 834A to C)?**
   (a) High left parasternal window.
   (b) RV inflow view.
   (c) Suprasternal/supraclavicular window.
   (d) Right parasternal window with the patient in the right lateral decubitus position.

Ans. (d)

Figure 252.1 and 833 could have also been taken from a high left parasternal window but the remaining views would need to involve the right parasternal approach. The asterisk in 834A points to crista terminalis which represents vestigial tissue at the SVC/RA junction. In 834B, the inter-atrial septum appears mobile and aneurysmal and bubble study was positive for a patent foramen ovale (PFO). Horizontal orientation of IAS in this view facilitates easy detection of ASDs since the ultrasonic beam would tend to be parallel to shunt flow. Also, in this view, SVC, IVC and coronary sinus (CS) entrance into RA are often imaged and, therefore, this is a good approach to assess for sinus venosus defects.

MOVIES 833 AND 834A TO C

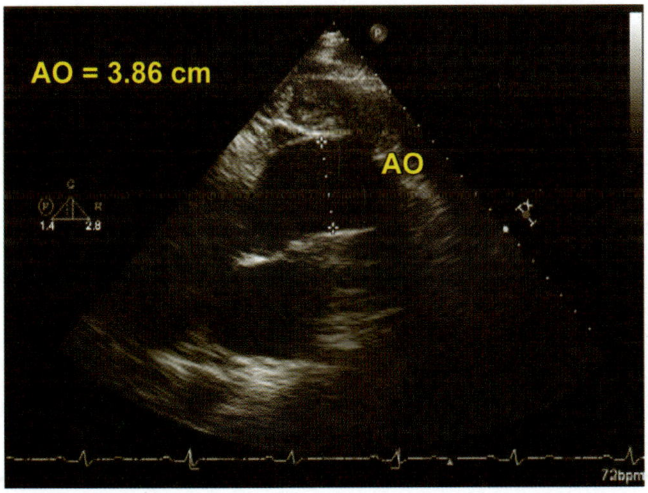

Fig. 252.1: Right parasternal examination. The ascending aorta (AO) is enlarged and measures 3.86 cm.

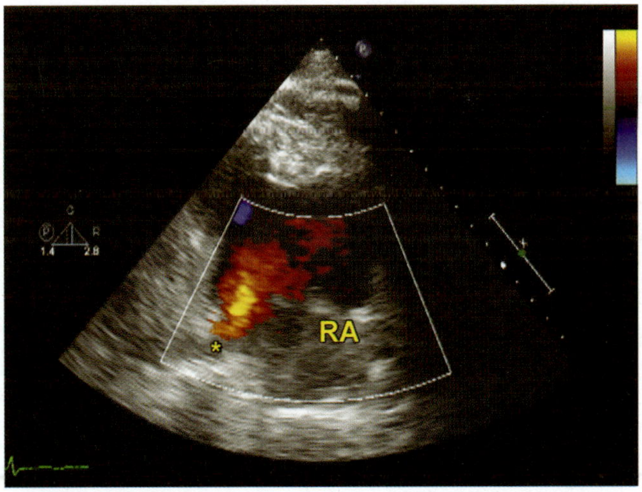

Fig. 252.2: Right parasternal examination. Flow signals are visualized moving from the coronary sinus (asterisk) into the RA.

CASE 253

Bulur S, Nanda NC

The patient is a 55-year-old female with shortness of breath and history of breast augmentation.

2D and 3D TTE right supraclavicular and suprasternal examinations were done.

1. **Supraclavicular approach (🎥 835) is generally used to view:**
   (a) Left pulmonary artery (LPA)
   (b) Left (LIV) and right (RIV) innominate veins which join to form the superior vena cava (SVC)
   (c) IVC
   (d) Coronary sinus

Ans. (b)

This is the best approach to study the proximal SVC by 2D echo and Doppler. SVC-RA junction is not visualized using this technique.

2. **In 🎥 836, the transducer is placed in the suprasternal notch and angled rightward and then leftward to view:**
   (a) Aortic arch (ACH)
   (b) Left common carotid artery (LCC)
   (c) Left subclavian artery (LSA)
   (d) Main (M), right (RPA) and left (LPA) pulmonary arteries
   (e) All of the above

Ans. (e)

This is a good maneuver to view and identify all the pulmonary arteries. The ascending aorta (AA) may also be visualized. The left pulmonary artery courses inferiorly (🎥 837). Right pulmonary artery (RPA) is visualized in Movie 838. 🎥 839-845 are 3D TTE images. 🎥 839 shows LPA, 🎥 840 M and LPA, 🎥 841 LPA in short axis, 🎥 842 a long segment of RPA with lobar branches (arrows), 🎥 843 SVC in addition to RPA and M, 🎥 844 RPA in short axis and 🎥 845 views SVC in short axis.

MOVIES 835 TO 845

CASE 254

Bulur S, Nanda NC

This is an 80-year-old female with atrial fibrillation. A subcostal view is shown (846).

1. **Which of the following statements is incorrect?**
   (a) It is easy to examine the SVC from the subcostal approach in an adult
   (b) SVC may be visualized adjacent to the ascending aorta in the apical 5-chamber view in some patients
   (c) SVC entrance into the RA may be observed during right parasternal examination
   (d) Right supraclavicular approach is useful in detecting SVC flow signals in its proximal portion

Ans. (a)

In 846, SVC is visualized entering RA in an adult patient using the subcostal approach. This is very uncommon in an adult but practically routine in children and infants.

MOVIE 846

CASE 255

Sourabh Prabhakar, Robert WW Biederman

CURIOUS CASE OF THREE CONTINUOUS-WAVE DOPPLER ENVELOPES; THE TRIPHASIC VALVE SIGN

A 71-year-old Caucasian male with a past medical history of CAD, s/p aortic and mitral mechanical (St. Jude) aortic valve replacement, HTN, atrial fibrillation on Coumadin, diabetes mellitus type 2, and HLD who presented to the hospital with headache, left sided weakness and numbness. A CT Head was performed and showed a right MCA stroke with petechial hemorrhage. A CTA of Head and Neck was negative except for a possible right M3 occlusion. A transthoracic echocardiogram was performed and showed normal left ventricular and right ventricular size and systolic function (LVEF 55%). His physical exam demonstrated reduced mechanical sounds and evidence for "muffled" clicks. There was severe pulmonary hypertension (PASP: 71 mm Hg). The mechanical aortic valve prosthesis appeared well-seated but gradients were elevated (peak gradient 117 mm Hg, mean gradient 67 mm Hg) consistent with severe prosthetic stenosis/obstruction. The mechanical mitral valve prosthesis was well seated and normal with a peak gradient 28 mm Hg and mean gradient 12 mm Hg. Given the elevated gradients across aortic valve, a transesophageal echocardiogram (TEE) was ordered.

The TEE showed normal left ventricular size and systolic function with normal wall motion. The right ventricular size and systolic function was normal. The mechanical aortic valve prosthesis was well-seated. There was restricted anterior hemi-disk mobility. The peak gradient of 69 mm Hg and mean gradient of 55 mm Hg consistent with severe prosthetic aortic valve stenosis. M-Mode demonstrated multiple shadows consistent with but not diagnostic for partial hemi-disk obstruction. However, in several CW acquisitions, subtle but unequivocal observation was made of 3 distinct CW velocity envelopes presumably indicating 3 levels of periaortic valvular flow (1) LVOT (2) pliable and (3) nonpliable leaflet (Figs. 255.1A to C). There was no evidence of mobile elements on either valve nor evidence of thrombus. The mechanical mitral valve prosthesis was well-seated.

DISCUSSION

CW Doppler records the velocities of all the red blood cells moving along the path of the sound beam. Consequently, a CW Doppler recording always consists of a full spectral envelope with the outer border corresponding to the fastest moving blood cells. But in our patient, we found that there were 3 distinct CW Doppler velocity envelopes indicating 3 levels of perivalvular flow: (1) LVOT; (2) pliable leaflet and (3) nonpliable leaflet; Interestingly, casual observation would have potentially missed such finding. Indeed, multiple attempts to capture higher quality imaging were repeatedly unsuccessful despite careful finite manipulation of the probe. Only at one extremely narrow probe position where the CW interrogated a precise junction exactly representing the junction of both the pliable and non-pliable leaflet was the triphasic CW envelope replicated. This is a very unusual finding, and to our knowledge, is the first such description in the literature. We believe this confirms that there was turbulence along the LVOT with differential velocities arising from the structures along the LVOT including a prosthetic valve which had one pliable leaflets while the other was mostly fixed and, thus, stenotic. Such a finding, the 'Triphasic Valve Sign', we propose is a CW equivalent for hemidisc stenosis and can be used by the astute clinician as a novel Echocardiographic marker for valve stenosis. We expect such a finding would be present independent of the valve replaced.

1. **The arrow is pointing to which of the following types of artifacts (Fig. 255.2):**
   (a) Refraction
   (b) Shadowing
   (c) Near-field clutter
   (d) Beam-width
   (e) Side lobes

Ans. (b)

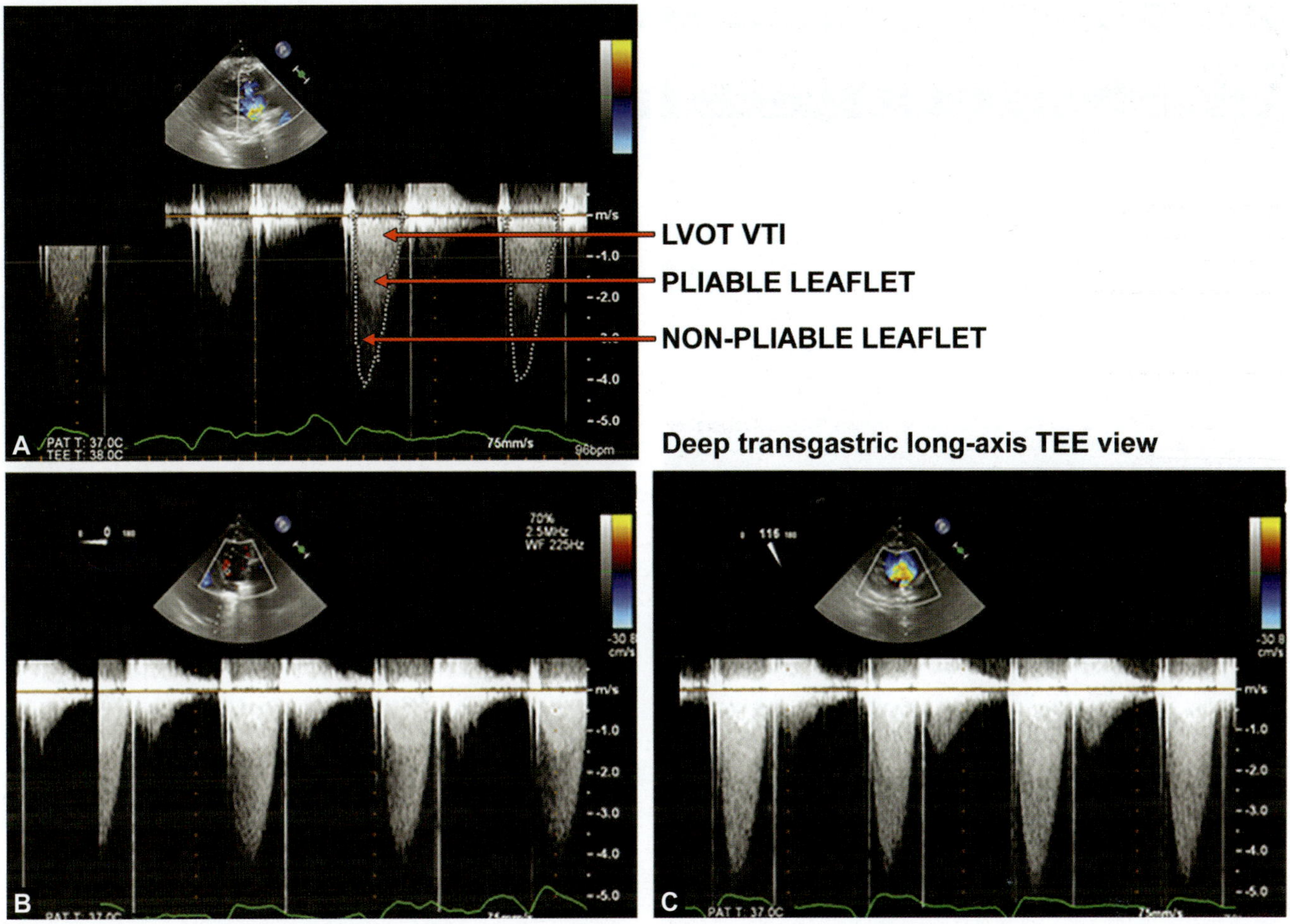

Figs. 255.1A to C: Deep transgastric 0° and 110° TEE view demonstrating the multiple levels of gradients; see insert.

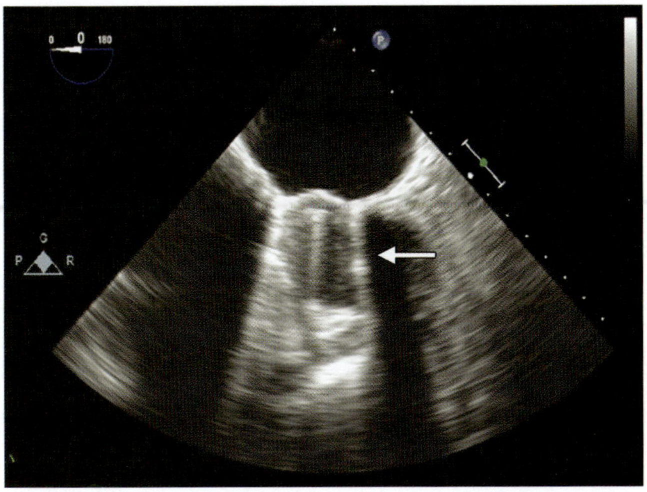

Fig. 255.2: TEE midesophageal 4-chamber view at 0 degrees

Shadowing from the acoustic interference of the non-penetrable ultrasound beam.

2. **The arrows are pointing to which of the following types of artifacts (Fig. 255.3)?**
   (a) Near-field clutter
   (b) Reverberation
   (c) Refraction
   (d) Ghosting

Ans. (b)

Reverberation is characterized as multiple horizontal lines that are equidistant with decreasing intensity and increasing depth.

3. **In the accompanying 847, which leaflet is immobile?**
   (a) Right coronary cusp

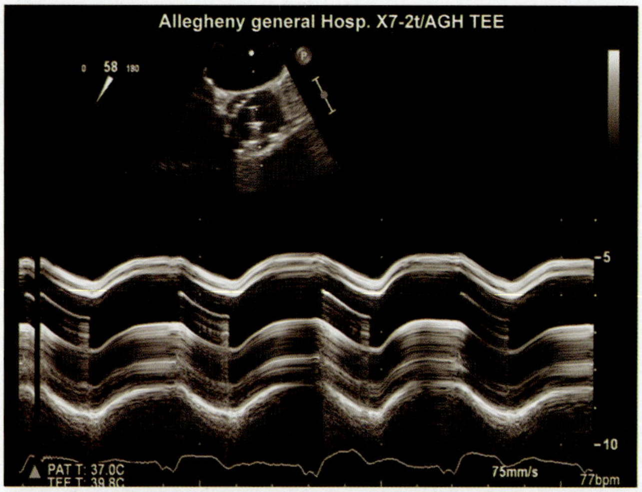

Fig. 255.3: M-mode through short-axis view of aortic valve

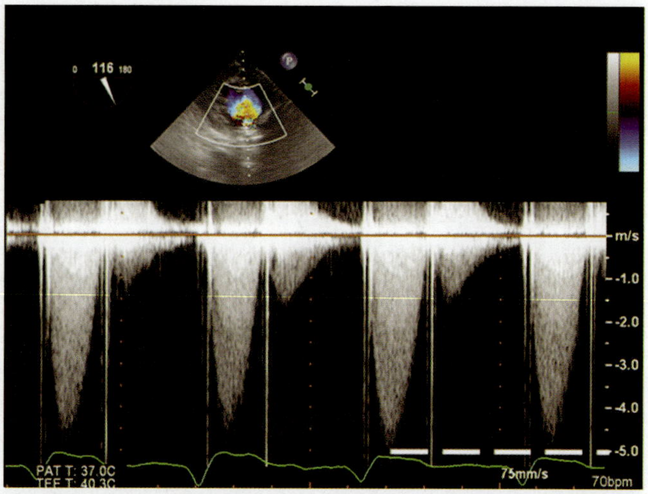

Fig. 255.4: Deep transgastric 116° TEE view again demonstrating the multiple levels of gradients albeit a bit more subtle.

(b) Left coronary cusp
(c) Anterior hemidisk
(d) Posterior hemidisk
(e) Noncoronary cusp

Ans. (c)

4. **Calculate the peak gradient across aortic valve from the CW Doppler velocities shown in Figure 255.4.**
   (a) 36 mm Hg
   (b) 64 mm Hg
   (c) 100 mm Hg
   (d) 144 mm Hg

Ans. (c)

Using modified Bernoulli's equation, ignoring acceleration, inertia and viscosity–4 $(V)^2 \times 4\ (5)^2 \times 100$ mm Hg.

MOVIE 847

CASE 256

Bulur S, Elsayed M, Alagic N, Uygur B, Turaga NSN, Chahwala JR, Adarna LG, Nanda NC

Shadowing produced by what appears to be calcification under the chest wall results in intermittent obliteration (A, artifact) of cardiac structures imaged in parasternal long-axis view (848 and 849).

MOVIES 848 AND 849

CASE 257

Taher A, Elsayed M, Alagic N, Uygur B, Turaga NSN, Chahwala JR, Adarna LG, Taher A, Mohamed A, Gupta N, Bulur S, Nanda NC

A 42-year-old female with cardiac transplantation. Pulsed wave Doppler examination of the descending thoracic aorta examined from the suprasternal notch shows artifacts which produce an unpleasant grating noise (Fig. 257.1). 850 shows color Doppler examination of the proximal descending aorta without any evidence of an artifact.

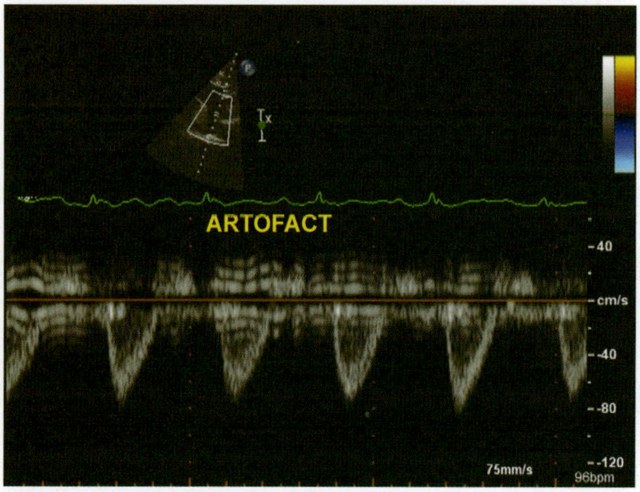

Fig. 257.1: Doppler artifact produced during pulsed wave interrogation of the proximal descending aorta.

MOVIE 850

CASE 258

Syed Arman Husain, Robert WW Biederman

CASE (FIGURES 258.1 AND 258.2)

A calm before the storm

A 57-year-old man with past medical history of HTN, HLD, CAD s/p PCI to LCX, ICM EF 25–30%, was admitted to the CCU 2 months prior to the index admission after suffering from a cardiac arrest. Left heart cath was done and showed an 80% distal LCX stenosis which was opened with a bare metal stent. During that admission he developed MSSA bacteremia and had a transesophageal echocardiogram (TEE) which showed severe left ventricular systolic dysfunction with EF 20–25%, a patent foramen ovale and moderate to severe aortic regurgitation with no evidence of endocarditis. He received a course of antibiotics for pneumonia and was discharged with a lifevest for secondary prevention of sudden cardiac death. He represents to the hospital for fever, hallucinations and painful left ankle, right wrist, and knees. Blood cultures drawn on admission were positive for MSSA bacteremia and orthopedics was consulted for possible septic joint. Arthocentesis was performed, and the patient was taken to the OR for the following right knee, left ankle and right wrist arthrotomy, irrigation and debridement for infection, left medial distal thigh abscess, irrigation and debridement left knee joint aspiration. Due to the recurrent bacteremia, a repeat TEE was requested.

On admission to the TEE suit, he was alert and oriented with stable vitals, BP 132/68, respiratory rate 17, HR 81 and pulse oximetry 99% on room air. His labs revealed normal coagulation profile and normal platelet count but H/H of

pH	↑	7.493
PaCO2	↓	26.6
PAO2	↑	436.0
Base excess		–2
HCO3	↓	20.2
SaO2		97.4
% O2Hb	* ↓	51.3
Hgb.	↓	8.6
Hematocrit, Calc.	↓	26.8
% Carboxyhemoglobin.		0.0
AaO2		229
% Methemoglobin.	* ↑	>31.0
Modified Allens test		
Barometric pressure		739.0
Comment.		TRRB 14...
EPAP		5
FiO2		100.0
Flow		
IPAP		10
Oxygen device		BIPAP

Fig. 258.1: Arterial blood gas prior to receiving Methylene blue.

pH		7.440
PaCO2	↓	32.9
PAO2	↑	114.0
Base excess		–1
HCO3		22.0
SaO2		98.3
% O2Hb		95.4
Hgb.	↓	7.6
Hematocrit, Calc.	↓	23.8
% Carboxyhemoglobin.		1.3
AaO2		43
% Methemoglobin.	↑	1.6
Modified Allens test		
Barometric pressure		739.0
Comment.		
EPAP		
FiO2		28.0
Flow		2.0
IPAP		
Oxygen device		NASAL...

Fig. 258.2: Arterial blood gas after receiving Methylene blue.

7.7/25.5. After a timeout was done, he received a total of 3 sprays of Cetacaine topical anesthetic spray of approximately 2 unwitnessed seconds in preparation for the procedure. Shortly after (<2 minutes), and prior to receiving any sedation, the patient started desaturating to 85–87% on the pulse-ox. Unusually, however, on physical exam and repeated questioning, he did not appear to be in distress but yet began developing cyanosis noticeable on his lips and nailbeds. His lungs were clear to auscultation with good respiratory effort. His hypoxia was not responsive to increasing supplemental O_2 up to 10L nasal re-breather. He avoided Ambu bagging remaining uncharacteristically calm and seemingly unaffected by the interest bestowed upon him. He was then transferred back to unit in company of our TEE team. There his O_2 sat remained at 85% despite supplemental O_2 and finally to a non-rebreather at 15L, all equally ineffective at improving his O_2. An arterial blood gas was obtained and while waiting for the results, the clinical scenario and judgment dictated a bedside diagnosis of methemoglobinemia. At this point 125 mg/dL of Methylene Blue was administered. With in a few minutes the arterial bleed was resulted: PH 7.49/PCO_2 27/PaO_2 436 and methhemoglobin of 47% (UNL<1%). Within 20–30 minutes the patients' cyanosis resolved and his pulse-oximetry showed 97% saturation on 6L via nasal cannula. A repeat ABG in 1 hr showed PH 7.45, PCO_2 28/PaO_2 131 and methhemoglobin of 4.8%. The patient remained equally nonplused; oblivious to the storm of activity surrounded him. Indeed, the following day on revisiting him, he curiously re-asked, "Why all the fuss about me yesterday?"

Discussion: Methemoglobin is an altered state of hemoglobin in which the ferrous state (Fe++) irons of heme are oxidized to the ferric (Fe+++) state. The ferric hemes of Methemoglobin are unable to bind oxygen, the oxygen affinity of any remaining ferrous hemes in the hemoglobin tetramer is increased resulting in impaired oxygen delivery to the tissues and the oxygen dissociation curve is shifted to the left. This creates a state of "functional anemia".

The molecular mechanism underlying the association between the use of topical anesthetics and methemoglobinemia is not clear and has been thought to be multifactorial such as the presence of an inconsistently present substance in the topical anesthetic solvent or infection in the affected subject along with alteration in hepatic metabolic from, favoring the production of metabolites with oxygen and potential.

Suspicion should rise when O_2 saturation remains <90% even after O_2 administration (typically around 85%; a clinical pearl), pale gray or blue-colored skin, lips and nail beds, chocolate-brown blood while drawing ABG lightheadedness, headache, tachycardia, fatigue, dyspnea and lethargy. However, often reported, as in our case is a particularly unusual state of 'calm' in the patient, unsettling normal relative to other clinical scenarios in which hypoxia is present. Indeed, this was our first clue and should be a clinical 'pearl'. However, not to be lulled into a false sense of security, at higher levels of methemoglobinemia, respiratory depression, altered sensorium, coma, shock, seizures ensue and death may occur. Preexisting conditions such as anemia, sepsis, heart and lung disease may and often exacerbate toxicity, particularly anemia now understood to reduce the oxygen carrying capacity of RBCs already so affected.

Methemoglobinemia can be congenital or acquired.

Congenital: Due to Cytochrome b5 reductase 3 deficiency which results in diminished enzymatic reduction of methemoglobin back to functional hemoglobin. Affected patients have lifelong cyanosis but are generally asymptomatic.

Acquired: results from ingestion of specific drugs or agents the cause an increase in the production of methemoglobin.

1. **Which enzyme is deficient in congenital methemoglobinemia?**
   (a) Cytochrome b5 reductase deficiency
   (b) Cytochrome p450 reductase
   (c) Cytochrome c oxidase
   (d) G6PD

Ans. (a)

2. **In methemoglobinemia the oxygen dissociation curve is:**
   (a) Shifted to the right
   (b) Shifted to the left
   (c) Remains the same

Ans. (a)

3. **What is the antidote for methemoglobinemia?**
   (a) Sodium bicarbonate
   (b) Pralidoxime
   (c) Deferoxamine
   (d) Methylene blue
   (e) Dimercaprol

Ans. (d)

At low concentrations: methylene blue → NADPH-dependent reduction to leucomethylene blue (due to action of methemoglobin reductase) → reduces methemoglobin → Hb.

4. **Methylene blue can cause methemoglobinemia:**
   (a) True
   (b) False

Ans. (a)

At high concentrations: methylene blue → converts ferrous iron of reduced Hb to ferric ion → forms methemoglobin

CASE 259

Nanda NC, Mohamed A, Arora G, Mahajan A, Sankhyan P, Joson M, Elsayed M

This is a 47-year-old male who presented with dyspnea on exertion and dizziness. He had a history of murmur for many years. The patient subsequently underwent an echocardiogram which demonstrated severe mitral valve prolapse with chordal rupture (arrow in 851) and severe mitral regurgitation (852). The estimated LV ejection fraction was 55%. He underwent MV repair with an annuloplasty band. He presented a few weeks after surgery with shortness of breath on exertion. 2D TTE was done (853 and 854).

1. **What is the most likely diagnosis?**
   (a) Mitral regurgitation
   (b) Mitral stenosis as a result of MV annuloplasty
   (c) Systolic anterior motion of mitral valve
   (d) Annuloplasty ring dehiscence

Ans. (c)

Occasionally, after MV annuloplasty systolic anterior movements (SAMs, arrow in 853) of anterior MV leaflet may develop causing significant LVOT obstruction and severe MR (854). These SAMs seem to occur when there is excessive MV tissue in comparison to the ring size. MV replacement may have to be performed if the obstruction is severe.

MOVIES 851 TO 854

CASE 260

Mohamed A, Arora G, Mahajan A, Sankhyan P, Joson M, Elsayed M, Nanda NC

A 30-year-old male with hypertrophic cardiomyopathy (HCM) and paroxysmal atrial fibrillation who underwent dual chamber ICD implantation presents with multiple episodes of palpitations associated with exertion. He underwent TTE (855-857).

1. **What is the diagnosis in this patient?**
   (a) Concentric hypertrophic cardiomyopathy (HCM)
   (b) Asymmetrical septal hypertrophy
   (c) Apical hypertrophy
   (d) Midcavity obstructive cardiomyopathy

Ans. (d)

There is asymmetrical septal hypertrophy at the level of mitral valve with interventricular septum (VS) thickness much greater than the proximal inferolateral (posterior) wall (PW, 855 and 856). At the level of papillary muscles the hypertrophy is practically concentric (857). Thus, in some patients with HCM, only the proximal portion of the PW shows much less hypertrophy compared to VS while the mid and distal portions of PW and other LV walls exhibit equal thickness to VS. In this patient, there is LV midcavity obliteration in systole at the papillary muscle level (arrow in 855).

MOVIES 855 TO 857

CASE 261

Mohamed A, Arora G, Mahajan A, Sankhyan P, Joson M, Elsayed M, Nanda NC

A 51-year-old male with shortness of breath. He underwent 2DTTE (Figs. 261.1, 261.2 and 858).

1. **What is the cause of this echo finding?**
    (a) Aorto-coronary fistula
    (b) Ventricular septal defect
    (c) Left ventricular assist device
    (d) Patent ductus arteriosus

Ans. (c)

This patient with LVAD placement has mild aortic regurgitation (AR). Note that AR (arrow) in this patient occurs throughout the cardiac cycle, shown by color M-mode in Figure 261.1 and by CW Doppler in Figure 261.2. This is because the LVAD cannula pumps out blood from the LV into the proximal ascending aorta practically continuously resulting in continuous AR through the incompetent AV. Also note essentially absence of AV opening (Fig. 261.1) during the cardiac cycle which is typical of LVAD patients.

MOVIE 858

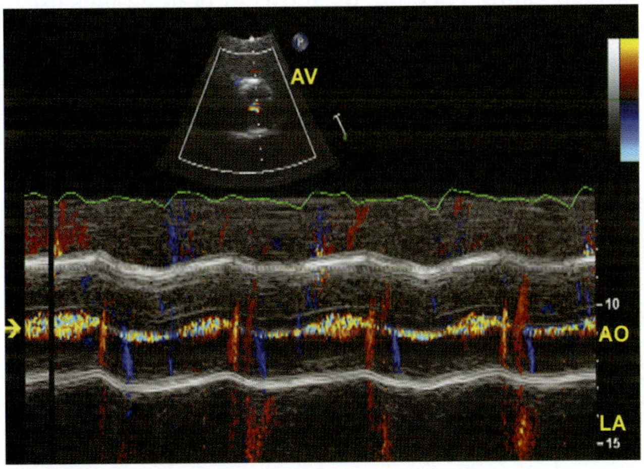

Fig. 261.1: Color M-mode examination demonstrating AR (arrow) throughout the cardiac cycle. The AV opens minimally if at all.

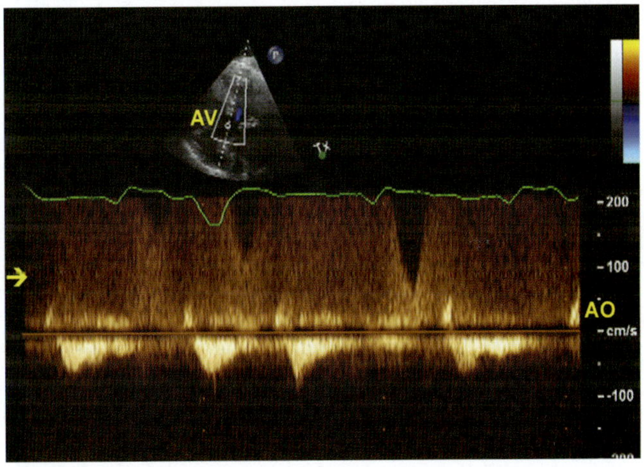

Fig. 261.2: Apical five chamber view. The arrow points to flow signals moving continuously towards the LV apex where the cannula is placed.

CASE 262

Nanda NC, Arora G, Mohamed A, Mahajan A, Sankhyan P, Joson M, Elsayed M

A 75-year-old female presented to cardiology clinic with dyspnea. The patient has history of hypertension and hyperlipidemia. She underwent 2DTEE and was found to have severe aortic stenosis (mean gradient 56 mm Hg, peak velocity 4.7m/s and AVA 0.7 cm^2), LVOT 19 mm, IVS 15 mm and posterior wall 14 mm (859-861).

1. **What should be considered in this patient? All are correct statements *except*:**
   (a) Coronary angiogram
   (b) Aortic valve replacement
   (c) Aortic valve replacement with myomectomy
   (d) CT scan

Ans. (d)

In a patient with aortic stenosis and significant ventricular hypertrophy (860) and narrow LVOT (less than 20 mm), co-existent hypertrophic cardiomyopathy (HCM) should be suspected and the surgeon alerted to look for a thick proximal septum bulging into the LVOT. If the surgeon notices this finding, concomitant myomectomy should be performed together with AV replacement. Distal stenosis such as severe AS can prevent development of typical SAMs of the MV because of the absence of a Venturi effect or "drag phenomenon". Thus, co-existing HCM is masked and may go undetected. A narrow LVOT in the presence of LVH may be the only finding suggestive of HCM. If this is not diagnosed and myomectomy not performed, correction of AS by AV replacement could result in unmasking of HCM with high LVOT gradients that sometimes may be higher than preop gradients from AS. Re-operation becomes difficult since to perform a myomectomy through the AV and LVOT would first require removal of the previously placed AV prosthesis.

In this patient, prominent SAMs (arrow in 859) indicative of HCM are well seen together with calcific AS (861) and hence the diagnosis of both entities existing together could be easily made by echocardiography. The patient successfully underwent AV replacement and myomectomy.

MOVIES 859 TO 861

CASE 263

Bulur S, Elsayed M, Nanda NC

This is an adult patient admitted with shortness of breath. 2DTTE was done.

1. **Echocardiograms show all of the following *except*:**
   (a) Late RV diastolic collapse (arrowhead in 867)
   (b) Minimal collapse of the IVC (arrowhead in 868)
   (c) Pericardial (arrowhead) and left pleural effusion (LPE) (862, 863 and 865)
   (d) Significant variation of MV inflow (arrow in 866)
   (e) Marked swinging of the heart (864)
   (f) Significant variation of TV inflow

Ans. (f)

A-E are consistent with cardiac tamponade. He presented with low cardiac output syndrome and BP 80/40 mm Hg. He improved dramatically after pericardiocentesis.

MOVIES 862 TO 868

CASE 264

Nanda NC, Keser N, Mohamed A, Arora G, Mahajan A, Sankhyan P, Joson M, Elsayed M

The patient is a 38-year-old female with acute myeloid leukemia (AML) that transformed from chronic myelomonocytic leukemia (CMML). She was admitted with dizziness and shortness of breath. Her BP was 72/53 mm Hg and HR in 130s on arrival. She underwent 2DTTE.

1. **What is unlikely to be seen in this patient?**
   (a) Pulsus paradoxus
   (b) Dilated IVC
   (c) Greater than 30% variability in tricuspid valve inflow
   (d) Normal mitral inflow
   (e) Right atrial wall collapse
   (f) RV diastolic collapse

Ans. (d)

In this patient, the most dramatic echo finding of cardiac tamponade is prominent RV diastolic collapse (arrow in 869), marked swinging of the heart in the short axis views toward the apex (872 and 873, arrow in 872 points to a fibrin band in the effusion) and a dilated non-collapsing IVC (875). Pericardial effusion is large and extends behind the LA wall (869). RA wall collapse is noted in the aortic short axis (870) and apical 4 chamber (871) views. 874 shows the subcostal view. The patient's clinical status improved and the BP normalized following pericardiocentesis which was urgently performed. 876, 877 and 878 show almost complete resolution of pericardial effusion with a collapsing normal-sized IVC. Ascites is noted in 876.

MOVIES 869 TO 878

CASE 265

Mohamed A, Arora G, Mahajan A, Sankhyan P, Joson M, Elsayed M, Nanda NC

A 77-year-old male with type 2 diabetes mellitus, systemic hypertension, hyperlipidemia and h/o gastric cancer s/p resection and chemotherapy presented to cardiology clinic with bradycardia (Figs. 265.1, 265.2 and 879 to 885).

1. **Where is this mass attached?**
   (a) Interatrial septum
   (b) Anterior leaflet of tricuspid valve
   (c) Posterior leaflet of tricuspid valve
   (d) Septal leaflet of tricuspid valve

Ans. (d)

2. **What is the likely diagnosis?**
   (a) Hemangioma
   (b) Myxoma
   (c) Papillary fibroelastoma
   (d) Metastasis from gastric carcinoma

Ans. (c)

Papillary fibroelastomas typically have frond-like structures on the surface (may look like a sea anemone). These are well seen on the 2D images (arrow in 879 to 882). 3D imaging was helpful in this case to identify the thin stalk (arrowhead in Fig. 265.2) of the fibroelastoma (arrow in Fig. 265.2 and 883) and point of attachment to the septal TV leaflet, both of which were not detected by 2D. 3D echo also gives more accurate measurements of dimensions since the mass can be acquired in its entirety in the three-dimensional data set. In addition, 3D provides assessment of volume of intracardiac masses which may be a more reliable parameter of size than dimensions.

3. **Does this patient also have a fibroelastoma on the AV (884)?**
   (a) Yes
   (b) No

Ans. (b)

The rounded mass or masses (884) seen in the parasternal long axis view could conceivably represent one or more fibroelsatomas on AV. However, in the aortic short axis view (885) they are observed without any visible stalk in the middle of each of the three cusps of the AV. These are typical locations for nodules of Arantius. These are normal findings and become thickened and calcified as the individual gets older.

MOVIES 879 TO 885

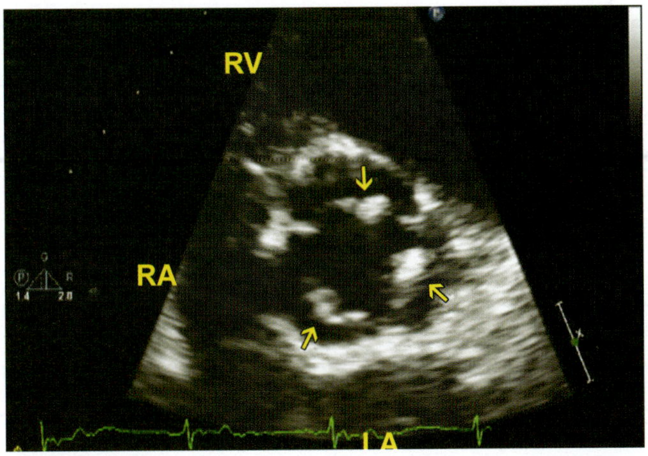

Fig. 265.1: 2DTTE. Aortic short axis view. Arrows represent nodules of Arantius.

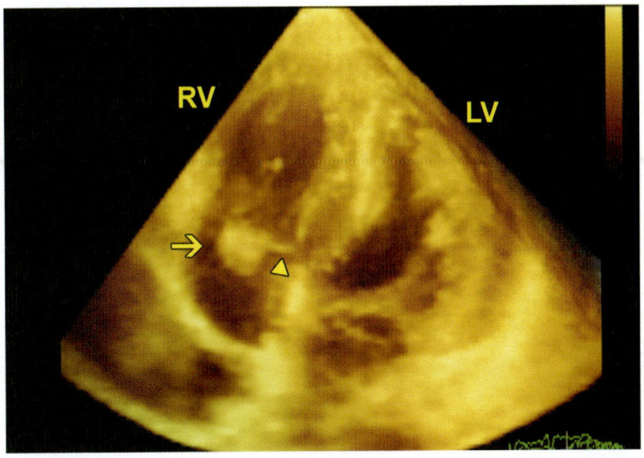

Fig. 265.2: Apical four chamber view. The arrow points to the TV fibroelastoma and the arrowhead its stalk.

CASE 266

Arora G, Mohamed A, Elsayed M, Nanda NC

A 66-year-old female with a history of renal cell carcinoma (RCC) s/p nephrectomy 10 years ago. She then had a cyst removed from the left kidney 6 years ago and a lung mass resected 3 years ago. Both were consistent with metastasis from RCC. She now presented with chest pain. There were no ECG changes and cardiac enzymes were negative. 2DTTE was performed (886 to 888). Arrows in the movies point to masses in RV wall. PE : pericardial effusion.

1. **What other tests would you perform to help in diagnosis?**
   (a) Cardiac MRI
   (b) 3D TEE
   (c) Cardiac CT
   (d) Coronary angiogram

Ans. (a)

Cardiac MRI was performed, which revealed a mass at the right atrioventricular groove. It encased the right coronary artery. It measured 3.8 cm × 4 cm. On T1 and T2 weighted sequence, the mass was slightly brighter as compared to the myocardium and less intense compared to fatty tissue. On triple IR sequences the mass was bright indicating that it was not lipomatous. Overall the mass had some signal heterogeneity. There was a large pericardial effusion.

2. **What is the most likely diagnosis?**
   (a) Primary cardiac tumor
   (b) Secondary cardiac tumor

Ans. (b)

The patient has not undergone right ventricular mass biospy. Given that she has had metastasis to lung, RCC is most likely. Though most cases of cardiac involvement are via direct extension through IVC and RA, in our case, the IVC was normal and no mass was seen in RA. Hence, the spread is most likely hematogenous.

MOVIES 886 TO 888

CASE 267

Arora G, Mohamed A, Elsayed M, Arisha MJ, Nanda NC

A 40-year-old female with history of type 1 diabetes mellitus and hypertension presents with right-sided weakness and expressive aphasia. She was found to have acute ischemic left middle cerebral artery (MCA) stroke on MRI. Further workup revealed:

Troponin: 0.052 ng/mL

Carotid ultrasound: <20% stenosis in right internal carotid artery (ICA). Normal left ICA

2D TTE done: Large 4 × 2.5 cm mass (arrows in 889-891) in LV with lateral wall hypokinesis and low normal systolic function were noted.

1. Which further test is less likely to be performed?

(a) TEE
(b) Cardiac MRI
(c) Coronary angiogram

Ans. (a)

The patient underwent cardiac MRI (Fig. 267.1), which revealed low normal to mildly reduced LV systolic function with regional wall motion abnormalities in lateral wall and apex. Aneurysmal LV apex and a long highly mobile serpiginous mass arising from apex were detected. Late gadolinium-enhanced images show transmural infarct in mid to distal lateral wall and apex.

Coronary angiogram revealed single vessel CAD in the large obtuse marginal (OM) branch of CFx with 60% stenosis and mild disease in other arteries.

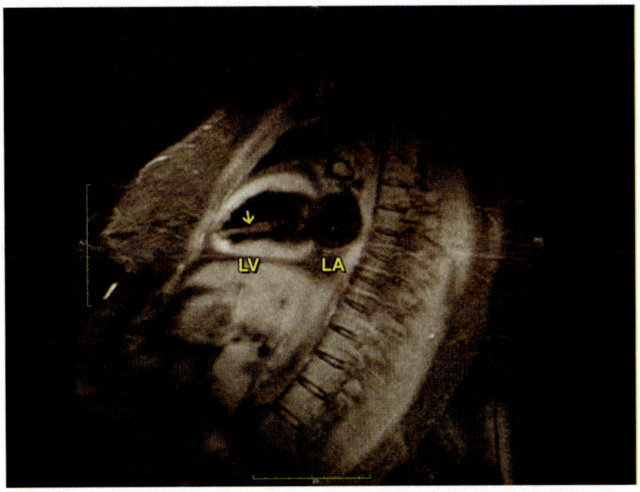

Fig. 267.1: Magnetic resonance imaging. Arrow points to the mass in LV.

2. How will you manage the patient?

(a) Start anticoagulation and treat coronary artery disease medically
(b) Start anticoagulation and treat coronary artery disease with placement of drug-eluting stent (DES)
(c) Refer to surgery for removal of LV mass

Ans. (c)

The patient underwent single vessel CABG with removal of LV mass. On histopathological examination the LV mass most likely represented an organized thrombus over a healed myocardial infarction.

MOVIES 889 TO 891

CASE 268

Nanda NC, Mohamed A, Elsayed M

This patient is a 38-year-old male with chronic kidney disease being evaluated for renal transplantation. 2D and 3D TTE were done (Figs. 268.1 to 268.11. 892-902 are 2D TTE, 903 and 904 are 3D TTE).

1. **What do the echo findings show? All the following statements are correct *except*:**
   (a) Changing position of AV closure (arrow) on M-mode so that in one view anterior cusp appears much smaller (Fig. 268.1) than the posterior cusp and vice versa in another view (Fig. 268.2). Because both cusps are practically equal in size, they need to have redundant folds otherwise significant stenosis will occur as the cusp diameters are much smaller than the circumference of the aortic root. The apparent change in the size of cusps depends on beat to beat variation in the position of redundant folds in relation to the ultrasound beam.
   (b) Obliquely oriented bicuspid AV without significant stenosis (893, parasternal short axis view and 904).
   (c) AV prolapse (892, parasternal long-axis view)
   (d) Intact atrial septum (Fig. 268.5 and 898 and 899 arrow in 898) imaged using the right parasternal approach. Since the atrial septum using this approach is also visualized in relation to both SVC and IVC, sinus venosus defects can be confidently excluded. A long segment of SVC together with right (RIV) and left (LIV) innominate veins joining to form the SVC are visualized in 897.
   (e) Normal RCA in the right atrioventricular annulus (arrow head in Figure 268.5, 898, right parasternal examination).
   (f) Absence of thrombus in RA and RA appendage imaged from the right parasternal window (RAA, 900 and 901, arrow head in 900 points to crista terminalis which is a linear vestigial fibromuscular tissue at the entrance of SVC into the RA). PE represents a small pericardial effusion in 901.
   (g) Moderately dilated ascending aorta (Figs. 268.3 and 268.4 and 892 and 894-897). Figure 268.3 and 892 are recorded using parasternal long axis view and Figure 268.4 and 894-897 are from the right parasternal approach.
   (h) Normal aortic arch and proximal descending aorta (ACH, Figs. 268.6 and 268.7, imaged from the suprasternal window).
   (i) Normal mid to distal descending aorta (Fig. 268.8, modified parasternal short-axis view) and proxi-

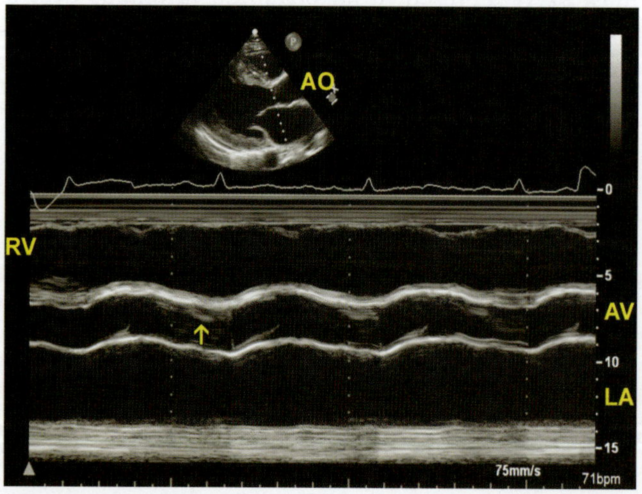

Fig. 268.1: M-mode examination. Arrow shows eccentric bicuspid AV closure with the posterior cusp apparently much larger than the anterior cusp.

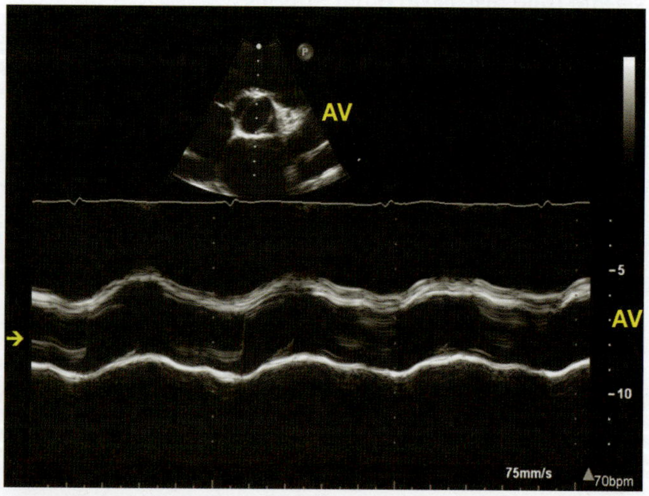

Fig. 268.2: Another M-mode recording from the same patient now shows the anterior cusp much larger than the posterior cusp. Arrow points to eccentric AV closure.

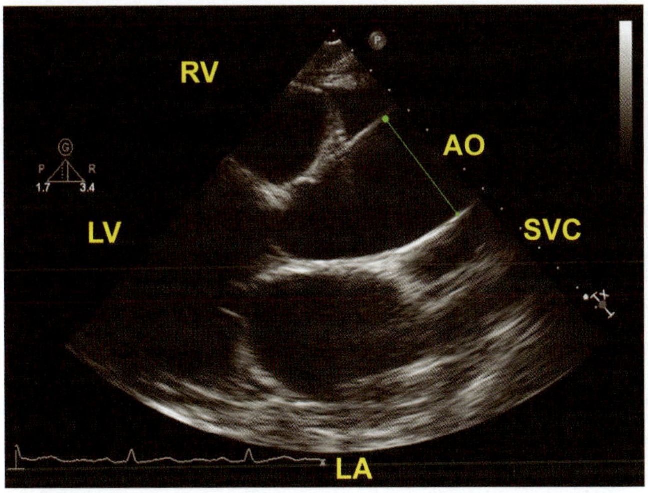

Fig. 268.3: Prarasternal long axis view. The ascending aorta is enlarged and measures 4.0 cm.

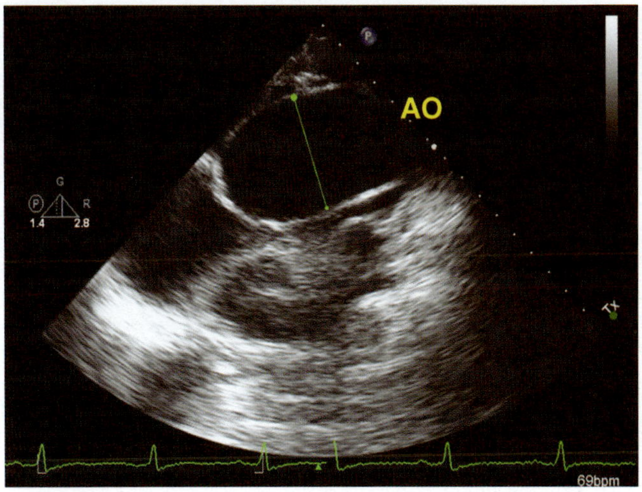

Fig. 268.4: Ascending aorta is examined from the right parasternal approach.

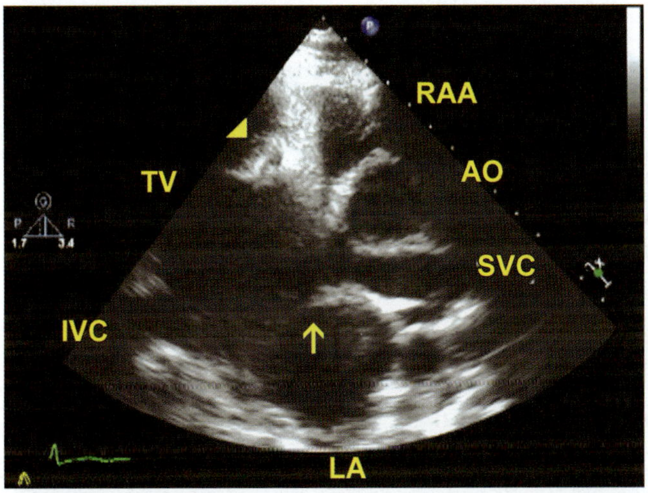

Fig. 268.5: Right parasternal examination. Arrowhead points to right coronary artery and arrow to interatrial septum.

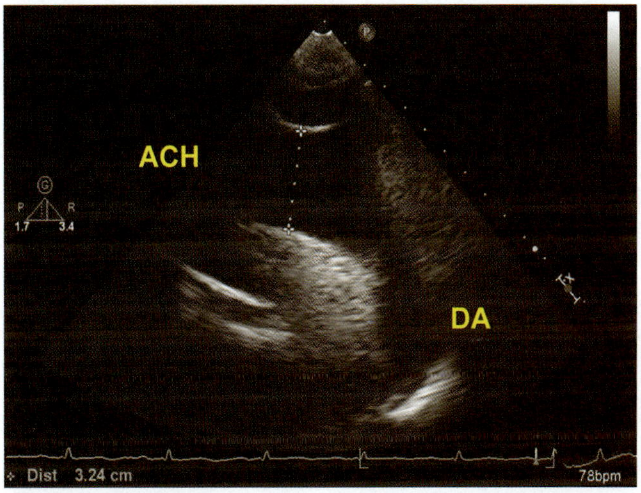

Fig. 268.6: Suprasternal examination. The aortic arch (ACH) and proximal thoracic descending aorta (DA) are imaged. The arch measures 3.24 cm.

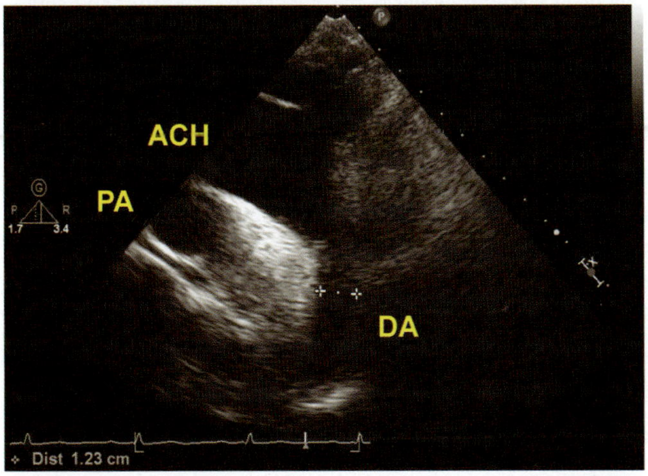

Fig. 268.7: Suprasternal examination. The proximal descending aorta (DA) measures 1.23 cm (normal).

mal abdominal aorta (AB AO, Fig. 268.9 and 902, subcostal examinattion).

(j) Color Doppler flow signals are visualized entering thc RΛ from both SVC and IVC (Fig. 268.10 and 899, right parasternal window).

(k) Because a bicuspid AV may be associated with pathological changes in the media of the aortic wall, aortic aneurysm formation and/or dissection are more likely to occur and these patients should have regular follow-up echocardiograms. Therefore, it is important to distinguish a bicuspid AV from a tricuspid AV (905 and 906 from a different patient, parasternal short axis views).

(l) Figure 268.11 represents a composite in this patient showing the aorta from its origin at the

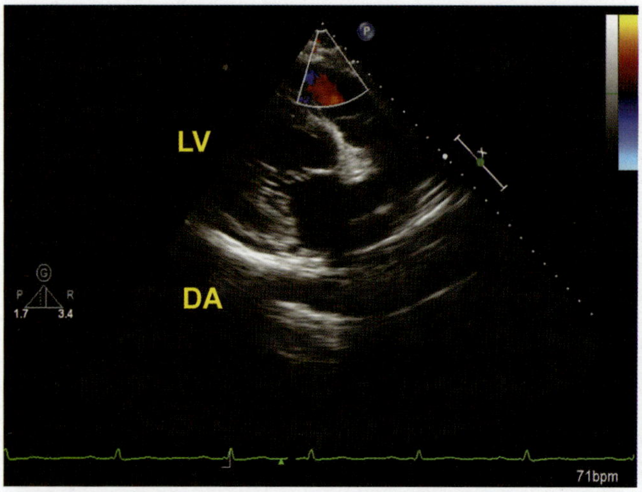

Fig. 268.8: Descending thoracic aorta (DA) viewed in long axis in the LV-pulmonic plane (modified parasternal short axis view).

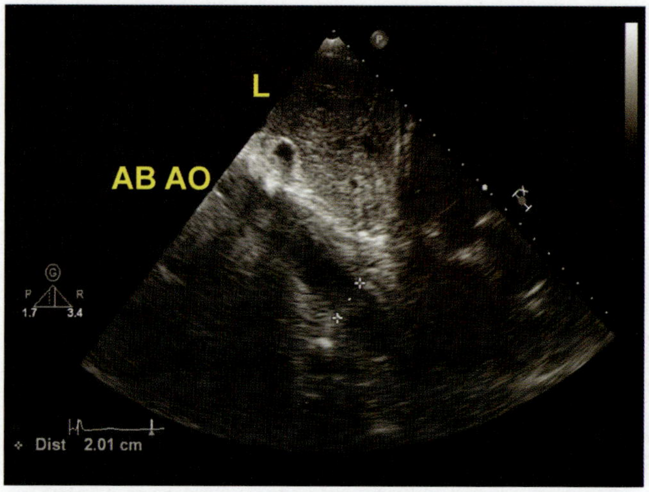

Fig. 268.9: Subcostal examination shows the proximal abdominal aorta (AB AO) which measures 2.01 cm (normal).

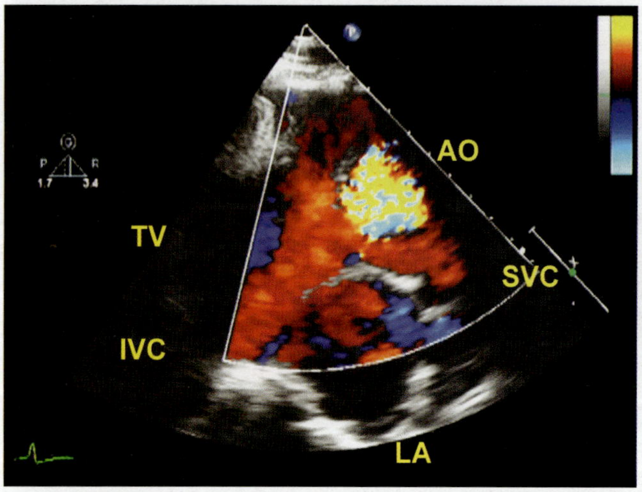

Fig. 268.10: Right parasternal examination. Color Doppler shows flow signals entering RA from both IVC and SVC.

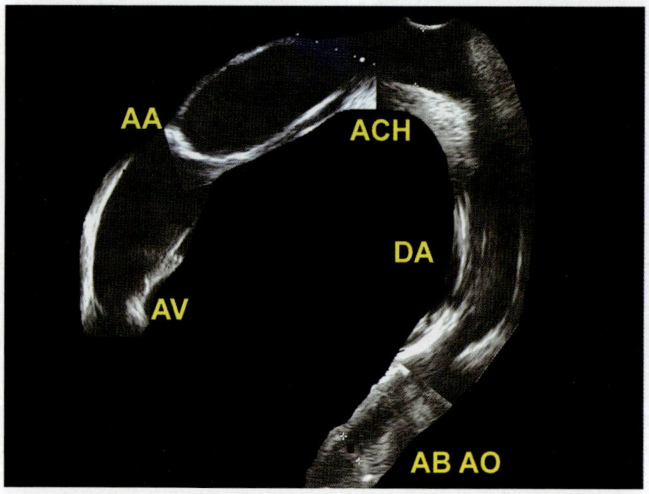

Fig. 268.11: Aortic segments obtained from various 2DTTE windows have been placed together in this patient to reconstruct the entire course of the aorta from the AV level to proximal abdominal aorta.

AV level to proximal abdominal aorta by splicing and pasting aortic segments obtained from various views. Figures 268.12 to 268.15 are composites prepared in the same manner as above from 4 different patients. Figure 268.16 is a schematic showing various echocardiographic windows used to image the aorta transthoracically.

(m) Right parasternal examination cannot be used to assess aortic stenosis.

Ans. (m)

It is recommended that right parasternal examination should be done in every patient with suspected aortic stenosis because maximum gradients may be obtained from this window and severity more accurately characterized. This is because the ultrasonic beam can be aligned parallel to the AS jet.

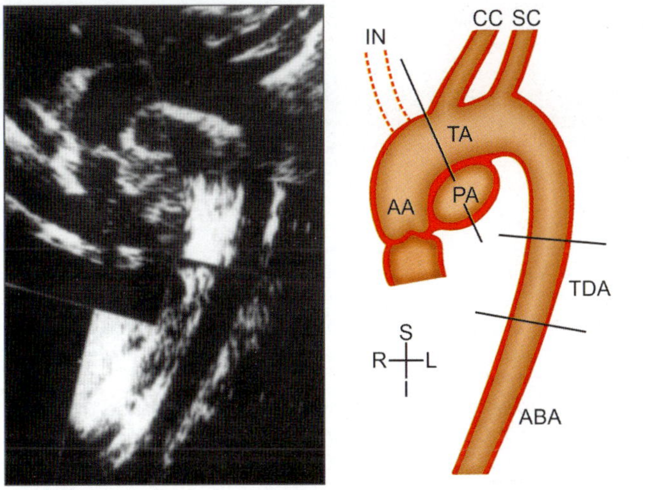

Fig. 268.12: The normal aorta reconstructed from the root level to the abdominal region by assembling 2D images of contiguous segments obtained from different transducer positions.

(AA: Ascending aorta: ABA: Abdominal aorta; CC: Common carotid artery; IN: Innominate artery; PA: Pulmonary artery; SC: Subclavian artery; TA: Transverse aorta (aortic arch); TDA: thoracic descending aorta).

Source: Reproduced with permission from Mathew T, Nanda NC. Two-dimensional and Doppler echocardiographic evaluation of aortic aneurysm and dissection. Am J Cardiol. 1984 Aug 1;54(3):379-85.

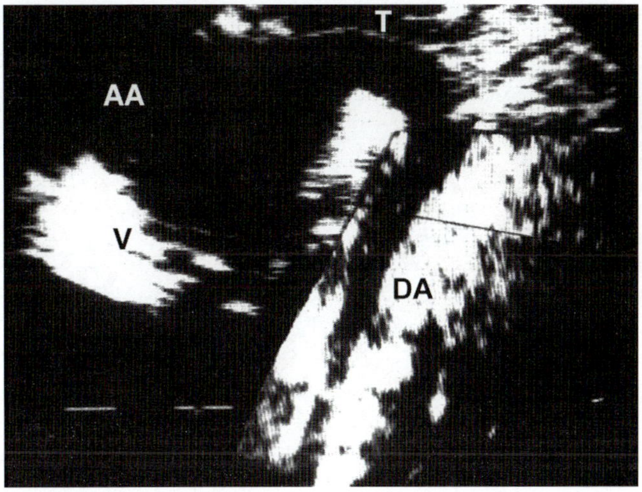

Fig. 268.13: Ascending aortic aneurysm. This composite illustration made by the reconstruction method as in Figure 268.12 to show the full extent of the aneurysm. The transverse aortic arch (T) and the descending thoracic aorta (DA) are not involved.

(AA: Ascending aorta; V: Aortic valve).

Source: Reproduced with permission from Mathew T, Nanda NC. Two-dimensional and Doppler echocardiographic evaluation of aortic aneurysm and dissection. Am J Cardiol. 1984 Aug 1;54(3):379-85.

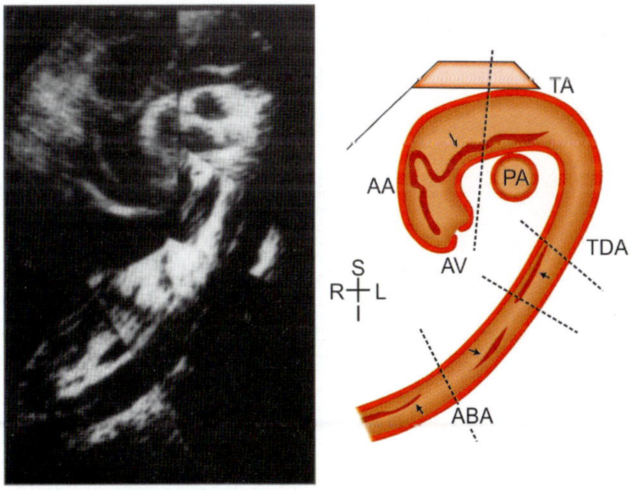

Fig. 268.14: Aortic dissection (DeBakey type I). This composite illustration was also made by the reconstruction method. The dissection flap (arrows) can be seen in the ascending aorta (AA), transverse aortic arch (TA), thoracic descending aorta (TDA) and in the abdominal segment (ABA).

(A: Aortic valve; PA: Pulmonary artery).

Source: Reproduced with permission from Mathew T, Nanda NC. Two-dimensional and Doppler echocardiographic evaluation of aortic aneurysm and dissection. Am J Cardiol. 1984 Aug 1;54(3):379-85.

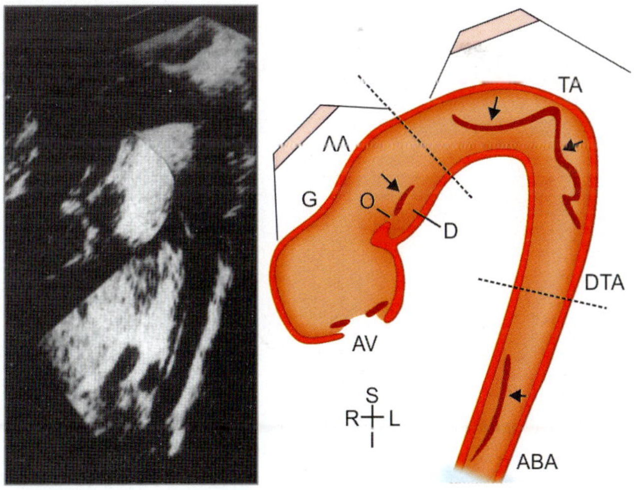

Fig. 268.15: Reopening of dissection in a patient previously treated by resection and graft replacement of the proximal ascending aorta. Top, dissection flap (arrows) in the ascending aorta (AA), transverse aortic arch (TA) and descending thoracic aorta (DTA). A small, constant area of discontinuity in the proximal flap suggests the presence of communication (0) between the false (D) and true lumen.

(ABA: Proximal abdominal aorta; AV: Aortic valve: G: Graft).

Source: Reproduced with permission from Mathew T, Nanda NC. Two-dimensional and Doppler echocardiographic evaluation of aortic aneurysm and dissection. Am J Cardiol. 1984 Aug 1;54(3):379-85.

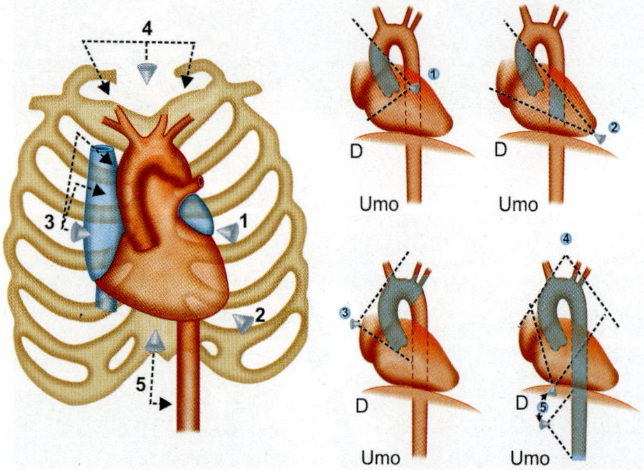

Fig. 268.16: Various transducer positions used to examine the aorta in our cases.
1: Precordial; 2: Apical: 3: Right parasternal including infraclavicular; 4: Suprasternal and supraclavicular; 5: Subcostal and abdominal. D: Diaphragm: Um: Umbilicus.
Source: Reproduced with permission from Mathew T, Nanda NC. Two-dimensional and Doppler echocardiographic evaluation of aortic aneurysm and dissection. Am J Cardiol. 1984 Aug 1;54(3):379-85.

MOVIES 892 TO 906

REFERENCES

1. Nanda NC, Gramiak R, Manning JA, Mahoney EB, Lipchik EO, DeWeese JA: Echocardiographic recognition of the congenital bicuspid aortic valve. Circulation 1974;49:870-875
2. Nanda NC, Karakus G, Degirmencioglu A (Editors). Manual of Echocardiography (2016). Jaypee Brothers. Philadelphia, New Delhi, London and Panama.

CASE 269

Mohamed A, Arora G, Kemaloglu Ozkt, Mahajan A, Sankhyan P, Joson M, Elsayed M, Arisha MJ, Nanda NC

A 60-year-old male with a history of cardiac murmur since childhood presents with worsening fatigue and shortness of breath. He underwent intraoperative 2DTEE (907-909).

1. **What is the diagnosis?**
   (a) Primum ASD/Partial atrioventricular septal defect
   (b) Secundum ASD
   (c) Complete AV canal defect/Complete atrioventricular septal defect
   (d) Sinus venosus ASD

Ans. (a)

In the complete form, both ASD and VSD as well as a common atrioventricular valve and ring are present. In the incomplete or partial form, as in this patient, the VSD is closed by a bridge of tissue so that only the ASD (arrows in 907 and 908) persists. The ASD is in the basal septum with no septal tissue between the defect and the two separate atrioventricular valves and rings. The arrow in 909 shows left to right shunt through the defect.

MOVIES 907 TO 909

CASE 270

Smadar Kort

CLINICAL PRESENTATION

A 75-year-old man presented for cardiac cath for evaluation of hypoxia.

History is significant for hypertension and remote stroke.

He is now s/p recent hip replacement.

Postoperative, the patient complained of shortness of breath upon sitting, standing and ambulating, but was completely asymptomatic lying down.

CARDIAC CATH

Revealed nonobstructive coronary artery disease normal LV systolic function and no evidence of shunting, as demonstrated in the oxygen saturation measurements in the table below.

SVC (superior vena cava)	64.5%
Mid-RA (right atrium)	61.8%
PCW (Pulmonary capillary wedge pressure)	66.2%
IVC (inferior vena cava)	69.8%
Main PA (pulmonary artery)	65.3%
Descending AO (aorta)	93.9%

ECHOCARDIOGRAM (REFER TO FIGS AND MOVIES)

1. **Are the images consistent and can explain the clinical presentation of this patient?**

Ans. Yes

2. **What is the clinical diagnosis?**

Ans. Platypnea orthodeoxia

PLATYPNEA ORTHODEOXIA

Platypnea—dyspnea induced by upright position.

Orthodeoxia—arterial desaturation in an upright position.

Two conditions must coexist in order to cause platypnea orthodeoxia—an anatomical component in the form of a intracardiac communication, most commonly a patent foramen ovale (PFO) or an atrial septal defect, and a functional component which redirects the shunt flow when assuming an upright position, such as pericardial effusion, emphysema, liver cirrhosis, ileus, aortic aneurysm or prominent Eustachian valve. Some of these conditions can externally compress the RA or change the relation of the IVC and the fossa ovalis. Upon standing up the interatrial septum and the patent foramen ovale are stretched and the IVC flow is preferentially directed across the patent foramen ovale. Compression of the RA will increase the RA pressure above that of the LA (left atrium), resulting in right to left shunt.

REVIEW OF THE QUESTIONS AND ANSWERS

910 and Figure 270.1 reveal the presence of a dilated aortic root as seen on TTE.

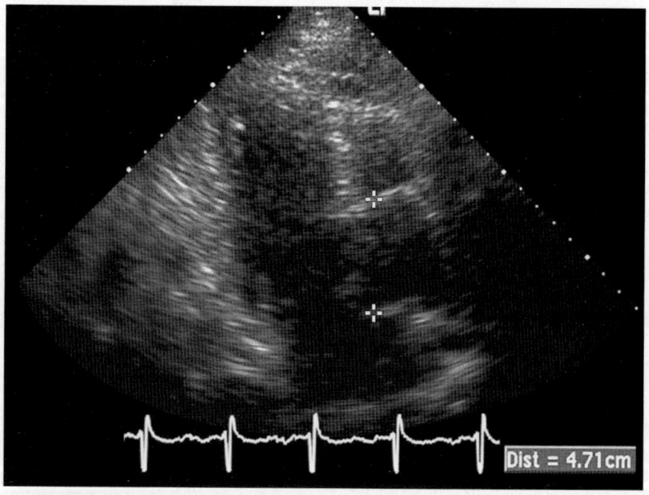

Fig. 270.1: Aortic root at the sinuses of Valsalva is dilated measuring 4.71 cm in diameter

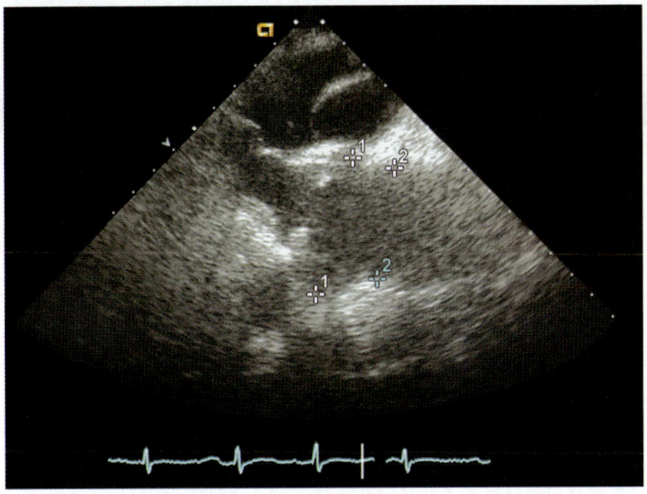

Fig. 270.2: Measurement of the aortic root obtained from a long axis of the aorta as seen on TEE. The aortic root at the sinuses of Valsalva is mildly dilated, measuring 4.76 cm in diameter. The proximal ascending aorta at the sinotubular junction measured 3.75 cm in diameter.

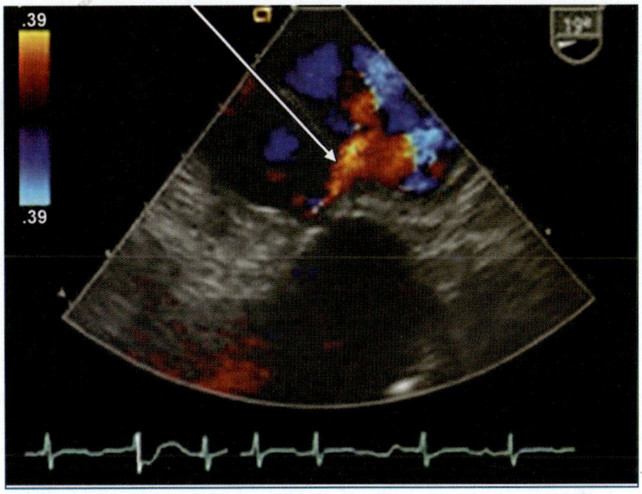

Fig. 270.3: Arrow points to a right to left shunt across a patent foramen ovale.

Figure 270.2 demonstrates additional images of the aortic root obtained using TEE. Figure 270.3 and the 910 to 917 demonstrate the presence of a PFO with a right to left shunt across it (arrow).

EXPLANATION OF THE MECHANISM

Our patient had a patent foramen ovale and a dilated aortic root, which externally compressed the right atrium, creating significant right to left shunting across the patent foramen ovale. However, the aortic root was only mildly dilated. The reason that the aortic root compressed the right atrium, was that it was pushed against it by an ileus that the patient developed following hip replacement surgery.

HAPPY ENDING

Our patient underwent a colonoscopy with placement of colonic decompression tube with resolution of symptoms and positional desaturation.

In summary, the diagnosis in this patient was established by echocardiography, while the treatment provided by colonoscopy.

MOVIES 910 TO 917

CASE 271

Virginia Michelis

A 54-year-old male, alcoholic until 10 years ago. Smoked 15 cigarettes daily until 12 years ago. Hepatitis C virus chronic infection, untreated.

- *Admitted in emergency*: Decompensated chronic obstructive pulmonary disease (COPD) dyspnea at rest. Normal lung examination; normal cardiovascular examination.
- *Abdominal ultrasound*: Liver with impaired morphostructure, portal hypertension, absence of ascites, 4 cm nodule in the left lobe.

Total bilirubin: 2.22 mg/dL, direct bilirubin 0.94 mg/dL, alkaline phosphatase 272 U/L, AST 139 U/L (33), ALT 97 U/L (30) albumin 3.4 g/dL, total protein 7.7 g/dL.

Prothrombin rate: 59% Hemoglobin 11.8 g/dL HCT 33%, mean corpuscular volume 99 fL, white blood cells 8100/cu.mm, platelets 102 × 10^9/L.

Fibrogastroscopy: Large esophageal variceal and subcardiales.

Abdominal magnetic resonance: Multiple nodules replaced most of the hepatic parenchyma (Fig. 271.2).

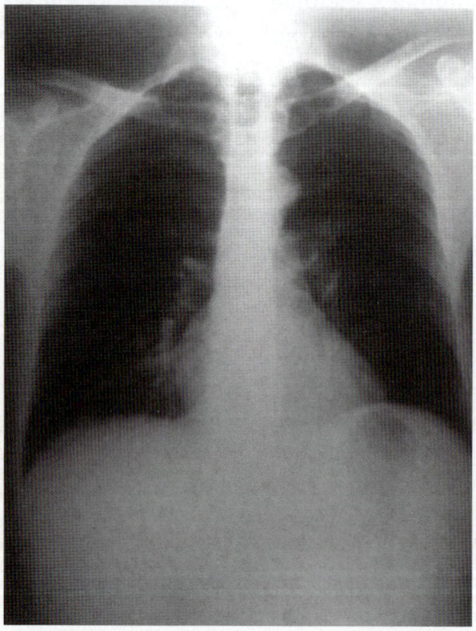

Fig. 271.1: Chest X-ray.

Mild splenomegaly, holder of 17 mm, permeable splenorenal collateral circulation.

No abdominal lymphadenopathy or ascites.

The patient is a candidate for liver transplantation.

The primary diagnosis of chronic obstructive pulmonary disease is a contraindication for transplant.

PRIMARY DIAGNOSIS: CHRONIC OBSTRUCTIVE PULMONARY DISEASE

COPD or differential diagnosis: hepatopulmonary syndrome (See Table 271.1 also).?

Can an echocardiogram, change the fate of this patient (Figs. 271.3 to 271.5 and 918 to 921?

Utility of agited saline contrast to unmask hepatopulmonary syndrome (Figs. 271.6 to 271.9 and 922).

DISCUSSION REGARDING HIS LUNG DISEASE

- Stopped smoking 12 years ago.
- Onset of respiratory symptoms 2 years ago.
- Onset of dyspnea on exertion 2 years ago which has progressed and currently dyspnic on minimal exertion
- Physical examination does not suggest chronic lung disease

  No clubbing and other stigma of chronic hypoxemia (Fig. 271.1).

Table 271.1: Consequences on lung of advanced liver disease arteriovenous fistulas → alteration in v/q.

Condition	*Usual findings*
Hepatopulmonary syndrome	Pulmonary vascular dilatations with varying degrees of hypoxemia
Portopulmonary hypertension	Pulmonary vasoconstriction, with eventual right heart failure
Alpha 1 antitrypsin deficiency	Panacinar emphysema with airflow obstruction
Hepatic hydrothorax	Pleural effusion, transudate type, with secondary atelectasis

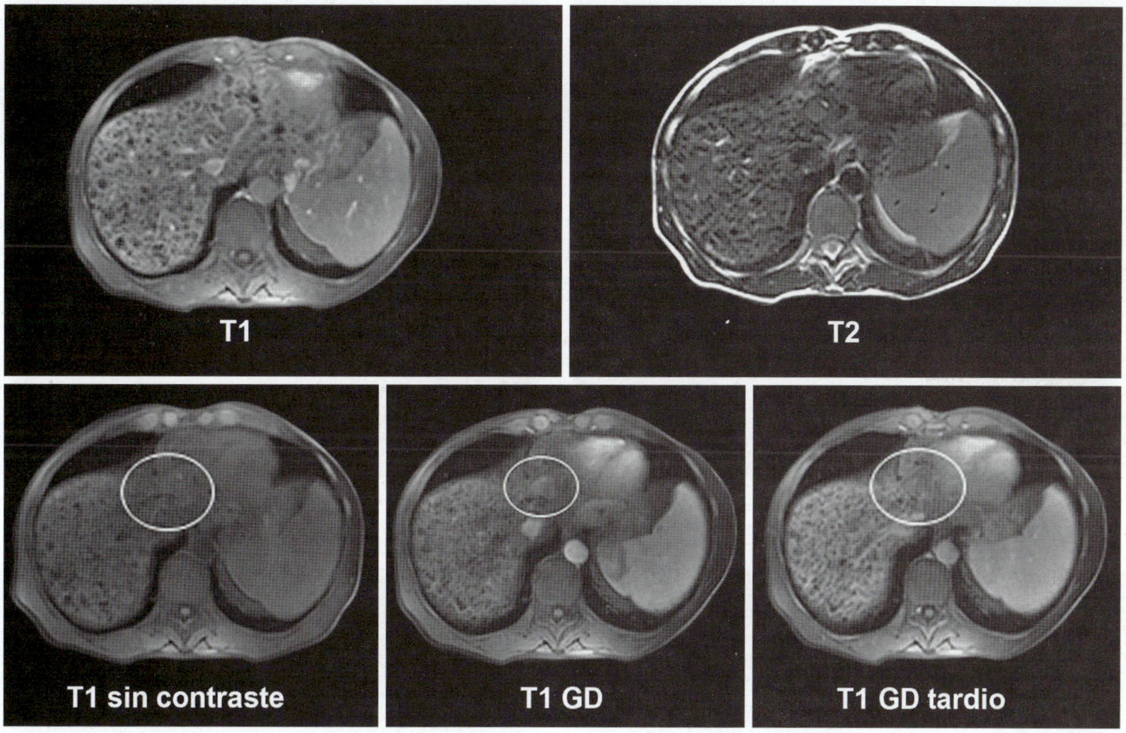

Fig. 271.2: Thoracoabdominal MRI scans.

With simple agitated saline contrast: The pathophysiology of symptoms became evident. Bubble study positive for intrapulmonary shunting. Bubbles (arrow in 922) appear in the LV and after a few beats in right chambers. The patient underwent a liver transplant with good evolution.

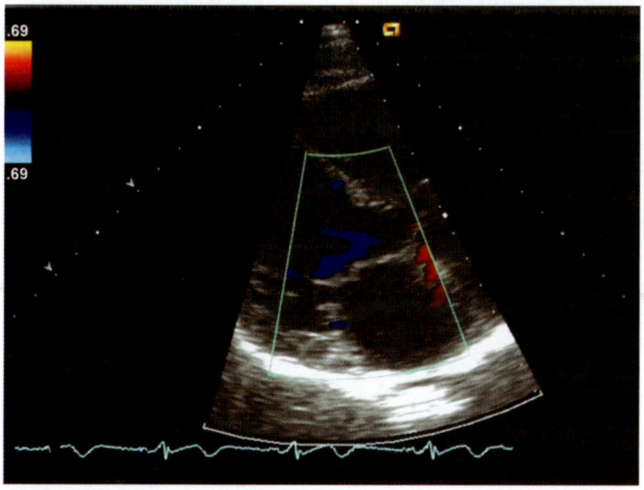

Fig. 271.3: Long axis view of LV.

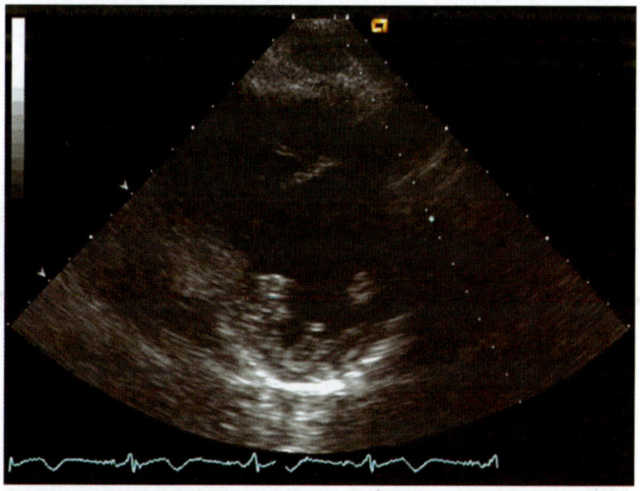

Fig. 271.4: Short axis view of LV.

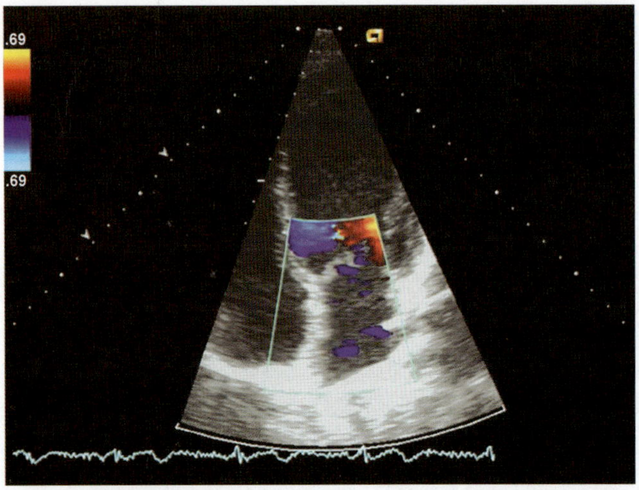

Fig. 271.5: Doppler of mitral valve.

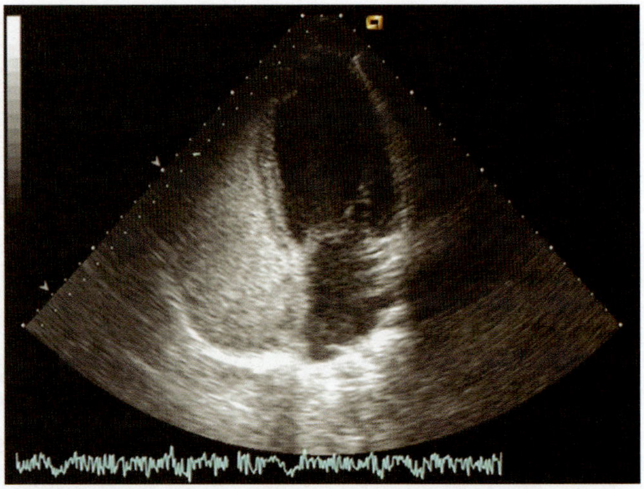

Fig. 271.6: Saline contrast only in right chambers. There is no intracardiac shunt.

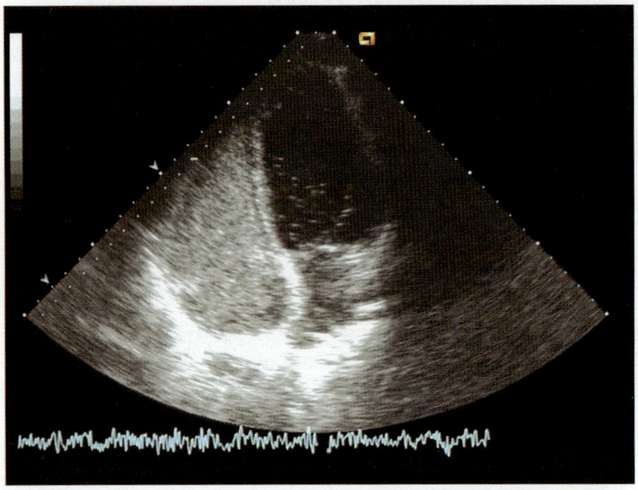

Fig. 271.7: After a few beats, microbubbles begin to appear in left chambers too.

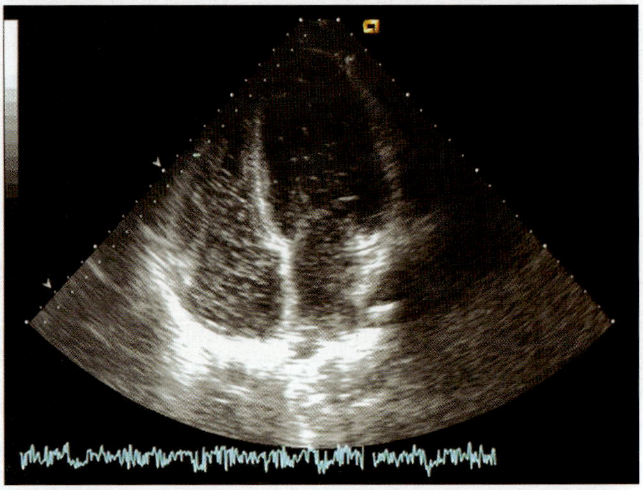

Fig. 271.8: Some beats later.

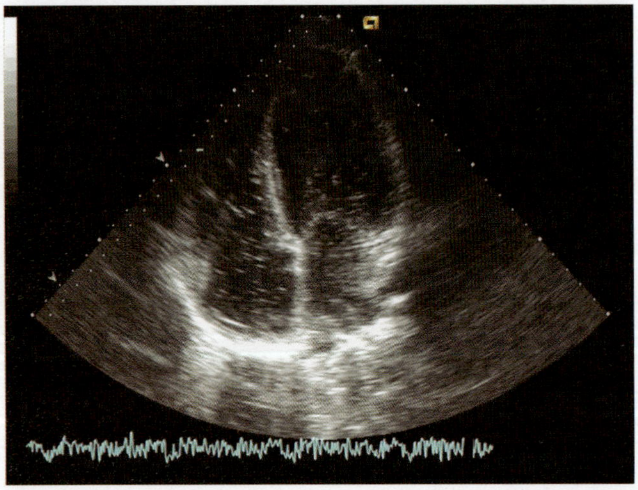

Fig. 271.9: After a few minutes, microbubbles persist. They cross pulmonary shunt and can be seen in right cavities.

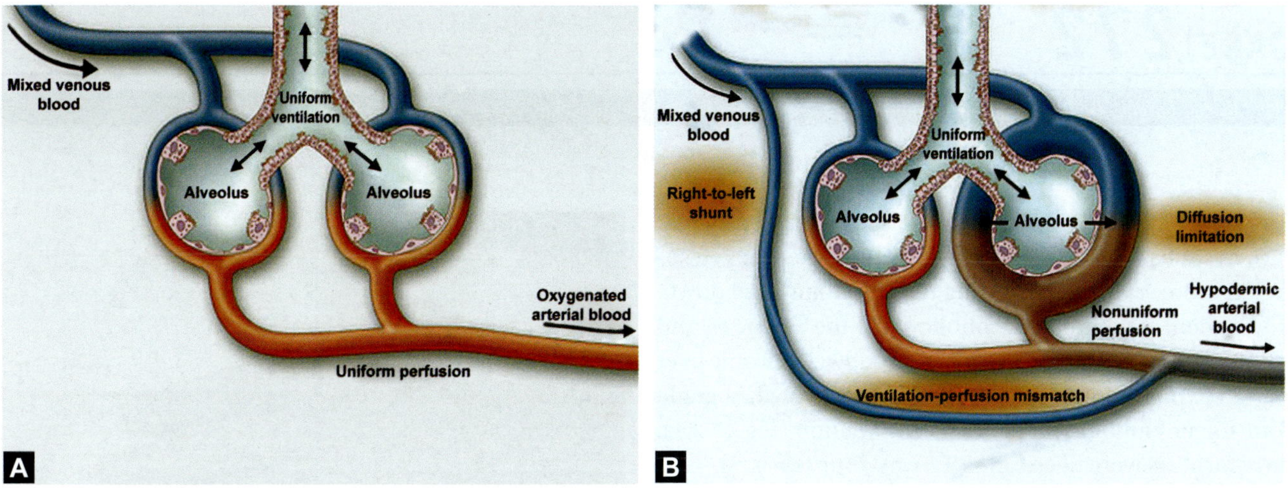

Figs. 271.10A and B: (A) Represents a healthy lung with uniform alveolar ventilation and homogenous blood flow. (B) shows 2 major reasons for shunting namely ventilation-perfusion mismatch and vascular dilation with diffusion limitation. (*Source*: Reproduced with permission Rodriguez-Roisin R, Krowka MJ. Hepatopulmonary syndrome—a liver-induced lung vascular disorder. N Engl J Med 2008;358(22):2384).

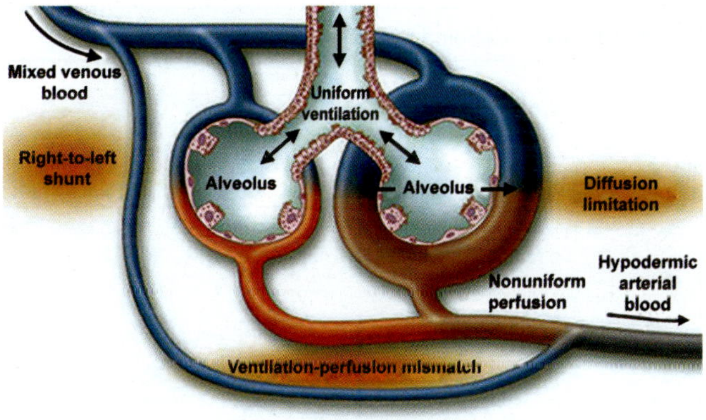

Fig. 271.11: Represents pathological lung.

MOVIES 918 TO 922

CASE 272

Rohit Tandon, Ravinder Pal Singh, Maninder Singh

The patient is a 34-year-old male with onset of progressive dyspnea 6 months ago. Over the past one week dyspnea is more severe in the sitting position than lying down. The patient is a chronic alcoholic since the age of 18 and ultrasound examination of abdomen showed chronic liver parenchymal changes suggestive of fibrosis. He has grade four finger clubbing on general examination (Fig. 272.1). No murmurs were heard. 2D TTE was done (923).

1. **What does the bubble study show?**
   (a) No significant intracardiac shunting. Bubbles can appear in the left heart normally.
   (b) Significant intrapulmonary shunting.
   (c) Significant shunt from RA to LA.

Ans. (b)

A large arteriovenous malformation was noted on the right side on the angiogram and the patient subsequently underwent coil repair. The patient is scheduled for liver transplantation. Arrow in 923 shows bubbles appearing in the LV following intravenous saline injection.

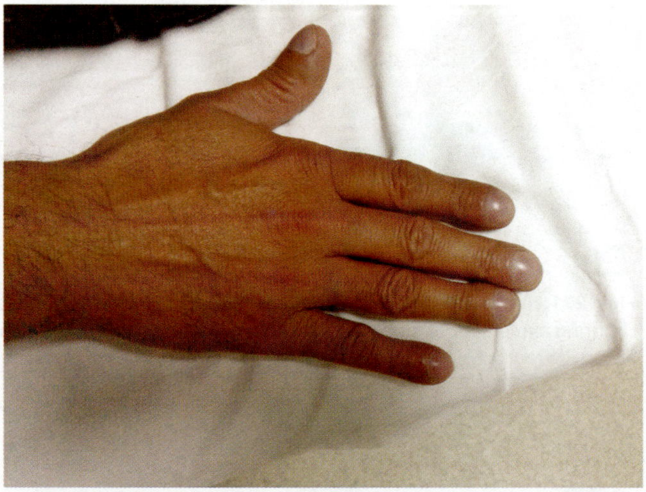

Fig. 272.1: Finger clubbing with cyanosis.

MOVIE 923

CASE 273

Nanda NC, Mohamed A, Keser N, Arora G, Mahajan A, Sankhyan P, Joson M, Gok G, Elsayed M

The patient is a 24-year-old female with a past medical history significant for tricuspid atresia and dexro-transposition of the great arteries (DTGA) s/p pulmonary artery band and classic Fontan repair who presents with chest pain and dizziness. She underwent TTE (924-931).

1. **What is the relationship of aorta and pulmonary artery (PA) in DTGA?**
   (a) Aorta anterior and to the left of the pulmonary artery
   (b) Aorta is anterior and to the right of the pulmonary artery
   (c) Aorta and pulmonary artery are side by side
   (d) Aorta to the right and posterior to the pulmonary artery

Ans. (b)

This is the most common presentation but we can also see aorta directly anterior to the pulmonary artery as in this patient (929 and 930). The arrows in 924 and 925 point to the VSD, arrow in 928 to the high velocity reverse shunt from LV to RV. This is because of PA banding (B). TA shows the atretic TV (931). Note the small RV.

MOVIES 924 TO 931

CASE 274

Elsayed M, Nanda NC

This was a 54-year-old female with drug refractory atrial fibrillation who was referred for catheter ablation. 2D TEE was done to rule out a thrombus in LA and LAA (932 and 933).

1. **What does 932 show?**
   (a) Large pulmonary vein
   (b) Blood cyst compressing LA
   (c) Pericardial cyst
   (d) Left sided SVC draining into coronary sinus (CS)
   (e) Loculated pericardial effusion

Ans. (d)

A dilated CS (932) into which a left sided SVC drains is generally imaged between the left upper pulmonary vein (LUPV) and the LAA. In 932, LAA is not visualized but the dilated CS is seen below the LUPV.

2. **933 was obtained by rotating the transesophageal probe posteriorly to image the descending thoracic aorta. What are the findings?**
   (a) Normal descending thoracic aorta.
   (b) Descending thoracic aorta dissection with true and false lumens
   (c) Cystic tumor behind the thoracic aorta
   (d) Dilated hemi-azygos vein

Ans. (d)

This patient also had an interrupted IVC with azygos continuation resulting in dilatation of the azygos vein which is noted posteriorly (lower arrow in 933).This finding can mimic aortic dissection. Color Doppler guided pulse Doppler interrogation would have been useful in this case because it would have shown venous type signals in the vein as opposed to arterial flow signals in the adjacent anteriorly located descending aorta (upper arrow in 933).[1,2]

MOVIES 932 AND 933

REFERENCES

1. Suthar, AL, Nanda, NC, Harris, PJ (1983), Two-dimensional and Doppler Echocardiographic Identification of Infrahepatic Interruption of Inferior Vena Cava with Azygos Continuation. Pacing and Clinical Electrophysiology, 6:963–971.
2. Hardwick T, Belcher E, Sabharwal T, King J. Interrupted inferior vena cava: high-risk anatomy for right thoracotomy. Interact Cardiovasc Thorac Surg. 2011 May;12(5):850-2.

CASE 275

Choudhary R, Gautam D, Mohamed A, Elsayed M, Nanda NC

This is an 8-year-old male child who presented with dyspnea on exertion of 2 years duration. On examination, a continuous murmur was heard at the lower left sternal border, more prominent in diastole. 2DTTE was done (Figs. 275.1A to D and 934).

1. **What do the echoes show?**
   (a) Sinus of Valsalva aneurysm with rupture
   (b) Dilated transverse sinus of the pericardium
   (c) Circumflex coronary artery to LA fistula
   (d) Cor triatriatum sinister

Ans. (c)

Arrows in Figures 275.1A to D show the dilated circumflex artery with turbulent flow and communication with LA (arrowhead in 934). His father has refused any further investigation and intervention.

MOVIE 934

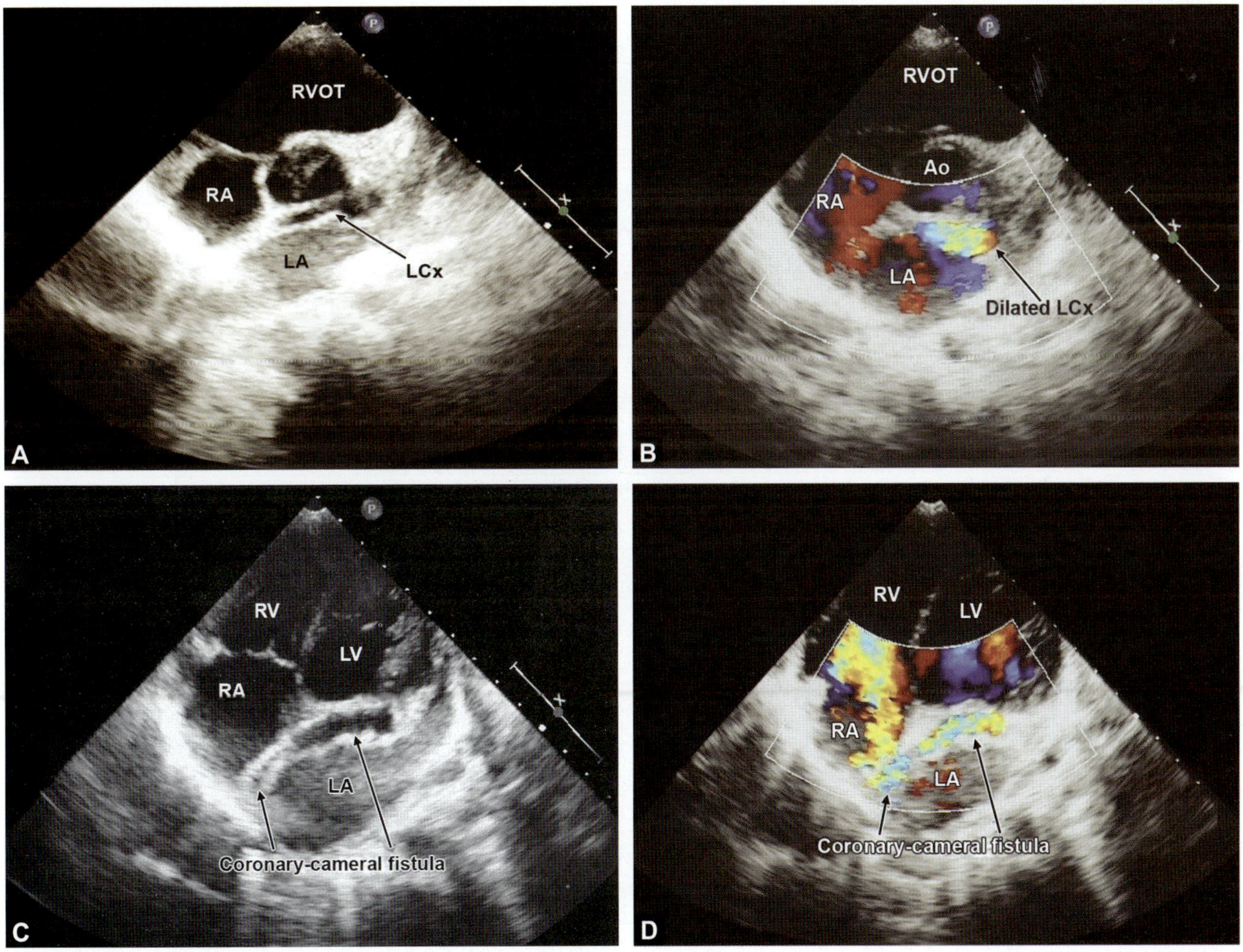

Figs. 275.1A to D: Coronary-cameral fistula. Parasternal views show a dilated left circumflex coronary artery (LCx) with turbulent flow communicating with the LA.

CASE 276

Virginia Michelis

The patient is a 57-year-old male, smoker with hypertension, type 2 diabetes mellitus and big hands. He presented with acute pulmonary edema and shock. Blood cultures were negative. EKG is shown below (Fig. 276.1).

Transthoracic echo was done (Figs. 276.2 to 276.4 and 935 to 937).

Coronary angiography was normal (Fig. 276.5).

Emergency surgery was performed for papillary muscle necrosis/rupture and biological mitral prosthesis was implanted.

1. **The following conditions could be considered in the differential diagnosis *except*:**
   (a) Papillary muscle necrosis
   (b) Large vegetation
   (c) Valvular/chordae tumor
   (d) Clot
   (e) Accessory papillary muscle

Ans. (e)

Accessory papillary muscle will not show hypermobility.

This patient had acromegaly with large hands and was later operated for pituitary adenoma.

2. **All the following statements regarding acromegaly are correct *except*:**
   (a) Prevalence is 50–70 cases per million individuals.
   (b) Coarse facial features, prominence of brow ridges, macroglossia, prognathism, large hands and toes.
   (c) Edema of fingers and toes and excessive sweating.
   (d) Very large ears and eyes.
   (e) Osteoarthritis, carpal tunnel syndrome and obstructive sleep apnea.

Ans. (d)

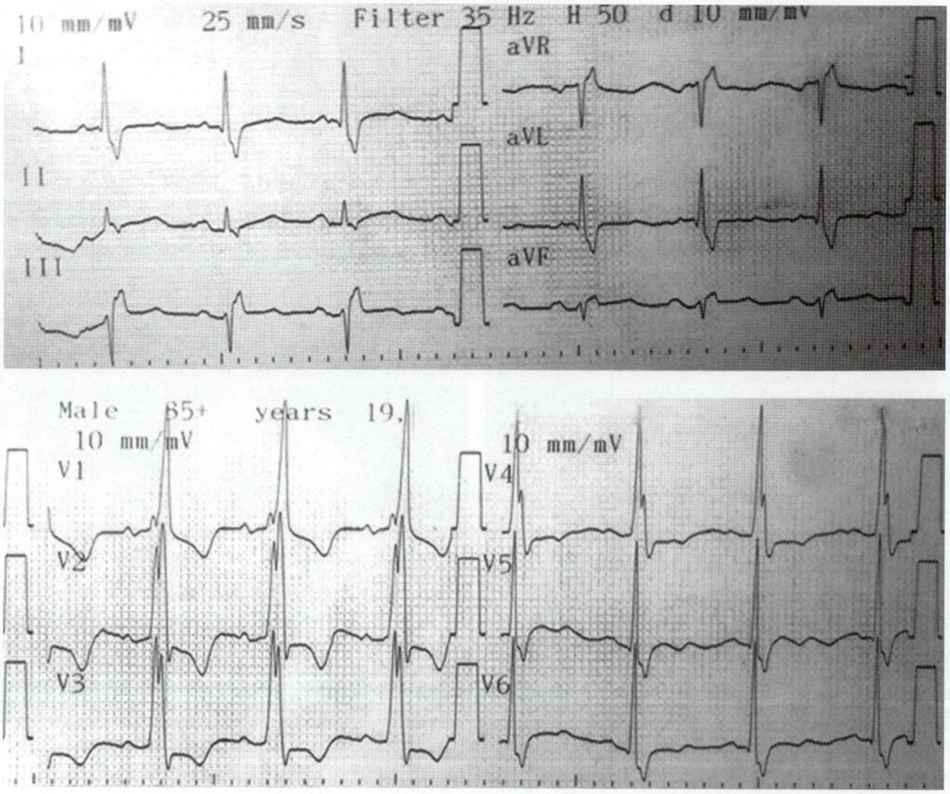

Fig. 276.1: Electrocardiogram.

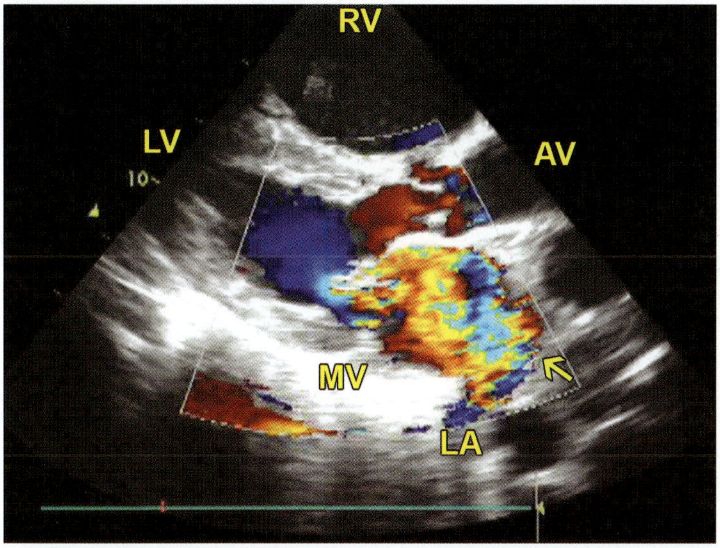

Fig. 276.2 and 935: TTE Parasternal long axis view. Arrow points to severe MR (also in 935).

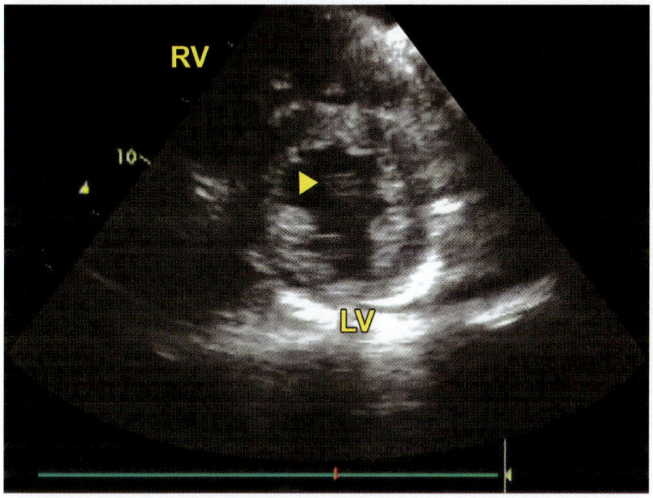

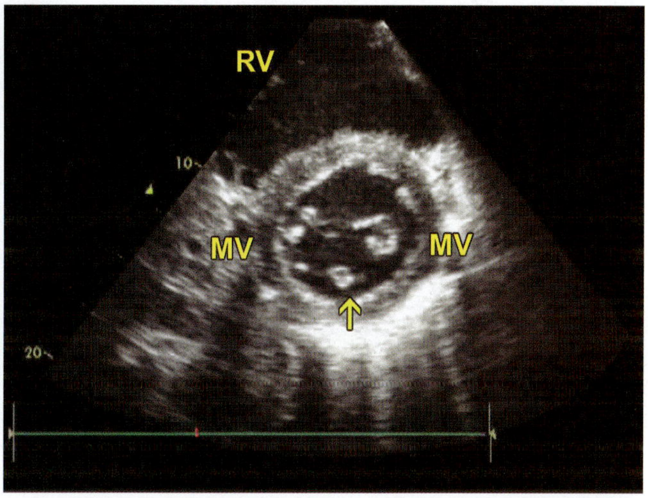

Figs. 276.3 and 276.4 and 936 and 937: TTE Parasternal short axis view. Arrowhead points to chordae (also in 936) and arrow points to a ruptured papillary muscle (also in 937).

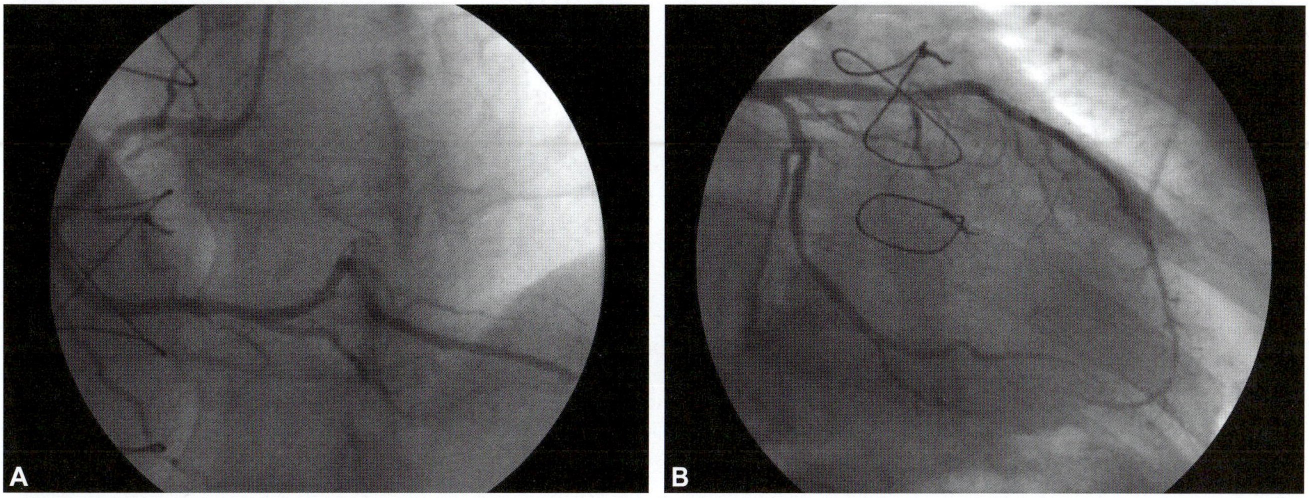

Figs. 276.5A and B: Coronary angiogram

The character of Shrek was inspired by a French fighter from the 1930s, Maurice Tillet, who suffered from acromegaly.

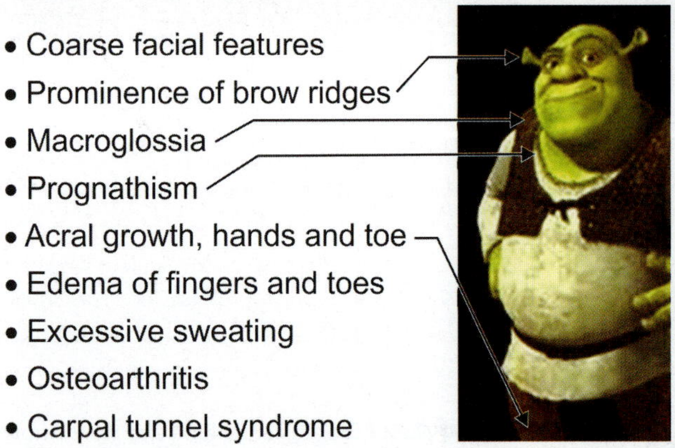

Fig. 276.6: Features of acromegaly.

MOVIES 935 TO 937

CASE 277

Roomi AU, Shah A, Siddiqui LI, Gupta N, Mohamed A, Arisha MJ, Nanda NC

The patient is a 63-year-old female with history of diabetes mellitus and hypertension, with a complaint of shortness of breath (NYHA class II). 2D TTE showed normal LV systolic function and moderate degenerative MR. She was referred for 2DTEE for further assessment of MR severity.

1. **What is the incidental finding on both 2D TTE (938, V = vertical hepatic vein) and 2D TEE (939-941)?**
   (a) RCA fistula
   (b) Hepatic vein flow
   (c) Abnormal pulmonary venous drainage
   (d) Budd-Chiari Syndrome

Ans. (b)

A hepatic vein (arrow) is seen directly entering the RA near the IVC-RA junction. Ultrasound and CT of the abdomen also confirmed the diagnosis. Generally, this is of no clinical significance.

MOVIES 938 TO 941

CASE 278

Shah A, Roomi AU, Siddiqui LI, Gupta N, Mohamed A, Nanda NC

This is an elderly patient with coronary artery disease. 2D TTE was done and showed normal LV and RV function. Valves were structurally normal with insignificant regurgitation (942 and 943).

1. **What abnormality is shown in the subcostal examination?**
   (a) Liver metastases
   (b) Fatty liver
   (c) Cirrhosis of liver
   (d) Normal liver texture

Ans. (b)

The liver displays generalized increase in parenchymal echogenicity which is compatible with diffuse hepatic steatosis (fatty liver).

2. **Ultrasound features of fatty liver include all of the following *except*:**
   (a) Hepatomegaly with smooth liver surface
   (b) Diffuse increased echogenicity
   (c) Acoustic penetration may be decreased, resulting in indistinctness of blood vessels and the diaphragm.
   (d) Large, localized, circumscribed echogenic areas

Ans. (d)

Localized, circumscribed echogenic areas may be seen in liver in cancer metastases. Fatty liver has been associated with several risk factors for coronary artery disease including obesity, diabetes mellitus and dyslipidemia. Therefore, this ultrasound finding may be of clinical importance to cardiologists.

Diffuse fatty liver has been graded as follows:

Grade I: Increased hepatic echogenicity with visible periportal and diaphragmatic echogenicity

Grade II: Increased hepatic echogenicity with imperceptible periportal echogenicity, without obscuration of diaphragm

Grade III: Increased hepatic echogenicity with imperceptible periportal echogenicity and obscuration of diaphragm.

MOVIES 942 AND 943

CASE 279

Nanda NC, Elsayed M

Subcostal images from two different adult patients are shown (944 and 945).

1. **What do the movies show?**
    (a) Stone in the gallbladder
    (b) Stone in the gallbladder plus thickened wall
    (c) Stone in a liver (L) cyst
    (d) Carcinoma of liver/gallbladder

Ans. (b)

The arrowhead in both movies shows a stone in the gallbladder and the arrow in 944 thickened walls of the gallbladder, suggestive of chronic inflammation. "S" represents shadowing from the calcified stones.

2. **What is the importance of these findings to the internist and cardiologist?**

Ans.

These findings may add valuable information in patients presenting with atypical chest pain and provide physicians with information which could be important in their future medical care. In some patients, cholecystitis resulting from a gallstone may present with severe low substernal pain clinically mimicking acute coronary syndrome and the echocardiogram has been helpful in detecting this finding and demonstrating no LV wall motion abnormalities.

MOVIE LEGEND

1. 944 and 945 are reproduced with permission from: Daly DD Jr, El-Shurafa H, Nanda NC, Dumaswala B, Dumaswala K, Kumar N, Mutluer FO. Does the routine echocardiographic exam have a role in the detection and evaluation of cholelithiasis and gallbladder wall thickening? Echocardiography. 2012 Sep;29(8):991-6.

CASE 280

Sangeeta Shah

A 55-year-old male with history of PVCs presents with intermittent palpitations.

- Physical exam: BP 110/70 mm Hg; HR 88 BPM; Pulse oximetry 100%
- EKG: NSR

Echocardiogram performed (946 to 948) shows an area of echodensity in the inferolateral wall (arrow).

1. **What additional CV imaging modality will assist with the diagnosis? What is the next best CV modality?**
   (a) Echocardiography with contrast
   (b) CT scan
   (c) Cardiac cath
   (d) Cardiac MRI

Ans. (d)

CARDIAC MRI (FIGS. 280.1, 280.2 AND 949 TO 952)

- Localization of mass
- Assess extent of mass and involvement of surrounding structures
- Tissue characterization

MRI

- T1, T2 weighted sequences
- Fat suppression
- Cine

} Tissue characteristics, Localization

- First pass perfusion
- Delayed perfusion
- Late Gadolinium enhancement

} Localization, Perfusion, Necrosis

2. **What is this mass (Table 280.1)?**
   (a) Area of infarct
   (b) Lipoma
   (c) Fibroma
   (d) Myxoma

Ans. (c)

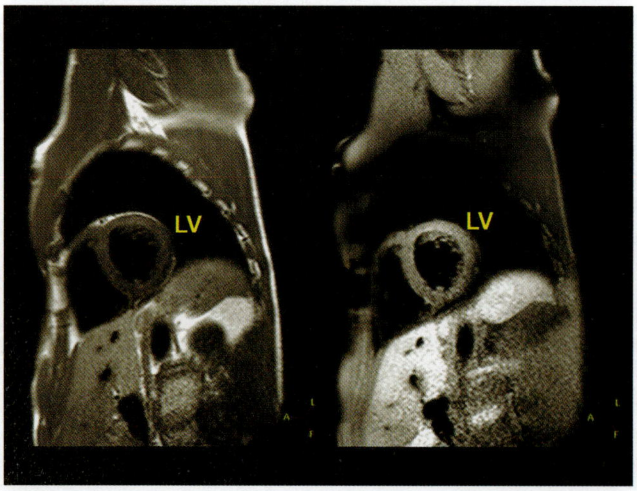

Fig. 280.1: The mass is not seen on black blood imaging with (left) or without (right) fat saturation.

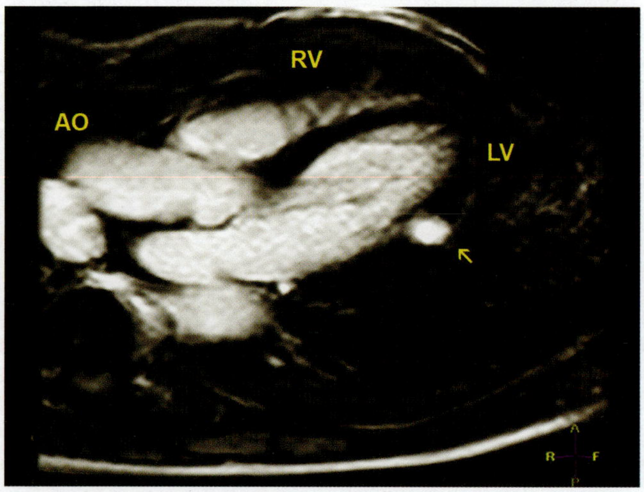

Fig. 280.2: Delayed hyperenhancement. Arrow points to the mass in the inferolateral wall in this figure and in 952.

CARDIAC MASSES OF LEFT VENTRICLE (TABLE 280.1)

Table 280.1: Likely causes of cardiac masses or masslike lesions in order of occurrence.

Size	*Causes of masses or masslike lesions*
Left atrium	Myxoma Thrombus Septal lipoma
Left ventricle	Thrombus Papillary muscle Rhabdomyoma Metastasis Fibroma
Right atrium	Thrombus Myxoma Hypernephroma Eustachian valve Chiari network Angiosarcoma
Right ventricle	Thrombus Rhabdomyoma Secondary deposit Angiosarcoma

Ref: MR imaging of Cardiac Tumors.
RadioGraphics 2005; 25:1255–1276. Published online 10.1148/rg.255045721.C.

- Thrombus would be black on delayed hyperenhancement
- Infarct would have wall motion abnormality
- Lipoma would be present on images with fat and suppressed on fat saturation images (Figs. 280.1 and 280.2)
- Rhabdomyoma: associated with tuberous sclerosis and found most frequently in children.

FIBROMA

- Benign tumors-composed of fibroblasts and collagen
- Intramyocardial
- Often associated with arrhythmia

MOVIE LEGENDS

946 and 947: Parasternal long-axis with a circumscribed echo bright mass (arrow) in the inferolateral wall.

948: Short-axis LV with an echo bright area (arrow) seen in the inferolateral wall.

949-951: Cardiac MRI Fast-Spine Echo. No mass is noted.

952: Cardiac perfusion with gadolinium. Arrow points to the mass.

CASE 281

Sridhar Venkatachalam, Masood Ahmad

This case is reproduced with permission from Echocardiography - Havins J., Lick S., Boor P., Arora H., Ahmad M., Real time three-dimensional transesophageal echocardiography in partial posteromedial papillary muscle rupture. Echocardiography 2013;30:E179–E181.

CASE

A 60-year-old Caucasian male presented to the emergency department with 2 days' history of shortness of breath on minimal exertion. He denied chest pain, palpitations, leg edema or fever. His past medical history was notable for well-controlled hypertension and asthma. On examination, he was in moderate distress with a respiratory rate of 22 per minute. His other vital signs were notable for a heart rate of 112 beats per minute, blood pressure of 95/60 mm Hg, and oxygen saturation of 92% on room air. A 2/6 systolic murmur was heard at the apex and he had bilateral basal crackles. Clinical exam was concerning for acute pulmonary edema. Twelve lead electrocardiogram demonstrated sinus tachycardia with 1 mm ST segment depression in leads II, III and aVF. Relevant laboratory data included serum troponin I of 10.9 ng/mL, creatine kinase-MB of 17.3 ng/mL, N-terminal pro brain natriuretic peptide of 15,200 pg/mL and creatinine of 1.83 mg/dL. Chest X ray revealed bilateral interstitial edema with no apparent cardiomegaly. Patient was initially managed with non-invasive ventilation but within an hour he required intubation and mechanical ventilation for progressive hypoxemia. He was also started on pressor support with norepinephrine infusion. A diagnosis of non-ST elevation myocardial infarction with cardiogenic shock was made.

A stat bedside two-dimensional transthoracic echocardiogram (TTE) revealed a normal left ventricular size with ejection fraction >65% and no evidence for regional wall motion abnormalities. Posterior mitral leaflet prolapse was seen with mild mitral regurgitation. Given the unstable hemodynamic picture, a two-dimensional transesophageal echocardiogram (2D-TEE) was performed without delay. Posterior mitral valve P2 and P3 scallop prolapse were noted (Fig. 281.1). The mitral regurgitation was found to be severe with an eccentric anteriorly directed jet noted in the mid-transesophageal short-axis view (Fig. 281.2 and 953). Transgastric views were suggestive for a partial posteromedial papillary muscle rupture (PMR) with no demonstrable systolic eversion into the left atrium.[1] In addition, three-dimensional transesophageal echocardiogram (3D-TEE) was performed for a thorough assessment of the mitral sub-valvular apparatus. P2 and P3 scallop

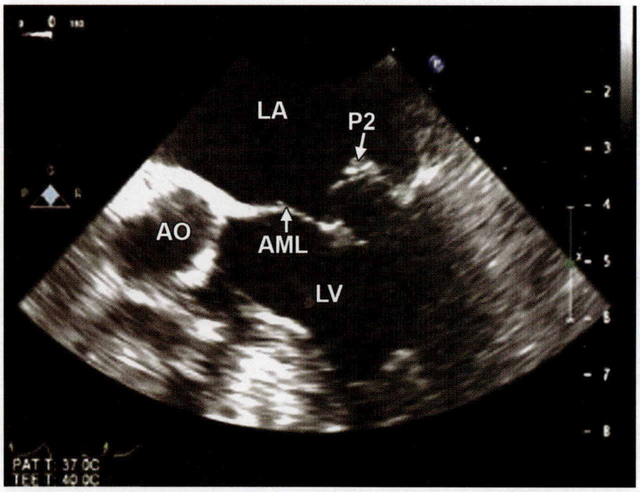

Fig. 281.1: Two-dimensional transesophageal echocardiogram at the mid-esophageal level demonstrating prolapse of the P2 scallop of the posterior mitral leaflet.

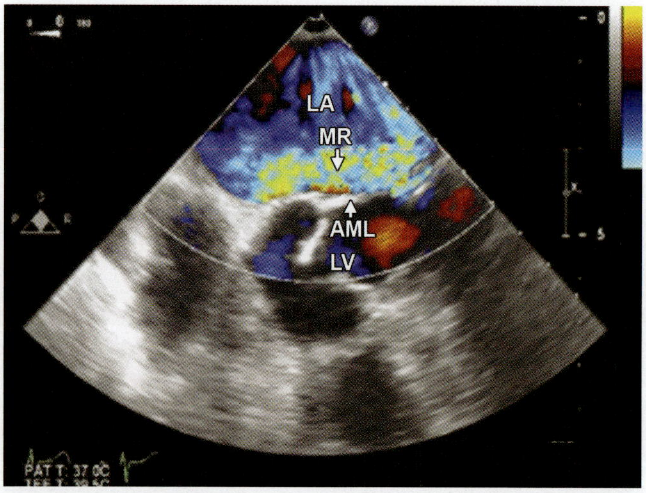

Fig. 281.2: Two-dimensional transesophageal echocardiogram with color Doppler imaging at the mid-esophageal level showing severe mitral regurgitation with an anteriorly directed eccentric jet from posterior mitral leaflet prolapse.

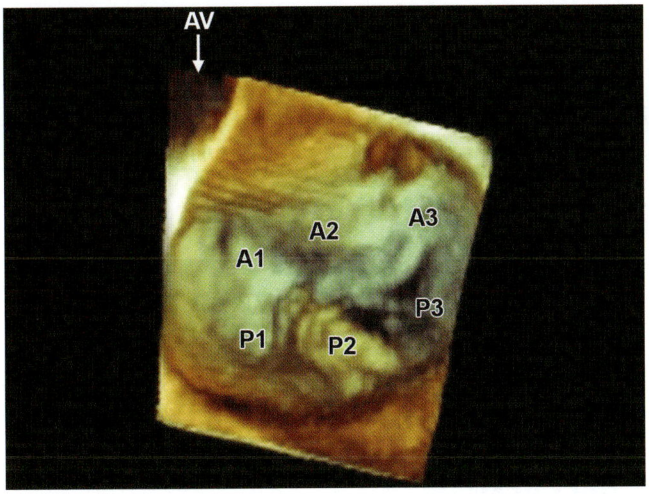

Fig. 281.3: Three-dimensional transesophageal echocardiographic view of the mitral valve demonstrating the mitral valve scallops in systole with P2 and P3 scallop prolapse. (AV: Aortic valve; A1, A2, A3: Scallops of the anterior mitral leaflet; P1, P2, P3: Scallops of the posterior mitral leaflet).

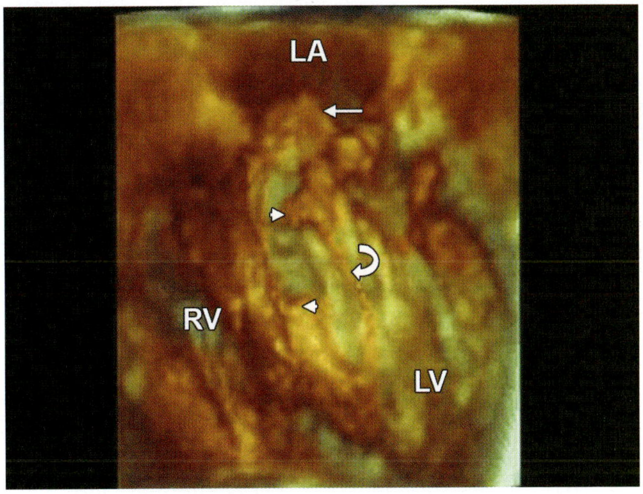

Fig. 281.4: Three-dimensional transesophageal echocardiogram with four-chamber view showing ruptured papillary muscle (arrowheads) with tissue strand tethering partially ruptured papillary muscle (curved arrow). P2 and P3 prolapse is seen (arrow). (LA: Left atrium; RV: Right ventricle; LV: Left ventricle).

prolapse of the posterior mitral valve were again identified (Fig. 281.3). A partially ruptured posteromedial papillary muscle (Fig. 281.4, 954) was clearly demonstrable on 3D-TEE, with only a thin string of tissue preventing its systolic eversion. Coronary angiography revealed severe three-vessel coronary artery disease. After placement of an intra-aortic balloon pump, patient underwent emergent coronary artery bypass graft surgery with mitral valve replacement. Surgical specimens revealed coagulative necrosis with inflammatory infiltrate and focal areas of fibrosis consistent with a recent myocardial infarction.

1. **All of the following are true regarding papillary muscles *except*:**
   (a) The posteromedial papillary muscle often comprises of two heads or trunks with each supporting one leaflet.
   (b) The anterolateral papillary muscle is frequently seen at 2-o'clock position in the short axis view on TTE.
   (c) Papillary muscle infarction is uncommon in the setting of non ST elevation myocardial infarction.
   (d) Rupture of posteromedial papillary muscle is more common because of its single blood supply.

Ans. (c)

More than 50% of PMR occurs in the setting of non-ST elevation myocardial infarction (sub-endocardial infarction), because the papillary muscle is a subendocardial structure.[2] The posteromedial papillary muscle is often composed of two heads or trunks with each supporting one leaflet while the anterolateral papillary muscle is usually a single trunk that supports both leaflets of the mitral valve. On TTE, the anterolateral papillary muscle is commonly seen at the 3-o'clock position and less frequently at 2-o'clock or 4-o'clock position. The posteromedial papillary muscle is commonly supplied by a branch of the right coronary artery. Therefore, it is more vulnerable to rupture in contrast to the anterolateral papillary muscle that receives dual blood supply from branches of both the left anterior descending and left circumflex coronary arteries.

2. **A diagnosis of PMR could be missed for the following reasons:**
   (a) Absence of a systolic murmur
   (b) Presence of mild to moderate mitral regurgitation on TTE or contrast ventriculography
   (c) No V waves on pulmonary capillary wedge pressure measurement
   (d) All of these

Ans. (d)

A diagnosis of PMR with severe mitral regurgitation could be missed on clinical exam, TTE and also on invasive testing with right heart catheterization in the absence of the typical findings. The systolic murmur tends to be softer in intensity and shorter in duration or may even be absent as a result of a reduced left ventricular to left atrial gradient. For similar reasons, TTE or contrast ventriculography may underestimate the severity of mitral regurgitation. Prominent V waves on pulmonary capillary wedge pressure measurement although suggestive of mitral regurgitation have poor sensitivity and specificity, and therefore should not be used to rule out the diagnosis.[3,4] A high index of suspicion is necessary in the appropriate clinical setting and further testing with TEE should be performed without delay.[5]

3. **The best echocardiographic views for the posteromedial papillary muscle include the following *except*:**
   (a) Parasternal long-axis view
   (b) Apical 3-chamber view
   (c) Apical 4-chamber view
   (d) Lower esophageal vertical 2-chamber view

Ans. (c)

The apical 4-chamber view cuts through the anterolateral wall of the left ventricle and hence images the anterolateral papillary muscle. Choices (a), (b) and (c) are suitable views for the posteromedial papillary muscle.

4. **The following is true regarding management of PMR in acute myocardial infarction:**
   (a) Surgical repair of PMR is associated with better outcomes in comparison to repair of ventricular septal rupture
   (b) Emergent or urgent surgical repair of PMR with severe mitral regurgitation is recommended
   (c) Intra-aortic balloon pump and vasodilators are often used to improve forward output
   (d) All of the above

Ans. (d)

With postinfarction PMR, operative mortality with surgical repair or replacement of the mitral valve combined with coronary artery bypass grafting have improved since the 1990s and long term outcome may be similar to patients without PMR.[6] Based on the Assessment of Pexelizumab in Acute Myocardial Infarction (APEX-AMI) trial data, ventricular septal rupture was associated with poor 30-day survival (20% vs. 73% respectively) when compared with patients that had acute mitral regurgitation with PMR.[7] In the subgroup with cardiogenic shock or heart failure, a similar trend was noted (17% vs. 64% respectively). Emergent CABG is a Class I recommendation for postinfarction PMR as per the 2011 guideline.[8] Vasodilator therapy and, if necessary, intra-aortic balloon counterpulsation are important for stabilizing patient prior to surgery.

MOVIES 953 AND 954

953: Two dimensional transthoracic echo showing posterior mitral valve P2 and P3 scallop prolapse with eccentric anteriorly directed mitral regurgitation jet.

954: 3D-TEE showing a partially ruptured posteromedial papillary muscle with a thin string of tissue preventing systolic eversion.

REFERENCES

1. Moursi MH, Bhatnagar SK, Vilacosta I, San Roman JA, Espinal MA, Nanda NC: Transesophageal echocardiographic assessment of papillary muscle rupture. Circulation 1996; 94:1003-9.
2. Nishimura RA, Schaff HV, Shub C, et al. Papillary muscle rupture complicating acute myocardial infarction: analysis of 17 patients. Am J Cardiol 1983;51:373-7.
3. Haskell RJ, French WJ: Accuracy of left atrial and pulmonary artery wedge pressure in pure mitral regurgitation in predicting left ventricular end diastolic pressure. Am J Cardiol 1988;61:136-41.
4. Hutchison, SJ. "Papillary Muscle Rupture and Postinfarction Mitral Insufficiency." Complications of Myocardial Infarction: Clinical Diagnostic Imaging Atlas. Saunders Elsevier, 2009. 231-75.
5. Havins J, Lick S, Boor P, et al: Real time three-dimensional transesophageal echocardiography in partial posteromedial papillary muscle rupture. Echocardiography 2013;30:E179–E81.
6. Russo A, Suri RM, Grigioni F, et al. Clinical outcome after surgical correction of mitral regurgitation due to papillary muscle rupture. Circulation 2008, 118:1528-34.
7. French, J.K., Hellkamp, A.S., Armstrong, P.W. et al, Mechanical complications after percutaneous coronary intervention in ST-elevation myocardial infarction (from APEX-AMI). Am J Cardiol. 2010;105:59–63.
8. Hillis LD, Smith PK, Anderson JL, et al. ACCF/AHA guideline for coronary artery bypass graft surgery: a report of the American College of Cardiology Foundation/American Heart Association Task Force on Practice Guidelines. J Am Coll Cardiol. 2011;58:e123–e210.

CASE 282

Elsayed Abo-Salem, Sherif Sakr

A 47-year-old female patient presented with a syncopal episode for 2 minutes witnessed by family members. Syncope occurred suddenly at rest without a prodrome. Consciousness was regained spontaneously without a residual neurological deficit. She had a history of deep vein thrombosis 15 years ago, during a postpartum period. There was not a prior history of cardiac disease. Examination was remarkable for regular tachycardia at 102 beats per minute and a short systolic murmur over the tricuspid area. Electrocardiography revealed sinus tachycardia. Chest X-ray was normal. Echocardiography was done (Fig. 282.1 and 955 are recorded from a modified parasternal window).

1. **What is the most likely diagnosis?**
   (a) Right atrial myxoma
   (b) Thrombus in transit
   (c) Chari network
   (d) Metastaic renal cancer
   (e) Infective endocarditis

Ans. (b)

DISCUSSION

The presence of warm-like hypermobile structure in the right atrium is consistent with a free-floating thrombus in right atrium (thrombus in transit). The patient had a history of deep vein thrombosis and presented with syncope, which is clinically consistent with echocardiographic diagnosis. Syncope is often secondary to an associated pulmonary embolism. In patients with patent foramen ovale or atrial septal defect, systemic embolization may occur. Treatment includes thrombolytic therapy, surgical or percutaneous removal, or heparin. Right atrial myxoma is more common in the left atrium, and typically appears as a mass attached to the interatrial septum. Chari network is a mobile net-like structure, with a little clinical significance, and often diagnosed incidentally. Advanced renal cancers can metastasize to the right atrium through inferior vena cava.

Our case had a chest computed tomography, which showed pulmonary embolism. Lower extremity venous

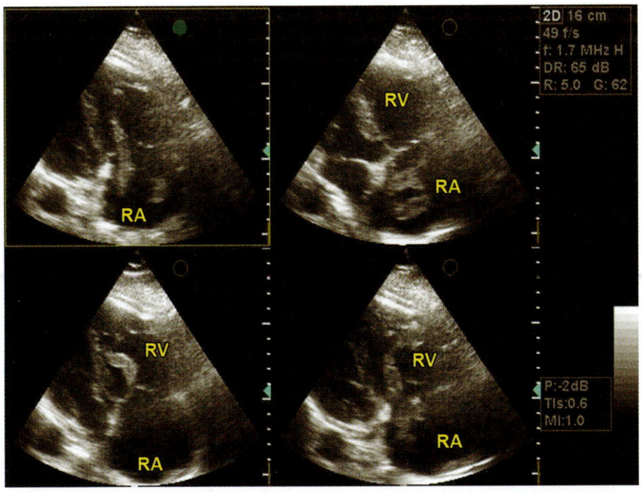

Fig. 282.1: Transthoracic echocardiography (modified parasternal right ventricular inflow view) shows a mobile mass in the right atrium.

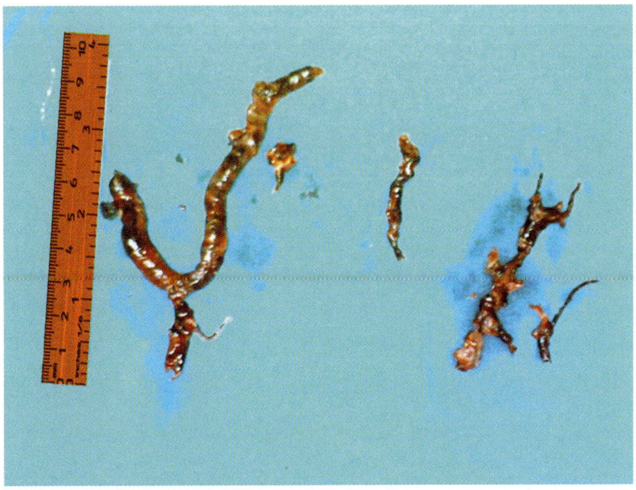

Fig. 282.2: Large branching thrombi were surgically removed from the right atrium and pulmonary artery.

Doppler revealed a left superficial femoral vein thrombosis. Systolic pulmonary artery pressure was estimated at 45 mm Hg. Anticoagulation was started immediately and urgent surgical removal of pulmonary embolism was performed successfully (Fig. 282.2). Patient improved significantly with no recurrent syncope. Follow-up echocardiography 3-months later revealed a normal pulmonary artery pressure.

MOVIE 955

REFERENCE

1. Chartier L1, Béra J, Delomez M, et al. Free-floating thrombi in the right heart: diagnosis, management, and prognostic indexes in 38 consecutive patients. Circulation. 1999;99(21):2779-83.

INDEX

Note: Page numbers followed by *f* refer to figure.

C

D

E

F

G

H

I

J

K

L

M

N

O

P

Q

R

S

T

U

V

W